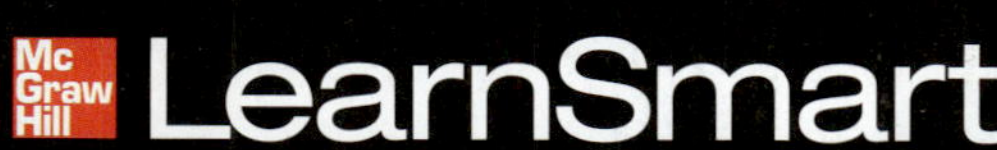

McGraw-Hill LearnSmart Student Quick Tips and FAQs

Use this *McGraw-Hill LearnSmart Student Quick Tips and FAQs* to get more out of this learning tool. Remember, LearnSmart is an adaptive learning system designed to help students learn faster, study more efficiently, and retain more knowledge for greater success.

Responding to a LearnSmart Assignment

TIP: Make an honest attempt to assess your confidence level on each probe. Doing so allows LearnSmart to more accurately direct you to the materials you need to study.

1) Click LearnSmart Assignment Title denoted by icon.

2) Click on a chapter module.

3) Read the probe & click your level of confidence in knowing the correct answer.

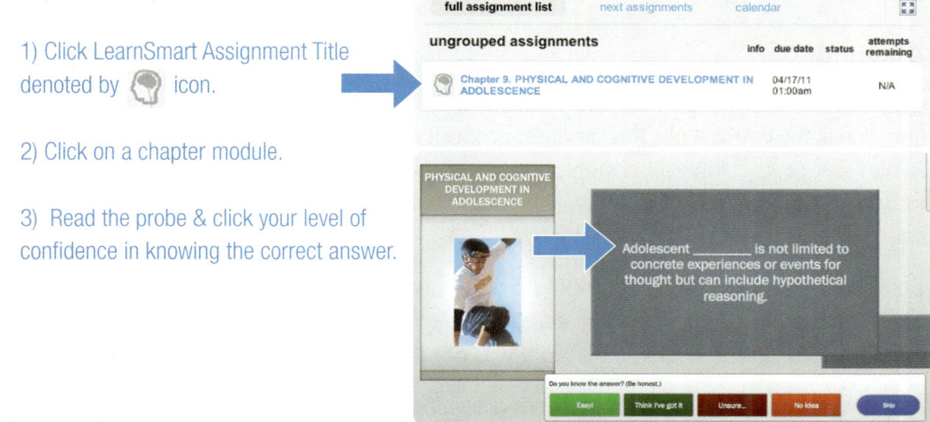

Help Yourself Succeed

TIP: We recommend completing all passive learning activities before you work on LearnSmart – such as reading the chapter, watching animations and videos available in Connect, etc.

Self-Assess

TIP: Before answering each question, click on the most appropriate confidence level to ensure you receive the most efficient learning experience.

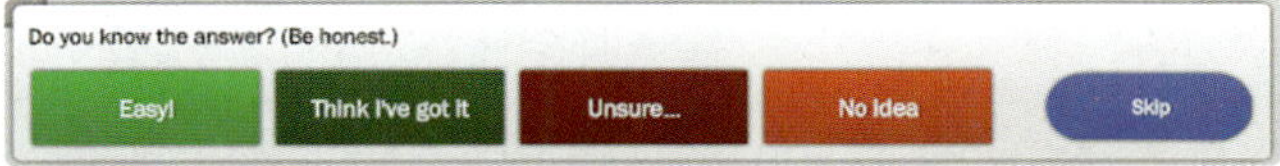

Take a Break!

TIP: Use Time-Out! readings to review topics you are struggling to learn.

Refresh Your Memory

TIP: Return to your completed assignments to rework material and refresh your memory before quizzes and tests. Don't be alarmed if you have forgotten some things – it's natural when learning a new subject!

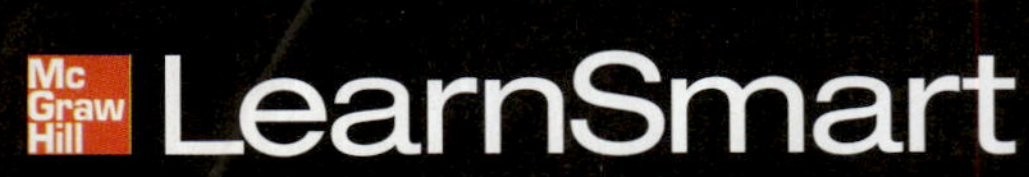

Share Your Feedback

TIP: Click the **Challenge Answer** button if you feel the content is incorrect or unclear.

Answers to Frequently Asked Questions (FAQs)

How is the percentage for each module calculated?

The percentage indicates the number of correctly answered questions within the module. In other words, the percentage indicates how much of the module you have learned so far. To learn more about your progress and overall status, click the 'Debriefing' button at the top of the screen.

How is my High Score calculated?

The amount of points you earn depends on how you assess your ability to answer a question. For instance, if you click 'Easy' and answer the question correctly, you will get the greatest amount of points. If you answer correctly after selecting one of the other buttons – 'Think I've got it,' 'Unsure,' and 'No idea' – you will also earn points. However, you will receive fewer points for the items you do not believe you know as well. If you select 'Unsure' and get the answer correct, you will get fewer points than if you selected 'Easy' or 'Think I've got it.'

The same applies if you get an answer incorrect. If you do not know the answer after clicking 'Easy,' points will be deducted from your score. Fewer points are deducted if you select 'Think I've got it' or 'Unsure,' and get the answer incorrect. If you click 'Unsure,' points will not be deducted even if you get the question wrong.

Spelling errors, nearly correct answers or partially correct answers also affect your score.

Of course, you can increase your score by going through the same module multiple times, rating your answers as honestly as possible. In essence, the more you learn, the better the score.

Why does the system repeat questions I have already answered?

If you answer a question incorrectly, it will be repeated later in the same session to give you a chance to learn. It might not be the exact same question, but rather a variant that represents the same learning objective. The system will adjust the difficulty of the questions according to your performance. In addition to this, the system will present the same questions the next day to help you remember the material over time. (For more information, see 'Why does it make me start all over on the module when I come back?')

The first day, you might see a 'multiple-choice question about a concept,' and the next day, a 'fill-in-the-blank' for the same concept to make it more difficult. This will assess whether you really know the subject. It closely monitors the exact questions you have been exposed to before, and will vary this in an attempt to match and improve your knowledge level.

Why am I only working on part of a module each day?

Instead of asking you to go through, say, 300 questions in one session, LearnSmart distributes the items and the review of these items over a period of time. Spreading the learning events over multiple sessions increases the likelihood of memory retention. If you are pressed for time, though, you can work ahead and do more questions one day, and LearnSmart will automatically adapt.

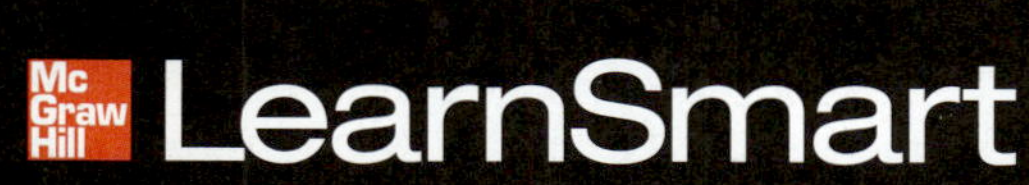

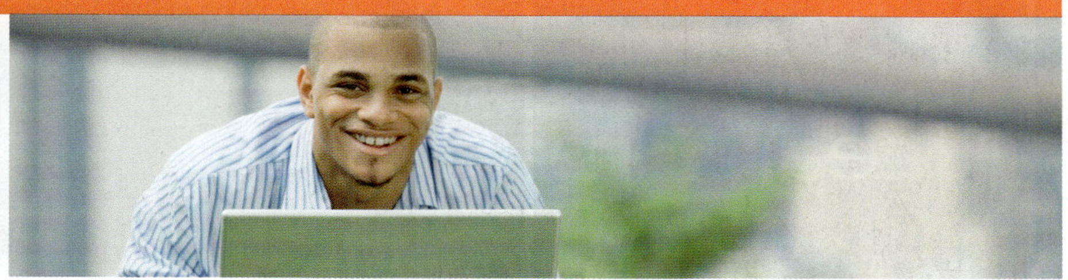

Why does it make me start the module again when I come back?

Research tells us frequency increases memory recall. The module seems to start over when logging in the next day in order to frequently assess your mastery of the material. So if you complete 100 flashcards the first day, you can expect about 25 of those to be repeated each of the next four days. If you answer all of these correctly, around 7 will be repeated each session for the next 14 days, and so on. The program automatically calculates the appropriate repetition interval for each student based on your individual 'forget curve' that is tracked in detail. The 'Learning Plan' feature in the LearnSmart Debriefing screen provides a daily estimate of how much you need to do on each module. This plan also adjusts if you skip a day or two or work ahead.

Why is it so strict about spelling?

If you make a small spelling error, the program will accept your answer. If you make a larger mistake, you will be prompted about the same topic again with a chance to improve your score (and your spelling). You might not see the exact same question, but the program allows another opportunity to demonstrate your knowledge.

'Fill-in-the-blank' questions are often the most difficult questions because they rely on active recall, rather than recognition. Once you master the 'fill-in-the-blank' questions, you are really learning!

Why do I need to click the Confidence buttons?

The 'Confidence' buttons are the self-assessment buttons that affect the high score as described above. In addition, rating your confidence also affects the schedule of questions. Simply put, this information is used to determine your awareness of your own knowledge level. It is applied to adjust your learning path. You can use the **Metacognitive Skills** report in the **LearnSmart Debriefing** to learn more about this. Click 'Debriefing' at the top of the screen to get access to this information.

Why are there so many questions?

This program is not just a testing system, but a *learning system*. The modules assess most of the material in the book. As you progress through the modules, you will learn most of the material assigned by your instructor for this course. LearnSmart presents the core or most critical material first. If you do not have time to complete the entire module, just work until you are out of time, and you can be assured your have tackled the most important items.

When you return, the system will recall the material for which you have demonstrated mastery and provide opportunities to practice material that still requires review. Again, LearnSmart presents the most important items first, which may include revisiting previous items or new material.

When the deadline has passed, why do I still have to work on the module?

The program prompts you to keep reviewing the same module to ensure recall and true mastery. Use the **Learning Plan** feature in the **LearnSmart Debriefing** screen to see the estimated time required for you to retain the information before the deadline approaches. You can also use the 'Status' feature in the 'Debriefing' screen for an estimate of when you are likely to forget what you have learned. If you follow the schedule proposed by the system, the workload for review will be minimal.

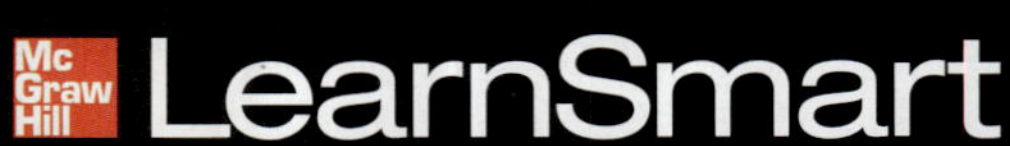

How can I change my name in the High Score list?

Just click your name within the list. You can change your name (to an alias) or become anonymous.

Should I continue to practice after my exam?

If you want to commit your new knowledge to long-term memory, we recommend that you keep working the modules even after the deadline. You have the option of setting a new deadline for your own purposes (e.g. 6 months in the future) as a target. The system will continuously monitor what you know and what you tend to forget. It will not prompt you to work on things you most likely remember, minimizing your workload. This will be the optimal way to learn the content and remember it.

What happens when I provide feedback?

We greatly appreciate your feedback. We do read it and use it to improve LearnSmart so that it better serves students like you. In cases where you have questions about the system, we will try to answer them. If you contest an answer or report incorrect markings, we will investigate and update the modules accordingly.

Need More Help with LearnSmart Assignments?

CONTACT US ONLINE:

Visit us at:

www.mhhe.com/learnsmart/support.html

Browse our most up-to-date support materials including tutorial videos and searchable knowledge base. If you cannot find an answer to your question, click on Contact Us to send us an email.

GIVE US A CALL

Call us at:

1-800-331-5094

Our live support is available:

Mon-Thurs:	8 am – 11 pm CT
Friday:	8 am – 6 pm CT
Sunday:	6 pm – 11 pm CT

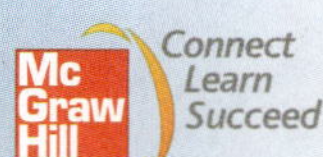

TOTAL WELLNESS

BROWARD COLLEGE

With Select Material from

Fit & Well: Core Concepts and Labs in Physical Fitness and Wellness
Tenth Edition, Alternate Edition

Thomas D. Fahey
California State University, Chico

Paul M. Insel
Stanford University

Walton T. Roth
Stanford University

with additional material from

Your Health Today
Third Edition, Brief Edition

Michael L. Teague | Sara L. C. Mackenzie | David M. Rosenthal

and

FitWell

Gary Liguori | Sandra Carroll-Cobb

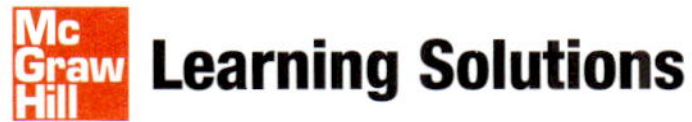

Boston Burr Ridge, IL Dubuque, IA New York San Francisco St. Louis
Bangkok Bogotá Caracas Lisbon London Madrid
Mexico City Milan New Delhi Seoul Singapore Sydney Taipei Toronto

The McGraw-Hill Companies

Total Wellness
Broward College
Tenth Edition

This book is a McGraw-Hill Learning Solutions textbook and contains select material from the following sources:
Fit & Well: Core Concepts and Labs in Physical Fitness and Wellness, Tenth Edition by Thomas D. Fahey, Paul M. Insel and Walton T. Roth. Copyright © 2013, 2011, 2009, 2007, 2005, 2003, 2001, 1999, 1997, 1994 by The McGraw-Hill Companies, Inc.
Your Health Today, Third Edition by Michael L. Teague, Sara L. C. Mackenzie and David M. Rosenthal. Copyright © 2011, 2009, 2007 by The McGraw-Hill Companies, Inc.
FitWell by Gary Liguori and Sandra Carroll-Cobb. Copyright © 2012 by The McGraw-Hill Companies, Inc.
All reprinted with permission of the publisher. Many custom published texts are modified versions or adaptations of our best-selling textbooks. Some adaptations are printed in black and white to keep prices at a minimum, while others are in color.

3 4 5 6 7 8 9 0 DOW DOW 16 15 14

ISBN-13: 978-0-07-769981-9
ISBN-10: 0-07-769981-5
PART OF:
ISBN-13: 978-0-07-769982-6
ISBN-10: 0-07-769982-3

Learning Solutions Consultant: Kimberly Wollschlager
Production Editor: Mia Burbach
Printer/Binder: R.R. Donnelley
Cover Photo Credits: © 2012 JupiterImages Corporation

BRIEF CONTENTS

CONTENTS

7

WEIGHT MANAGEMENT *191*

8

MUSCULAR STRENGTH AND ENDURANCE *219*

BOXES

TAKE CHARGE

CRITICAL CONSUMER

IN FOCUS

DIMENSIONS OF DIVERSITY

THE EVIDENCE FOR EXERCISE

PERSONAL CHALLENGE

WELLNESS IN THE DIGITAL AGE

LABORATORY ACTIVITIES

The laboratory activities are also found in an interactive format in Connect (www.mcgrawhillconnect.com).

CHAPTER 1

Introduction to Wellness, Fitness, and Lifestyle Management

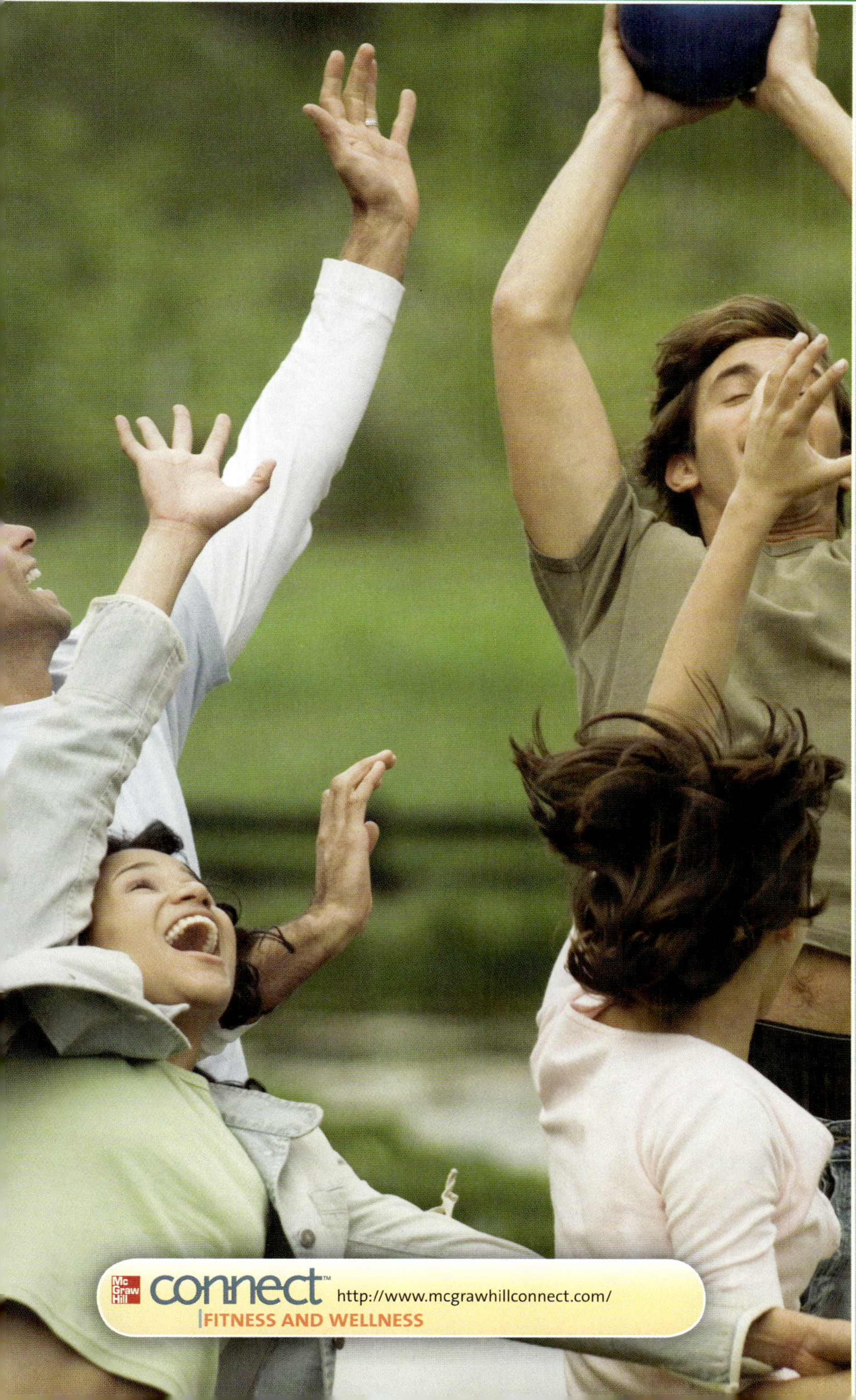

LOOKING AHEAD...

After reading this chapter, you should be able to:

- Describe the dimensions of wellness
- Identify the major health problems in the United States today, and discuss their causes
- Describe the behaviors that are part of a wellness lifestyle
- Explain the steps in creating a behavior management plan to change a wellness-related behavior
- List some of the available sources of wellness information and explain how to think critically about them

TEST YOUR KNOWLEDGE

1. Which of the following lifestyle factors is the leading preventable cause of death for Americans?
   a. excess alcohol consumption
   b. cigarette smoking
   c. obesity
2. The terms *health* and *wellness* mean the same thing. True or false?
3. A person's genetic makeup determines whether he or she will develop certain diseases (such as breast cancer), regardless of that person's health habits. True or false?

ANSWERS

1. **b.** Smoking causes about 440,000 deaths per year. Obesity is responsible for more than 100,000 premature deaths, and alcohol is a factor in as many as 85,000 deaths.
2. **False.** Although the words are used interchangeably, they actually have different meanings. The term *health* refers to the overall condition of the body or mind and to the presence or absence of illness or injury. The term *wellness* refers to optimal health and vitality, encompassing all the dimensions of well-being.
3. **False.** In many cases, behavior can tip the balance toward good health even when heredity or environment is a negative factor.

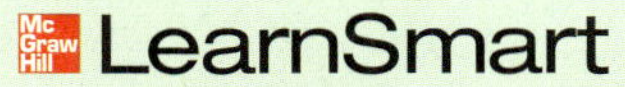

A college sophomore sets the following goals for herself:

- To join new social circles and make new friends whenever possible
- To exercise every day
- To clean up trash and plant trees in blighted neighborhoods in her community

These goals may differ, but they have one thing in common. Each contributes, in its own way, to this student's health and well-being. Not satisfied merely to be free of illness, she wants more. She has decided to live actively and fully—not just to be healthy, but to pursue a state of overall wellness.

WELLNESS: NEW HEALTH GOALS

Generations of people have viewed health simply as the absence of disease, and that view largely prevails today. The word **health** typically refers to the overall condition of a person's body or mind and to the presence or absence of illness or injury. **Wellness** is a relatively new concept that expands our idea of health to include our ability to achieve optimal health. Beyond the simple presence or absence of disease, wellness refers to optimal health and vitality—to living life to its fullest. Although we use the terms *health* and *wellness* interchangeably, there are two important differences between them:

- Health—or some aspects of it—can be determined or influenced by factors beyond your control, such as your genes, age, and family history. For example, consider a man with a strong family history of prostate cancer. These factors place this man at a higher-than-average risk for developing prostate cancer himself.
- Wellness is largely determined by the decisions you make about how you live. That same man can reduce his risk of cancer by eating sensibly, exercising, and having regular screening tests. Even if he develops the disease, he may still rise above its effects to live a rich, meaningful life. This means choosing not only to care for himself physically but also to maintain a positive outlook, keep up his relationships with others, challenge himself intellectually, and nurture other aspects of his life.

KEY TERMS

health The overall condition of body or mind and the presence or absence of illness or injury.

wellness Optimal health and vitality, encompassing all the dimensions of well-being.

Enhanced wellness, therefore, involves making conscious decisions to control **risk factors** that contribute to disease or injury. Age and family history are risk factors you cannot control. Behaviors such as choosing not to smoke, exercising, and eating a healthy diet are well within your control.

The Dimensions of Wellness

Experts have defined six dimensions of wellness:

- Physical
- Emotional
- Intellectual
- Interpersonal
- Spiritual
- Environmental

Each dimension of wellness affects the others. Further, the process of achieving wellness is constant and dynamic (Figure 1.1), involving change and growth. Ignoring any dimension of wellness can have harmful effects on your life. The following sections briefly introduce the dimensions of wellness. Table 1.1 lists some of the specific qualities and behaviors associated with each dimension. Lab 1.1 will help you learn what wellness means to you and where you fall on the wellness continuum.

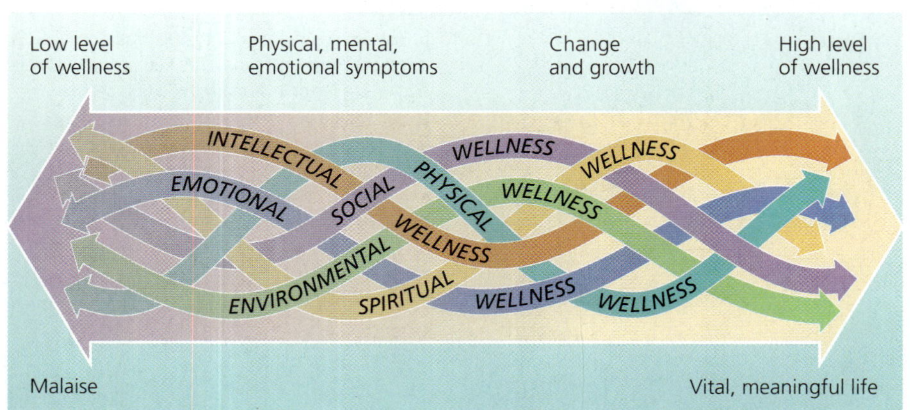

FIGURE 1.1 The wellness continuum. The concept of wellness includes vitality in six interrelated dimensions, all of which contribute to overall wellness.

Table 1.1 Examples of Qualities and Behaviors Associated with the Dimensions of Wellness

PHYSICAL	EMOTIONAL	INTELLECTUAL	INTERPERSONAL	SPIRITUAL	ENVIRONMENTAL
• Eating well	• Optimism	• Openness to new ideas	• Communication skills	• Capacity for love	• Having abundant, clean natural resources
• Exercising	• Trust	• Capacity to question	• Capacity for intimacy	• Compassion	• Maintaining sustainable development
• Avoiding harmful habits	• Self-esteem	• Ability to think critically	• Ability to establish and maintain satisfying relationships	• Forgiveness	• Recycling whenever possible
• Practicing safer sex	• Self-acceptance	• Motivation to master new skills	• Ability to cultivate a support system of friends and family	• Altruism	• Reducing pollution and waste
• Recognizing symptoms of disease	• Self-confidence	• Sense of humor		• Joy	
• Getting regular checkups	• Ability to understand and accept one's feelings	• Creativity		• Fulfillment	
• Avoiding injuries	• Ability to share feelings with others	• Curiosity		• Caring for others	
		• Lifelong learning		• Sense of meaning and purpose	
				• Sense of belonging to something greater than oneself	

Physical Wellness Your physical wellness includes not just your body's overall condition and the absence of disease, but your fitness level and your ability to care for yourself. The higher your fitness level (which is discussed throughout this book), the higher your level of physical wellness will be. Similarly, as you become more able to care for your own physical needs, you ensure greater physical wellness. To achieve optimum physical wellness, you need to make choices that help you avoid illnesses and injuries. The decisions you make now—and the habits you develop over your lifetime—will largely determine the length and quality of your life.

Emotional Wellness Your emotional wellness reflects your ability to understand and deal with your feelings. Emotional wellness involves attending to your own thoughts and feelings, monitoring your reactions, and identifying obstacles to emotional stability. Achieving this type of wellness means finding solutions to emotional problems, with professional help if necessary.

Intellectual Wellness Those who enjoy intellectual wellness constantly challenge their minds. An active mind is essential to wellness because it detects problems, finds solutions, and directs behavior. People who enjoy intellectual wellness never stop learning; they continue trying to learn new things throughout their lifetime. They seek out and relish new experiences and challenges.

Interpersonal Wellness Your interpersonal (or social) wellness is defined by your ability to develop and maintain satisfying and supportive relationships. Such relationships are essential to physical and emotional health. Social wellness requires participating in and contributing to your community and to society.

Spiritual Wellness To enjoy spiritual wellness is to possess a set of guiding beliefs, principles, or values that give meaning and purpose to your life, especially in difficult times. The spiritually well person focuses on the positive aspects of life and finds spirituality to be an antidote for negative feelings such as cynicism, anger, and pessimism. Organized religions help many people develop spiritual health. Religion, however, is not the only source or form of spiritual wellness. Many people find meaning and purpose in their lives on their own—through nature, art, meditation, or good works—or with their loved ones.

Environmental Wellness Your environmental wellness is defined by the livability of your surroundings. Personal health depends on the health of the planet—from the

risk factor A condition that increases one's chances of disease or injury.

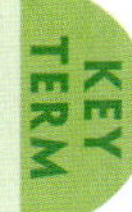

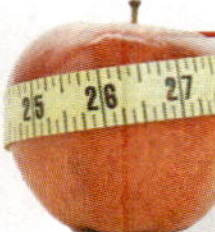

Wellness Tip

Enhancing one dimension of wellness can have positive effects on others. Joining a meditation group can help you enhance your spiritual well-being, for example, but can also affect the emotional and interpersonal dimensions of wellness by enabling you to meet new people and develop new friendships.

safety of the food supply to the degree of violence in society. Your physical environment either supports your wellness or diminishes it. To improve your environmental wellness, you can learn about and protect yourself against hazards in your surroundings and work to make your world a cleaner and safer place.

Other Aspects of Wellness Many experts consider occupational wellness and financial wellness to be additional important dimensions of wellness. *Occupational wellness* refers to the level of happiness and fulfillment you gain through your work. Although high salaries and prestigious titles are nice, they alone generally do not bring about occupational wellness. An occupationally well person truly likes his or her work, feels a connection with others in the workplace, and has opportunities to learn and be challenged. Other aspects of occupational wellness include enjoyable work, job satisfaction, and recognition from managers and colleagues. An ideal job draws on your interests and passions, as well as your vocational or professional skills, and allows you to feel that you are contributing to society in your everyday work.

To achieve occupational wellness, set career goals that reflect your personal values. For example, a career in sales might be a good choice for someone who values financial security, whereas a career in teaching or nursing might be a good choice for someone who values service to others.

Financial wellness refers to your ability to live within your means and manage your money in a way that gives you peace of mind. It includes balancing your income and expenditures, staying out of debt, saving for the future, and understanding your emotions about money. For more on this topic, see the box "Financial Wellness."

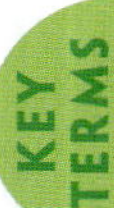

KEY TERMS

infectious disease A disease that can spread from person to person; caused by microorganisms such as bacteria and viruses.

chronic disease A disease that develops and continues over a long period of time, such as heart disease or cancer.

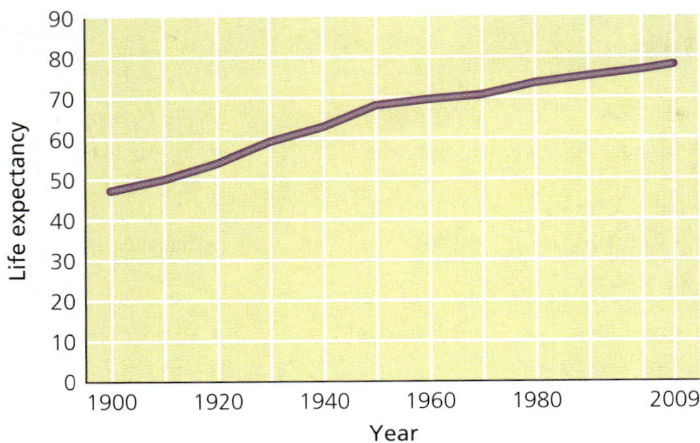

FIGURE 1.2 Life expectancy of Americans from birth, 1900–2009.
SOURCE: National Center for Health Statistics. 2011. Deaths: Preliminary data for 2009. *National Vital Statistics Reports* 59(4).

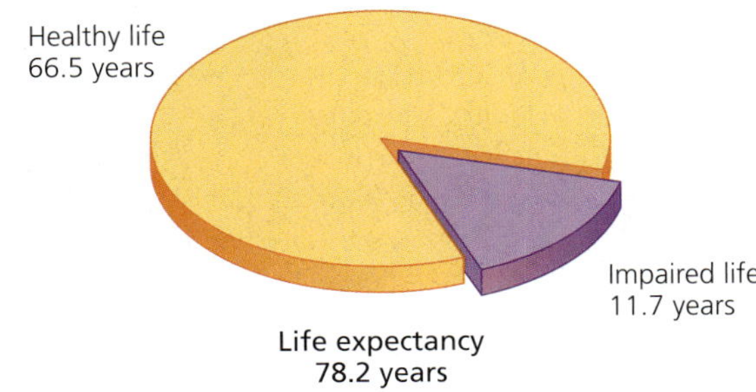

FIGURE 1.3 Quantity of life versus quality of life. Years of healthy life as a proportion of life expectancy in the U.S. population.
SOURCES: National Center for Health Statistics. 2011. Deaths: Preliminary data for 2009. *National Vital Statistics Reports.* 59(4); National Center for Health Statistics. *Healthy People* 2010; Midcourse Review. Hyattsville, Md.: Public Health Service.

New Opportunities for Taking Charge

Wellness is a fairly new concept. A century ago, Americans considered themselves lucky just to survive to adulthood (Figure 1.2). A child born in 1900, for example, could expect to live only about 47 years. Many people died from common **infectious diseases** (such as pneumonia, tuberculosis, or diarrhea) and poor environmental conditions (such as water pollution and poor sanitation).

Since 1900, however, life expectancy has nearly doubled, and as of 2009, the average American's life expectancy was 78.2 years. This increase in life span is due largely to the development of vaccines and antibiotics to fight infections, and to public health measures to improve living conditions. But even though life expectancy has increased, poor health limits most Americans' activities during the last 15% of their lives, resulting in some sort of impaired life (Figure 1.3). Today, a different set of diseases has emerged as our major health threat, and heart disease, cancer, and chronic lower respiratory diseases are now the three leading causes of death for Americans (Table 1.2). Treating such **chronic diseases** is costly and difficult.

Financial Wellness

With the news full of stories of home foreclosures, credit card debt, and personal bankruptcies, it has become painfully clear that many Americans do not know how to manage their finances. You can avoid such stress—and gain financial peace of mind—by developing skills that contribute to financial wellness.

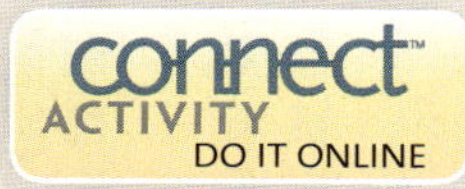

Financial wellness means having a healthy relationship with money. It involves knowing how to manage your money, using self-discipline to live within your means, using credit cards wisely, staying out of debt, meeting your financial obligations, having a long-range financial plan, and saving.

Learn to Budget

Although the word *budget* may conjure up thoughts of deprivation, a budget is really just a way of tracking where your money goes and making sure you're spending it on the things that are most important to you. To start one, list your monthly income and your expenditures. If you aren't sure where you spend your money, track your expenses for a few weeks or a month. Then organize them into categories, such as housing, food, transportation, entertainment, services, personal care, clothes, books and school supplies, health care, credit card and loan payments, and miscellaneous. Use categories that reflect the way you actually spend your money. Knowing where your money goes is the first step in gaining control of it.

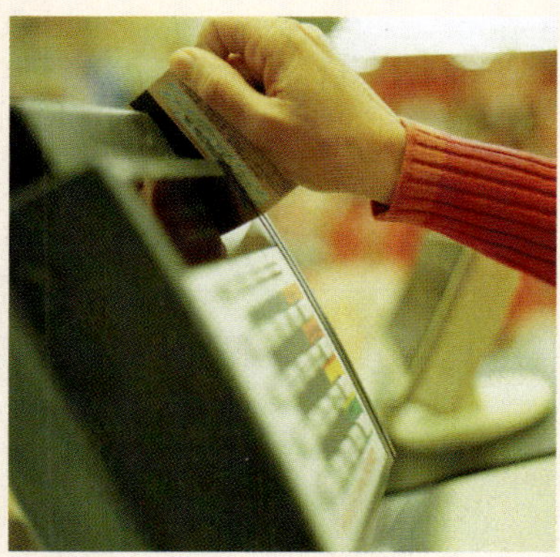

Now total your income and expenditures. Are you taking in more than you spend, or vice versa? Are you surprised by your spending patterns? Use this information to set guidelines and goals for yourself. If your expenses exceed your income, identify ways to make some cuts. If you have both a cell phone and a land line, for example, consider whether you can give one up. If you spend money on movies and restaurants, consider less expensive options like having a weekly game night with friends or organizing an occasional potluck.

Be Wary of Credit Cards

College students are prime targets for credit card companies, and most undergraduates have at least one card. In fact, many college students use credit cards to live beyond their means, not just for convenience. According a recent report, half of all students have four or more cards, and the average outstanding balance on undergraduate credit cards is over $3000.

The best way to avoid credit card debt is to have just one card, to use it only when necessary, and to pay off the entire balance every month. Make sure you understand terms like *APR* (annual percentage rate—the interest you're charged on your balance), *credit limit* (the maximum amount you can borrow at any one time), *minimum monthly payment* (the smallest payment your creditor will accept each month), *grace period* (the number of days you have to pay your bill before interest or penalties are charged), and *over-the-limit* and *late fees* (the amount you'll be charged if your payment is late or you go over your credit limit).

Get Out of Debt

If you have credit card debt, stop using your cards and start paying them off. If you can't pay the whole balance, at least try to pay more than the minimum payment each month. It can take a very long time to pay off a loan by making only the minimum payments. For example, to pay off a credit card balance of $2000 at 10% interest with monthly payments of $20 would take 203 months—17 years. To see for yourself, check out an online credit card calculator like http://www.bankrate.com/calculators/credit-cards/credit-card-payoff-calculator.aspx. And remember: By carrying a balance and incurring finance charges, you are also paying back much more than your initial loan.

Start Saving

The same miracle of compound interest that locks you into years of credit card debt can work to your benefit if you start saving early (for an online compound interest calculator, visit http://www.moneychimp.com/calculator/compound_interest_calculator.htm). Experts recommend "paying yourself first" every month—that is, putting some money into savings before you start paying your bills, depending on what your budget allows. You may want to save for a large purchase, or you may even be looking ahead to retirement. If you work for a company with a 401(k) retirement plan, contribute as much as you can every pay period.

Become Financially Literate

Although modern life requires financial literacy, most Americans have not received any kind of basic financial training. Even before the economic meltdown that began in 2008, the U.S. government had established the Financial Literacy and Education Commission (www.MyMoney.gov) to help Americans develop financial literacy and learn how to save, invest, and manage their money better. The consensus is that developing lifelong financial skills should begin in early adulthood, during the college years, if not earlier.

SOURCES: Federal Deposit Insurance Corporation. 2010. *Money Smart: A Financial Education Program* (http://www.fdic.gov/consumers/consumer/moneysmart/young.html; retrieved June 23, 2011); Plymouth State University. 2011. *Student Monetary Awareness and Responsibility Today!* (http://www.plymouth.edu/finaid/smart; retrieved June 23, 2011); U.S. Financial Literacy and Education Commission. 2010. *Do You Want to Learn How to Save, Manage, and Invest Your Money Better?* (http://www.mymoney.gov; retrieved June 23, 2011).

VITAL STATISTICS

Table 1.2 Leading Causes of Death in the United States, 2009

RANK	CAUSE OF DEATH	NUMBER OF DEATHS	PERCENTAGE OF TOTAL DEATHS*	DEATH RATE†	LIFESTYLE FACTORS
	All causes	2,436,652	100.0	741.0	
1	Heart disease	598,607	24.5	179.8	D I S A
2	Cancer	568,668	23.3	173.6	D I S A
3	Chronic lower respiratory diseases	137,082	5.6	42.2	S
4	Stroke	128,603	5.3	38.9	D I S A
5	Unintentional injuries (accidents)	117,176	4.8	37.0	D I S A
6	Alzheimer's disease	78,889	3.2	23.4	
7	Diabetes mellitus	68,504	2.8	20.9	D I S
8	Influenza and pneumonia	53,582	2.2	16.2	S
9	Kidney disease	48,714	2.0	14.8	D I S A
10	Intentional self-harm (suicide)	36,547	1.5	11.7	A
11	Septicemia (systemic blood infection)	35,587	1.5	10.9	A
12	Chronic liver disease and cirrhosis	30,444	1.2	9.2	A
13	Hypertension (high blood pressure)	25,651	1.0	7.7	D I S A
14	Parkinson's disease	20,552	0.8	6.4	
15	Assault (homicide)	16,591	0.6	5.5	A
	All other causes	471,455			

Key
D Diet plays a part
I Inactive lifestyle plays a part
S Smoking plays a part
A Excessive alcohol use plays a part

*Percentages may not total 100% due to rounding.

†Age-adjusted death rate per 100,000 persons.

NOTE: Although not among the overall top 15 causes of death, HIV/AIDS is a major killer. In 2009, HIV/AIDS was the twelfth leading cause of death for Americans age 15–24 years and the sixth leading cause of death for those age 25–44 years.

SOURCE: National Center for Health Statistics. 2011. Deaths: Preliminary data for 2009. *National Vital Statistics Report* 59(4).

The good news is that people have some control over whether they develop chronic diseases. People make choices every day that increase or decrease their risks for such diseases. These **lifestyle choices** include behaviors such as smoking, diet, exercise, and alcohol use. As Table 1.3 makes clear, lifestyle factors contribute to many deaths in the United States, and people can influence their own health risks. The need to make good choices is especially true for teens and young adults. For Americans age 15–24, for example, the top three causes of death are accidents, homicide, and suicide (Table 1.4).

The Healthy People Initiative

Wellness is a personal concern, but the U.S. government has financial and humanitarian interests in it, too. A healthy population is the nation's source of vitality, creativity, and wealth. Poor health drains the nation's resources and raises health care costs for all.

The national Healthy People initiative aims to prevent disease and improve Americans' quality of life. Healthy People reports, published each decade since 1980, set national health goals based on 10-year agendas. The initiative's most recent iteration, *Healthy People 2020,* was developed in 2008–2009 and released to the public in 2010. *Healthy People 2020* envisions "a society in which all people

KEY TERM **lifestyle choice** A conscious behavior that can increase or decrease a person's risk of disease or injury; such behaviors include smoking, exercising, eating a healthy diet, and others.

Fitness Tip

In Table 1.2, notice how many causes of death are related to lifestyle. This is an excellent motivator for adopting healthy habits and staying in good condition. Maintaining physical fitness and a healthy diet can lead to a longer life. It's a fact!

VITAL STATISTICS

Table 1.3 Key Contributors to Death Among Americans

	NUMBER OF DEATHS PER YEAR	PERCENTAGE OF TOTAL DEATHS PER YEAR
Tobacco	440,000	18.1
Obesity*	112,000	4.6
Alcohol consumption	85,000	3.5
Microbial agents	75,000	3.1
Toxic agents	55,000	2.3
Motor vehicles	43,000	1.8
Firearms	29,000	1.2
Sexual behavior	20,000	0.8
Illicit drug use	17,000	0.7

NOTE: The factors listed here are defined as lifestyle and environmental factors that contribute to the leading killers of Americans (health experts often refer to these as the *actual causes of death).* Microbial agents include bacterial and viral infections like influenza and pneumonia; toxic agents include environmental pollutants and chemical agents such as asbestos.

*The number of deaths due to obesity is an area of ongoing controversy and research. Recent estimates have ranged from 112,000 to 365,000.

SOURCES: Centers for Disease Control and Prevention. 2005. *Frequently Asked Questions About Calculating Obesity-Related Risk.* Atlanta, Ga.: Centers for Disease Control and Prevention. Mokdad, A. H., et al. 2005. Correction: Actual causes of death in the United States, 2000. *Journal of the American Medical Association* 293(3): 293–294. Mokdad, A. H., et al. 2004. Actual causes of death in the United States, 2000. *Journal of the American Medical Association* 291(10): 1238–1245.

VITAL STATISTICS

Table 1.4 Leading Causes of Death Among Americans Age 15–24, 2008

RANK	CAUSE OF DEATH	NUMBER OF DEATHS	PERCENTAGE OF TOTAL DEATHS
1	Accidents:	12,351	40.8
	Motor vehicle	7,648	25.2
	All other accidents	4,703	15.5
2	Homicide	4,820	15.9
3	Suicide	4,341	14.3
4	Cancer	1,659	5.4
5	Heart disease	1,010	3.3
	All causes	30,252	100.0

SOURCE: National Center for Health Statistics. 2011. Deaths: Preliminary data for 2009. *National Vital Statistics Report* 59(4).

live long, healthy lives" and proposes the eventual achievement of the following broad national health objectives:

- ***Eliminate preventable disease, disability, injury, and premature death.*** This objective involves activities such as taking more concrete steps to prevent diseases and injuries among individuals and groups, promoting healthy lifestyle choices, improving the nation's preparedness for emergencies, and strengthening the public health infrastructure.
- ***Achieve health equity, eliminate disparities, and improve the health of all groups.*** This objective involves identifying, measuring, and addressing health differences between individuals or groups that result from a social or economic disadvantage. (See the box "Wellness Issues for Diverse Populations.")
- ***Create social and physical environments that promote good health for all.*** This objective involves the use of health interventions at many different levels (such as anti-smoking campaigns by schools, workplaces, and local agencies), improving the situation of undereducated and poor Americans by providing a broader array of educational and job opportunities, and actively developing healthier living and natural environments for everyone.
- ***Promote healthy development and healthy behaviors across every stage of life.*** This goal involves taking a cradle-to-grave approach to health promotion by encouraging disease prevention and healthy behaviors in Americans of all ages.

In a shift from the past, *Healthy People 2020* emphasizes the importance of health determinants—factors that affect the health of individuals, demographic groups, or entire populations. Health determinants are social (including factors such as ethnicity, education level, and economic status) and environmental (including natural and human-made environments). Thus, one goal is to improve living conditions in ways that reduce the impact of negative health determinants.

Examples of individual health promotion goals from *Healthy People 2020,* along with estimates of how well Americans are tracking toward achieving those goals, appear in Table 1.5.

Behaviors That Contribute to Wellness

A lifestyle based on good choices and healthy behaviors maximizes quality of life. It helps people avoid disease, remain strong and fit, and maintain their physical and mental health as long as they live.

Be Physically Active The human body is designed to work best when it is active. It readily adapts to nearly any level of activity and exertion. **Physical fitness** is a set of physical attributes that allow the body to respond or adapt to the demands and stress of physical effort. The more we ask of our bodies, the stronger and more fit they become.

physical fitness A set of physical attributes that allows the body to respond or adapt to the demands and stress of physical effort.

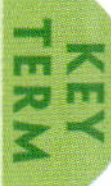

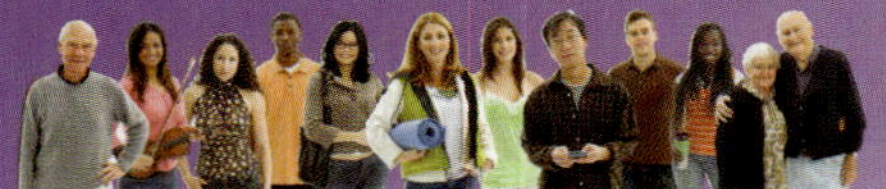

Wellness Issues for Diverse Populations

DIMENSIONS OF DIVERSITY

When it comes to striving for wellness, most differences among people are insignificant. We all need to exercise, eat well, and manage stress. We all need to know how to protect ourselves from disease and injuries.

But some of our differences—both as individuals and as members of groups—have important implications for wellness. Some of us, for example, have grown up with eating habits that increase our risk of obesity or heart disease. Some of us have inherited predispositions for certain health problems, such as osteoporosis or high cholesterol levels. These health-related differences among individuals and groups can be biological (determined genetically) or cultural (acquired as patterns of behavior through daily interactions with family, community, and society). Many health conditions are a function of biology and culture combined.

Every person is an individual with her or his own unique genetic endowment as well as unique experiences in life. However, many of these influences are shared with others of similar genetic and cultural backgrounds. Information about group similarities relating to wellness issues can be useful. For example, it can alert people to areas that may be of special concern for them and their families.

Wellness-related differences among groups can be described along several dimensions, including the following:

- ***Gender.*** Men and women have different life expectancies and different incidences of many diseases, including heart disease, cancer, and osteoporosis. Men have higher rates of death from injuries, suicide, and homicide, whereas women are at greater risk for Alzheimer's disease and depression. Men and women also differ in body composition and certain aspects of physical performance.

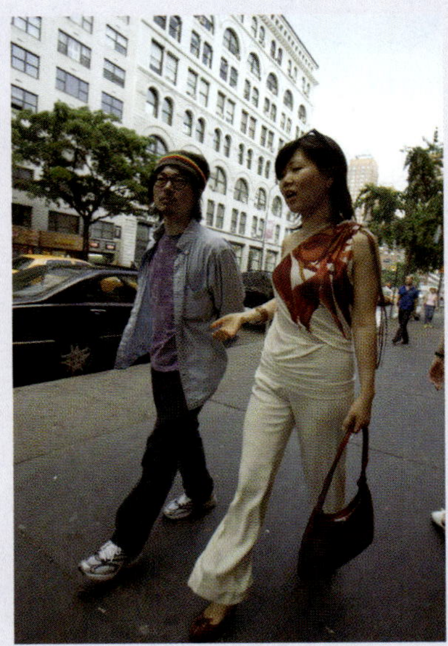

- ***Race and ethnicity.*** A genetic predisposition for a particular health problem can be linked to race or ethnicity as a result of each group's relatively distinct history. Diabetes is more prevalent among individuals of Native American or Latino heritage, for example, and African Americans have higher rates of hypertension. Racial or ethnic groups may also vary in other ways that relate to wellness: traditional diets; patterns of family and interpersonal relationships; and attitudes toward using tobacco, alcohol, and other drugs, to name just a few.

- ***Income and education.*** Inequalities in income and education underlie many of the health disparities among Americans. People with low incomes (low *socioeconomic status,* or *SES*) and less education have higher rates of injury and many diseases, are more likely to smoke, and have less access to health care. Poverty and low educational attainment are far more important predictors of poor health than any racial or ethnic factor.

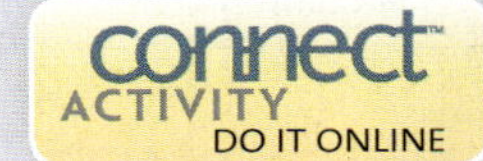

Table 1.5 Selected *Healthy People 2020* Objectives

OBJECTIVE	ESTIMATE OF CURRENT STATUS*	GOAL*
Reduce the proportion of adults who engage in no leisure-time physical activity	36.2	32.6
Increase the proportion of adults who are at a healthy weight	30.8	33.9
Reduce tobacco use (cigarette smoking) among adults	20.6	12.0
Increase the proportion of adults with mental health disorders who receive treatment	58.7	64.6
Reduce the proportion of adults with hypertension	29.9	26.9
Increase the proportion of adults who get sufficient sleep	69.6	70.9
Reduce the proportion of adults who drank excessively in the previous 30 days	28.1	25.3
Increase the proportion of persons who use the Internet to communicate with their health care provider	13	15

*Percentage of adult Americans

SOURCE: U.S. Department of Health and Human Services. 2011. *Healthy People 2010* (http://www.healthypeople.gov; retrieved April 15, 2011).

How Active Are You?

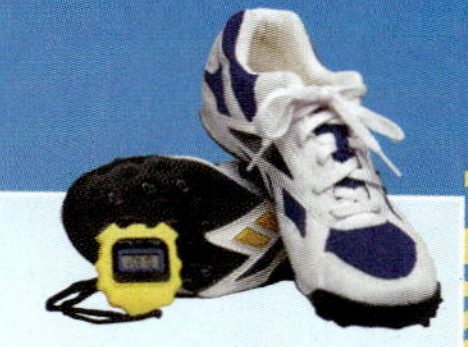

PERSONAL CHALLENGE

How much of your leisure time do you spend doing nothing? It's easy to figure out: Just keep a simple log (like the one shown here) for a full week. Log the number of minutes of free time you have each day, and list your activities during those times. For our purposes, "free time" means exactly that; it doesn't include time you spend studying.

Day 1: ______________________ (minutes) ______________________ (activities)

Day 2: ______________________ (minutes) ______________________ (activities)

Day 3: ______________________ (minutes) ______________________ (activities)

Day 4: ______________________ (minutes) ______________________ (activities)

Day 5: ______________________ (minutes) ______________________ (activities)

Day 6: ______________________ (minutes) ______________________ (activities)

Day 7: ______________________ (minutes) ______________________ (activities)

Based on this information, do you spend less than 30 minutes of your daily free time engaged in some type of physical activity? If so, look at your log and consider switching some of your current leisure-time activities for moderate-intensity exercise (like a brisk walk or a short bike ride).

Remember: you don't need to exercise for 30 minutes at a time to get the benefits of daily activity. You can break your exercise routine into three 10-minute chunks to make exercise fit your schedule and still enjoy all the health benefits of daily activity.

When our bodies are not kept active, however, they deteriorate. Bones lose their density, joints stiffen, muscles become weak, and cellular energy systems degenerate. To be truly well, human beings must be active.

Unfortunately, a **sedentary** lifestyle is common among Americans. According to recent estmates from the Healthy People program, fewer than one-third of adult Americans regularly engage in some sort of moderate physical activity. A recent study by the National Center for Health Statistics (NCHS) found that nearly 40% of adult Americans get no leisure-time activity at all.

The benefits of physical activity are both physical and mental, immediate and long term (Figure 1.4). In the short term, being physically fit makes it easier to do everyday tasks, such as lifting; it provides reserve strength for emergencies; and it helps people look and feel good. In the long term, being physically fit confers protection against chronic diseases and lowers the risk of dying prematurely. (See the box "Does Being Physically Active Make a Difference in How Long You Live?") Physically active people are less likely to develop or die from heart diease, respiratory disease, high blood pressure, cancer,

- Increased endurance, strength, and flexibility
- Healthier muscles, bones, and joints
- Increased energy (calorie) expenditure
- Improved body composition
- More energy
- Improved ability to cope with stress
- Improved mood, higher self-esteem, and a greater sense of well-being
- Improved ability to fall asleep and sleep well

- Reduced risk of dying prematurely from all causes
- Reduced risk of developing and/or dying from heart disease, diabetes, high blood pressure, and colon cancer
- Reduced risk of becoming obese
- Reduced anxiety, tension, and depression
- Reduced risk of falls and fractures
- Reduced spending for health care

FIGURE 1.4 Benefits of regular physical activity.

sedentary Physically inactive; literally, "sitting."

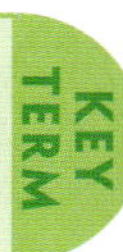

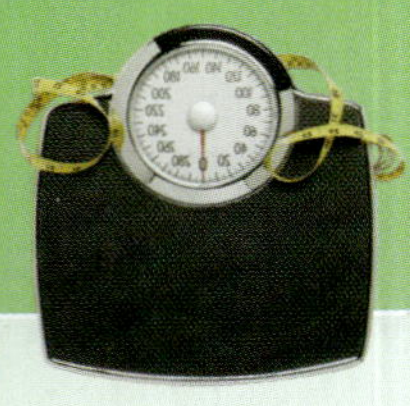

THE EVIDENCE FOR EXERCISE

Does Being Physically Active Make a Difference in How Long You Live?

How can we be sure that physical activity and exercise are good for our health? To answer this question, the U.S. Department of Health and Human Services asked a committee to review scientific literature. The committee's mission was to determine if enough evidence exists to warrant the government making physical activity recommendations to the public. The committee's report, the *Physical Activity Guidelines Advisory Committee Report, 2008*, summarizes the scientific evidence for the health benefits of regular physical activity and the risks of sedentary behavior. The report provides the rationale for the federal government's physical activity guidelines.

The committee started by asking whether physical activity actually helps people live longer. The committee investigated the link between physical activity and all-cause mortality—deaths from all causes—by looking at 73 studies dating from 1995 to 2008. The studies included men and women from all age groups (16 to 65 +) and from different racial and ethnic groups.

The data from these studies strongly support an *inverse relation* between physical activity and all-cause mortality; that is, physically active people were less likely to die during a study's follow-up period (ranging from 10 months to 28 years). The review found that active people have about a 30% lower risk of dying compared with inactive people. These inverse associations were found not just for healthy adults but also for older adults (age 65 and older), for people with coronary artery disease and diabetes, for people with impaired mobility, and for people who were overweight or obese. Poor fitness and low physical activity levels were found to be better predictors of premature death than smoking, diabetes, or obesity. Based on the evidence, the committee determined that about 150 minutes (2.5 hours) of physical activity per week is enough to reduce all-cause mortality (see Chapter 2 for more details). It appears that it is the overall volume of energy expended, no matter what kinds of activities are done, that makes a difference in risk of premature death.

The committee also looked at whether there is a *dose-response* relation between physical activity and all-cause mortality—that is, whether more activity reduces death rates even further. Again, the studies showed an inverse relation between these two variables. So, more activity above and beyond 150 minutes per week produces greater benefits. Surprisingly, for inactive people, benefits are seen at levels below 150 minutes per week. In fact, *any* increase in physical activity resulted in reduced risk of death. The committee refers to this as the "some is good; more is better" message. A target of 150 minutes per week is recommended, but any level of activity below the target is encouraged for inactive people.

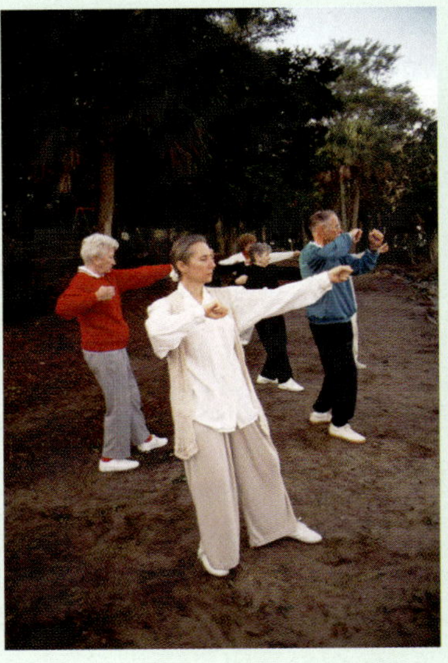

Looking more closely at this relationship, the committee found that the greatest risk reduction is seen at the lower end of the physical activity spectrum (30 to 90 minutes per week). In fact, sedentary people who become more active have the greatest potential for improving health and reducing the risk of premature death. Additional risk reduction occurs as physical activity increases, but at a slower rate. For example, people who engaged in physical activity 90 minutes per week had a 20% reduction in mortality risk compared with inactive people, and those who were active 150 minutes per week, as noted earlier, had a 30% reduction in risk. But to achieve a 40% reduction in mortality risk, study participants had to be physically active 420 minutes per week (7 hours).

The message from the research is clear: It doesn't matter what activity you choose or even how much time you can devote to it per week, as long as you get moving!

SOURCE: Physical Activity Guidelines Advisory Committee. 2008. *Physical Activity Guidelines Advisory Committee Report, 2008*. Washington, D.C.: U.S. Department of Health and Human Services.

osteoporosis, and type 2 diabetes (the most common form of diabetes). As they get older, they may be able to avoid weight gain, muscle and bone loss, fatigue, and other problems associated with aging.

Choose a Healthy Diet In addition to being sedentary, many Americans have a diet that is too high in calories, unhealthy fats, and added sugars and too low in fiber, complex carbohydrates, fruits, and vegetables. Like physical inactivity, this diet is linked to a number of chronic diseases. A healthy diet provides necessary nutrients and sufficient energy without also providing too much of the dietary substances linked to diseases.

Maintain a Healthy Body Weight Overweight and obesity are associated with a number of disabling and potentially fatal conditions and diseases, including heart disease, cancer, and type 2 diabetes. The Centers for Disease Control and Prevention (CDC) estimates that obesity kills 112,000 Americans each year. Healthy body weight is an important part of wellness—but short-term dieting is not part of fitness or wellness. Maintaining a healthy body

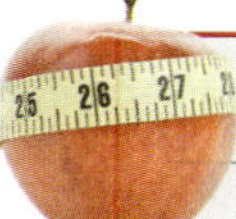

Wellness Tip

If you're overweight, losing as little as 5 pounds can significantly reduce your risk of developing diabetes. To learn more, visit the American Diabetes Association's Web site at http://www.diabetes.org.

weight requires a lifelong commitment to regular exercise, a healthy diet, and effective stress management.

Manage Stress Effectively Many people cope with stress by eating, drinking, or smoking too much. Others don't deal with it at all. In the short term, inappropriate stress management can lead to fatigue, sleep disturbances, and other symptoms. Over longer periods of time, poor stress management can lead to less efficient functioning of the immune system and increased susceptibility to disease. Learning to incorporate effective stress management techniques into daily life is an important part of a fit and well lifestyle.

Avoid Tobacco and Drug Use and Limit Alcohol Consumption Tobacco use is associated with 8 of the top 10 causes of death in the United States; personal tobacco use and second-hand smoke kill about 440,000 Americans each year, more than any other behavioral or environmental factor. With 21% of adult Americans describing themselves as current smokers as of 2009, lung cancer is the most common cause of cancer death among both men and women and one of the leading causes of death overall. On average, the direct health care costs associated with smoking exceed $100 billion per year. If the cost of lost productivity from sickness, disability, and premature death is included, the total is closer to $193 billion.

Excessive alcohol consumption is linked to 6 of the top 10 causes of death and results in about 85,000 deaths a year in the United States. The social, economic, and medical costs of alcohol abuse are estimated at over $185 billion per year. Alcohol or drug intoxication is an especially notable factor in the death and disability of young people, particularly through **unintentional injuries** (such as drownings and car crashes caused by drunken driving) and violence.

Protect Yourself from Disease and Injury The most effective way of dealing with disease and injury is to prevent them. Many of the lifestyle strategies discussed here help protect you against chronic illnesses. In addition, you can take specific steps to avoid infectious diseases, particularly those that are sexually transmitted.

Take Other Steps Toward Wellness Other important behaviors contribute to wellness, including these:

- Developing meaningful relationships
- Planning for successful aging
- Learning about the health care system
- Acting responsibly toward the environment

Labs 1.1 and 1.2 will help you evaluate your behaviors as they relate to wellness.

Ask Yourself

QUESTIONS FOR CRITICAL THINKING AND REFLECTION

How often do you feel exuberant? Vital? Joyful? What makes you feel that way? Conversely, how often do you feel downhearted, de-energized, or depressed? What makes you feel that way? Have you ever thought about how you might increase experiences of vitality and decrease experiences of discouragement?

The Role of Other Factors in Wellness

Heredity, the environment, and adequate health care are other important influences on health and wellness. These factors can interact in ways that raise or lower the quality of a person's life and the risk of developing particular diseases. For example, a sedentary lifestyle combined with a genetic predisposition for diabetes can greatly increase one's risk for developing the disease. If this person also lacks adequate health care, he or she is much more likely to suffer dangerous complications from diabetes.

But in many cases, behavior can tip the balance toward health even if heredity or environment is a negative factor. Breast cancer, for example, can run in families, but it is also associated with overweight and a sedentary lifestyle. A woman with a family history of breast cancer is less likely to die from the disease if she controls her weight, exercises, performs regular breast self-exams, and consults with her physician about mammograms.

REACHING WELLNESS THROUGH LIFESTYLE MANAGEMENT

As you consider this description of behaviors that contribute to wellness—being physically active, choosing a healthy diet, and so on—you may be doing a mental comparison with your own behaviors. If you are like most young adults, you probably have some healthy habits and some habits that place your health at risk. For example, you may be physically active and have a healthy diet but indulge in binge drinking on weekends. You may be careful to wear your seat belt in your car but smoke cigarettes or use chewing tobacco. Moving in the direction of

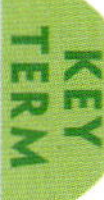

KEY TERM

unintentional injury An injury that occurs without harm being intended.

wellness means cultivating healthy behaviors and working to overcome unhealthy ones. This approach to lifestyle management is called **behavior change.**

As you may already know from experience, changing an unhealthy habit can be harder than it sounds. When you embark on a behavior change plan, it may seem like too much work at first. But as you make progress, you will gain confidence in your ability to take charge of your life. You will also experience the benefits of wellness—more energy, greater vitality, deeper feelings of appreciation and curiosity, and a higher quality of life.

The rest of this chapter outlines a general process for changing unhealthy behaviors that is backed by research and that has worked for many people. You will also find many specific strategies and tips for change. For additional support, work through the activities in the Behavior Change Workbook at the end of the text.

Getting Serious About Your Health

Before you can start changing a wellness-related behavior, you have to know that the behavior is problematic and that you *can* change it. To make good decisions, you need information about relevant topics and issues, including what resources are available to help you change.

Examine Your Current Health Habits Have you considered how your current lifestyle is affecting your health today and how it will affect your health in the future? Do you know which of your current habits enhance your health and which ones may be harmful? Begin your journey toward wellness with self-assessment: Think about your own behavior, complete the self-assessment in Lab 1.2, and talk with friends and family members about what they've noticed about your lifestyle and your health.

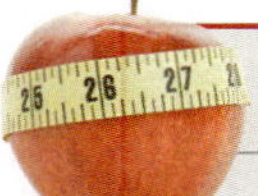

Wellness Tip

When it comes to behavior change, you can win big by starting small, so pick a habit that will be easy to fix. Good examples are drinking more water every day or brushing your teeth for 2 minutes, twice a day. Each time you adopt a healthy new behavior, it's a stepping stone toward a bigger goal.

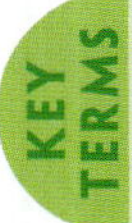

KEY TERMS

behavior change A lifestyle management process that involves cultivating healthy behaviors and working to overcome unhealthy ones.

target behavior An isolated behavior selected as the object of a behavior change program.

Choose a Target Behavior Changing any behavior can be demanding. This is why it's a good idea to start small, by choosing one behavior you want to change—called a **target behavior**—and working on it until you succeed. Your chances of success will be greater if your first goal is simple, such as resisting the urge to snack between classes. As you change one behavior, make your next goal a little more significant, and build on your success over time.

Learn About Your Target Behavior Once you've chosen a target behavior, you need to learn its risks and benefits for you—both now and in the future. Ask these questions:

- How is your target behavior affecting your level of wellness today?
- What diseases or conditions does this behavior place you at risk for?
- What effect would changing your behavior have on your health?

As a starting point, use this text and the resources listed in the For Further Exploration section at the end of

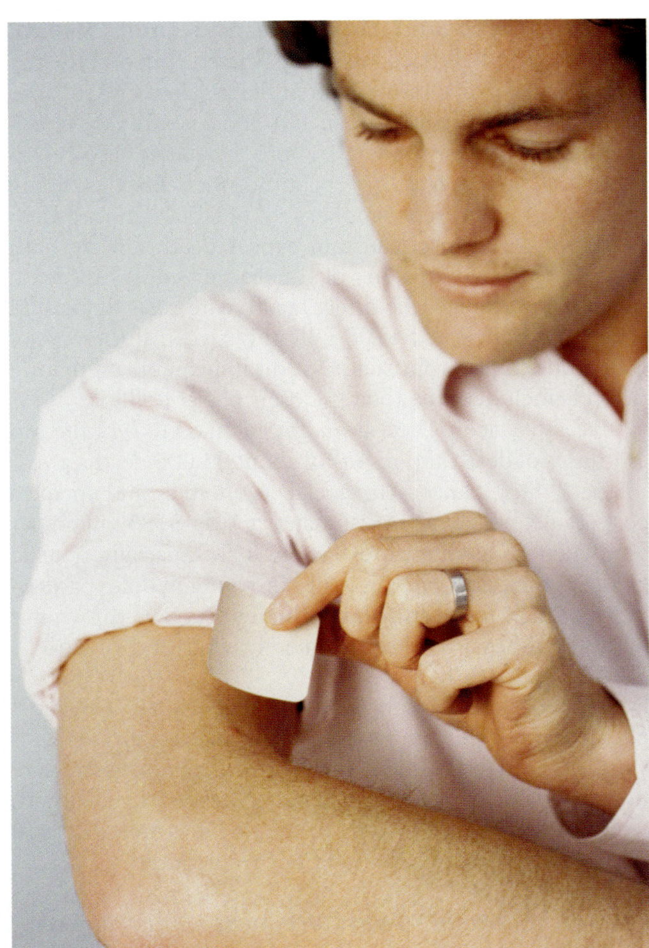

Certain health behaviors are exceptionally difficult to change. Some people can quit smoking on their own; others get help from a smoking cessation program or a nicotine replacement product.

Evaluating Sources of Health Information

CRITICAL CONSUMER

Believability of Health Information Sources

Surveys indicate that college students are smart about evaluating health information. They trust the health information they receive from health professionals and educators and are skeptical about popular information sources, such as magazine articles and Web sites.

How smart are you about evaluating health information? Here are some tips.

General Strategies

Whenever you encounter health-related information, take the following steps to make sure it is credible:

- ***Go to the original source.*** Media reports often simplify the results of medical research. Find out for yourself what a study really reported, and determine whether it was based on good science. What type of study was it? Was it published in a recognized medical journal? Was it an animal study, or did it involve people? Did the study include a large number of people? What did the study's authors actually report?
- ***Watch for misleading language.*** Reports that tout "breakthroughs" or "dramatic proof" are probably hype. A study may state that a behavior "contributes to" or is "associated with" an outcome, but this does not prove a cause-and-effect relationship.
- ***Distinguish between research reports and public health advice.*** Do not change your behavior based on the results of a single report or study. If an agency such as the National Cancer Institute urges a behavior change, however, you should follow its advice. Large, publicly funded organizations issue such advice based on many studies, not a single report.
- ***Remember that anecdotes are not facts.*** A friend may tell you he lost weight on some new diet, but individual success stories do not mean the plan is truly safe or effective. Check with your doctor before making any serious lifestyle changes.
- ***Be skeptical.*** If a report seems too good to be true, it probably is. Be wary of information contained in advertisements. An ad's goal is to sell a product, even if there is no need for it, and sometimes even if the product has not been proven to be safe or effective.
- ***Make choices that are right for you.*** Friends and family members can be a great source of ideas and inspiration, but you need to make health-related choices that work best for you.

Internet Resources

Online information sources pose special challenges. When reviewing a health-related Web site, ask these questions:

- ***What is the source of the information?*** Web sites maintained by government agencies, professional associations, or established academic or medical institutions are likely to present trustworthy information. Many other groups and individuals post accurate information, but it is important to look at the qualifications of the people who are behind the site. (Check the home page or click the "About Us" link.)
- ***How often is the site updated?*** Look for sites that are updated frequently. Check the "last modified" date of any Web page.
- ***Is the site promotional?*** Be wary of information from sites that sell specific products, use testimonials as evidence, appear to have a social or political agenda, or ask for money.
- ***What do other sources say about a topic?*** Be wary of claims and information that appear at only one site or come from a chat room, bulletin board, or blog.
- ***Does the site conform to any set of guidelines or criteria for quality and accuracy?*** Look for sites that identify themselves as conforming to some code or set of principles, such as those set forth by the Health on the Net Foundation or the American Medical Association. These codes include criteria such as use of information from respected sources and disclosure of the site's sponsors.

each chapter; see the box "Evaluating Sources of Health Information" for additional guidelines.

Find Help Have you identified a particularly challenging target behavior or mood—something like alcohol addiction, binge eating, or depression—that interferes with your ability to function or places you at a serious health risk? Help may be needed to change behaviors or conditions that are too deeply rooted or too serious for self-management. Don't be discouraged by the seriousness or extent of the problem; many resources are available to help you solve it. On campus, the student health center or campus counseling center can provide assistance. To locate community resources, consult the yellow pages, your physician, or the Internet.

Building Motivation to Change

Knowledge is necessary for behavior change, but it isn't usually enough to make people act. Millions of people have sedentary lifestyles, for example, even though they know it's bad for their health. This is particularly true of young adults, who may not be motivated to change because they feel healthy in spite of their unhealthy behaviors (see the box "Wellness Matters for College Students"). To succeed at behavior change, you need strong motivation.

IN FOCUS

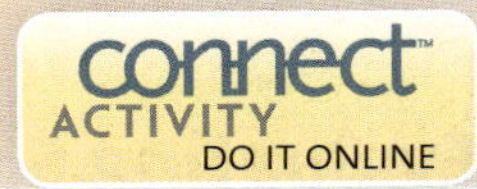

Wellness Matters for College Students

If you are like most college students, you probably feel pretty good about your health right now. Most college students are in their late teens or early twenties, lead active lives, have plenty of friends, and look forward to a future filled with opportunity. With all these things going for you, why shouldn't you feel good?

A Closer Look

Although most college-age people look healthy, appearances can be deceiving. Each year, thousands of students lose productive academic time to physical and emotional health problems—some of which can continue to plague them for life.

The following table shows the top 10 health issues affecting students' academic performance, according to the Fall 2010 American College Health Association National College Health Assessment II.

HEALTH ISSUE	STUDENTS AFFECTED (%)
Stress	25.4
Sleep difficulties	17.8
Anxiety	16.4
Cold/flu/sore throat	13.8
Internet use/computer games	11.6
Work	11.4
Concern for a friend/ family member	10.1
Depression	10.0
Relationship difficulties	9.6
Extracurricular activities	8.8

Each of these issues is related to one or more of the six dimensions of wellness, and most can be influenced by choices students make daily. Although some troubles—such as the death of a friend—cannot be controlled, other physical and emotional concerns can be minimized by choosing healthy behaviors. For example, there are many ways to manage stress, the top health issue affecting students. By reducing unhealthy choices (such as using alcohol to relax) and by increasing healthy choices (such as using time management techniques), even busy students can reduce the impact of stress on their life.

The survey also estimated that, based on students' reporting of their height and weight, more than 33% of college students are either overweight or obese. Although heredity plays a role in determining one's weight, lifestyle is also a factor in weight and weight management. In many studies over the past few decades, a large percentage of students have reported behaviors such as these:

- Overeating
- Snacking on junk food
- Frequently eating high-fat foods
- Using alcohol and binge drinking

Clearly, eating behaviors are often a matter of choice. Although students may not see (or feel) the effects of their dietary habits today, the long-term health risks are significant. Overweight and obese persons run a higher-than-normal risk of developing diabetes, heart disease, and cancer later in life. We now know with certainty that improving one's eating habits, even a little, can lead to weight loss and improved overall health.

Other Choices, Other Problems

Students commonly make other unhealthy choices. Here are some examples from the Fall 2010 National College Health Assessment II:

- About 50% of students reported that they did not use a contraceptive the last time they had vaginal intercourse.
- About 16% of students had 7 or more drinks the last time they partied.
- Almost 15% of students had smoked cigarettes at least once during the past month.

What choices do you make in these situations? Remember: It's never too late to change. The sooner you trade an unhealthy behavior for a healthy one, the longer you'll be around to enjoy the benefits.

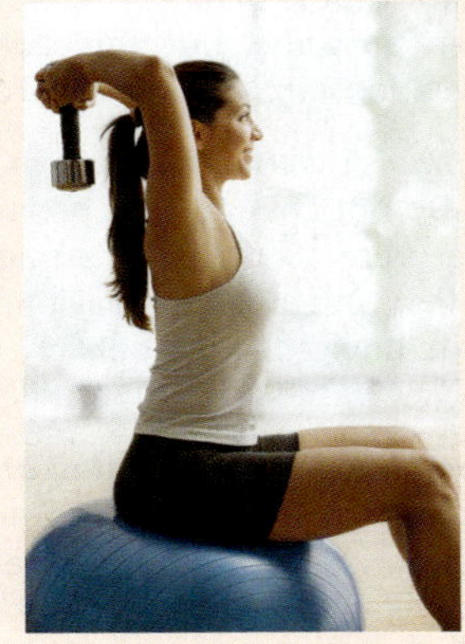

SOURCE: American College Health Association. 2011. *American College Health Association National College Health Assessment II: Reference Group Executive Summary Fall 2010.* Linthicum, Md.: American College Health Association.

Examine the Pros and Cons of Change Health behaviors have short-term and long-term benefits and costs. Consider the benefits and costs of an inactive lifestyle:

- Short-term, such a lifestyle allows you more time to watch TV and hang out with friends, but it leaves you less physically fit and less able to participate in recreational activities.
- Long-term, it increases the risk of heart disease, cancer, stroke, and premature death.

To successfully change your behavior, you must believe that the benefits of change outweigh the costs.

Carefully examine the pros and cons of continuing your current behavior and of changing to a healthier one. Focus on the effects that are most meaningful to you, including those that are tied to your personal identity and values. For example, if you see yourself as an active person who is a good role model for others, then adopting behaviors such as engaging in regular physical activity and getting adequate sleep will support your personal identity.

If you value independence and control over your life, then quitting smoking will be consistent with your values and goals. To complete your analysis, ask friends and family members about the effects of your behavior on them. For example, a younger sister may tell you that your smoking habit influenced her decision to take up smoking.

The short-term benefits of behavior change can be an important motivating force. Although some people are motivated by long-term goals, such as avoiding a disease that may hit them in 30 years, most are more likely to be moved to action by shorter-term, more personal goals. Feeling better, doing better in school, improving at a sport, reducing stress, and increasing self-esteem are common short-term benefits of health behavior change. Many wellness behaviors are associated with immediate improvements in quality of life. For example, surveys of Americans have found that nonsmokers feel healthy and full of energy more days each month than do smokers, and they report fewer days of sadness and troubled sleep. The same is true when physically active people are compared with sedentary people. Over time, these types of differences add up to a substantially higher quality of life for people who engage in healthy behaviors.

Boost Self-Efficacy When you start thinking about changing a health behavior, a big factor in your eventual success is whether you have confidence in yourself and in your ability to change. **Self-efficacy** refers to your belief in your ability to successfully take action and perform a specific task. Strategies for boosting self-efficacy include developing an internal locus of control, using visualization and self-talk, and getting encouragement from supportive people.

LOCUS OF CONTROL Who do you believe is controlling your life? Is it your parents, friends, or school? Is it "fate"? Or is it you? **Locus of control** refers to the figurative "place" a person designates as the source of responsibility for the events in his or her life. People who believe they are in control of their own lives are said to have an *internal locus of control*. Those who believe that factors beyond their control determine the course of their lives are said to have an *external locus of control*.

For lifestyle management, an internal locus of control is an advantage because it reinforces motivation and commitment. An external locus of control can sabotage efforts to change behavior. For example, if you believe that you are destined to die of breast cancer because your mother died from the disease, you may view monthly breast self-exams and regular checkups as a waste of time. In contrast, if you believe that you can take action to reduce your risk of breast cancer in spite of hereditary factors, you will be motivated to follow guidelines for early detection of the disease.

If you find yourself attributing too much influence to outside forces, gather more information about your wellness-related behaviors. List all the ways that making lifestyle changes will improve your health. If you believe you'll succeed, and if you recognize that you are in charge of your life, you're on your way to wellness.

> **Fitness Tip**
>
> Visualization is such a powerful technique that Olympic athletes learn how to harness it for peak performance. It works for average people, too. Set a small fitness goal, then imagine yourself doing it—as clearly and as often as you can. Visualization can help you believe in yourself, and belief can be a step toward success!

VISUALIZATION AND SELF-TALK One of the best ways to boost your confidence and self-efficacy is to visualize yourself successfully engaging in a new, healthier behavior. Imagine yourself going for an afternoon run 3 days a week or no longer smoking cigarettes. Also visualize yourself enjoying all the short-term and long-term benefits that your lifestyle change will bring. Create a new self-image: What will you and your life be like when you become a regular exerciser or a nonsmoker?

You can also use **self-talk,** the internal dialogue you carry on with yourself, to increase your confidence in your ability to change. Counter any self-defeating patterns of thought with more positive or realistic thoughts: "I am a strong, capable person, and I can maintain my commitment to change." See Chapter 10 for more on self-talk.

ROLE MODELS AND OTHER SUPPORTIVE INDIVIDUALS Social support can make a big difference in your level of motivation and your chances of success. Perhaps you know people who have reached the goal you are striving for; they could be role models or mentors for you, providing information and support for your efforts. Gain strength from their experiences, and tell yourself, "If they can do it, so can I." In addition, find a buddy who wants to make the same changes you do and who can take an active role in your behavior change program. For example, an exercise buddy can provide companionship and encouragement when you might be tempted to skip your workout.

Identify and Overcome Barriers to Change Don't let past failures at behavior change discourage you; they can be a great source of information you can use to boost your chances of future success. Make a list of the problems and challenges you faced in any previous behavior change attempts. To this list, add the short-term costs of behavior

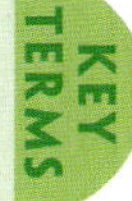

self-efficacy The belief in one's ability to take action and perform a specific task.

locus of control The figurative "place" a person designates as the source of responsibility for the events in his or her life.

self-talk A person's internal dialogue.

change that you identified in your analysis of the pros and cons of change. Once you've listed these key barriers to change, develop a practical plan for overcoming each one. For example, if you always smoke when you're with certain friends, decide in advance how you will turn down the next cigarette you are offered.

Enhancing Your Readiness to Change

The transtheoretical, or "stages-of-change," model is an effective approach to lifestyle self-management. According to this model, you move through distinct stages as you work to change your target behavior. It is important to determine what stage you are in now so that you can choose appropriate strategies for progressing through the cycle of change. This approach can help you enhance your readiness and intention to change. Read the following sections to determine what stage you are in for your target behavior. For ideas on changing stages, see the box "Tips for Moving Forward in the Cycle of Behavior Change."

Precontemplation People at this stage do not think they have a problem and do not intend to change their behavior. They may be unaware of the risks associated with their behavior or may deny them. They may have tried unsuccessfully to change in the past and may now think the situation is hopeless. They may also blame other people or external factors for their problems. People in the precontemplation stage believe that there are more reasons or more important reasons not to change than there are reasons to change.

Contemplation People at this stage know they have a problem and intend to take action within 6 months. They acknowledge the benefits of behavior change but are also aware of the costs of changing. To be successful, people must believe that the benefits of change outweigh the costs. People in the contemplation stage wonder about possible courses of action but don't know how to proceed. There may also be specific barriers to change that appear too difficult to overcome.

Preparation People at this stage plan to take action within a month or may already have begun to make small changes in their behavior. They may be engaging in their new, healthier behavior but not yet regularly or consistently. They may have created a plan for change but may be worried about failing.

Action During the action stage, people outwardly modify their behavior and their environment. The action stage requires the greatest commitment of time and energy, and people in this stage are at risk for reverting to old, unhealthy patterns of behavior.

Maintenance People at this stage have maintained their new, healthier lifestyle for at least 6 months. Lapses may have occurred, but people in maintenance have been successful in quickly reestablishing the desired behavior. The maintenance stage can last for months or years.

Termination For some behaviors, a person may reach the sixth and final stage of termination. People at this stage have exited the cycle of change and are no longer tempted to lapse back into their old behavior. They have a new self-image and total self-efficacy with regard to their target behavior.

Dealing with Relapse

People seldom progress through the stages of change in a straightforward, linear way. Rather, they tend to move to a certain stage and then slip back to a previous stage before resuming their forward progress. Research suggests that most people make several attempts before they successfully change a behavior; 4 out of 5 people experience some degree of backsliding. For this reason, the stages of change are best conceptualized as a spiral, in which people cycle back through previous stages but are farther along in the process each time they renew their commitment (Figure 1.5).

If you experience a lapse—a single slip—or a relapse—a return to old habits—don't give up. Relapse can be demoralizing, but it is not the same as failure. Failure means stopping before you reach your goal and never changing your target behavior. During the early stages of

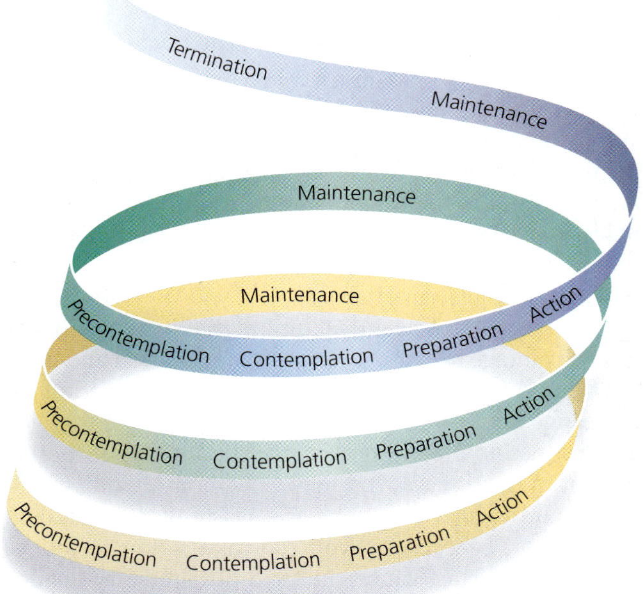

FIGURE 1.5 The stages of change: A spiral model.
SOURCE: Adapted from Prochaska, J. O., C. C. Diclemente, and J. C. Norcross. 1992. In search of how people change. *American Psychologist* 47(9): 1102–1114. Copyright © 1992 by the American Psychological Association. Reprinted by permission.

Tips for Moving Forward in the Cycle of Behavior Change

TAKE CHARGE

Precontemplation

- ***Raise your awareness.*** Research your target behavior and its effects.
- ***Be self-aware.*** Look at the mechanisms you use to resist change, such as denial or rationalization. Find ways to counteract these mechanisms.
- ***Seek social support.*** Friends and family members can help you identify target behaviors and understand their impact on the people around you.
- ***Identify helpful resources.*** These might include exercise classes or stress-management workshops offered by your school.

Contemplation

- ***Keep a journal.*** A record of your target behavior and the circumstances that elicit the behavior can help you plan a change program.
- ***Do a cost-benefit analysis.*** Identify the costs and benefits (both current and future) of maintaining your behavior and of changing it. Costs can be monetary, social, emotional, and so on.
- ***Identify barriers to change.*** Knowing these obstacles can help you overcome them.
- ***Engage your emotions.*** Watch movies or read books about people with your target behavior. Imagine what your life will be like if you don't change.
- ***Create a new self-image.*** Imagine what you'll be like after changing your target behavior. Try to think of yourself in new terms right now.
- ***Think before you act.*** Learn why you engage in the target behavior. Determine what "sets you off," and train yourself not to act reflexively.

Preparation

- ***Create a plan.*** Include a start date, goals, rewards, and specific steps you will take to change your behavior.
- ***Make change a priority.*** Create and sign a contract with yourself.
- ***Practice visualization and self-talk.*** These techniques can help prepare you mentally for challenging situations.
- ***Take short steps.*** Successfully practicing your new behavior for a short time—even a single day—can boost your confidence and motivation.

Action

- ***Monitor your progress.*** Keep up with your journal entries.
- ***Change your environment.*** Make changes that will discourage the target behavior—for example, getting rid of snack foods or not stocking the refrigerator with beer.
- ***Find alternatives to your target behavior.*** Make a list of things you can do to replace the behavior.
- ***Reward yourself.*** Rewards should be identified in your change plan. Give yourself lots of praise, and focus on your success.
- ***Involve your friends.*** Tell them you want to change, and ask for their help.
- ***Don't get discouraged.*** Real change is difficult.

Maintenance

- ***Keep going.*** Continue using the positive strategies that worked in earlier stages.
- ***Be prepared for lapses.*** Don't let slip-ups set you back.
- ***Be a role model.*** Once you have successfully changed your behavior, you may be able to help someone else do the same thing.

the change process, it's a good idea to plan for relapse so you can avoid guilt and self-blame and get back on track quickly. Follow these steps:

1. **Forgive yourself.** A single setback isn't the end of the world, but abandoning your efforts to change could have negative effects on your life.
2. **Give yourself credit for the progress you have already made**. You can use that success as motivation to continue.
3. **Move on.** You can learn from a relapse and use that knowledge to deal with potential setbacks in the future.

If relapses keep occurring or if you can't seem to control them, you may need to return to a previous stage of the behavior change process. If this is necessary, reevaluate your goals and your strategy. A different or less stressful approach may help you avoid setbacks when you try again.

Developing Skills for Change: Creating a Personalized Plan

Once you are committed to making a change, it's time to put together a plan of action. Your key to success is a well-thought-out plan that sets goals, anticipates problems, and includes rewards.

PERSONAL CHALLENGE

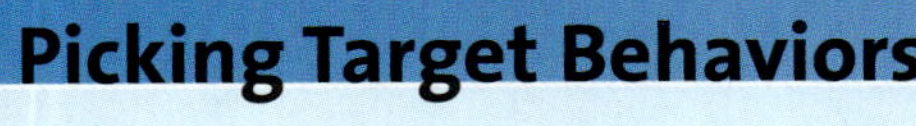

Picking Target Behaviors

When starting out on any behavior change plan, the hardest part can be deciding what behavior you want to change. But it doesn't have to be hard; as mentioned in the chapter, you'll probably have the greatest success if you start small. Use the following list to identify five health-related behaviors that you would like to change. List them in order, starting with the behavior you think would be easiest to change and ending with the most difficult.

1. ______________________________
2. ______________________________
3. ______________________________
4. ______________________________
5. ______________________________

The real challenge of this activity is thinking. Examine your lifestyle thoroughly, and consider the things you do (or don't do) every day that may be having a negative effect on your health or wellness. Don't worry if it takes some time to come up with a list, and don't be surprised if you shuffle the items around a few times. The goal is to come up with a list that is doable and realistic for you.

1. Monitor Your Behavior and Gather Data Keep a record of your target behavior and the circumstances surrounding it. Record this information for at least a week or two. Keep your notes in a health journal or notebook or on your computer (see the sample journal entries in Figure 1.6). Record each occurrence of your behavior, noting the following:

- What the activity was
- When and where it happened
- What you were doing
- How you felt at that time

If your goal is to start an exercise program, track your activities to determine how to make time for workouts. A blank log is provided in Activity 3 in the Behavior Change Workbook at the end of this text.

2. Analyze the Data and Identify Patterns After you have collected data on the behavior, analyze the data to identify patterns. When are you most likely to overeat? What events trigger your appetite? Perhaps you are especially hungry at midmorning or when you put off eating dinner until 9:00 P.M. Perhaps you overindulge in food and drink when you go to a particular restaurant or when you're with certain friends. Note the connections between your feelings and such external cues as time of day, location, situation, and the actions of others around you.

3. Be "SMART" About Setting Goals If your goals are too challenging, you will have trouble making steady progress and will be more likely to give up altogether. If, for example, you are in poor physical condition, it will not make sense to set a goal of being ready to run a marathon within 2 months. If you set goals you can live with, it will be easier to stick with your behavior change plan and be successful.

Experts suggest that your goals meet the "SMART" criteria. That is, your behavior change goals should be:

- *Specific.* Avoid vague goals like "eat more fruits and vegetables." Instead, state your objectives in specific terms, such as "eat 2 cups of fruit and 3 cups of vegetables every day."
- *Measurable.* Recognize that your progress will be easier to track if your goals are quantifiable, so give your goal a number. You might measure your goal in terms of time (such as "walk briskly for 20 minutes a day"), distance ("run 2 miles, 3 days per week"), or some other amount ("drink 8 glasses of water every day").
- *Attainable.* Set goals that are within your physical limits. For example, if you are a poor swimmer, it might not be possible for you to meet a short-term fitness goal by swimming laps. Walking or biking might be better options.
- *Realistic.* Manage your expectations when you set goals. For example, it may not be possible for a long-time smoker to quit cold turkey. A more realistic approach might be to use nicotine replacement patches or gum for several weeks while getting help from a support group.
- *Time frame–specific.* Give yourself a reasonable amount of time to reach your goal, state the time frame in your behavior change plan, and set your agenda to meet the goal within the given time frame.

Using these criteria, a sedentary person who wants to improve his health and build fitness might set a goal of being able to run 3 miles in 30 minutes, to be achieved within a time frame of 6 months. To work toward that goal, he might set a number of smaller, intermediate goals that are easier to achieve. For example, his list of goals might look like this:

WEEK	FREQUENCY (DAYS/WEEK)	ACTIVITY	DURATION (MINUTES)
1	3	Walk < 1 mile	10–15
2	3	Walk 1 mile	15–20
3	4	Walk 1–2 miles	20–25
4	4	Walk 2–3 miles	25–30
5–7	3–4	Walk/run 1 mile	15–20
~			
21–24	4–5	Run 2–3 miles	25–30

Of course, it may not be possible to meet these goals, but you never know until you try. As you work toward meeting your long-term goal, you may find it necessary to adjust your short-term goals. For example, you may find that you can start running sooner than you thought, or you may be able to run farther than you originally estimated. In such cases, it may be reasonable to make your goals more challenging. Otherwise, you may want to make them easier in order to stay motivated.

For some goals and situations, it may make more sense to focus on something other than your outcome goal. If you are in an early stage of change, for example, your goal may be to learn more about the risks associated with your target behavior or to complete a cost-benefit analysis. If your goal involves a long-term lifestyle change, such as reaching a healthy weight, it is better to focus on developing healthy habits than to target a specific weight loss. Your goal in this case might be exercising for 30 minutes every day, reducing portion sizes, or eliminating late-night snacks.

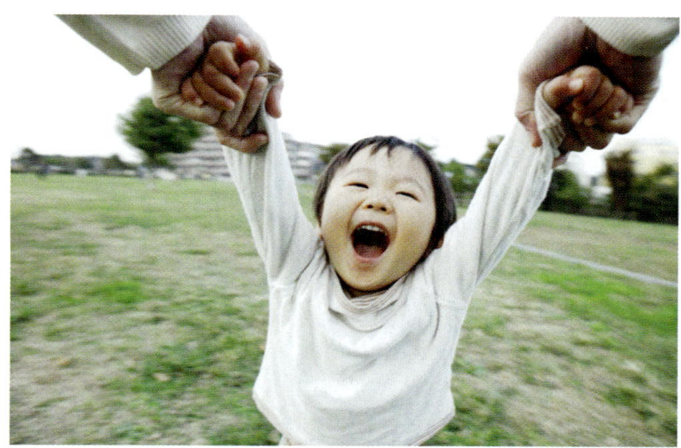

Your environment contains powerful cues for both positive and negative lifestyle choices. The presence of parks and running/bike paths encourages physical activity, even in an urban setting.

4. Devise a Plan of Action Develop a strategy that will support your efforts to change. Your plan of action should include the following steps:

- ***Get what you need.*** Identify resources that can help you. For example, you can join a community walking club or sign up for a smoking cessation program. You may also need to buy some new running shoes or nicotine replacement patches. Get the items you need right away; waiting can delay your progress.
- ***Modify your environment.*** If there are cues in your environment that trigger your target behavior, try to control them. For example, if you normally have alcohol at home, getting rid of it can help prevent you from indulging. If you usually study with a group of friends in an environment that allows smoking, try moving to a nonsmoking area. If you always buy a snack at a certain vending machine, change your route to avoid it.

Date November 5 Day M [TU] W TH F SA SU

Time of day	*M/S*	*Food eaten*	*Cals.*	*H*	*Where did you eat?*	*What else were you doing?*	*How did someone else influence you?*	*What made you want to eat what you did?*	*Emotions and feelings?*	*Thoughts and concerns?*
7:30	M	1 C Crispix cereal 1/2 C skim milk coffee, black 1 C orange juice	110 40 — 120	3	home	reading newspaper	alone	I always eat cereal in the morning	a little keyed up & worried	thinking about quiz in class today
10:30	S	1 apple	90	1	hall outside classroom	studying	alone	felt tired & wanted to wake up	tired	worried about next class
12:30	M	1 C chili 1 roll 1 pat butter 1 orange 2 oatmeal cookies 1 soda	290 120 35 60 120 150	2	campus food court	talking	eating w/ friends; we decided to eat at the food court	wanted to be part of group	excited and happy	interested in hearing everyone's plans for the weekend

M/S = Meal or snack H = Hunger rating (0–3)

FIGURE 1.6 Sample health journal entries.

• ***Control related habits.*** You may have habits that contribute to your target behavior; modifying these habits can help change the behavior. For example, if you usually plop down on the sofa while watching TV, try putting an exercise bike in front of the set so you can burn calories while watching your favorite programs.

• ***Reward yourself.*** Giving yourself instant, real rewards for good behavior will reinforce your efforts. Plan your rewards; decide in advance what each one will be and how you will earn it. Tie rewards to achieving specific goals or subgoals. For example, you might treat yourself to a movie after a week of avoiding snacks. Make a list of items or events to use as rewards. They should be special to you and preferably unrelated to food or alcohol.

• ***Involve the people around you.*** Tell family and friends about your plan, and ask them to help. To help them respond appropriately to your needs, create a specific list of dos and don'ts. For example, ask them to support you when you set aside time to exercise or avoid second helpings at dinner.

• ***Plan for challenges.*** Think about situations and people that might derail your program, and develop ways to cope with them. For example, if you think it will be hard to stick to your usual exercise program during exams, schedule short bouts of physical activity (such as a brisk walk) as stress-reducing study breaks.

5. Make a Personal Contract A serious personal contract—one that commits you to your word—can result in a higher chance of follow-through than a casual, offhand promise. Your contract can help prevent procrastination by specifying important dates and can also serve as a reminder of your personal commitment to change.

Your contract should include a statement of your goal and your commitment to reaching it. The contract should also include details, such as the following:

- The date you will start
- The steps you will take to measure your progress
- The strategies you plan to use to promote change
- The date you expect to reach your final goal

Have someone—preferably someone who will be actively helping you with your program—sign your contract as a witness.

Figure 1.7 shows a sample behavior change contract for someone committing to eating more fruit every day. A blank contract is included as Activity 8 in the Behavior Change Workbook at the end of this text.

Behavior Change Contract

1. I, Tammy Lau, agree to increase my consumption of fruit from 1 cup per week to 2 cups per day.
2. I will begin on 10/5 and plan to reach my goal of 2 cups of fruit per day by 12/7
3. To reach my final goal, I have devised the following schedule of mini-goals. For each step in my program, I will give myself the reward listed.

I will begin to have ½ cup of fruit with breakfast	10/5	see movie
I will begin to have ½ cup of fruit with lunch	10/26	new cd
I will begin to substitute fruit juice for soda 1 time per day	11/16	concert

   My overall reward for reaching my goal will be trip to beach
4. I have gathered and analyzed data on my target behavior and have identified the following strategies for changing my behavior: Keep the fridge stocked with easy-to-carry fruit. Pack fruit in my backpack every day. Buy lunch at place that serves fruit.
5. I will use the following tools to monitor my progress toward my final goal:
   Chart on fridge door
   Health journal

   I sign this contract as an indication of my personal commitment to reach my goal: Tammy Lau 9/28

   I have recruited a helper who will witness my contract and also increase his consumption of fruit; eat lunch with me twice a week.

   Eric March 9/28

FIGURE 1.7 A sample behavior change contract.

Putting Your Plan into Action

The starting date has arrived, and you are ready to put your plan into action. This stage requires commitment, the resolve to stick with the plan no matter what temptations you encounter. Remember all the reasons you have to make the change—and remember that *you* are the boss. Use all your strategies to make your plan work. Make sure your environment is change-friendly, and get as much support and encouragement from others as possible. Keep track of your progress in your health journal, and give yourself regular rewards. And don't forget to give yourself a pat on the back—congratulate yourself, notice how much better you look or feel, and feel good about how far you've come and how you've gained control of your behavior.

Staying with It

As you continue with your program, don't be surprised when you run up against obstacles; they're inevitable. In fact, it's a good idea to expect problems and give yourself time to step back, see how you're doing, and make some changes before going on. If your program is grinding to a halt, identify what is blocking your progress. It may come from one of the sources described in the following sections.

Social Influences Take a hard look at the reactions of the people you're counting on, and see if they're really supporting you. If they come up short, connect with others who will be more supportive.

A related trap is trying to get your friends or family members to change *their* behaviors. The decision to make a major behavior change is something people come to only after intensive self-examination. You may be able to influence someone by tactfully providing facts or support, but that's all. Focus on yourself. When you succeed, you may become a role model for others.

Levels of Motivation and Commitment You won't make real progress until an inner drive leads you to the stage of change at which you are ready to make a personal commitment to the goal. If commitment is your problem, you may need to wait until the behavior you're dealing with makes you unhappier or unhealthier; then your desire to change it will be stronger. Or you may find that changing your goal will inspire you to keep going. For more ideas, refer to Activity 9 in the Behavior Change Workbook.

Choice of Techniques and Level of Effort If your plan is not working as well as you thought it would, make changes where you're having the most trouble. If you've lagged on your running schedule, for example, maybe it's because you don't like running. An aerobics class might suit you better. There are many ways to move toward your goal. Or you may not be trying hard enough. You do have to push toward your goal. If it were easy, you wouldn't need a plan.

Stress Barrier If you hit a wall in your program, look at the sources of stress in your life. If the stress is temporary, such as catching a cold or having a term paper due, you may want to wait until it passes before strengthening your efforts. If the stress is ongoing, find healthy ways to manage it (see Chapter 10). You may even want to make stress management your highest priority for behavior change.

Procrastinating, Rationalizing, and Blaming Be alert to games you might be playing with yourself, so you can stop them. Such games include the following:

- ***Procrastinating.*** If you tell yourself, "It's Friday already; I might as well wait until Monday to start," you're procrastinating. Break your plan into smaller steps that you can accomplish one day at a time.
- ***Rationalizing.*** If you tell yourself, "I wanted to go swimming today but wouldn't have had time to wash my hair afterward," you're making excuses.
- ***Blaming.*** If you tell yourself, "I couldn't exercise because Dave was hogging the elliptical trainer," you're blaming others for your own failure to follow through. Blaming is a way of taking your focus off the real problem and denying responsibility for your own actions.

Being Fit and Well for Life

Your first attempts at making behavior changes may never go beyond the contemplation or preparation stage. Those that do may not all succeed. But as you experience some success, you'll start to have more positive feelings about yourself. You may discover new physical activities and sports you enjoy, and you may encounter new situations and meet new people. Perhaps you'll surprise yourself by accomplishing things you didn't think were possible—breaking a long-standing nicotine habit, competing in a race, climbing a mountain, or developing a leaner body. Most of all, you'll discover the feeling of empowerment that comes from taking charge of your health. Being healthy takes effort, but the paybacks in energy and vitality are priceless.

Once you've started, don't stop. Assume that health improvement is forever. Take on the easier problems first, and then use what you learn to tackle more difficult problems later. When you feel challenged, remind yourself that you are creating a lifestyle that minimizes your health risks and maximizes your enjoyment of life. You *can* take charge of your health in a dramatic and meaningful way. *Fit and Well* will show you how.

Ask Yourself

QUESTIONS FOR CRITICAL THINKING AND REFLECTION

Think about the last time you made an unhealthy choice instead of a healthy one. How could you have changed the situation, the people in the situation, or your own thoughts, feelings, or intentions to avoid making that choice? What can you do in similar situations in the future to produce a different outcome?

TIPS FOR TODAY AND THE FUTURE

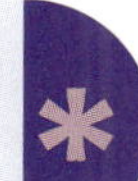

You are in charge of your health. Many of the decisions you make every day have an impact on the quality of your life, both now and in the future.

RIGHT NOW YOU CAN

- Go for a 15-minute walk.
- Have a piece of fruit for a snack.
- Call a friend and arrange for a time to catch up with each other.
- Start thinking about whether you have a health behavior you'd like to change. If you do, consider the elements of a behavior change strategy. For example, begin a mental list of the pros and cons of the behavior, or talk to someone who can support you in your attempts to change.

IN THE FUTURE YOU CAN

- Stay current on health- and wellness-related news and issues.
- Participate in health awareness and promotion campaigns in your community—for example, support smoking restrictions in local venues.
- Be a role model for someone else who is working on a health behavior you have successfully changed.

SUMMARY

- Wellness is the ability to live life fully, with vitality and meaning. Wellness is dynamic and multidimensional; it incorporates physical, emotional, intellectual, spiritual, interpersonal, and environmental dimensions.
- People today have greater control over and greater responsibility for their health than ever before.
- Behaviors that promote wellness include being physically active, choosing a healthy diet, maintaining a healthy body weight, managing stress effectively, avoiding tobacco and limiting alcohol use, and protecting yourself from disease and injury.
- Although heredity, environment, and health care all play roles in wellness and disease, behavior can mitigate their effects.
- To make lifestyle changes, you need information about yourself, your health habits, and resources available to help you change.
- You can increase your motivation for behavior change by examining the benefits and costs of change, boosting self-efficacy, and identifying and overcoming key barriers to change.
- The stages-of-change model describes six stages that people may move through as they try to change their behavior: precontemplation, contemplation, preparation, action, maintenance, and termination.
- A specific plan for change can be developed by (1) collecting data on your behavior and recording it in a journal; (2) analyzing the recorded data; (3) setting specific goals; (4) devising strategies for modifying the environment, rewarding yourself, and involving others; and (5) making a personal contract.
- To start and maintain a behavior change program, you need commitment, a well-developed and manageable plan, social support, and strong stress-management techniques. It is also important to monitor the progress of your program, revising it as necessary.

FOR FURTHER EXPLORATION

BOOKS

American Medical Association. 2006. *American Medical Association Concise Medical Encyclopedia.* New York: Random House. *Includes more than 3000 entries on health and wellness topics, symptoms, conditions, and treatments.*

Claiborn, J., and C. Pedrick. 2009. *The Habit Change Workbook: How to Break Bad Habits and Form Good Ones.* Oakland, Ca.: New Harbinger Publications. *Provides step-by-step instructions for identifying and overcoming a variety of unhealthy behaviors, such as poor eating habits, reluctance to exercise, and addictive behavior.*

Komaroff, A. L., ed. 2005. *Harvard Medical School Family Health Guide.* New York: Free Press. *Provides consumer-oriented advice for the prevention and treatment of common health concerns.*

Krueger, H., et al. 2007. *The Health Impact of Smoking and Obesity and What to Do About It.* Toronto: University of Toronto Press. *Examines the effects of smoking and sedentary lifestyle, the costs to individuals and society, and strategies for overcoming these behaviors.*

Litin, S. C., ed. 2009. *Mayo Clinic Family Health Book,* 4th ed. New York: HarperCollins Publishers. *A complete health reference for every stage of life, covering thousands of conditions, symptoms, and treatments.*

Murat, B., and G. Stewart. 2009. *Do I Need to See the Doctor? The Home-Treatment Encyclopedia—Written by Medical Doctors—That Lets You Decide,* 2nd ed. New York: John Wiley & Sons. *Fully illustrated, easy-to-read guide to hundreds of common symptoms and ailments, designed to help consumers determine whether they can treat themselves or should seek professional medical attention.*

NEWSLETTERS

Center for Science in the Public Interest Nutrition Action Health Letter
(http://www.cspinet.org/nah/index.htm)
Consumer Reports on Health (800-274-7596;
http://www.consumerreports.org/oh/index.htm)
Harvard Health Publications (877-649-9457;
http://www.health.harvard.edu)
Harvard Men's Health Watch (877-649-9457)
Harvard Women's Health Watch (877-649-9457)
Mayo Clinic Health Letter (800-291-1128)
Tufts University Health & Nutrition Newsletter
(http://www.tuftshealthletter.com)
University of California at Berkeley Wellness Letter
(800-829-9170; http://www.wellnessletter.com)

ORGANIZATIONS, HOTLINES, AND WEB SITES

The Internet addresses listed here were accurate at the time of publication.

Centers for Disease Control and Prevention. Through phone, fax, and the Internet, the CDC provides a wide variety of health information.
http://www.cdc.gov

Federal Trade Commission: Consumer Protection—Health. Includes online brochures about a variety of consumer health topics, including fitness equipment, generic drugs, and fraudulent health claims.
http://www.ftc.gov/bcp/menus/consumer/health.shtm

FirstGov for Consumers: Health. Provides links to online brochures from a variety of government agencies.
http://consumer.gov/ncpw/category/health

Healthfinder. A gateway to online publications, Web sites, support and self-help groups, and agencies and organizations that produce reliable health information.
http://www.healthfinder.gov

Healthy Campus. The American College Health Association's introduction to the Healthy Campus program.
http://www.acha.org/info_resources/hc2010.cfm

Healthy People. Provides information on Healthy People objectives and priority areas.
http://www.healthypeople.gov

MedlinePlus. Provides links to news and reliable information about health from government agencies and professional associations; also includes a health encyclopedia and information on prescription and over-the-counter drugs.
http://www.medlineplus.gov

National Health Information Center (NHIC). Puts consumers in touch with the organizations that are best able to provide answers to health-related questions.

http://www.health.gov/nhic

National Institutes of Health. Provides information about all NIH activities as well as consumer publications, hotline information, and an A-to-Z listing of health issues with links to the appropriate NIH institute.

http://www.nih.gov

National Wellness Institute. Serves professionals and organizations that promote optimal health and wellness.

http://www.nationalwellness.org

National Women's Health Information Center. Provides information and answers to frequently asked questions.

http://www.womenshealth.gov

Office of Minority Health. Promotes improved health among racial and ethnic minority populations.

http://minorityhealth.hhs.gov

Surgeon General. Includes information on activities of the Surgeon General and the text of many key reports on such topics as tobacco use, physical activity, and mental health.

http://www.surgeongeneral.gov

World Health Organization (WHO). Provides information about health topics and issues affecting people around the world.

http://www.who.int

The following are just a few of the many sites that provide consumer-oriented information on a variety of health issues:

CNN Health: http://www.cnn.com/health

FamilyDoctor.Org: http://familydoctor.org/online/famdocen/home.html

InteliHealth: http://www.intelihealth.com

MayoClinic.com: http://www.mayoclinic.com

SELECTED BIBLIOGRAPHY

American Cancer Society. 2011. *Cancer Facts and Figures—2011.* Atlanta: American Cancer Society.

American Heart Association. 2011. *Heart Disease and Stroke Statistics—2011 Update.* Dallas: American Heart Association.

Banks, J., et al. 2006. Disease and disadvantage in the United States and in England. *Journal of the American Medical Association* 295(17): 2037–2045.

Barr, D. A. 2008. *Health Disparities in the United States: Social Class, Race, Ethnicity, and Health.* Baltimore: The Johns Hopkins University Press.

Beckman, M. 2007. Help wanted: In the pursuit of a healthy lifestyle, sheer grit only takes you so far. *Stanford Medicine Magazine* 24(3).

Centers for Disease Control and Prevention. 2008. Racial/Ethnic Disparities in Self-Rated Health Status among Adults with and without Disabilities—United States, 2004–2006. *Morbidity and Mortality Weekly Report* 57(39): 1069–1073.

Centers for Disease Control and Prevention. 2011. *Racial and Ethnic Approaches to Community Health (REACH)* (http://www.cdc.gov/reach; retrieved June 26, 2010).

Finkelstein, E. A., et al. 2008. Do obese persons comprehend their personal health risks? *American Journal of Health Behavior* 32(5): 508–516.

Flegal, K. M., et al. 2005. Excess deaths associated with underweight, overweight, and obesity. *Journal of the American Medical Association* 293(15): 1861–1867.

Flegal, K. M., et al. 2007. Cause-specific excess deaths associated with underweight, overweight, and obesity. *Journal of the American Medical Association* 298(17): 2028–2037.

Flegal, K. M., et al. 2010. Prevalence and Trends in Obesity Among U.S. Adults, 1999–2008. *Journal of the American Medical Association* 303(3): 235–241.

Gorman, B. K., and J. G. Read. 2006. Gender disparities in adult health: An examination of three measures of morbidity. *Journal of Health and Social Behavior* 47(2): 95–110.

Herd, P., et al. 2007. Socioeconomic position and health: The differential effects of education versus income on the onset versus progression of health problems. *Journal of Health and Social Behavior* 48(3): 223–238.

Horneffer-Ginter, K. 2008. Stages of change and possible selves: Two tools for promoting college health. *Journal of American College Health* 56(4): 351–358.

Martin, G., and J. Pear. 2007. *Behaviour Modification: What It Is and How to Do It,* 8th ed. Upper Saddle River, N.J.: Prentice-Hall.

Mokdad, A. H., et al. 2004. Actual causes of death in the United States, 2000. *Journal of the American Medical Association* 291(10): 1238–1245.

Mokdad, A. H., et al. 2005. Correction: Actual causes of death in the United States, 2000. *Journal of the American Medical Association* 293(3): 293–294.

National Center for Health Statistics. 2010. *Health, United States, 2010.* Hyattsville, Md.: National Center for Health Statistics.

National Center for Health Statistics. 2010. Health behaviors of adults: United States, 2005–07. *Vital and Health Statistics* 10(245).

National Center for Health Statistics. 2011. Deaths: Preliminary data for 2009. *National Vital Statistics Report* 59(4).

Nothwehr, F., et al. 2008. Age group differences in diet and physical activity–related behaviors among rural men and women. *Journal of Nutrition, Health and Aging* 12(3): 169–174.

O'Loughlin, J., et al. 2007. Lifestyle risk factors for chronic disease across family origin among adults in multiethnic, low-income, urban neighborhoods. *Ethnicity and Disease* 17(4): 657–663.

Participants at the 6th Global Conference on Health Promotion. The Bangkok Charter for health promotion in a globalized world. Geneva: World Health Organization, August 11, 2005.

Pinkhasov, R. M., et al. 2010. Are men shortchanged on health? Perspective on health care utilization and health risk behavior in men and women in the United States. *International Journal of Clinical Practice* 64(4): 475–487.

Song, J., et al. 2006. Gender differences across race/ethnicity in use of health care among Medicare–aged Americans. *Journal of Women's Health* 15(10): 1205–1213.

U.C. Berkeley. 2010 Update. *Evaluating Web Pages: Techniques to Apply and Questions to Ask* (http://www.lib.berkeley.edu/TeachingLib/Guides/Internet/Evaluate.html; retrieved June 26, 2011).

Walker, B., and C. P. Mouton. 2008. Environmental influences on cardiovascular health. *Journal of the National Medical Association* 100(1): 98–102.

World Health Organization. 2011. *Why Gender and Health?* (http://www.who.int/gender/genderandhealth/en; retrieved June 26, 2011).

Name ______________________ Section ____________ Date ____________

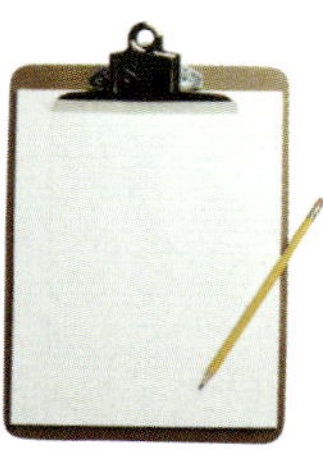

LAB 1.1 Your Wellness Profile

Consider how your lifestyle, attitudes, and characteristics relate to each of the six dimensions of wellness. Fill in your strengths for each dimension (examples of strengths are listed with each dimension). Once you've completed your lists, choose what you believe are your five most important strengths, and circle them.

Physical wellness: To maintain overall physical health and engage in appropriate physical activity (e.g., stamina, strength, flexibility, healthy body composition).

____

____

____

Emotional wellness: To have a positive self-concept, deal constructively with your feelings, and develop positive qualities (e.g., optimism, trust, self-confidence, determination).

____

____

____

Intellectual wellness: To pursue and retain knowledge, think critically about issues, make sound decisions, identify problems, and find solutions (e.g., common sense, creativity, curiosity).

____

____

____

Interpersonal/social wellness: To develop and maintain meaningful relationships with a network of friends and family members, and to contribute to your community (e.g., friendly, good-natured, compassionate, supportive, good listener).

____

____

____

Spiritual wellness: To develop a set of beliefs, principles, or values that gives meaning or purpose to your life; to develop faith in something beyond yourself (e.g., religious faith, service to others).

____

____

____

Environmental wellness: To protect yourself from environmental hazards and to minimize the negative impact of your behavior on the environment (e.g., carpooling, recycling).

____

____

____

Next, think about where you fall on the wellness continuum for each of the dimensions of wellness. Indicate your placement for each—physical, emotional, intellectual, interpersonal/social, spiritual, and environmental—by placing Xs on the continuum below.

Low level of wellness ⟵ Physical, psychological, emotional symptoms — Change and growth ⟶ High level of wellness

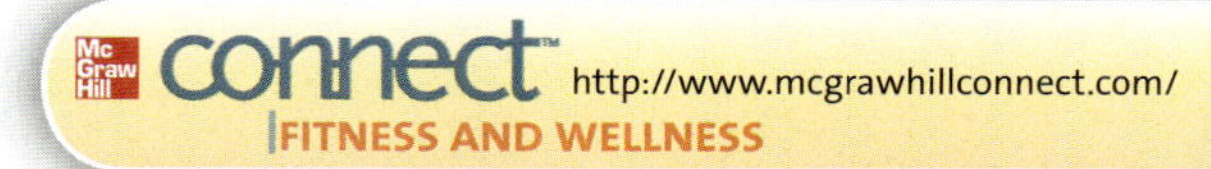

Based on both your current lifestyle and your goals for the future, what do you think your placement on the wellness continuum will be in 10 years? What new health behaviors will you have to adopt to achieve your goals? Which of your current behaviors will you need to change to maintain or improve your level of wellness in the future?

Does the description of wellness given in this chapter encompass everything you believe is part of wellness for you? Write your own definition of wellness, including any additional dimensions that are important to you. Then rate your level of wellness based on your own definition.

Using Your Results

How did you score? Are you satisfied with your current level of wellness—overall and in each dimension? In which dimension(s) would you most like to increase your level of wellness?

What should you do next? As you consider possible target behaviors for a behavior change program, choose things that will maintain or increase your level of wellness in one of the dimensions you listed as an area of concern. Remember to consider health behaviors such as smoking or eating a high-fat diet that may threaten your level of wellness in the future. Below, list several possible target behaviors and the wellness dimensions that they influence.

For additional guidance in choosing a target behavior, complete the lifestyle self-assessment in Lab 1.2.

Name ______________________ Section ______________ Date ____________

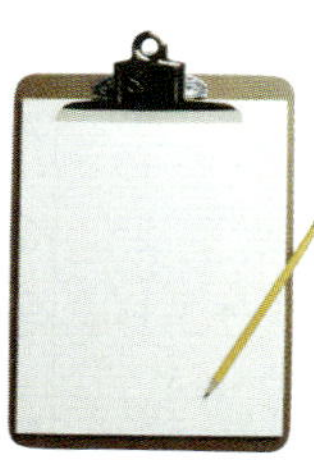

LAB 1.2 Lifestyle Evaluation

How does your current lifestyle compare with the lifestyle recommended for wellness? For each question, choose the answer that best describes your behavior. Then add up your score for each section.

Exercise/Fitness

	Almost Always	Sometimes	Never
1. I engage in moderate exercise, such as brisk walking or swimming, for 20–60 minutes, three to five times a week.	4	1	0
2. I do exercises to develop muscular strength and endurance at least twice a week.	2	1	0
3. I spend some of my leisure time participating in individual, family, or team activities, such as gardening, bowling, or softball.	2	1	0
4. I maintain a healthy body weight, avoiding overweight and underweight.	2	1	0

Exercise/Fitness Score: ____________

Nutrition

1. I eat a variety of foods each day, including seven or more servings of fruits and/or vegetables.	3	1	0
2. I limit the amount of total fat and saturated and trans fat in my diet.	3	1	0
3. I avoid skipping meals.	2	1	0
4. I limit the amount of salt and sugar I eat.	2	1	0

Nutrition Score: ____________

Tobacco Use

If you never or no longer use tobacco, enter a score of 10 for this section and go to the next section.

1. I avoid using tobacco.	2	1	0
2. I smoke only a pipe or cigars, *or* I use smokeless tobacco.	2	1	0

Tobacco Use Score: ____________

Alcohol and Drugs

1. I avoid alcohol, or I drink no more than one (women) or two (men) drinks a day.	4	1	0
2. I avoid using alcohol or other drugs as a way of handling stressful situations or the problems in my life.	2	1	0
3. I am careful not to drink alcohol when taking medications (such as cold or allergy medications) or when pregnant.	2	1	0
4. I read and follow the label directions when using prescribed and over-the-counter drugs.	2	1	0

Alcohol and Drugs Score: ____________

Emotional Health

1. I enjoy being a student, and I have a job or do other work that I enjoy.	2	1	0
2. I find it easy to relax and express my feelings freely.	2	1	0
3. I manage stress well.	2	1	0
4. I have close friends, relatives, or others whom I can talk to about personal matters and call on for help when needed.	2	1	0
5. I participate in group activities (such as community or church organizations) or hobbies that I enjoy	2	1	0

Emotional Health Score: ____________

Safety

	Almost Always	Sometimes	Never
1. I wear a safety belt while riding in a car.	2	1	0
2. I avoid driving while under the influence of alcohol or other drugs.	2	1	0
3. I obey traffic rules and the speed limit when driving.	2	1	0
4. I read and follow instructions on the labels of potentially harmful products or substances, such as household cleaners, poisons, and electrical appliances.	2	1	0
5. I avoid smoking in bed.	2	1	0

Safety Score: ______________

Disease Prevention

1. I know the warning signs of cancer, heart attack, and stroke.	2	1	0
2. I avoid overexposure to the sun and use sunscreen.	2	1	0
3. I get recommended medical screening tests (such as blood pressure and cholesterol checks and Pap tests), immunizations, and booster shots.	2	1	0
4. I practice monthly skin and breast/testicle self-exams.	2	1	0
5. I am not sexually active, *or* I have sex with only one mutually faithful, uninfected partner, *or* I always engage in safer sex (using condoms), and I do not share needles to inject drugs.	2	1	0

Disease Prevention Score: ______________

Scores of 9 and 10 Excellent! Your answers show that you are aware of the importance of this area to your health. More important, you are putting your knowledge to work for you by practicing good health habits. As long as you continue to do so, this area should not pose a serious health risk.
Scores of 6 to 8 Your health practices in this area are good, but there is room for improvement.
Scores of 3 to 5 Your health risks are showing.
Scores of 0 to 2 You may be taking serious and unnecessary risks with your health.

Using Your Results

How did you score? In which areas did you score the lowest? Are you satisfied with your scores in each area? In which areas would you most like to improve your scores?

What should you do next? To improve your scores, look closely at any item to which you answered "sometimes" or "never." Identify and list at least three possible targets for a health behavior change program. (If you are aware of other risky health behaviors you currently engage in, but that were not covered by this assessment, you may include those in your list.) For each item on your list, identify your current "stage of change" and one strategy you could adopt to move forward (see pp. 16–21). Possible strategies might be obtaining information about the behavior, completing an analysis of the pros and cons of change, or beginning a written record of your target behavior.

Behavior	Stage	Strategy
1. ______________	______________	______________
2. ______________	______________	______________
3. ______________	______________	______________

SOURCE: Adapted from *Healthstyle: A Self-Test,* developed by the U.S. Public Health Service. The behaviors covered in this test are recommended for most Americans, but some may not apply to people with certain chronic diseases or disabilities or to pregnant women, who may require special advice from their physician.

CHAPTER 2

Principles of Physical Fitness

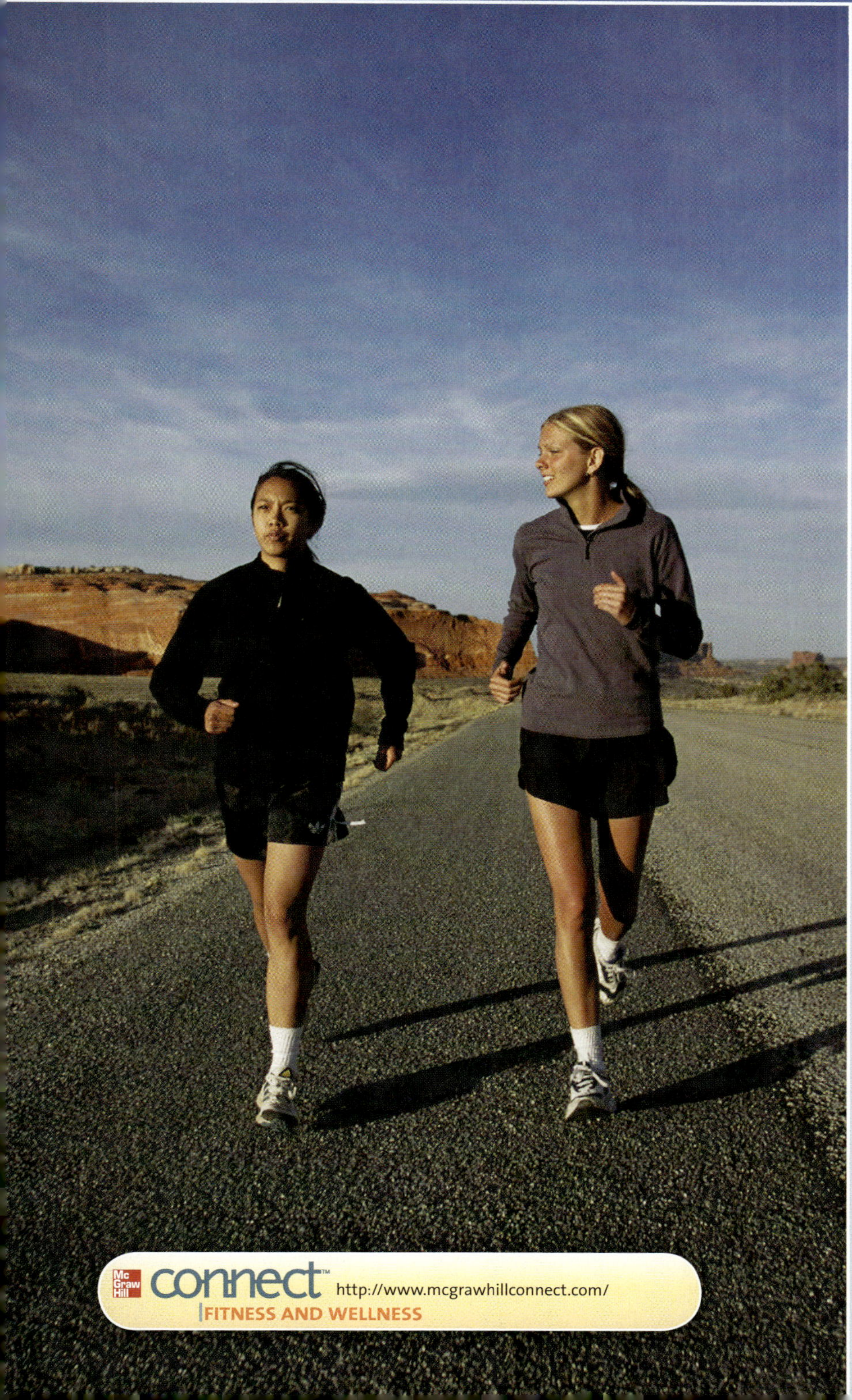

LOOKING AHEAD...

After reading this chapter, you should be able to:

- Describe how much physical activity is recommended for developing health and fitness
- Identify the components of physical fitness and the way each component affects wellness
- Explain the goal of physical training and the basic principles of training
- Describe the principles involved in designing a well-rounded exercise program
- List the steps that can be taken to make an exercise program safe, effective, and successful

TEST YOUR KNOWLEDGE

1. To improve your health, you must exercise vigorously for at least 30 minutes straight, 5 or more days per week. True or false?
2. Which of the following activities uses about 150 calories?
   a. washing a car for 45–60 minutes
   b. shooting a basketball for 30 minutes
   c. jumping rope for 15 minutes
3. Regular exercise can make a person smarter. True or false?

Answers

1. **False.** Experts recommend 150 minutes of moderate-intensity physical activity per week, but activity can be done in short bouts—10-minute sessions, for example—spread out over the course of the day.
2. **All three.** The more intense an activity is, the more calories it burns in a given amount of time. This is one reason that people who exercise vigorously can get the same benefits in less time than people who exercise longer at a moderate intensity.
3. **True.** Regular exercise (even moderate-intensity exercise) benefits the human brain and nervous system in a variety of ways. For example, exercise improves cognitive function—that is, the brain's ability to learn, remember, think, and reason.

Any list of the benefits of physical activity is impressive. Although people vary greatly in physical fitness and performance ability, the benefits of regular physical activity are available to everyone.

This chapter provides an overview of physical fitness. It explains how both lifestyle physical activity and more formal exercise programs contribute to wellness. It also describes the components of fitness, the basic principles of physical training, and the essential elements of a well-rounded exercise program. Chapters 4, 6, 8 and 9 provide an in-depth look at each of the elements of a fitness program.

PHYSICAL ACTIVITY AND EXERCISE FOR HEALTH AND FITNESS

Despite the many benefits of an active lifestyle, levels of physical activity remain low for all populations of Americans (Figure 2.1). However, there is some good news. In August 2010, the Centers for Disease Control and Prevention (CDC) reported the following statistics about the physical activity levels of adult Americans:

- About 33% participate in some leisure-time physical activity, 35% engage in leisure-time physical activity on a regular basis, and 28% participate in vigorous leisure-time physical activity lasting at least 10 minutes three or more times per week.
- The percentage of people reporting no leisure-time physical activity decreased by nearly 6% between 1988 and 2009. Physical activity levels decline with age; are higher in men than in women; and are lower in Hispanics, American Indians, and blacks than in whites. Approximately 25% of Americans participate in no leisure-time physical activity—a level that has remained steady for a decade.

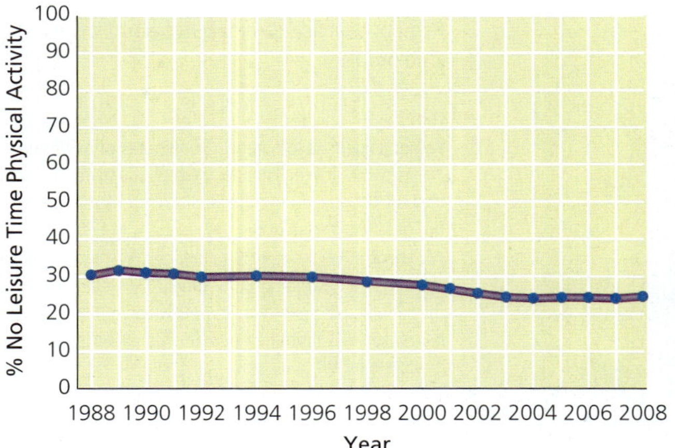

FIGURE 2.1 Percentage of adult Americans reporting no leisure-time physical activity.

SOURCE: Centers for Disease Control and Prevention. 2010. *Physical Activity Statistics* (http://www.cdc.gov/nccdphp/dnpa/physical/stats/leisure_time.htm; retrieved June 26, 2011).

- People with higher levels of education exercise vigorously more often than people with less education. For example, 78% of high school dropouts never exercise vigorously, compared with 39% of college graduates.
- People living in large urban areas are less active than those living in smaller communities, and those living in the South and Northeast were less active than people living in other areas of the country.

Possible barriers to increased activity include lack of time and resources, social and environmental influences, and—most important—lack of motivation and commitment (see Lab 2.2 for more on barriers). Some people also fear injury. Although physical activity carries some risks, the risks from inactivity are far greater. Increased physical activity may be the single most important lifestyle behavior for promoting health and well-being.

Physical Activity on a Continuum

Physical activity is movement carried out by the skeletal muscles that requires energy. Different types of physical activity can vary by ease or intensity. Standing up or walking down a hallway require little energy or effort. More intense, sustained activities, such as cycling five miles or running in a race, require considerably more.

Exercise refers to planned, structured, repetitive movement intended specifically to improve or maintain physical fitness. As discussed in Chapter 1, physical fitness is a set of physical attributes that allows the body to respond or adapt to the demands and stress of physical effort—to perform moderate to vigorous levels of physical activity without becoming overly tired. Levels of fitness depend on such physiological factors as the heart's ability to pump blood and the energy-generating capacity of the cells. These factors depend on genetics—a person's inborn potential for physical fitness—and behavior—getting enough physical activity to stress the body and cause long-term physiological changes.

Physical activity is essential to health and confers wide-ranging health benefits, but exercise is necessary to significantly improve physical fitness. This important distinction between physical activity, which improves health and wellness, and exercise, which improves fitness, is a key concept in understanding the guidelines discussed in this section.

Increasing Physical Activity to Improve Health and Wellness In 2010, the U.S. Surgeon General issued *The Surgeon General's Vision for a Healthy and Fit Nation*, following up the U.S. Department of Health and Human Services' landmark 2008 report, titled *Physical Activity Guidelines for Americans,* which made specific recommendations for promoting exercise and health. (You can read these reports at www.surgeongeneral.gov/library/obesityvision/obesityvision2010.pdf and www.health.gov/paguidelines.) Also, in 2011 the ACSM released its

Is Exercise Good for Your Brain?

THE EVIDENCE FOR EXERCISE

Some scientists are now calling exercise the new "brain food." A variety of studies show that even moderate physical activity can improve brain health and function and may delay the decline in cognitive function that occurs for many people as they age. Recent evidence shows that regular physical activity has the following positive effects on the brain:

- Exercise improves cognitive function—the brain's ability to learn, remember, think, and reason.
- Exercise can help overcome the negative effects of a poor diet on brain health.
- Exercise promotes the creation of new nerve cells (neurons) throughout the nervous system. By promoting this process (called *neurogenesis*), exercise provides protection against injury and degenerative conditions that destroy neurons.
- Exercise enhances the nervous system's *plasticity*—its ability to change and adapt. In the brain, spinal cord, and nerves, this can mean developing new pathways for transmitting sensory information or motor commands.
- Exercise appears to have a protective effect on the brain as people age, helping to delay or even prevent the onset of neurodegenerative disorders such as Alzheimer's disease.

Although most people consider brain health to be a concern for the elderly, it is vital to wellness throughout life. For this reason, many studies on exercise and brain health include children as well as older adults. Targeted research has also focused on the impact of exercise on people with disorders such as cerebral palsy, multiple sclerosis, and developmental disabilities. Generally speaking, these studies all reach a similar conclusion: Exercise enhances brain health, at least to some degree, in people of all ages and a wide range of health statuses.

Along with the brain's physical health, mental health is enhanced by exercise. Even modest activity, such as taking a daily walk, can help combat a variety of mental health disorders.

It's hard to understate the impact of physical and mental disorders related to brain health. According to the Alzheimer's Association, 5.3 million Americans currently suffer from Alzheimer's disease, and the number is increasing at a rate of 70 people per second. People with depression, anxiety, or other mental disorders are more likely to suffer from chronic physical conditions. Taken together, these and other brain-related disorders cost untold millions of dollars in health care costs and lost productivity, as well as thousands of years of productive lifetime lost.

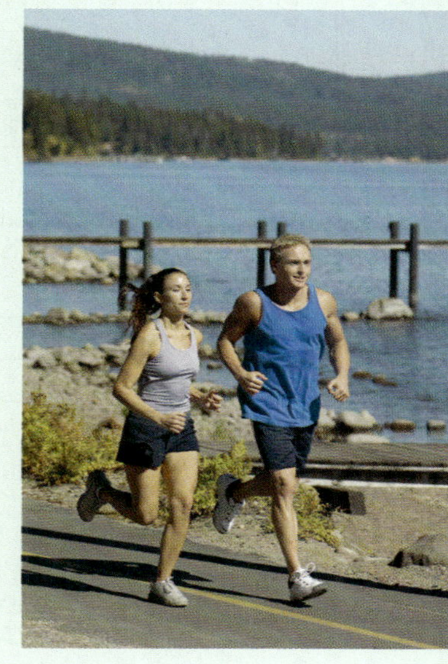

So, for the sake of your brain—as well as your muscles, bones, and heart—start creating your exercise program soon. You'll be healthier, and you may even feel a little smarter.

SOURCES: Garber, C. E., et al. 2011. Quantity and quality of exercise for developing and maintaining cardiorespiratory, musculoskeletal, and neuromotor fitness in apparently healthy adults: guidance for prescribing exercise. *Medicine and Science in Sports and Exercise* 43(7): 1334–1359; Physical Activity Guidelines Advisory Committee. 2008. *Physical Activity Guidelines Advisory Committee Report, 2008*. Washington, D.C.: U.S. Department of Health and Human Services; Stranahan, A. M., and M. P. Mattson. 2011. Bidirectional metabolic regulation of neurocognitive function. *Neurobiology of Learning and Memory* January (epub); Ploughman, M. 2008. Exercise is brain food: The effects of physical activity on cognitive function. *Developmental Neurorehabilitation* 11(3): 236–240; van Praag, H. 2009. Exercise and the brain: Something to chew on. *Trends in Neurosciences* 32(5): 283–290.

exercise guidelines for healthy adults titled, "Quantity and quality of exercise for developing and maintaining cardiorespiratory, musculoskeletal, and neuromotor fitness in apparently healthy adults: guidance for prescribing exercise." These reports stress the importance of regular physical activity and emphasize that some physical activity is better than none. They also present evidence that regular activity promotes health and prevents premature death and a variety of diseases (see the box "Is Exercise Good for Your Brain?"). The guidelines follow previous recommendations from the Surgeon General (issued in 1996), the Department of Health and Human Services (2005 and 2008), and the American College of Sports Medicine and American Heart Association (2007). *Physical Activity Guidelines for Americans* and the Surgeon General's recommendations include the following key guidelines for adults:

- For substantial health benefits, adults should do at least 150 minutes (2 and a half hours) a week of moderate-intensity aerobic physical activity, or 75 minutes (1 hour and 15 minutes) a week of vigorous-intensity aerobic physical activity, or an equivalent combination of moderate- and

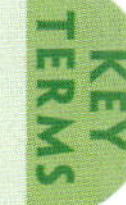

physical activity Body movement carried out by the skeletal muscles that requires energy.

exercise Planned, structured, repetitive movement intended to improve or maintain physical fitness.

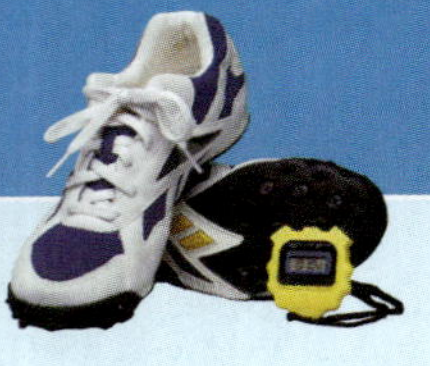

PERSONAL CHALLENGE

To Work Out. . . Or Not to Work Out?

What reasons do you have for not exercising—or not exercising more? Forget about superficial excuses such as "I couldn't run today because a SpongeBob marathon was on." Focus on *real* reasons that consistently interfere with your ability to be physically active. List the top three reasons, in order of significance:

Reason #1: ______________________________

Reason #2: ______________________________

Reason #3: ______________________________

Now, focus on a real solution to each of the three problems. What can you do to prevent these issues from interfering with your ability to exercise in the future? Don't worry about one-time solutions; think about real, permanent solutions that will make these reasons for not exercising go away. List the solutions in the same order as the reasons you listed above:

Solution #1: ______________________________

Solution #2: ______________________________

Solution #3: ______________________________

Think of this as more than just a list. Think of it as a commitment to resolve issues that keep you from meeting your fitness goals. That's the challenging part: Apply your solutions and stay active!

vigorous-intensity aerobic activity. Activity should preferably be spread throughout the week.

- For additional and more extensive health benefits, adults should increase their aerobic physical activity to 300 minutes (5 hours) a week of moderate-intensity activity, or 150 minutes a week of vigorous-intensity activity, or an equivalent combination of moderate- and vigorous-intensity activity. Adults can enjoy additional health benefits by engaging in physical activity beyond this amount.
- Adults should also do muscle-strengthening activities that are moderate or high intensity and involve all major muscle groups on two or more days a week, as these activities provide additional health benefits.
- Everyone should avoid inactivity. Adults, teenagers, and children should spend less time in front of a television or computer screen because it decreases metabolic health and contributes to a sedentary lifestyle and increases the risk of obesity.

The reports state that physical activity benefits people of all ages and of all racial and ethnic groups, including people with disabilities. The reports emphasize that the benefits of activity outweigh the dangers.

These levels of physical activity promote health and wellness by lowering the risk of high blood pressure, stroke, heart disease, type 2 diabetes, colon cancer, and osteoporosis and by reducing feelings of mild to moderate depression and anxiety.

What exactly is moderate physical activity? Activities such as brisk walking, dancing, swimming, cycling, and yard work can all count toward the daily total. A moderate amount of activity uses about 150 calories of energy and causes a noticeable increase in heart rate, such as would occur with a brisk walk. Examples of activities that use about 150 calories are shown in Figure 2.2. You

Common Activities	Duration (min.)	
Washing and waxing a car	45–60	***Less Vigorous, More Time***
Washing windows or floors	45–60	
Gardening	30–45	
Wheeling self in wheelchair	30–40	
Pushing a stroller 1½ miles	30	
Raking leaves	30	
Walking 2 miles	30 (15 min/mile)	
Shoveling snow	15	
Stairwalking	15	
Sporting Activities		
Playing volleyball	45–60	
Playing touch football	45	
Walking 1¾ miles	35 (20 min/mile)	
Basketball (shooting baskets)	30	
Bicycling 5 miles	30	
Dancing fast (social)	30	
Water aerobics	30	
Swimming laps	20	
Basketball (playing game)	15–20	
Bicycling 4 miles	15	***More Vigorous, Less Time***
Jumping rope	15	
Running 1½ miles	15 (10 min/mile)	

FIGURE 2.2 Examples of moderate-intensity physical activity. Each example uses about 150 calories.

SOURCE: National Heart, Lung, and Blood Institute. 2010. *Why Is Exercise Important?* (www.nhlbi.nih.gov/health/public/heart/obesity/lose_wt/physical.htm; retrieved June 26, 2011).

Classifying Activity Levels

IN FOCUS

Assessing your physical activity level is easier if you know how to classify different kinds of activities. Fitness experts categorize activities into the following three levels:

- *Light activity* includes the routine tasks associated with typical day-to-day life, such as vacuuming, walking slowly, shopping, or stretching. You probably perform dozens of light activities every day without even thinking about it. You can gain significant health benefits by turning light activities into moderate activities—by walking briskly instead of slowly, for example.
- *Moderate activity*, such as walking at 3–4 miles per hour, causes your breathing and heart rate to accelerate but still allows for comfortable conversation. It is sometimes described as activity that can be performed comfortably for about 45 minutes. Examples of moderate physical activity include brisk walking, social dancing, and cycling moderately on level terrain.
- *Vigorous activity* elevates your heart and breathing rates considerably and has other physical effects that improve your fitness level. Examples include jogging, hiking uphill, swimming laps, and playing most competitive sports.

can burn the same number of calories by doing a lower-intensity activity for a longer time or a higher-intensity activity for a shorter time. College-age people are more likely to participate in physical activities they enjoy, such as dancing.

In contrast to moderate-intensity activity, ***vigorous*** physical activity causes rapid breathing and a substantial increase in heart rate, as exemplified by jogging. Physical activity and exercise recommendations for promoting general health, fitness, and weight management are shown in Table 2.1. Examples of light, moderate, and vigorous activities are given in the box "Classifying Activity Levels."

The daily total of physical activity can be accumulated in multiple bouts of 10 or more minutes per day—for example, two 10-minute bike rides to and from class and

Fitness Tip

To make your workouts more effective, find an exercise buddy. You can help each other set goals, stay on track, keep time, and count reps. Exercising with a friend makes working out more enjoyable, too.

Table 2.1 Physical Activity and Exercise Recommendations for Promoting General Health, Fitness, and Weight Management

GOAL	RECOMMENDATION
General health	Perform moderate-intensity aerobic physical activity for at least 150 minutes per week or 75 minutes of vigorous-intensity physical activity per week. Examples of moderate-intensity physical activity include brisk walking, water aerobics, tennis (doubles), dancing, and cycling less than 10 miles per hour. Examples of vigorous-intensity physical activity include jogging, power-walking, tennis (singles), jumping rope, hiking uphill, and cycling faster than 10 miles per hour. Also, be more active in your daily life: Walk instead of driving, take the stairs instead of the elevator, and watch less television.
Increased health benefits	Exercise at moderate intensity for 300 minutes per week or at vigorous intensity for 150 minutes per week.
Achieve or maintain weight loss	Exercise moderately for 60–90 minutes per day on most days of the week.
Muscle strength and endurance	Perform 1 or more sets of resistance exercises that work the major muscle groups for 8–12 repetitions (10–15 reps for older adults) on at least 2 nonconsecutive days per week. Examples include weight training and exercises that use body weight as resistance (such as core stabilizing exercises, pull-ups, push-ups, lunges, and squats).
Flexibility	Perform range-of-motion (stretching) exercises at least 2 days per week. Hold each stretch for 10–30 seconds.
Neuromuscular training	Older adults should do balance training 2–3 days per week. Examples include yoga, tai chi, and balance exercises (standing on one foot, step-ups, and walking lunges). These exercises are probably beneficial for young and middle-aged adults, as well.

SOURCES: Garber, C. E., et al. 2011. Quantity and quality of exercise for developing and maintaining cardiorespiratory, musculoskeletal, and neuromotor fitness in apparently health adults: Guidance for prescribing exercise. *Medicine and Science in Sports and Exercise* 43(7): 1334–1359; Physical Activity Guidelines Advisory Committee. 2008. *Physical Activity Guidelines Advisory Committee Report, 2008.* Washington, D.C.: U.S. Department of Health and Human Services; U.S. Department of Health and Human Services. 2010. *The Surgeon General's Vision for a Healthy and Fit Nation.* Rockville, Md: U.S. Department of Health and Human Services, Office of the Surgeon General.

a brisk 10-minute walk to the store. In this lifestyle approach to physical activity, people can choose activities that they find enjoyable and that fit into their daily routine; everyday tasks at school, work, and home can be structured to contribute to the daily activity total. If all Americans who are currently sedentary were to increase their lifestyle physical activity to 30 minutes per day, there would be an enormous benefit to public health and to individual well-being.

Increasing Physical Activity to Manage Weight Because two-thirds of Americans are overweight, the U.S. Department of Health and Human Services has also published physical activity guidelines focusing on weight management. These guidelines recognize that for people who need to prevent weight gain, lose weight, or maintain weight loss, 150 minutes per week of physical activity may not be enough. Instead, they recommend up to 90 minutes of physical activity per day.

Exercising to Improve Physical Fitness As mentioned earlier, moderate physical activity confers significant health and wellness benefits, especially for those who are currently sedentary and become moderately active. However, people can obtain even greater health and wellness benefits by increasing the duration and intensity of physical activity. With increased activity, they will see more improvements in quality of life and greater reductions in disease and mortality risk.

More vigorous activity, as in a structured, systematic exercise program, is also needed to improve physical fitness; moderate physical activity alone is not enough. Physical fitness requires more intense movement that poses a substantially greater challenge to the body. The American College of Sports Medicine issued guidelines in 2006 and again in 2011 for creating a formal exercise program that will develop physical fitness. These guidelines are described in detail later in the chapter.

How Much Physical Activity Is Enough?

Some experts feel that people get most of the health benefits of physical activity simply by becoming more active over the course of the day; the amount of activity needed depends on an individual's health status and goals. Other experts feel that leisure-time physical activity is not enough; they argue that people should exercise long enough and intensely enough to improve the body's capacity for exercise—that is, to improve physical fitness. There is probably some truth in both of these positions.

Regular physical activity, regardless of the intensity, makes you healthier and can help protect you from many chronic diseases. Although you get many of the health benefits of exercise simply by being more active, you obtain even more benefits when you are physically fit. In addition to long-term health benefits, fitness also contributes significantly to quality of life. Fitness can give you freedom to move your body the way you want. Fit people have more energy and better body control. They can enjoy a more active lifestyle than their more sedentary counterparts. Even if you don't like sports, you need physical energy and stamina in your daily life and for many nonsport leisure activities such as visiting museums, playing with children, gardening, and so on.

Where does this leave you? Most experts agree that some physical activity is better than none, but that more—as long as it does not result in injury—is better than some. To set a personal goal for physical activity and exercise, consider your current activity level, your health status, and your overall goals. At the very least, strive to become more active and do 30 minutes of moderate-intensity activity at least 5 days per week. Choose to be active whenever you can. If weight management is a concern for you, begin by achieving the goal of 30 minutes of activity per day and then try to raise your activity level further, to 60–90 minutes per day or more. For even better health and well-being, participate in a structured exercise program that develops physical fitness. Any increase in physical activity will contribute to your health and well-being, now and in the future.

Wellness Tip

Do you set aside blocks of time every day for studying? If so, your schedule probably makes it easier to get your work done. The same is true of exercising, so make it a part of your daily routine, like studying.

HEALTH-RELATED COMPONENTS OF PHYSICAL FITNESS

Some components of fitness are related to specific activities, and others relate to general health. **Health-related fitness** includes the following components:

- Cardiorespiratory endurance
- Muscular strength

Ask Yourself

QUESTIONS FOR CRITICAL THINKING AND REFLECTION

Does your current lifestyle include enough physical activity—30 minutes of moderate-intensity activity 5 or more days a week—to support health and wellness? Does your lifestyle go beyond this level to include enough vigorous physical activity and exercise to build physical fitness? What changes could you make in your lifestyle to develop physical fitness?

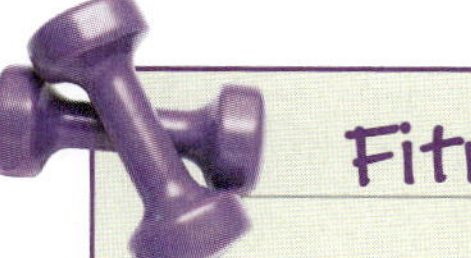

Fitness Tip

Very few activities build all the health-related components of fitness at the same time. This is why variety is important. Create a routine that lets you build one or two fitness components every day. Variety also keeps your workouts enjoyable.

- Muscular endurance
- Flexibility
- Body composition

Health-related fitness helps you withstand physical challenges and protects you from diseases.

Cardiorespiratory Endurance

Cardiorespiratory endurance is the ability to perform prolonged, large-muscle, dynamic exercise at moderate to high levels of intensity. It depends on such factors as the ability of the lungs to deliver oxygen from the environment to the bloodstream, the capacity of the heart to pump blood, the ability of the nervous system and blood vessels to regulate blood flow, and the capability of the cells' chemical systems to use oxygen and process fuels for exercise.

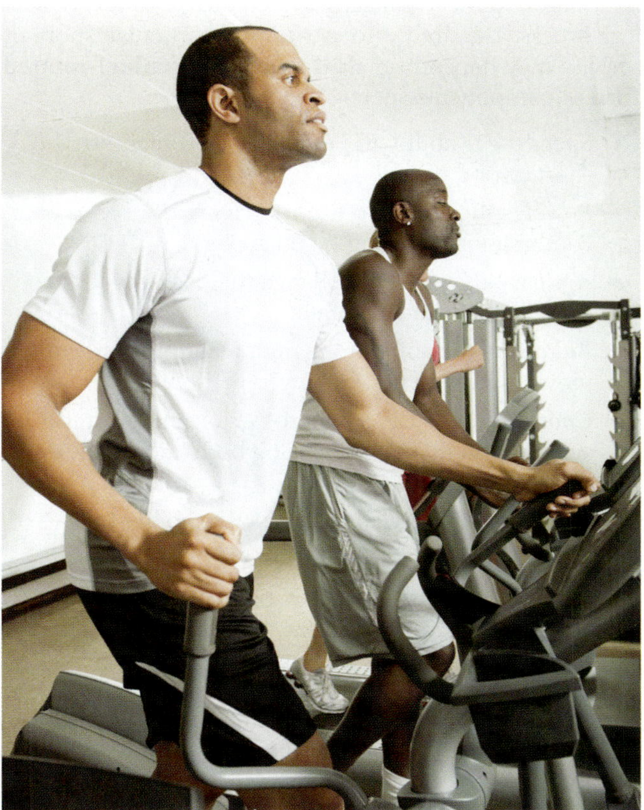

Cardiorespiratory endurance is a key component of health-related fitness.

When cardiorespiratory fitness is low, the heart has to work hard during normal daily activities and may not be able to work hard enough to sustain high-intensity physical activity in an emergency. As cardiorespiratory fitness improves, related physical functions also improve. For example:

- The heart pumps more blood per heartbeat.
- Resting heart rate slows.
- Blood volume increases.
- Blood supply to tissues improves.
- The body can cool itself better.
- Resting blood pressure decreases.
- Metabolism in skeletal muscle is enhanced, which improves fuel use.
- Resistance and aerobic training increases the level of antioxidant chemicals in the body and lowers oxidative stress.

A healthy heart can better withstand the strains of everyday life, the stress of occasional emergencies, and the wear and tear of time.

Endurance training also improves the functioning of the body's chemical systems, particularly in the muscles and liver. These changes enhance the body's ability to derive energy from food, allow the body to perform more exercise with less effort, increase sensitivity to insulin, and prevent type 2 diabetes.

Cardiorespiratory endurance is a central component of health-related fitness because heart and lung function is so essential to overall good health. A person can't live very long or very well without a healthy heart. Poor cardiorespiratory fitness is linked with heart disease, type 2 diabetes, colon cancer, stroke, depression, and anxiety. A moderate level of cardiorespiratory fitness can help compensate for certain health risks, including excess body fat: People who are lean but have low cardiorespiratory fitness have been found to have higher death rates than people with higher levels of body fat who are otherwise fit.

You can develop cardiorespiratory endurance through activities that involve continuous, rhythmic movements of large-muscle groups, such as the legs. Such activities include walking, jogging, cycling, and group aerobics.

Muscular Strength

Muscular strength is the amount of force a muscle can produce with a single maximum effort. It depends on

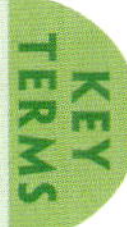

health-related fitness Physical capacities that contribute to health: cardiorespiratory endurance, muscular strength, muscular endurance, flexibility, and body composition.

cardiorespiratory endurance The ability of the body to perform prolonged, large-muscle, dynamic exercise at moderate to high levels of intensity.

muscular strength The amount of force a muscle can produce with a single maximum effort.

such factors as the size of muscle cells and the ability of nerves to activate muscle cells. Strong muscles are important for everyday activities, such as climbing stairs, as well as for emergency situations. They help keep the skeleton in proper alignment, preventing back and leg pain and providing the support necessary for good posture. Muscular strength has obvious importance in recreational activities. Strong people can hit a tennis ball harder, kick a soccer ball farther, and ride a bicycle uphill more easily.

Muscle tissue is an important element of overall body composition. Greater muscle mass means a higher rate of **metabolism** and faster energy use. Greater muscle mass reduces markers of oxidative stress and maintains mitochondria (the "powerhouses" of the cell), both of which are important for metabolic health and longevity. Training to build muscular strength can also help people manage stress and boost their self-confidence.

Maintaining strength and muscle mass is vital for healthy aging. Older people tend to experience a decrease in both number and size of muscle cells, a condition called *sarcopenia.* Many of the remaining muscle cells become slower, and some become nonfunctional because they lose their attachment to the nervous system. Strength training (also known as *resistance training* or *weight training)* increases antioxidant enzymes and lowers oxidative stress. It also helps maintain muscle mass and function and possibly helps decrease the risk of osteoporosis (bone loss) in older people, which greatly enhances their quality of life and prevents life-threatening injuries.

Muscular Endurance

Muscular endurance is the ability to resist fatigue and sustain a given level of muscle tension—that is, to hold a muscle contraction for a long time or to contract a muscle over and over again. It depends on such factors as the size of muscle cells, the ability of muscles to store fuel, and the blood supply to muscles.

Muscular endurance is important for good posture and for injury prevention. For example, if abdominal and back muscles cannot support the spine correctly when sitting or standing for long periods, the chances of low-back pain and back injury are increased. Good muscular endurance in the trunk muscles is more important than muscular strength for preventing back pain. Muscular endurance helps people cope with daily physical demands and enhances performance in sports and work.

Flexibility

Flexibility is the ability to move the joints through their full range of motion. It depends on joint structure, the length and elasticity of connective tissue, and nervous system activity. Flexible, pain-free joints are important for good health and well-being. Inactivity causes the joints to become stiffer with age. Stiffness, in turn, often causes people to assume unnatural body postures that can stress joints and muscles. Stretching exercises can help ensure a healthy range of motion for all major joints.

Body Composition

Body composition refers to the proportion of fat and **fat-free mass** (muscle, bone, and water) in the body. Healthy body composition involves a high proportion of fat-free mass and an acceptably low level of body fat, adjusted for age and gender. A person with excessive body fat—especially excess fat in the abdomen—is more likely to experience health problems, including heart disease, insulin resistance, high blood pressure, stroke, joint problems, type 2 diabetes, gallbladder disease, blood vessel inflammation, some types of cancer, back pain, and premature death.

The best way to lose fat is through a lifestyle that includes a sensible diet and exercise. The best way to add muscle mass is through strength training. Large changes in body composition are not necessary to improve health; even a small increase in physical activity and a small decrease in body fat can lead to substantial health improvements.

Skill (Neuromuscular)-Related Components of Fitness

In addition to the five health-related components of physical fitness, the ability to perform a particular sport or activity may depend on **skill (neuromuscular)-related fitness** components such as the following:

- *Speed*—the ability to perform a movement in a short period of time
- *Power*—the ability to exert force rapidly, based on a combination of strength and speed
- *Agility*—the ability to change the position of the body quickly and accurately
- *Balance*—the ability to maintain equilibrium while moving or while stationary
- *Coordination*—the ability to perform motor tasks accurately and smoothly using body movements and the senses
- *Reaction and movement time*—the ability to respond and react quickly to a stimulus

Skill-related fitness tends to be sport-specific and is best developed through practice. For example, the speed, coordination, and agility needed to play basketball can be developed by playing basketball. These activities are particularly important for older adults for preventing life-threatening falls. Participating in sports is fun, can help you build fitness, and contributes to other areas of wellness. Young adults often find it easier to exercise regularly when they participate in sports and activities they enjoy, such as dancing, tennis, snowboarding, or basketball.

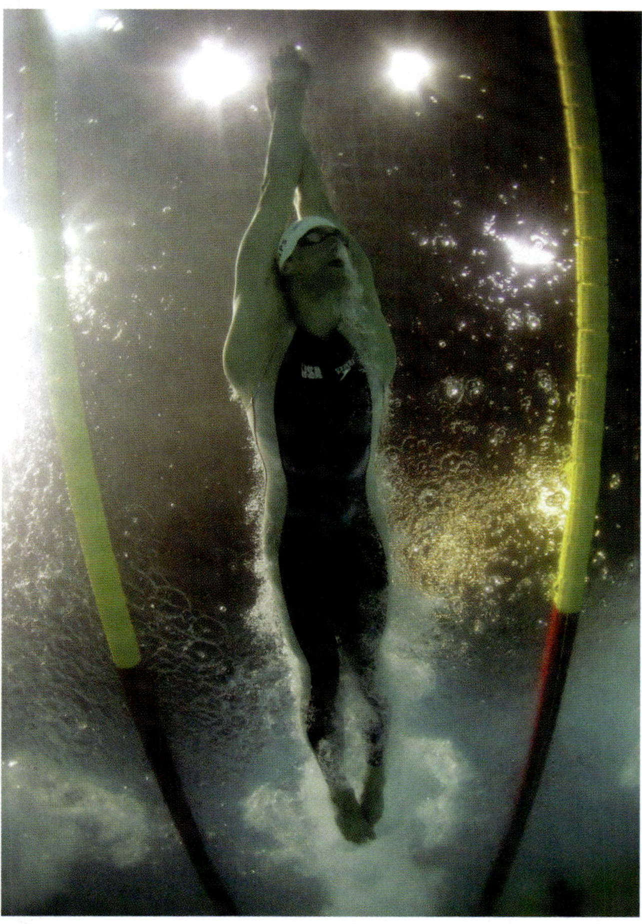

Elite athletes demonstrate sport-specific skills such as speed, power, agility, coordination, and reaction time.

Older adults can develop balance by practicing exercises such as yoga and tai chi.

PRINCIPLES OF PHYSICAL TRAINING: ADAPTATION TO STRESS

The human body is very adaptable. The greater the demands made on it, the more it adjusts to meet those demands. Over time, immediate, short-term adjustments translate into long-term changes and improvements. When breathing and heart rate increase during exercise, for example, the heart gradually develops the ability to pump more blood with each beat. Then, during exercise, it doesn't have to beat as fast to meet the cells' demands for oxygen. The goal of **physical training** is to produce these long-term changes and improvements in the body's functioning. Although people differ in the maximum levels of physical fitness and performance they can achieve through training, the wellness benefits of exercise are available to everyone (see the box "Fitness and Disability").

Particular types and amounts of exercise are most effective in developing the various components of fitness. To put together an effective exercise program, you should first understand the basic principles of physical training, including the following:

- Specificity
- Progressive overload
- Reversibility
- Individual differences

All of these rest on the larger principle of adaptation.

Wellness Tip

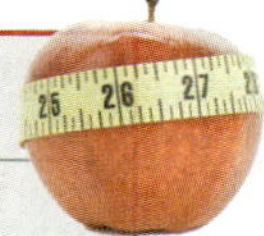

The words "over time" are key to realizing the benefits of physical activity. If you get in the habit of being active, you'll notice the benefits over time. After a few workouts, you'll breathe with less effort and recover faster, feel stronger and more flexible. In a few weeks your clothes will fit differently, and you'll notice changes in the mirror. Practice patience and watch the rewards pile up!

? Ask Yourself

QUESTIONS FOR CRITICAL THINKING AND REFLECTION

When you think about exercise, do you think of only one or two of the five components of health-related fitness, such as muscular strength or body composition? If so, where do you think your ideas come from? What role do the media play in shaping your ideas about fitness?

KEY TERMS

metabolism The sum of all the vital processes by which food energy and nutrients are made available to and used by the body.

muscular endurance The ability of a muscle to remain contracted or to contract repeatedly for a long period of time.

flexibility The ability to move joints through their full range of motion.

body composition The proportion of fat and fat-free mass (muscle, bone, and water) in the body.

fat-free mass The nonfat component of the human body, consisting of skeletal muscle, bone, and water.

skill (neuromuscular)-related fitness Physical capacities that contribute to performance in a sport or an activity: speed, power, agility, balance, coordination, and reaction time; neuromuscular fitness refers to specific fitness related to maintaining performance levels of balance, agility, coordination, and gait.

physical training The performance of different types of activities that cause the body to adapt and improve its level of fitness.

DIMENSIONS OF DIVERSITY

Fitness and Disability

Physical fitness and athletic achievement are not limited to the able-bodied. People with disabilities can also attain high levels of fitness and performance, as shown by the elite athletes who compete in the Paralympics. The premier event for athletes with disabilities, the Paralympics are held in the same year and city as the Olympics. The performance of these skilled athletes makes it clear that people with disabilities can be active, healthy, and extraordinarily fit. Just like able-bodied athletes, athletes with disabilities strive for excellence and can serve as role models.

According to the U.S. Census Bureau, about 54 million Americans have some type of chronic disability. Some disabilities are the result of injury, such as spinal cord injuries sustained in car crashes or war. Other disabilities result from illness, such as the blindness that sometimes occurs as a complication of diabetes or the joint stiffness that accompanies arthritis. And some disabilities are present at birth, as in the case of congenital limb deformities or cerebral palsy.

Exercise and physical activity are as important for people with disabilities as for able-bodied individuals—if not *more* important. Being active helps prevent secondary conditions that may result from prolonged inactivity, such as circulatory or muscular problems. Currently, about 19% of people with disabilities engage in regular moderate-intensity activity.

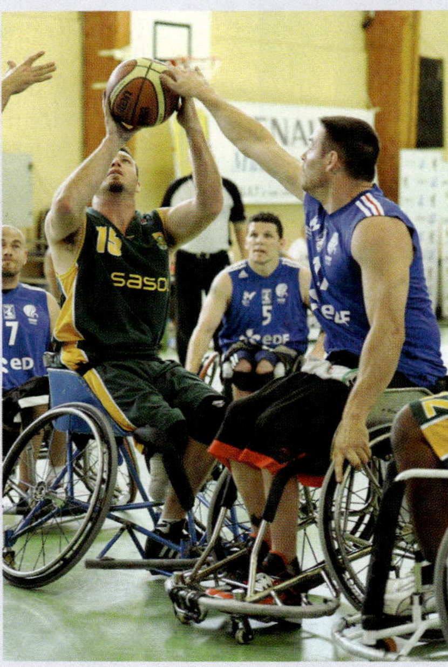

People with disabilities don't have to be elite athletes to participate in sports and lead an active life. Some health clubs, fitness centers, city recreation centers, and universities offer activities and events geared for people of all ages and types of disabilities. They may have modified aerobics classes, special weight training machines, classes involving mild exercise in warm water, and other activities adapted for people with disabilities. Popular sports and recreational activities include adapted horseback riding, golf, swimming, and skiing. Competitive sports are also available—for example, there are wheelchair versions of billiards, tennis, weight lifting, hockey, and basketball, as well as sports for people with hearing, visual, or mental impairments. For those who prefer to get their exercise at home, special videos are available geared to individuals who use wheelchairs or who have arthritis, hearing impairments, metabolic diseases, or many other disabilities.

If you have a disability and want to be more active, check with your physician about what's appropriate for you. Call your local community center, university, YMCA/YWCA, hospital, independent living center, or fitness center to locate facilities. Look for a facility with experienced personnel and appropriate adaptive equipment. For specialized videos, check with hospitals and health associations that are geared to specific disabilities, such as the Arthritis Foundation.

Specificity—Adapting to Type of Training

To develop a particular fitness component, you must perform exercises designed specifically for that component. This is the principle of **specificity.** Weight training, for example, develops muscular strength but is less effective for developing cardiorespiratory endurance or flexibility. Specificity also applies to the skill-related fitness components (to improve at tennis, you must practice tennis) and to the different parts of the body (to develop stronger arms, you must exercise your arms). A well-rounded exercise program includes exercises geared to each component of fitness, to different parts of the body, and to specific activities or sports.

Progressive Overload—Adapting to the Amount of Training and the FITT Principle

The body adapts to the demands of exercise by improving its functioning. When the amount of exercise (also called *overload* or *stress*) is increased progressively, fitness continues to improve. This is the principle of **progressive overload.**

The amount of overload is important. Too little exercise will have no effect on fitness (although it may improve health); too much may cause injury and problems with the body's immune or endocrine (hormone) systems. The point at which exercise becomes excessive is highly individual; it occurs at a much higher level in an Olympic athlete than in a sedentary person. For every type of exercise, there is a training threshold at which fitness benefits begin to occur, a zone within which maximum fitness benefits occur, and an upper limit of safe training.

The amount of exercise needed depends on the individual's current level of fitness, the person's genetically determined capacity to adapt to training, his or her fitness goals, and the component being developed. A novice, for example, might experience fitness benefits from jogging a mile in 10 minutes, but this level of exercise would cause no physical adaptations in a trained distance runner. Beginners should start at the lower end of the fitness benefit zone; fitter individuals will make more rapid gains by exercising at the higher end of the fitness benefit zone. Progression is critical because fitness increases only if the volume and intensity of workouts increase. Exercising at the same intensity every training session will maintain fitness but will not increase it, because the training stress is below the threshold required to produce adaptation.

The amount of overload needed to maintain or improve a particular level of fitness for a particular fitness component is determined through four dimensions, represented by the acronym FITT:

- *Frequency*—how often
- *Intensity*—how hard
- *Time*—how long (duration)
- *Type*—mode of activity

Chapters 4, 8, and 9 show you how to apply the FITT principle to exercise programs for cardiorespiratory endurance, muscular strength and endurance, and flexibility, respectively.

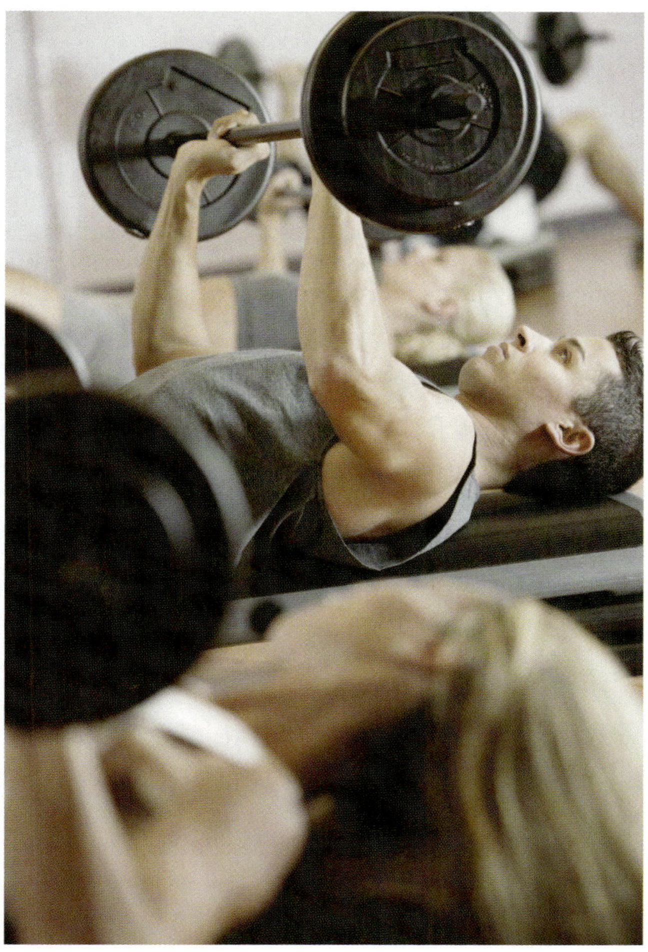

Progressive overload is important because fitness increases only when the volume and intensity of exercise increase. The body adapts to overload by becoming more fit.

Frequency Developing fitness requires regular exercise. Optimum exercise frequency, expressed in number of days per week, varies with the component being developed and the individual's fitness goals. For most people, a frequency of 3–5 days per week for cardiorespiratory endurance exercise and 2 or more days per week for resistance and flexibility training is appropriate for a general fitness program.

An important consideration in determining appropriate exercise frequency is recovery time, which is also highly individual and depends on factors such as training experience, age, and intensity of training. For example, 24 hours of rest between highly intense workouts involving heavy weights or track sprints is not enough recovery time for safe and effective training. Intense workouts need to be spaced out during the week to allow for sufficient recovery time. On the other hand, you can exercise every day if your program consists of moderate-intensity walking or cycling. Learn to "listen to your body" to get enough rest between workouts. Chapters 4, 8, and 9 provide more detailed information about training techniques and recovery periods for workouts focused on different fitness components.

Intensity Fitness benefits occur when a person exercises harder than his or her normal level of activity. The appropriate exercise intensity varies with each fitness component. To develop cardiorespiratory endurance, for example, you must raise your heart rate above normal. To develop muscular strength, you must lift a heavier weight than normal. To develop flexibility, you must stretch muscles beyond their normal length.

Time (Duration) Fitness benefits occur when you exercise for an extended period of time. For cardiorespiratory endurance exercise, 20–60 minutes is recommended. Exercise can take place in a single session or in several sessions of 10 or more minutes. The greater the intensity of exercise, the less time needed to obtain fitness benefits. For high-intensity exercise, such as running, 20–30 minutes is appropriate. For moderate-intensity exercise, such as walking, 45–60 minutes may be needed. High-intensity exercise poses a greater risk of injury than low-intensity exercise, so if you are a nonathletic adult, it's best to first emphasize low- to moderate-intensity activity of longer duration.

To build muscular strength, muscular endurance, and flexibility, similar amounts of time are advisable, but these exercises are more commonly organized in terms of a

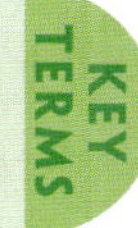

specificity The training principle that the body adapts to the particular type and amount of stress placed on it.

progressive overload The training principle that placing increasing amounts of stress on the body causes adaptations that improve fitness.

specific number of repetitions of particular exercises. For resistance training, for example, a recommended program includes one or more sets of 8–12 repetitions of 8–10 different exercises that work the major muscle groups. Older adults should do 10–15 repetitions per set.

Type (Mode of Activity) The type of exercise in which you should engage varies with each fitness component and with your personal fitness goals. To develop cardiorespiratory endurance, you need to engage in continuous activities involving large-muscle groups—walking, jogging, cycling, or swimming, for example. Resistance exercises develop muscular strength and endurance, while stretching exercises build flexibility. The frequency, intensity, and time of the exercise will be different for each type of activity. (See pp. 41–44 for more on choosing appropriate activities for your fitness program.)

Reversibility—Adapting to a Reduction in Training

Fitness is a reversible adaptation. The body adjusts to lower levels of physical activity the same way it adjusts to higher levels. This is the principle of **reversibility.** When a person stops exercising, up to 50% of fitness improvements are lost within 2 months. However, not all fitness levels reverse at the same rate. Strength fitness is very resilient, so a person can maintain strength fitness by doing resistance exercise as infrequently as once a week. On the other hand, cardiovascular and cellular fitness reverse themselves more quickly—sometimes within just a few days or weeks. If you must temporarily curtail your training, you can maintain your fitness improvements by keeping the intensity of your workouts constant while reducing their frequency or duration.

Individual Differences—Limits on Adaptability

Anyone watching the Olympics can see that, from a physical standpoint, we are not all created equal. There are large individual differences in our ability to improve fitness, achieve a desirable body composition, and learn and perform sports skills. Some people are able to run longer distances, or lift more weight, or kick a soccer ball more skillfully than others will ever be able to, no matter how much they train. People respond to training at different rates, so a program that works for one person may not be right for another person.

There are limits on the adaptability—the potential for improvement—of any human body. The body's ability to transport and use oxygen, for example, can be improved by only about 5–30% through training. An endurance athlete must therefore inherit a large metabolic capacity in order to reach competitive performance levels. In the past few years, scientists have identified specific genes that influence body fat, strength, and endurance. For example, they have identified more than 800 genes associated with endurance performance, and 100 of those determine individual differences in exercise capacity. However, physical training improves fitness regardless of heredity. For the average person, the body's adaptability is enough to achieve reasonable fitness goals.

Fitness Tip

At the gym, it can be intimidating to find yourself surrounded by people who seem to be in better shape than you are. But remember: They got in shape by focusing on themselves, not by worrying about what other people thought about them. You can avoid feeling intimidated by doing the same thing. Focus on ***you***, and let others worry about themselves.

Ask Yourself

QUESTIONS FOR CRITICAL THINKING AND REFLECTION

Many people who play sports have had the experience of realizing that they are not as physically gifted as a teammate or that they are never going to be in the Olympics. What can you say to encourage someone who is discouraged by this realization? What benefits of physical activity, exercise, and sports might you point out?

DESIGNING YOUR OWN EXERCISE PROGRAM

Physical training works best when you have a plan. A plan helps you make gradual but steady progress toward your goals. Once you've determined that exercise is safe for you, planning for physical fitness consists of assessing how fit you are now, determining where you want to be, and choosing the right activities to help you get there.

Getting Medical Clearance

People of any age who are not at high risk for serious health problems can safely exercise at a moderate intensity (60% or less of maximum heart rate) without a prior medical evaluation (see Chapter 4 for a discussion of maximum heart rate). Likewise, if you are male and under 40 or female and under 50 and in good health, exercise is probably safe for you. If you do not fit into these age groups, or if you have health problems—especially high blood pressure, heart disease, muscle or joint problems,

Are You Healthy Enough for Exercise?

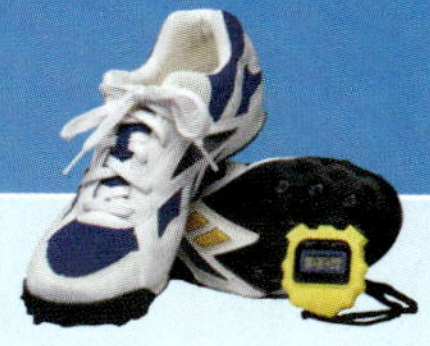

PERSONAL CHALLENGE

Heart disease and diabetes aren't the only reasons to get a doctor's approval before starting an exercise program. If you are severely overweight, have a family history of some chronic disease, or have just never exercised before, it could be advisable to talk to your doctor before becoming physically active.

Think about your current health status and your family history. If you think of any issues that might interfere with being physically active—or that might make exercise dangerous for you—list them below:

____

____

____

____

____

If you write down anything, even *one* thing, make an appointment to see your doctor as soon as possible. Ask your doctor for an overall health evaluation, review your family history, and make sure the doctor knows you want to start being physically active on a regular basis. Then address the specific issues you listed above.

If your physician offers any specific advice, follow it. But if you can be physically active, even with some restrictions, make a commitment and get started on your exercise plan. And see your doctor regularly to make sure physical activity is working for you.

or obesity—see your physician before starting a vigorous exercise program. The Canadian Society for Exercise Physiology has developed the Physical Activity Readiness Questionnaire (PAR-Q) to help evaluate exercise safety; it is included in Lab 2.1. Completing it should alert you to any potential problems you may have. If a physician isn't sure whether exercise is safe for you, she or he may recommend an **exercise stress test** or a **graded exercise test (GXT)** to see whether you show symptoms of heart disease during exercise. For most people, however, it's far safer to exercise than to remain sedentary. For more information, see the box "Exercise and Cardiac Risk."

Assessing Yourself

The first step in creating a successful fitness program is to assess your current level of physical activity and fitness for each of the five health-related fitness components. The results of the assessment tests will help you set specific fitness goals and plan your fitness program. Lab 2.3 gives you the opportunity to assess your current overall level of activity and determine if it is appropriate. Assessment tests in Chapters 4, 6, 8 and 9 will help you evaluate your cardiorespiratory endurance, muscular strength, muscular endurance, flexibility, and body composition.

Setting Goals

The ultimate general goal of every health-related fitness program is the same—wellness that lasts a lifetime. Whatever your specific goals, they must be important enough to you to keep you motivated. Most sports psychologists believe that setting and achieving goals is the most effective way to stay motivated about exercise. (Refer to Chapter 1 for more on goal setting, as well as Common Questions Answered at the end of this chapter.) After you complete the assessment tests in Chapters 4, 6, 8 and 9 you will be able to set goals directly related to each fitness component, such as working toward a 3-mile jog or doing 20 push-ups. First, though, think carefully about your overall goals, and be clear about why you are starting a program.

Choosing Activities for a Balanced Program

An ideal fitness program combines a physically active lifestyle with a systematic exercise program to develop and maintain physical fitness. This overall program is

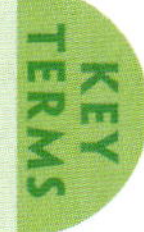

reversibility The training principle that fitness improvements are lost when demands on the body are lowered.

exercise stress test A test usually administered on a treadmill or cycle ergometer that involves analysis of the changes in electrical activity in the heart from an electrocardiogram (EKG or ECG) taken during exercise; used to determine if any heart disease is present and to assess current fitness level.

graded exercise test (GXT) An exercise test that starts at an easy intensity and progresses to maximum capacity.

IN FOCUS

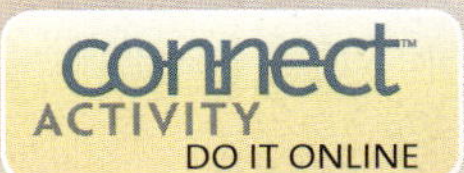

Exercise and Cardiac Risk

Participating in exercise and sports is usually a wonderful experience that improves wellness in both the short and long term. In rare instances, however, vigorous exertion is associated with sudden death. It may seem difficult to understand that although regular exercise protects people from heart disease, it also increases the risk of sudden death.

Congenital heart defects (heart abnormalities present at birth) are the most common cause of exercise-related sudden death in people under 35. In nearly all other cases, coronary artery disease is responsible. In this condition, fat and other substances build up in the arteries that supply blood to the heart. Death can result if an artery becomes blocked or if the heart's rhythm and pumping action are disrupted. Exercise, particularly intense exercise, may trigger a heart attack in someone with underlying heart disease.

A study of jogging deaths in Rhode Island found that there was one death per 396,000 hours of jogging, or about one death per 7620 joggers per year—an extremely low risk for each individual jogger. Another study of men involved in a variety of physical activities found one death per 1.51 million hours of exercise. This 12-year study of more than 21,000 men found that those who didn't exercise vigorously were 74 times more likely to die suddenly from cardiac arrest during or shortly after exercise. It is also important to note that people are much safer exercising than engaging in many other common activities, including driving a car.

Although quite small, the risk does exist and may lead some people to wonder why exercise is considered such an important part of a wellness lifestyle. Exercise causes many positive changes in the body—in healthy people as well as those with heart disease—that more than make up for the slightly increased short-term risk of sudden death. Training slows or reverses the fatty buildup in arteries, helps protect people from deadly heart rhythm abnormalities, and enhances blood sugar regulation. People who exercise regularly have an overall risk of sudden death only about two-thirds that of nonexercisers. Active people who stop exercising can expect their heart attack risk to increase by 300%.

Obviously, someone with underlying coronary artery disease is at greater risk than someone who is free from the condition. However, many cases of heart disease go undiagnosed. The riskiest scenario may involve the middle-aged or older individual who suddenly begins participating in a vigorous sport or activity after being sedentary for a long time. This finding provides strong evidence for the recommendation that people increase their level of physical activity gradually and engage in regular, rather than sporadic, activity. Fortunately, the risk of heart-related sudden death in middle-aged and older adults is least in people who exercise approximately 150 minutes per week—the activity level recommended by the U.S. Department of Health and Human Services.

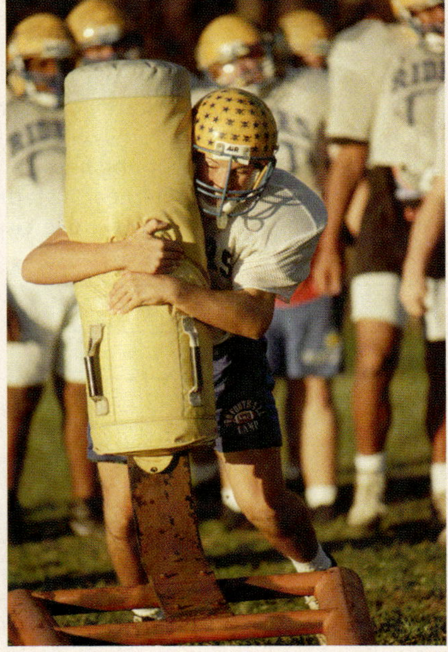

SOURCES: Fahey, T. D., and G. D. Swanson. 2008. A model for defining the optimal amount of exercise contributing to health and avoiding sudden cardiac death. *Medicina Sportiva* 12(4): 124–128; Albert, C. M., et al. 2000. Trigger of sudden death from cardiac causes by vigorous exertion. *New England Journal of Medicine* 343(19): 1355–1361.

shown in the physical activity pyramid in Figure 2.3. If you are currently sedentary, your goal should be to focus on activities at the bottom of the pyramid and gradually increase the amount of moderate-intensity physical activity in your daily life. Appropriate activities include walking briskly, climbing stairs, doing yard work, and washing your car. You don't have to exercise vigorously, but you should experience a moderate increase in your heart and breathing rates. As described earlier, your activity time can be broken up into small blocks over the course of a day.

The next two levels of the pyramid illustrate parts of a formal exercise program. The principles of this program are consistent with those of the American College of Sports Medicine (ACSM), the professional organization for people involved in sports medicine and exercise science. The ACSM has established guidelines for creating an exercise program that will develop physical fitness (Table 2.2). A balanced program includes activities to develop all the health-related components of fitness:

- *Cardiorespiratory endurance* is developed by continuous rhythmic movements of large-muscle groups in activities such as walking, jogging, cycling, swimming, and aerobic dance and other forms of group exercise. Choose activities that you enjoy and that are convenient. Other popular choices are in-line skating, dancing, and backpacking. Start-and-stop activities such as tennis, racquetball, and soccer can also develop cardiorespiratory endurance if your skill level is sufficient to enable periods of continuous play. Training for cardiorespiratory endurance is discussed in Chapter 4.

Sedentary Activities
Do infrequently
Watching television, surfing the Internet, talking on the telephone

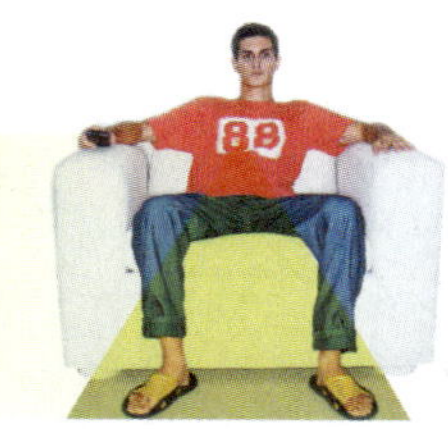

Strength Training
2–3 nonconsecutive days per week (all major muscle groups)
Bicep curls, push-ups, abdominal curls, bench press, calf raises

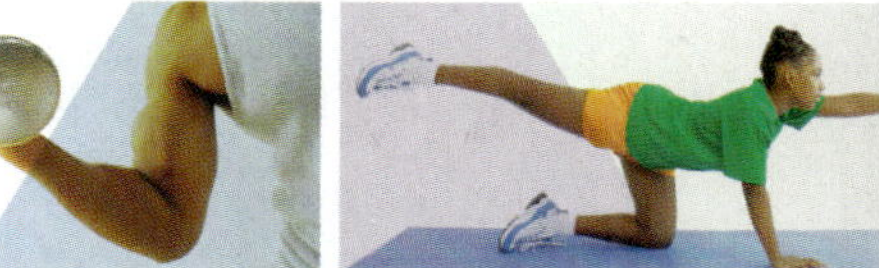

Flexibility Training
At least 2–3 days per week, ideally 5–7 days per week (all major joints)
Calf stretch, side lunge, step stretch, hurdler stretch

Cardiorespiratory Endurance Exercise
3–5 days per week (20–60 minutes per day)
Walking, jogging, bicycling, swimming, aerobic dancing, in-line skating, cross-country skiing, dancing, basketball

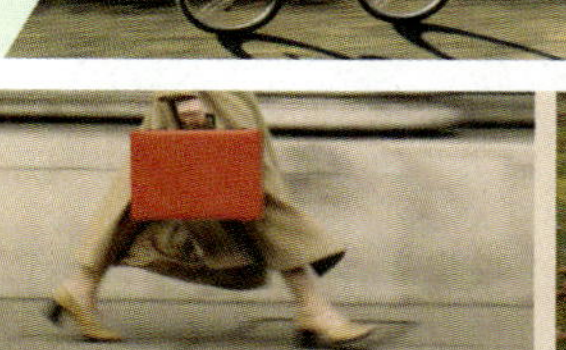

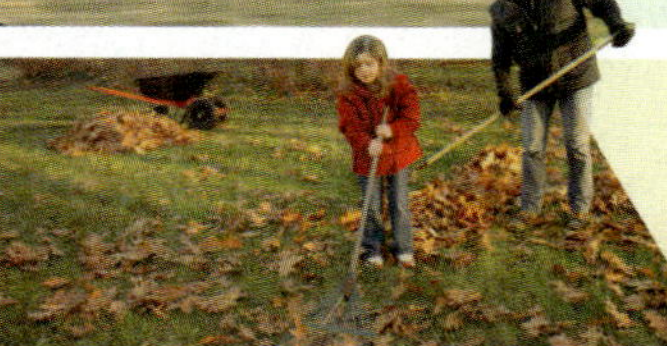

Moderate-Intensity Physical Activity
150 minutes per week; for weight loss or prevention of weight regain following weight loss, 60–90 minutes per day
Walking to the store or bank, washing windows or your car, climbing stairs, working in your yard, walking your dog, cleaning your room

FIGURE 2.3 Physical activity pyramid.

Table 2.2 ACSM Exercise Recommendations for Fitness Development in Healthy Adults

EXERCISE TO DEVELOP AND MAINTAIN CARDIORESPIRATORY ENDURANCE AND BODY COMPOSITION	
Frequency of training	3–5 days per week.
Intensity of training	55/65–90% of maximum heart rate or 40/50–85% of heart rate reserve or maximum oxygen uptake reserve.* The lower-intensity values (55–64% of maximum heart rate and 40–49% of heart rate reserve) are most applicable to unfit individuals. For average individuals, intensities of 70–85% of maximum heart rate or 60–80% of heart rate reserve are appropriate.
Time (duration) of training	20–60 total minutes per day of continuous or intermittent (in sessions lasting 10 or more minutes) aerobic activity. Duration depends on the intensity of activity; thus, low-intensity activity should be conducted over a longer period of time (30 minutes or more). Low to moderate-intensity activity of longer duration is recommended for nonathletic adults.
Type (mode) of activity	Any activity that uses large-muscle groups, can be maintained continuously, and is rhythmic and aerobic in nature—for example, walking-hiking, running-jogging, bicycling, cross-country skiing, aerobic dancing and other forms of group exercise, rope skipping, rowing, stair climbing, swimming, skating, and endurance game activities.
EXERCISE TO DEVELOP AND MAINTAIN MUSCULAR STRENGTH AND ENDURANCE, FLEXIBILITY, AND BODY COMPOSITION	
Resistance training	One set of 8–10 exercises that condition the major muscle groups, performed at least 2 days per week. Most people should complete 8–12 repetitions of each exercise to the point of fatigue; practicing other repetition ranges (for example, 3–5 or 12–15) also builds strength and endurance; for older and frailer people (approximately 50–60 and older), 10–15 repetitions with a lighter weight may be more appropriate. Multiple-set regimens will provide greater benefits if time allows. Any mode of exercise that is comfortable throughout the full range of motion is appropriate (for example, free weights, elastic bands, or machines).
Flexibility training	Static stretches, performed for the major muscle groups at least 2–3 days per week, ideally 5–7 days per week. Stretch to the point of tightness, holding each stretch for 10–30 seconds; perform 2–4 repetitions of each stretch.

*Instructions for calculating target heart rate intensity for cardiorespiratory endurance exercise are presented in Chapter 4.

SOURCE: Adapted from American College of Sports Medicine. 2009. *ACSM's Guidelines for Exercise Testing and Prescription*, 8th ed. Philadelphia: Lippincott Williams and Wilkins; Garber, C. E., et al. 2011. Quantity and quality of exercise for developing and maintaining cardiorespiratory, musculoskeletal, and neuromotor fitness in apparently healthy adults: guidance for prescribing exercise. *Medicine and Science in Sports and Exercise* 43(7): 1334–1359.

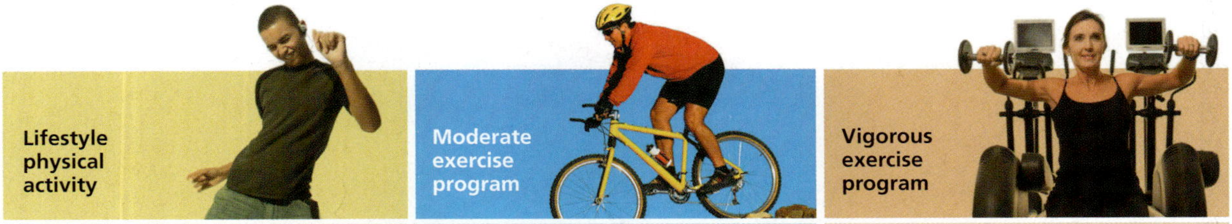

	Lifestyle physical activity	Moderate exercise program	Vigorous exercise program
Description	Moderate physical activity (150 minutes per week; muscle-strengthening exercises 2 or more days per week)	Cardiorespiratory endurance exercise (20–60 minutes, 3–5 days per week); strength training (2–3 nonconsecutive days per week); and stretching exercises (2 or more days per week)	Cardiorespiratory endurance exercise (20–60 minutes, 3–5 days per week); interval training; strength training (3–4 nonconsecutive days per week); and stretching exercises (5–7 days per week)
Sample activities or program	• Walking to and from work, 15 minutes each way • Cycling to and from class, 10 minutes each way • Doing yard work for 30 minutes • Dancing (fast) for 30 minutes • Playing basketball for 20 minutes • Muscle exercises such as push-ups, squats, or back exercises	• Jogging for 30 minutes, 3 days per week • Weight training, 1 set of 8 exercises, 2 days per week • Stretching exercises, 3 days per week	• Running for 45 minutes, 3 days per week • Intervals, running 400 m at high effort, 4 sets, 2 days per week • Weight training, 3 sets of 10 exercises, 3 days per week • Stretching exercises, 6 days per week
Health and fitness benefits	Better blood cholesterol levels, reduced body fat, better control of blood pressure, improved metabolic health, and enhanced glucose metabolism; improved quality of life; reduced risk of some chronic diseases Greater amounts of activity can help prevent weight gain and promote weight loss	All the benefits of lifestyle physical activity, plus improved physical fitness (increased cardiorespiratory endurance, muscular strength and endurance, and flexibility) and even greater improvements in health and quality of life and reductions in chronic disease risk	All the benefits of lifestyle physical activity and a moderate exercise program, with greater increases in fitness and somewhat greater reductions in chronic disease risk Participating in a vigorous exercise program may increase risk of injury and overtraining

FIGURE 2.4 Health and fitness benefits of different amounts of physical activity and exercise.

• *Muscular strength and endurance* can be developed through resistance training—training with weights or performing calisthenic exercises such as push-ups and curl-ups. Training for muscular strength and endurance is discussed in Chapter 8.

• *Flexibility* is developed by stretching the major muscle groups regularly and with proper technique. Flexibility is discussed in Chapter 9.

• *Healthy body composition* can be developed through a sensible diet and a program of regular exercise. Cardiorespiratory endurance exercise is best for reducing body fat; resistance training builds muscle mass, which, to a small extent, helps increase metabolism. Body composition is discussed in Chapter 6.

(Refer to Figure 2.4 for a summary of the health and fitness benefits of different levels of physical activity.)

What about the tip of the activity pyramid? Although sedentary activities are often unavoidable—attending class, studying, working in an office, and so on—many people choose inactivity over activity during their leisure time. Change sedentary patterns by becoming more active whenever you can. Move more and sit less.

Guidelines for Training

The following guidelines will make your exercise program more effective and successful.

Train the Way You Want Your Body to Change

Stress your body so it adapts in the desired manner. To have a more muscular build, lift weights. To be more flexible, do stretching exercises. To improve performance in a particular sport, practice that sport or its movements.

Train Regularly Consistency is the key to improving fitness. Fitness improvements are lost if too much time passes between exercise sessions.

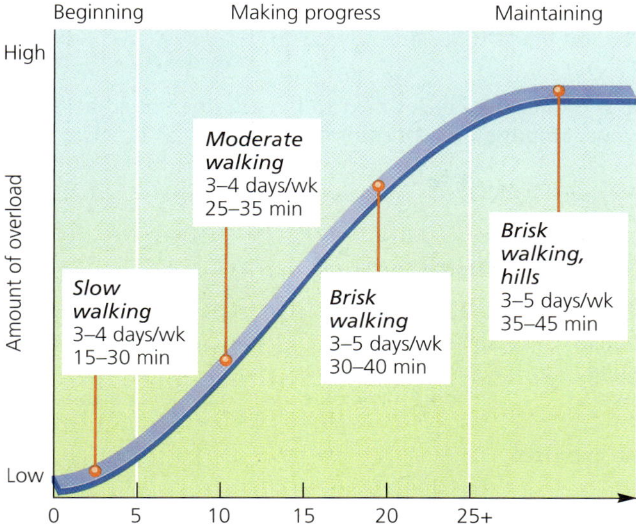

FIGURE 2.5 Progression of an exercise program.
This figure shows how the amount of overload is increased gradually over time in a sample walking program. Regardless of the activity chosen, it is important that an exercise program begin slowly and progress gradually. Once you achieve the desired level of fitness, you can maintain it by exercising 3–5 days a week.
SOURCE: Progression data from American College of Sports Medicine. 2009. *ACSM's Guidelines for Exercise Testing and Prescription,* 8th ed. Philadelphia: Lippincott Williams and Wilkins.

Start Slowly, and Get in Shape Gradually As Figure 2.5 shows, an exercise program can be divided into three phases:

- ***Beginning phase.*** The body adjusts to the new type and level of activity.
- ***Progress phase.*** Fitness increases.
- ***Maintenance phase.*** The targeted level of fitness is sustained over the long term.

When beginning a program, start slowly to give your body time to adapt to the stress of exercise. Choose activities carefully according to your fitness status. If you have been sedentary or are overweight, try an activity such as walking or swimming that won't jar the body or strain the joints.

As you progress, increase duration and frequency before increasing intensity. If you train too much or too intensely, you are more likely to suffer injuries or become **overtrained**, a condition characterized by lack of energy, aching muscles and joints, and decreased physical performance. Injuries and overtraining slow down an exercise program and impede motivation. The goal is not to get in shape as quickly as possible but to gradually become and then remain physically fit.

Warm Up Before Exercise Warming up can decrease your chances of injury by helping your body gradually progress from rest to activity. A good warm-up can increase muscle temperature, reduce joint stiffness, bathe the joint surfaces in lubricating fluid, and increase blood flow to the muscles, including the heart. Some studies suggest that warming up may also enhance muscle metabolism and mentally prepare you for a workout.

A warm-up should include low-intensity, whole-body movements similar to those used in the activity that will follow. For example, runners may walk and jog slowly prior to running at full speed. A tennis player might hit forehands and backhands at a low intensity before playing a vigorous set of tennis. A warm-up is not the same as a stretching workout. For safety and effectiveness, it is best to stretch *after* an endurance or strength training workout, when muscles are warm—and not as part of a warm-up. (Appropriate and effective warm-ups are discussed in greater detail in Chapters 4, 8 and 9.)

Wellness Tip

Moderation is important, especially if you're just starting to get physically active. Work at a pace that's comfortable and enjoyable, with a goal of making gradual improvements. This will help you get into the habit of being active, and will help you avoid burnout.

Cool Down After Exercise During exercise, as much as 90% of circulating blood is directed to the muscles and skin, up from as little as 20% during rest. If you suddenly stop moving after exercise, the amount of blood returning to your heart and brain may be insufficient, and you may experience dizziness, a drop in blood pressure, or other problems. Cooling down at the end of a workout helps safely restore circulation to its normal resting condition. So, after you exercise, cool down before you sit or lie down or jump into the shower. Cool down by continuing to move at a slow pace—walking for 5–10 minutes, for example, as your heart and breathing rate and blood pressure slowly return to normal. At the end of the cool-down period, do stretching exercises while your muscles are still warm. Cool down longer after intense exercise sessions.

Exercise Safely Physical activity can cause injury or even death if you don't consider safety. For example, you should always:

- Wear a helmet when biking, skiing, or rock climbing.
- Wear eye protection when playing racquetball or squash.

KEY TERM

overtraining A condition caused by training too much or too intensely, characterized by lack of energy, decreased physical performance, and aching muscles and joints.

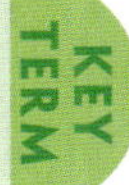

TAKE CHARGE

Vary Your Activities

Do you have a hard time thinking of new activities to try? Check the boxes next to the activities listed here that interest you. Then look for resources and facilities on your campus or in your community.

Outdoor Exercises

- ❑ Walking
- ❑ Running
- ❑ Cycling
- ❑ Swimming
- ❑ In-line skating
- ❑ Skateboarding
- ❑ Rowing
- ❑ Horseback riding
- ❑ Hiking
- ❑ Backpacking
- ❑ Ice skating
- ❑ Fly fishing

Exercises You Can Do at Home and Work

- ❑ Desk exercises
- ❑ Calisthenics
- ❑ Gardening
- ❑ Housework
- ❑ Yard work
- ❑ Sweeping
- ❑ Exploring on foot
- ❑ Doing a walk-a-thon
- ❑ Painting walls
- ❑ Walking the dog
- ❑ Shopping
- ❑ Doing errands

Sports and Games

- ❑ Basketball
- ❑ Tennis
- ❑ Volleyball
- ❑ Golf
- ❑ Soccer
- ❑ Softball
- ❑ Water skiing
- ❑ Windsurfing
- ❑ Badminton
- ❑ Ultimate Frisbee
- ❑ Bowling
- ❑ Surfing
- ❑ Dancing
- ❑ Snow skiing
- ❑ Gymnastics

Health Club Exercises

- ❑ Weight training
- ❑ Circuit training
- ❑ Group exercise
- ❑ Treadmill
- ❑ Stationary bike
- ❑ Ski machine
- ❑ Supine bike
- ❑ Rowing machine
- ❑ Plyometrics
- ❑ Water aerobics
- ❑ Elliptical trainer
- ❑ Medicine ball
- ❑ Rope skipping
- ❑ Punching bag
- ❑ Racquetball

- Wear bright clothing when exercising on a public street.
- Walk or run with a partner on a deserted track or in a park.
- Give vehicles plenty of leeway, even when you have the right of way.
- In the weight room, be aware of people exercising near you, and use spotters when appropriate.

Overloading your muscles and joints can lead to serious injury, so train within your capacity. Use high-quality equipment and keep it in good repair. Report broken gym equipment to the health club manager. (See Appendix A for more information on personal safety.)

Listen to Your Body and Get Adequate Rest Rest can be as important as exercise for improving fitness. Fitness reflects an adaptation to the stress of exercise. Building fitness involves a series of exercise stresses, recuperation, and adaptation leading to improved fitness, followed by further stresses. Build rest into your training program, and don't exercise if it doesn't feel right. Sometimes you need a few days of rest to recover enough to train with the intensity required for improving fitness. Getting enough sleep is an important part of the recovery process. On the other hand, you can't train sporadically, either. If you listen to your body and it always tells you to rest, you won't make any progress.

Cycle the Volume and Intensity of Your Workouts To add enjoyment and variety to your program and to further improve fitness, don't train at the same intensity during every workout. Train intensely on some days and train lightly on others. Proper management of workout intensity is a key to improving physical fitness. Use cycle training, also known as *periodization*, to provide enough recovery for intense training: By training lightly one workout, you can train harder the next. However, take care to increase the volume and intensity of your program gradually—never more than 10% per week.

Vary Your Activities Change your exercise program from time to time to keep things fresh and help develop a higher degree of fitness. The body adapts quickly to an exercise stress, such as walking, cycling, or swimming. Gains in fitness in a particular activity become more difficult with time. Varying the exercises in your program allows you to adapt to many types of exercise and develops fitness in a variety of activities (see the box "Vary Your Activities"). Changing activities may also help reduce your risk of injury.

Train with a Partner Training partners can motivate and encourage each other through rough spots and help each other develop proper exercise techniques. Training with a partner can make exercising seem easier and more fun. It can also help you keep motivated and on track. A commitment to a friend is a powerful motivator. If you can afford it, you may benefit from a personal trainer who can give you instruction in exercise techniques and help provide motivation.

Train Your Mind Becoming fit requires commitment, discipline, and patience. These qualities come from understanding the importance of exercise and having clear and reachable goals. Use the lifestyle management

Digital Workout Aids

WELLNESS IN THE DIGITAL AGE

When you're just starting to get physically active, you can wind up with a lot of questions. How many miles did I walk? How many sit-ups did I do? How many minutes did I run? When your mind is completely focused on just *doing* an activity, it's easy to lose count of time, distance, and reps. But it's important to keep track of these things: Move too little and you won't see any progress; move too much and you run the risk of injury or burnout. Either outcome is bad news for your exercise program.

Luckily, we live in a digital age, and the fitness industry is providing an ever-growing array of tools that can track your progress for you. If you like to walk or run, digital pedometers can track your distance and the number of steps you take. Advanced trackers can even record any hills you encounter during your workout. If calisthenics are your choice, there are gaming systems and smartphone apps that work for specific exercises to count reps, assess your form, and challenge you to push yourself harder.

You can track more than just your exercise habits with digital assistance. Electronic devices and smart programs are available to help with many aspects of wellness, including the following:

- Dietary habits
- Calories consumed and burned
- Stress management
- Meditation and spirituality
- Heart rate and respiration
- Menstrual cycles
- Family medical history
- Journaling

And that's just to name a few. We'll introduce a variety of these digital devices and apps in later chapters, in the new "Wellness in the Digital Age" feature box like this one. You may find one or more digital apps (many of which are free) that appeal to you and can help you make progress toward your own fitness and wellness goals.

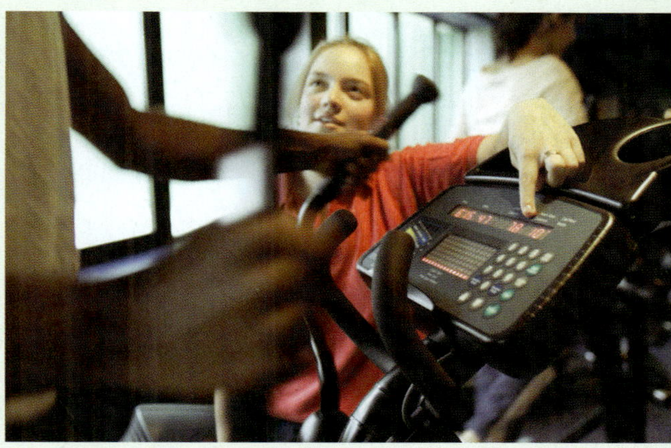

techniques discussed in Chapter 1 to keep your program on track.

Fuel Your Activity Appropriately Good nutrition, including rehydration and resynthesis of liver and muscle carbohydrate stores, is part of optimal recuperation from exercise. Consume enough calories to support your exercise program without gaining body fat. Many studies show that consuming carbohydrates and protein before or after exercise promotes restoration of stored fuels and helps heal injured tissues so that you can exercise intensely again shortly. Nutrition for exercise is discussed in greater detail in Chapters 4 and 3.

Have Fun You are more likely to stick with an exercise program if it's fun. Choose a variety of activities that you enjoy. Some people like to play competitive sports, such as tennis, golf, or volleyball. Competition can boost motivation, but remember: Sports are competitive, whereas training for fitness is not. Other people like more solitary activities, such as jogging, walking, or swimming. Still others like high-skill individual sports, such as skiing, surfing, or skateboarding. Many activities can help you get fit, so choose the ones you enjoy. You can also boost

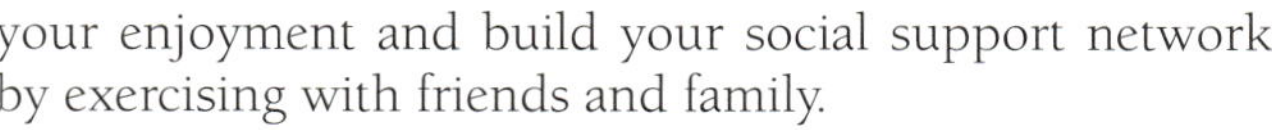

your enjoyment and build your social support network by exercising with friends and family.

Track Your Progress Monitoring the progress of your program can help keep you motivated and on track. Depending on the activities you've included in your program, you may track different measures of your program—minutes of jogging, miles of cycling, laps of swimming, number of push-ups, amount of weight lifted, and so on. If your program focuses on increasing daily physical activity, consider using an inexpensive pedometer to monitor the number of steps you take each day. (See Lab 2.3 for more information on setting goals and monitoring activity with a pedometer; see the box "Digital Workout Aids" for an introduction to products and apps that can help you track your progress.) Specific examples of program monitoring can be found in the labs for Chapters 4, 8 and 9.

Keep Your Exercise Program in Perspective As important as physical fitness is, it is only part of a well-rounded life. You need time for work and school, family and friends, relaxation and hobbies. Some people become overinvolved in exercise and neglect other parts of their lives. They think of themselves as runners, dancers,

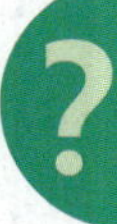

Ask yourself

QUESTIONS FOR CRITICAL THINKING AND REFLECTION

If you were to start planning a program, what would be your three most important long-term goals? What would you set as short-term goals? What rewards would be meaningful to you?

swimmers, or triathletes rather than as people who participate in those activities. Balance and moderation are the key ingredients of a fit and well life.

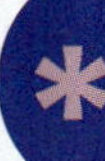

TIPS FOR TODAY AND THE FUTURE

Physical activity and exercise offer benefits in nearly every area of wellness. Even a low to moderate level of activity provides valuable health benefits. The important thing is to get moving!

RIGHT NOW YOU CAN

- Look at your calendar for the rest of the week and write in some physical activity—such as walking, running, biking, skating, swimming, hiking, or playing Frisbee—on as many days as you can. Schedule the activity for a specific time and stick to it.
- Call a friend and invite her or him to start planning a regular exercise program with you.

IN THE FUTURE YOU CAN

- Schedule a session with a qualified personal trainer who can evaluate your current fitness level and help you set personalized fitness goals.
- Create seasonal workout programs for the spring, summer, fall, and winter. Develop programs that are varied but consistent with your overall fitness goals.

SUMMARY

- Moderate daily physical activity contributes substantially to good health. Even without a formal, vigorous exercise program, you can get many of the same health benefits by becoming more physically active.
- If you are already active, you benefit even more by increasing the intensity or duration of your activities.
- The five components of physical fitness most important for health are cardiorespiratory endurance, muscular strength, muscular endurance, flexibility, and body composition.
- Physical training is the process of producing long-term improvements in the body's functioning through exercise. All training is based on the fact that the body adapts to physical stress.
- According to the principle of specificity, bodies change specifically in response to the type of training received.
- Bodies also adapt to progressive overload. When you progressively increase the frequency, intensity, and time (duration) of the right type of exercise, you become increasingly fit.
- Bodies adjust to lower levels of activity by losing fitness, a principle known as reversibility. To counter the effects of reversibility, it's important to keep training at the same intensity, even if you have to reduce the number or length of sessions.
- According to the principle of individual differences, people vary in the maximum level of fitness they can achieve and in the rate of change they can expect from an exercise program.
- When designing an exercise program, determine if medical clearance is needed, assess your current level of fitness, set realistic goals, and choose activities that develop all the components of fitness.
- Train regularly, get in shape gradually, warm up and cool down, maintain a structured but flexible program, exercise safely, consider training with a partner or personal trainer, train your mind, have fun, and keep exercise in perspective.

FOR FURTHER EXPLORATION

BOOKS

American College of Sports Medicine. 2009. *ACSM's Guidelines for Exercise Testing and Prescription,* 8th ed. Philadelphia: Lippincott Williams and Wilkins. *Includes the ACSM guidelines for safety of exercising, a basic discussion of exercise physiology, and information about fitness testing and prescription.*

Earle, R. W., and T. R. Baechle, eds. 2008. *NSCA's Essentials of Personal Training,* 3rd ed. Champaign, Ill.: Human Kinetics. *Comprehensive discussions of fitness testing, exercise and disease, nutrition and physical performance, and exercise prescription.*

Marcus, B. H., and L. A. Forsyth. 2009. *Motivating People to Be Physically Active,* 2nd ed. Champaign, Ill.: Human Kinetics. *Describes methods for helping people increase physical activity levels.*

Page, P. 2011. *Pilates Illustrated.* Champaign, Ill.: Human Kinetics. *A guide to improving muscle fitness, while improving posture, flexibility, and balance.*

JOURNALS

ACSM Health and Fitness Journal (401 West Michigan Street, Indianapolis, In. 46202; http://journals.lww.com/acsm-healthfitness/pages/default.aspx)

Physician and Sportsmedicine (1235 Westlakes Drive, Suite 220, Berwyn, Pa. 19312; https://physsportsmed.com)

COMMON QUESTIONS ANSWERED

Q I have asthma. Is it OK for me to start an exercise program?

A Probably, but you should see your doctor before you start exercising, especially if you have been sedentary up to this point. Your personal physician can advise you on the type of exercise program that is best for you, given the severity of your condition, and how to avoid suffering exercise-related asthma attacks.

Q What should my fitness goals be?

A Begin by thinking about your general overall goals—the benefits you want to obtain by increasing your activity level and/or beginning a formal exercise program. Examples of long-term goals include reducing your risk of chronic diseases, increasing your energy level, and maintaining a healthy body weight.

To help shape your fitness program, you need to set specific, short-term goals based on measurable factors. These specific goals should be an extension of your overall goals—the specific changes to your current activity and exercise habits needed to achieve your general goals. In setting short-term goals, be sure to use the SMART criteria described in Chapter 1. As noted there, your goals should be **S**pecific, **M**easurable, **A**ttainable, **R**ealistic, and **T**ime frame–specific (SMART).

You need information about your current levels of physical activity and physical fitness in order to set appropriate goals. The labs in this chapter will help you determine your physical activity level—for example, how many minutes per day you engage in moderate or vigorous activity or how many daily steps you take. Using this information, you can set goals for lifestyle physical activity to help you meet your overall goals. For example, if your general long-term goals are to reduce the risk of chronic disease and prevent weight gain, the Dietary Guidelines recommend 60 minutes of moderate physical activity daily. If you currently engage in 30 minutes of moderate activity daily, then your behavior change goal would be to add 30 minutes of daily physical activity (or an equivalent number of additional daily steps—about 3500–4000); your time frame for the change might be 8–12 weeks.

Labs in Chapters 4, 6, 8 and 9 provide opportunities to assess your fitness status for all the health-related components of fitness. The results of these assessments can guide you in setting specific fitness goals. For instance, if the labs in Chapter 8 indicate that you have good muscular strength and endurance in your lower body but poor strength and endurance in your upper body, then setting a specific goal for improving upper-body muscle fitness would be an appropriate goal—increasing the number of push-ups you can do from 22 to 30, for example. Chapters 4, 6, 8 and 9 include additional advice for setting appropriate goals.

Once you start your behavior change program, you may discover that your goals aren't quite appropriate; perhaps you were overly optimistic, or maybe you set the bar too low. There are limits to the amount of fitness you can achieve, but within the limits of your genes, health status, and motivation, you can make significant improvements in fitness. Adjust your goals as needed.

Q How can I fit a workout into my day?

A Good time management is an important skill in creating and maintaining an exercise program. Choose a regular time to exercise, preferably the same time every day. Don't tell yourself you'll exercise "sometime during the day when you have free time." That free time may never come. Schedule your workout, and make it a priority. Include alternative plans in your program to account for circumstances like bad weather or vacations.

Q Where can I get help and advice about exercise?

A One of the best places to get help is an exercise class. If you join a health club or fitness center, follow the guidelines in the box "Choosing a Fitness Center." There, expert instructors can help you learn the basics of training and answer your questions. Make sure the instructor is certified by a recognized professional organization and/or has formal training in exercise physiology. Read articles by credible experts in fitness magazines (such as *Fitness Rx for Women* and *Fitness Rx for Men*). Many of these magazines include articles by leading experts in exercise science written at a layperson's level.

A qualified personal trainer can also help you get started in an exercise program or a new form of training. Make sure this person has proper qualifications, such as certification by the ACSM, National Strength and Conditioning Association (NSCA), or International Sports Sciences Association (ISSA). Don't seek out a person for advice simply because he or she looks fit. UCLA researchers found that 60% of the personal trainers in their study couldn't pass a basic exam on training methods, exercise physiology, or biomechanics. Trainers who performed best had college degrees in exercise physiology, physical education, or physical therapy. So choose your trainer carefully and don't get caught up with fads or appearances.

Q Should I follow my exercise program if I'm sick?

A If you have a mild head cold or feel one coming on, it is probably OK to exercise moderately. Just begin slowly and see how you feel. However, if you have symptoms of a more serious illness—fever, swollen glands, nausea, extreme tiredness, muscle aches—wait until you have recovered fully before resuming your exercise program. Continuing to exercise while suffering from an illness more serious than a cold can compromise your recovery and may even be dangerous.

For more Common Questions Answered about fitness, visit the Online Learning Center at www.mhhe.com/fahey.

CRITICAL CONSUMER

Choosing a Fitness Center

Fitness centers can provide you with many benefits—motivation and companionship are among the most important. A fitness center may also offer expert instruction and supervision as well as access to better equipment than you could afford on your own. All fitness centers, however, are not of the same overall quality, and every fitness center is not for every person. If you're thinking of joining a fitness center, here are some guidelines to help you choose a club that's right for you.

Convenience

- Look for an established facility that's within 10–15 minutes of your home or work. If it's farther away, your chances of sticking to an exercise regimen start to diminish.
- Visit the facility at the time you would normally exercise. Is there adequate parking? Will you have easy access to equipment and classes at that time?
- What child care services are available, and how are they supervised?

Atmosphere

- Look around to see if there are other members who are your age and at about your fitness level. Some clubs cater to a certain age group or lifestyle, such as hard-core bodybuilders.
- Observe how the members dress. Will you fit in, or will you be uncomfortable?
- Observe the staff. Are they easy to identify? Are they friendly, professional, and helpful?
- Check to see that the facility is clean, including showers and lockers. Make sure the facility is climate controlled, well ventilated, and well lit.

Safety

- Find out if the facility offers some type of preactivity screening as well as basic fitness testing that includes cardiovascular screening.
- Determine if personnel are trained in CPR and if there is emergency equipment such as automated external defibrillators (AEDs) on the premises. An AED can help someone who has a cardiac arrest.
- Ask if at least one staff member on each shift is trained in first aid.

Trained Personnel

- Determine if the personal trainers and fitness instructors are certified by a recognized professional association such as the American College of Sports Medicine (ACSM), Aerobics and Fitness Association of America (AFAA), National Strength and Conditioning Association (NSCA), or International Sports Sciences Association (ISSA). All personal trainers are not equal; more than 100 organizations certify trainers, and few of these require much formal training.
- Find out if the club has a trained exercise physiologist on staff, such as someone with a degree in exercise physiology, kinesiology, or exercise science. If the facility offers nutritional counseling, it should employ someone who is a registered dietitian (RD) or has similar formal training.
- Ask how much experience the instructors have. Ideally, trainers should have both academic preparation and practical experience.

Cost

- Buy only what you need and can afford. If you want to use only workout equipment, you may not need a club that has racquetball courts and saunas.
- Check the contract. Choose the one that covers the shortest period of time possible, especially if it's your first fitness club experience. Don't feel pressured to sign a long-term contract.
- Make sure the contract permits you to extend your membership if you have a prolonged illness or go on vacation. Some clubs have exchange agreements that allow you to train in other cities while on vacation or business.
- Try out the club. Ask for a free trial workout, or a 1-day pass, or an inexpensive 1- or 2-week trial membership.
- Find out whether there is an extra charge for the particular services you want. Get any special offers in writing.

Effectiveness

- Tour the facility. Does it offer what the brochure says it does? Does it offer the activities and equipment you want?
- Check the equipment. A good club will have treadmills, bikes, stair-climbers, resistance machines, and weights. Make sure these machines are up to date and well maintained.
- Find out if new members get a formal orientation and instruction on how to safely use the equipment. Will a staff member help you develop a program that is appropriate for your current fitness level and goals?
- Make sure the facility is certified. Look for the displayed names American College of Sports Medicine (ACSM), American Council on Exercise (ACE), Aerobics and Fitness Association of America (AFAA), or International Health, Racquet, and Sports club Association (IHRSA).

ORGANIZATIONS, HOTLINES, AND WEB SITES

American Alliance for Health, Physical Education, Recreation, and Dance (AAHPERD). A professional organization dedicated to promoting quality health and physical education programs.

http://www.aahperd.org

American College of Sports Medicine (ACSM). The principal professional organization for sports medicine and exercise science. Provides brochures, publications, and audio- and videotapes.

http://www.acsm.org

American Council on Exercise (ACE). Promotes exercise and fitness; the Web site features fact sheets on many consumer topics, including choosing shoes, cross-training, and steroids.

http://www.acefitness.org

American Heart Association: Start! Walking for a Healthier Lifestyle. Provides practical advice for people of all fitness levels plus an online fitness diary.

http://startwalkingnow.org

CDC Physical Activity Information. Provides information on the benefits of physical activity and suggestions for incorporating moderate physical activity into daily life.

http://www.cdc.gov/physicalactivity

Disabled Sports USA. Provides sports and recreation services to people with physical or mobility disorders.

http://www.dsusa.org

International Health, Racquet, and Sportsclub Association (IHRSA): Health Clubs. Provides guidelines for choosing a health or fitness facility and links to clubs that belong to IHRSA.

http://www.healthclubs.com

International Sports Sciences Association (ISSA). Trains and certifies personal trainers.

http://www.issaonline.com

MedlinePlus: Exercise and Physical Fitness. Provides links to news and reliable information about fitness and exercise from government agencies and professional associations.

http://www.nlm.nih.gov/medlineplus/exerciseandphysicalfitness.html

President's Council on Fitness, Sports and Nutrition. Provides information on programs and publications, including fitness guides and fact sheets.

http://www.fitness.gov

http://www.presidentschallenge.org

Shape Up America! A nonprofit organization that provides information and resources on exercise, nutrition, and weight loss.

http://www.shapeup.org

SmallStep.Gov. Provides resources for increasing activity and improving diet through small changes in daily habits.

http://www.smallstep.gov

SELECTED BIBLIOGRAPHY

Alzheimer's Association. 2011. *Generation Alzheimer's: The Defining Disease of the Baby Boomers.* Chicago: Alzheimer's Association.

American College of Sports Medicine. 1998. The recommended quantity and quality of exercise for developing and maintaining cardiorespiratory and muscular fitness, and flexibility in healthy adults. ACSM position paper. *Medicine and Science in Sports and Exercise* 30(6): 975–991.

American College of Sports Medicine. 2007. *ACSM's Health/Fitness Facility Standards and Guidelines,* 3rd ed. Champaign, Ill.: Human Kinetics.

American College of Sports Medicine. 2009. *ACSM's Guidelines for Exercise Testing and Prescription,* 8th ed. Philadelphia: Lippincott Williams and Wilkins.

American College of Sports Medicine. 2009. *ACSM's Resource Manual for Guidelines for Exercise Testing and Prescription,* 6th ed. Philadelphia: Lippincott Williams and Wilkins.

American Heart Association. 2007. Resistance exercise in individuals with and without cardiovascular disease, 2007 update: A scientific statement from the American Heart Association Council on Clinical Cardiology and Council on Nutrition, Physical Activity, and Metabolism. *Circulation* 116(5): 572–584.

Ascensao, A., et al. 2011. Mitochondria as a target for exercise-induced cardioprotection. *Current Drug Targets* 12(6): 860–871.

Bouchard, C., et al. 2007. *Physical Activity and Health.* Champaign, Ill.: Human Kinetics.

Centers for Disease Control and Prevention. 2008. Prevalence of self-reported physically active adults—United States, 2007. *Morbidity and Mortality Weekly Report* 57(48): 1297–1300.

Dietary Guidelines Advisory Committee. 2011. *Report of the Dietary Guidelines Advisory Committee on the Dietary Guidelines for Americans, 2010, to the Secretary of Agriculture and the Secretary of Health and Human Services.* Washington, D.C.: U.S. Department of Agriculture, Agricultural Research Service.

Cooper, K. H. 2010. The benefits of exercise in promoting long and healthy lives—my observations. *Methodist DeBakey Cardiovascular Journal* 6(4): 10–12.

Courneya, K. S., and C. M. Friedenreich. 2011. Physical activity and cancer: an introduction. *Recent Results Cancer Research* 186: 1–10.

Donnelly, J. E., et al. 2009. Appropriate physical activity intervention strategies for weight loss and prevention of weight regain for adults (ACSM position stand). *Medicine and Science in Sports and Exercise.* 41(2): 459–471.

Duke University Medical Health News. 2010. Exercise! The anti-aging weapon. 4 new studies affirm the multiple benefits of exercise—at any age, even starting in midlife. *Duke Medical Health News* 16(5): 5–6.

Garber, C. E., et al. 2011. Quantity and quality of exercise for developing and maintaining cardiorespiratory, musculoskeletal, and neuromotor fitness in apparently healthy adults: Guidance for prescribing exercise. *Medicine and Science in Sports and Exercise* 43(7): 1334–1359.

Haskell, W. L., et al. 2007. Physical activity and public health: Updated recommendation for adults from the American College of Sports Medicine and the American Heart Association. *Medicine and Science in Sports and Exercise* 39(8): 1423–1434.

Hobson, K. 2010. How exercise can boost longevity. *US News World Report* 147(2): 30.

Hughes, E., et al. 2010. Surveillance for Certain Health Behaviors Among States and Selected Local Areas — United States, 2008. *Morbidity and Mortality Weekly Report* 597(ss1044): 1203–1205.

Keller, P., et al. 2011. A transcriptional map of the impact of endurance exercise training on skeletal muscle phenotype. *Journal of Applied Physiology* 110(1): 46–59.

Kushi, L. H., et al. 2006. American Cancer Society guidelines on nutrition and physical activity for cancer prevention: Reducing the risk of cancer with healthy food choices and physical activity. *Cancer Journal for Clinicians* 56(5): 254–281.

Lanza, I. R., and K. S. Nair. 2010. Mitochondrial function as a determinant of life span. *Pflugers Archives* 459(2): 277–289.

Masley, S., et al. 2009. Aerobic exercise enhances cognitive flexibility. *Journal Clinical Psychology in Medical Settings* 16(2): 186–193.

Muscari, A., et al. 2010. Chronic endurance exercise training prevents aging-related cognitive decline in healthy older adults: a randomized controlled trial. *International Journal of Geriatric Psychiatry* 25(10): 1055–1064.

National Center for Health Statistics. 2010. *Summary Health Statistics for U.S. Adults: National Health Interview Survey, 2009.* Series 10 (249). Hyattsville, Md.: National Center for Health Statistics.

Nelson, M. E., et al. 2007. Physical activity and public health in older adults: Recommendation from the American College of Sports Medicine and the American Heart Association. *Medicine and Science in Sports and Exercise* 39(8): 1435–1445.

Physical Activity Guidelines Advisory Committee. 2008. *Physical Activity Guidelines Advisory Committee Report, 2008.* Washington, D.C.: U.S. Department of Health and Human Services.

Rhyu, I. J., et al. 2010. Effects of aerobic exercise training on cognitive function and cortical vascularity in monkeys. *Neuroscience* 167(4): 1239–1248.

Richardson, C. R., et al. 2008. A meta-analysis of pedometer-based walking interventions and weight loss. *Annals of Family Medicine* 6(1): 69–77.

Sailors, M. H., et al. 2010. Exposing college students to exercise: the Training Interventions and Genetics of Exercise Response (TIGER) study. *Journal American College of Health* 59(1): 13–20.

Smith, J. K. 2010. Exercise and cardiovascular disease. *Cardiovascular Hematologic Disorders Drug Targets* 10(4): 269–272.

Stranahan, A. M., and M. P. Mattson. 2011. Bidirectional metabolic regulation of neurocognitive function. *Neurobiology Learning Memory*. Published online January 11, 2011.

Tarnopolsky, M. A. 2009. Mitochondrial DNA shifting in older adults following resistance exercise training. *Applied Physiology, Nutrition, and Metabolism* 34(3): 348–354.

Teixeira-Lemos, E., et al. 2011. Regular physical exercise training assists in preventing type 2 diabetes development: focus on its antioxidant and anti-inflammatory properties. *Cardiovascular Diabetology* 10(1): 12.

U.S. Department of Health and Human Services. 1996. *Physical Activity and Health: A Report of the Surgeon General*. Atlanta: U.S. Department of Health and Human Services.

U.S. Department of Health and Human Services. 2008. *Physical Activity Guidelines for Americans.* Washington, D.C.: U.S. Department of Health and Human Services.

U.S. Department of Health and Human Services. 2010. *The Surgeon General's Vision for a Healthy and Fit Nation*. Rockville, Md.: U.S. Department of Health and Human Services, Office of the Surgeon General.

World Health Organization. 2010. *World Health Statistics 2010*. Geneva: World Health Organization.

Name ______________________ Section ______________ Date ____________

Physical Activity Readiness Questionnaire - PAR-Q (revised 2002)

LAB 2.1 Safety of Exercise Participation

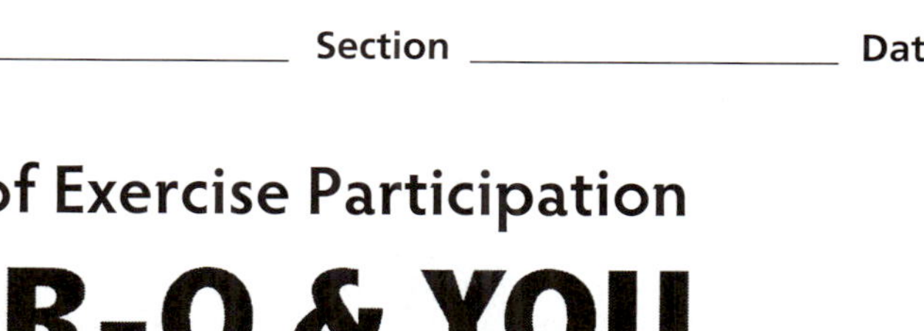

(A Questionnaire for People Aged 15 to 69)

Regular physical activity is fun and healthy, and increasingly more people are starting to become more active every day. Being more active is very safe for most people. However, some people should check with their doctor before they start becoming much more physically active.

If you are planning to become much more physically active than you are now, start by answering the seven questions in the box below. If you are between the ages of 15 and 69, the PAR-Q will tell you if you should check with your doctor before you start. If you are over 69 years of age, and you are not used to being very active, check with your doctor.

Common sense is your best guide when you answer these questions. Please read the questions carefully and answer each one honestly: check YES or NO.

YES	NO		
☐	☐	1.	**Has your doctor ever said that you have a heart condition and that you should only do physical activity recommended by a doctor?**
☐	☐	2.	**Do you feel pain in your chest when you do physical activity?**
☐	☐	3.	**In the past month, have you had chest pain when you were not doing physical activity?**
☐	☐	4.	**Do you lose your balance because of dizziness or do you ever lose consciousness?**
☐	☐	5.	**Do you have a bone or joint problem (for example, back, knee or hip) that could be made worse by a change in your physical activity?**
☐	☐	6.	**Is your doctor currently prescribing drugs (for example, water pills) for your blood pressure or heart condition?**
☐	☐	7.	**Do you know of any other reason why you should not do physical activity?**

If you answered

YES to one or more questions

Talk with your doctor by phone or in person BEFORE you start becoming much more physically active or BEFORE you have a fitness appraisal. Tell your doctor about the PAR-Q and which questions you answered YES.

- You may be able to do any activity you want — as long as you start slowly and build up gradually. Or, you may need to restrict your activities to those which are safe for you. Talk with your doctor about the kinds of activities you wish to participate in and follow his/her advice.
- Find out which community programs are safe and helpful for you.

NO to all questions

If you answered NO honestly to all PAR-Q questions, you can be reasonably sure that you can:

- start becoming much more physically active – begin slowly and build up gradually. This is the safest and easiest way to go.
- take part in a fitness appraisal – this is an excellent way to determine your basic fitness so that you can plan the best way for you to live actively. It is also highly recommended that you have your blood pressure evaluated. If your reading is over 144/94, talk with your doctor before you start becoming much more physically active.

DELAY BECOMING MUCH MORE ACTIVE:

- if you are not feeling well because of a temporary illness such as a cold or a fever – wait until you feel better; or
- if you are or may be pregnant – talk to your doctor before you start becoming more active.

PLEASE NOTE: If your health changes so that you then answer YES to any of the above questions, tell your fitness or health professional. Ask whether you should change your physical activity plan.

Informed Use of the PAR-Q: The Canadian Society for Exercise Physiology, Health Canada, and their agents assume no liability for persons who undertake physical activity, and if in doubt after completing this questionnaire, consult your doctor prior to physical activity.

No changes permitted. You are encouraged to photocopy the PAR-Q but only if you use the entire form.

NOTE: If the PAR-Q is being given to a person before he or she participates in a physical activity program or a fitness appraisal, this section may be used for legal or administrative purposes.

"I have read, understood and completed this questionnaire. Any questions I had were answered to my full satisfaction."

NAME ______________________

SIGNATURE ______________________ DATE ______________________

SIGNATURE OF PARENT ______________________ WITNESS ______________________
or GUARDIAN (for participants under the age of majority)

Note: This physical activity clearance is valid for a maximum of 12 months from the date it is completed and becomes invalid if your condition changes so that you would answer YES to any of the seven questions.

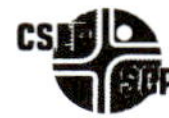

Supported by: 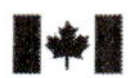 Health Canada Santé Canada

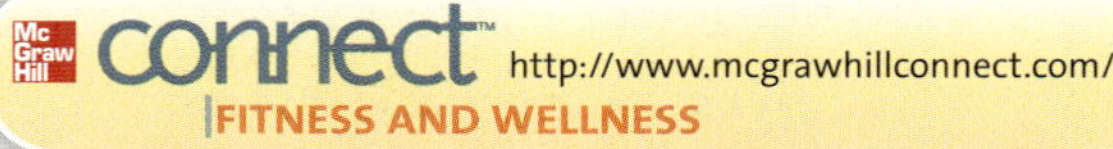

General Health Profile

To help further assess the safety of exercise for you, complete as much of this health profile as possible.

General Information

Age: _________ Total cholesterol: _________ Blood pressure: _________ / _________

Height: _________ HDL: _________ Triglycerides: _________

Weight: _________ LDL: _________ Blood glucose: _________

Are you currently trying to _________ gain or _________ lose weight? (check one if appropriate)

Medical Conditions/Treatments

Check any of the following that apply to you, and add any other conditions that might affect your ability to exercise safely.

_________ heart disease
_________ lung disease
_________ diabetes
_________ allegies
_________ asthma
_________ depression, anxiety, or other psychological disorder
_________ eating disorder
_________ back pain
_________ arthritis
_________ other injury to joint problem: ___________
_________ substance abuse problem
_________ other: ___________________________
_________ other: ___________________________
_________ other: ___________________________

_________ Do you have a family history of cardiovascular disease (CVD) (a parent, sibling, or child who had a heart attack or stroke before age 55 for men or 65 for women)?

List any medications or supplements you are taking or any medical treatments you are undergoing. Include the name of the substance or treatment and its purpose. Include both prescription and over-the-counter drugs and supplements.

____ ____

____ ____

Lifestyle Information

Check any of the following that is true for you, and fill in the requested information.

_________ I usually eat high-fat foods (fatty meats, cheese, fried foods, butter, full-fat dairy products) every day.
_________ I consume fewer than 5 servings of fruits and vegetables on most days.
_________ I smoke cigarettes or use other tobacco products. If true, describe your use of tobacco (type and frequency): ____
_________ I regularly drink alcohol. If true, describe your typical weekly consumption pattern: ___________________________
_________ I often feel as if I need more sleep. (I need about ____ hours per day; I get about ____ hours per day.)
_________ I feel as though stress has adversely affected my level of wellness during the past year.

Describe your current activity pattern. What types of moderate physical activity do you engage in on a daily basis? Are you involved in a formal exercise program, or do you regularly participate in sports or recreational activities?

____

____

Using Your Results

How did you score? Did the PAR-Q indicate that exercise is likely to be safe for you? Is there anything in your health profile that you think may affect your ability to exercise safely? Have you had any problems with exercise in the past?

What should you do next? If the assessments in this lab indicate that you should see your physician before beginning an exercise program, or if you have any questions about the safety of exercise for you, make an appointment to talk with your health care provider to address your concerns.

Name ______________________ Section ____________ Date ____________

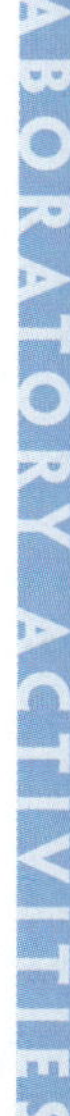

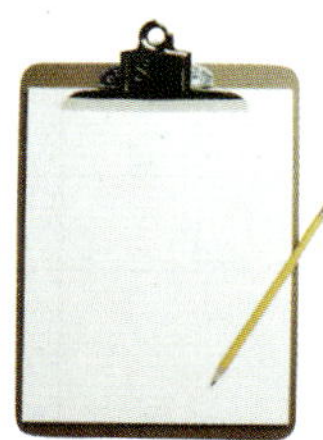

LAB 2.2 Overcoming Barriers to Being Active

Barriers to Being Active Quiz

Directions: Listed below are reasons that people give to describe why they do not get as much physical activity as they think they should. Please read each statement and indicate how likely you are to say each of the following statements.

How likely are you to say this?	Very likely	Somewhat likely	Somewhat unlikely	Very unlikely
1. My day is so busy now, I just don't think I can make the time to include physical activity in my regular schedule.	3	2	1	0
2. None of my family members or friends like to do anything active, so I don't have a chance to exercise.	3	2	1	0
3. I'm just too tired after work to get any exercise.	3	2	1	0
4. I've been thinking about getting more exercise, but I just can't seem to get started.	3	2	1	0
5. I'm getting older so exercise can be risky.	3	2	1	0
6. I don't get enough exercise because I have never learned the skills for any sport.	3	2	1	0
7. I don't have access to jogging trails, swimming pools, bike paths, etc.	3	2	1	0
8. Physical activity takes too much time away from other commitments—like work, family, etc.	3	2	1	0
9. I'm embarrassed about how I will look when I exercise with others.	3	2	1	0
10. I don't get enough sleep as it is. I just couldn't get up early or stay up late to get some exercise.	3	2	1	0
11. It's easier for me to find excuses not to exercise than to go out and do something.	3	2	1	0
12. I know of too many people who have hurt themselves by overdoing it with exercise.	3	2	1	0
13. I really can't see learning a new sport at my age.	3	2	1	0
14. It's just too expensive. You have to take a class or join a club or buy the right equipment.	3	2	1	0
15. My free times during the day are too short to include exercise.	3	2	1	0
16. My usual social activities with family or friends do not include physical activity.	3	2	1	0
17. I'm too tired during the week and I need the weekend to catch up on my rest.	3	2	1	0

How likely are you to say this?	Very likely	Somewhat likely	Somewhat unlikely	Very unlikely
18. I want to get more exercise, but I just can't seem to make myself stick to anything.	3	2	1	0
19. I'm afraid I might injure myself or have a heart attack.	3	2	1	0
20. I'm not good enough at any physical activity to make it fun.	3	2	1	0
21. If we had exercise facilities and showers at work, then I would be more likely to exercise.	3	2	1	0

Scoring

- Enter the circled numbers in the spaces provided, putting the number for statement 1 on line 1, statement 2 on line 2, and so on.
- Add the three scores on each line. Your barriers to physical activity fall into one or more of seven categories: lack of time, social influences, lack of energy, lack of willpower, fear of injury, lack of skill, and lack of resources. A score of 5 or above in any category shows that this is an important barrier for you to overcome.

____ 1	+	____ 8	+	____ 15	=	________ Lack of time
____ 2	+	____ 9	+	____ 16	=	________ Social influences
____ 3	+	____ 10	+	____ 17	=	________ Lack of energy
____ 4	+	____ 11	+	____ 18	=	________ Lack of willpower
____ 5	+	____ 12	+	____ 19	=	________ Fear of injury
____ 6	+	____ 13	+	____ 20	=	________ Lack of skill
____ 7	+	____ 14	+	____ 21	=	________ Lack of resources

Using Your Results

How did you score? How many key barriers did you identify? Are they what you expected?

What should you do next? For your key barriers, try the strategies listed on the following pages and/or develop additional strategies that work for you. Check off any strategy that you try.

Suggestions for Overcoming Physical Activity Barriers

Lack of Time

_______ Identify available time slots. Monitor your daily activities for 1 week. Identify at least three 30-minute time slots you could use for physical activity.

_______ Add physical activity to your daily routine. For example, walk or ride your bike to work or shopping, organize social activities around physical activity, walk the dog, exercise while you watch TV, park farther from your destination, etc.

_______ Make time for physical activity. For example, walk, jog, or swim during your lunch hour, or take fitness breaks instead of coffee breaks.

_______ Select activities requiring minimal time, such as walking, jogging, or stair climbing.

_______ Other: ____________________

Social Influences

_______ Explain your interest in physical activity to friends and family. Ask them to support your efforts.

_______ Invite friends and family members to exercise with you. Plan social activities involving exercise.

_______ Develop new friendships with physically active people. Join a group, such as the YMCA or a hiking club.

_______ Other: ____________________

Lack of Energy

_______ Schedule physical activity for times in the day or week when you feel energetic.

_______ Convince yourself that if you give it a chance, exercise will increase your energy level. Then try it.

_______ Other: ____________________

Lack of Willpower

_______ Plan ahead. Make physical activity a regular part of your daily or weekly schedule and write it on your calendar.

_______ Invite a friend to exercise with you on a regular basis and write it on *both* your calendars.

_______ Join an exercise group or class.

_______ Other: ____________________

Fear of Injury

_______ Learn how to warm up and cool down to prevent injury.

_______ Learn how to exercise appropriately considering your age, fitness level, skill level, and health status.

_______ Choose activities involving minimal risk.

_______ Other: ____________________

Lack of Skill

_______ Select activities requiring no new skills, such as walking, jogging, or stair climbing.

_______ Exercise with friends who are at the same skill level as you are.

_______ Find a friend who is willing to teach you some new skills.

_______ Take a class to develop new skills.

_______ Other: ____________________

Lack of Resources

_______ Select activities that require minimal facilities or equipment, such as walking, jogging, jumping rope, or calisthenics.

_______ Identify inexpensive, convenient resources available in your community (community education programs, park and recreation programs, worksite programs, etc.).

_______ Other: ____________________

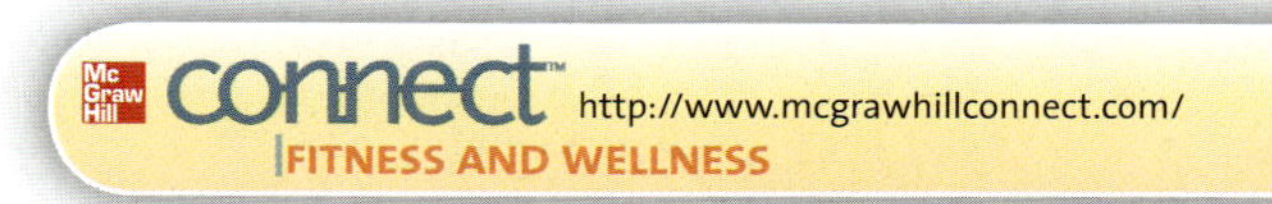

Are any of the following additional barriers important for you? If so, try some of the strategies listed here or invent your own.

Weather Conditions

_______ Develop a set of regular activities that are always available regardless of weather (indoor cycling, aerobic dance, indoor swimming, calisthenics, stair climbing, rope skipping, mall walking, dancing, gymnasium games, etc.).

_______ Look on outdoor activities that depend on weather conditions (cross-country skiing, outdoor swimming, outdoor tennis, etc.) as "bonuses"—extra activities possible when weather and circumstances permit.

_______ Other: ____

Travel

_______ Put a jump rope in your suitcase and jump rope.

_______ Walk the halls and climb the stairs in hotels.

_______ Stay in places with swimming pools or exercise facilities.

_______ Join the YMCA or YWCA (ask about reciprocal membership agreements).

_______ Visit the local shopping mall and walk for half an hour or more.

_______ Bring a personal music player loaded with your favorite workout music.

_______ Other: ____

Family Obligations

_______ Trade babysitting time with a friend, neighbor, or family member who also has small children.

_______ Exercise *with* the kids—go for a walk together, play tag or other running games, or get an aerobic dance or exercise DVD for kids (there are several on the market) and exercise together. You can spend time together and still get your exercise.

_______ Hire a babysitter and look at the cost as a worthwhile investment in your physical and mental health.

_______ Jump rope, do calisthenics, ride a stationary bicycle, or use other home gymnasium equipment while the kids watch TV or when they are sleeping.

_______ Try to exercise when the kids are not around (e.g., during school hours or their nap time).

_______ Other: ____

Retirement Years

_______ Look on your retirement as an opportunity to become more active instead of less. Spend more time gardening, walking the dog, and playing with your grandchildren. Children with short legs and grandparents with slower gaits are often great walking partners.

_______ Learn a new skill you've always been interested in, such as ballroom dancing, square dancing, or swimming.

_______ Now that you have the time, make regular physical activity a part of every day. Go for a walk every morning or every evening before dinner. Treat yourself to an exercycle and ride every day during a favorite TV show.

_______ Other: ____

SOURCE: Adapted from CDC Division of Nutrition and Physical Activity. 1999. *Promoting Physical Activity: A Guide for Community Action*. Champaign, Ill.: Human Kinetics.

Name ______________________ Section ____________ Date ____________

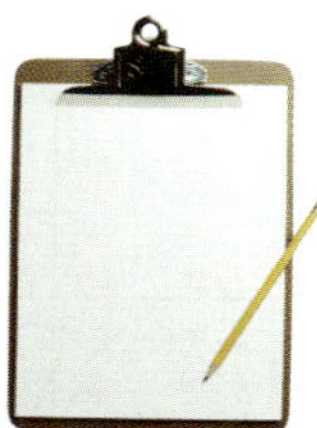

LAB 2.3 Using a Pedometer to Track Physical Activity

How physically active are you? Would you be more motivated to increase daily physical activity if you had an easy way to monitor your level of activity? If so, consider wearing a pedometer to track the number of steps you take each day—a rough but easily obtainable reflection of daily physical activity.

Determine Your Baseline

Wear the pedometer for a week to obtain a baseline average daily number of steps.

	M	T	W	Th	F	Sa	Su	Average
Steps								

Set Goals

Set an appropriate goal for increasing steps. The goal of 10,000 steps per day is widely recommended, but your personal goal should reflect your baseline level of steps. For example, if your current daily steps are far below 10,000, a goal of walking 2000 additional steps each day might be appropriate. If you are already close to 10,000 steps per day, choose a higher goal. Also consider the following guidelines from health experts:

- To reduce the risk of chronic disease, aim to accumulate at least 150 minutes of moderate physical activity per week.
- To help manage body weight and prevent gradual, unhealthy weight gain, engage in 60 minutes of moderate to vigorous-intensity activity on most days of the week.
- To sustain weight loss, engage daily in at least 60–90 minutes of moderate-intensity physical activity.

To help gauge how close you are to meeting these time-based physical activity goals, you might walk for 10–15 minutes while wearing your pedometer to determine how many steps correspond with the time-based goals.

Once you have set your overall goal, break it down into several steps. For example, if your goal is to increase daily steps by 2000, set mini-goals of increasing daily steps by 500, allowing 2 weeks to reach each mini-goal. Smaller goals are easier to achieve and can help keep you motivated and on track. Having several interim goals also gives you the opportunity to reward yourself more frequently. Note your goals below:

Mini-goal 1: ______________ Target date: ______________ Reward: ______________
Mini-goal 2: ______________ Target date: ______________ Reward: ______________
Mini-goal 3: ______________ Target date: ______________ Reward: ______________
Overall goal: ______________ Target date: ______________ Reward: ______________

Develop Strategies for Increasing Steps

What can you do to become more active? The possibilities include walking when you do errands, getting off one stop from your destination on public transportation, parking an extra block or two away from your destination, and doing at least one chore every day that requires physical activity. If weather or neighborhood safety is an issue, look for alternative locations to walk. For example, find an indoor gym or shopping mall or even a long hallway. Check out locations that are near or on the way to your campus, workplace, or residence. If you think walking indoors will be dull, walk with friends or family members or wear headphones (if safe) and listen to music or audiobooks.

Are there any days of the week for which your baseline steps are particularly low and/or it will be especially difficult because of your schedule to increase your number of steps? Be sure to develop specific strategies for difficult situations.

Below, list at least five strategies for increasing daily steps:

______________________ ______________________

______________________ ______________________

______________________ ______________________

Track Your Progress

Based on the goals you set, fill in your goal portion of the progress chart with your target average daily steps for each week. Then wear your pedometer every day and note your total daily steps. Track your progress toward each mini-goal and your final goal. Every few weeks, stop and evaluate your progress. If needed, adjust your plan and develop additional strategies for increasing steps. In addition to the chart in this worksheet, you might also want to graph your daily steps to provide a visual reminder of how you are progressing toward your goals. Make as many copies of this chart as you need.

Week	Goal	M	Tu	W	Th	F	Sa	Su	Average
1									
2									
3									
4									

Progress Checkup

How close are you to meeting your goal? How do you feel about your program and your progress?

If needed, describe changes to your plan and additional strategies for increasing steps:

Week	Goal	M	Tu	W	Th	F	Sa	Su	Average
5									
6									
7									
8									

Progress Checkup

How close are you to meeting your goal? How do you feel about your program and your progress?

If needed, describe changes to your plan and additional strategies for increasing steps:

Week	Goal	M	Tu	W	Th	F	Sa	Su	Average
9									
10									
11									
12									

Progress Checkup

How close are you to meeting your goal? How do you feel about your program and your progress?

If needed, describe changes to your plan and additional strategies for increasing steps in the space below.

CHAPTER 3

Nutrition

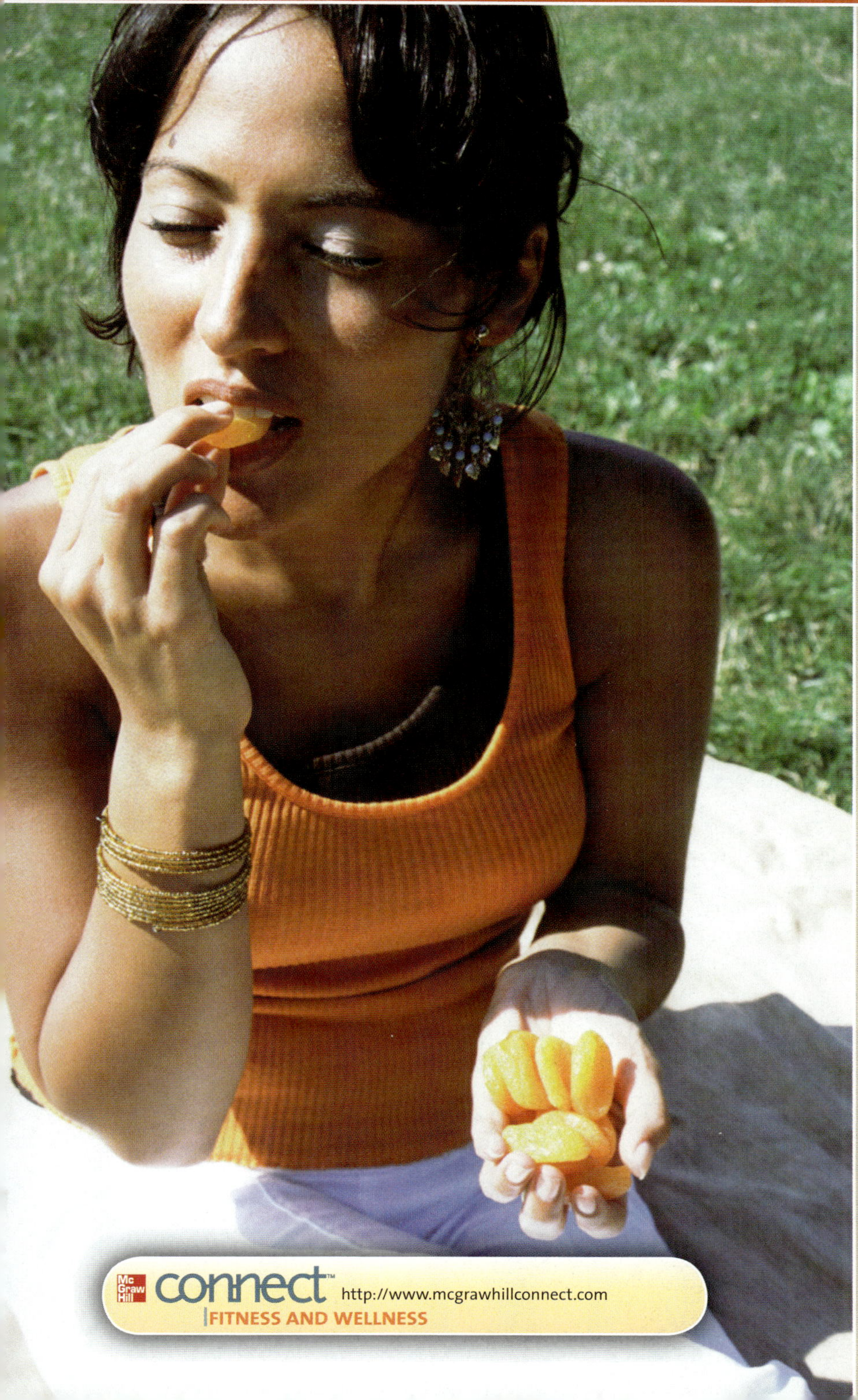

LOOKING AHEAD...

After reading this chapter, you should be able to:

- List the essential nutrients and describe the functions they perform in the body
- Describe the guidelines that have been developed to help people choose a healthy diet, avoid nutritional deficiencies, and reduce their risk of diet-related chronic diseases
- Describe nutritional guidelines for vegetarians and for special population groups
- Explain how to use food labels and other consumer tools to make informed choices about foods
- Put together a personal nutrition plan based on affordable foods that you enjoy and that will promote wellness, today and in the future

TEST YOUR KNOWLEDGE

1. It is recommended that all adults consume 1–2 servings each of fruits and vegetables every day. True or false?
2. Candy is the leading source of added sugars in the American diet. True or false?
3. Which of the following is not a whole grain?
   a. brown rice
   b. wheat flour
   c. popcorn

Answers

1. **False.** For someone consuming 2000 calories per day, a minimum of 9 servings per day—4 of fruits and 5 of vegetables—is recommended. This is the equivalent of 4 1/2 cups per day.
2. **False.** Regular (nondiet) sodas are the leading source of added sugars. Together with energy drinks and sports drinks, they account for 36% of the added sugars in the American diet, and added sugars contribute an average of 16% of the total calories in American diets. Each 12-ounce soda supplies about 10 teaspoons of sugar, or nearly 10% of the calories in a 2000-calorie diet.
3. **b.** Unless labeled "whole wheat," wheat flour is processed to remove the bran and germ and is not a whole grain.

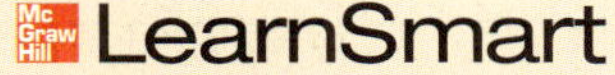

In your lifetime, you will spend about 6 years eating—about 70,000 meals and 60 tons of food. What you eat affects your energy level, well-being, and overall health. Your nutritional habits help determine your risk of major chronic diseases, including heart disease, cancer, stroke, and diabetes. Choosing foods that provide the nutrients you need while limiting the substances linked to disease should be an important part of your daily life.

Choosing a healthy diet is a two-part process. First, you have to know which nutrients you need and in what amounts. Second, you have to translate those requirements into a diet consisting of foods you like that are both available and affordable. Once you know what constitutes a healthy diet for you, you can adjust your current diet to bring it into line with your goals.

This chapter explains the basic principles of **nutrition.** It introduces the six classes of essential nutrients, explaining their role in the functioning of the body. It also provides guidelines that you can use to design a healthy eating plan. Finally, it offers practical tools and advice to help you apply the guidelines to your life.

NUTRITIONAL REQUIREMENTS: COMPONENTS OF A HEALTHY DIET

You probably think about your diet in terms of the foods you like to eat. More important for your health, though, are the nutrients contained in those foods. Your body requires proteins, fats, carbohydrates, vitamins, minerals, and water—about 45 **essential nutrients.** In this context, the word *essential* means that you must get these substances from food because your body is unable to manufacture them, or at least not fast enough to meet your physiological needs. The six classes of nutrients, along with their functions and major sources, are listed in Table 3.1

The body needs some essential nutrients in relatively large amounts; these **macronutrients** include protein, fat, carbohydrate, and water. **Micronutrients,** such as vitamins and minerals, are required in much smaller amounts. Your body obtains nutrients through the process of **digestion,** which breaks down food into compounds that the gastrointestinal tract can absorb and the body can use (Figure 3.1, p. 64). A diet that provides enough essential nutrients is vital because they provide energy, help build and maintain body tissues, and help regulate body functions.

Calories

The energy in foods is expressed as **kilocalories.** One kilocalorie represents the amount of heat it takes to raise the temperature of one liter of water 1°C. A person needs about 2000 kilocalories a day to meet his or her energy needs. In common usage, people refer to kilocalories as *calories,* which is a much smaller energy unit: 1 kilocalorie contains 1000 calories. This text uses the familiar word *calorie* to stand for the larger energy unit; you'll also find *calorie* used on food labels.

Of the six classes of essential nutrients, three supply energy:

- Fat = 9 calories per gram
- Protein = 4 calories per gram
- Carbohydrate = 4 calories per gram

Alcohol, though not an essential nutrient, also supplies energy, providing 7 calories per gram. (One gram equals a little less than 0.04 ounce.) The high caloric content of fat is one reason experts often advise against high fat consumption; most of us do not need the extra calories to meet energy needs. Regardless of their source, calories consumed in excess of energy needs can be converted to fat and stored in the body.

Table 3.1 The Six Classes of Essential Nutrients

NUTRIENT	FUNCTION	MAJOR SOURCES
Proteins products, (4 calories/gram)	Form important parts of muscles, bone, blood, enzymes, some hormones, and cell membranes; repair tissue; regulate water and acid-base balance; help in growth; supply energy	Meat, fish, poultry, eggs, milk legumes, nuts
Carbohydrates (4 calories/gram)	Supply energy to cells in brain, nervous system, and blood; supply energy to muscles during exercise	Grains (breads and cereals), fruits, vegetables, milk
Fats (9 calories/gram)	Supply energy; insulate, support, and cushion organs; provide medium for absorption of fat-soluble vitamins	Animal foods, grains, nuts, seeds, fish, vegetables
Vitamins	Promote (initiate or speed up) specific chemical reactions within cells	Abundant in fruits, vegetables, and grains; also found in meat and dairy products
Minerals	Help regulate body functions; aid in growth and maintenance of body tissues; act as catalysts for release of energy	Found in most food groups
Water	Makes up 50–60% of body weight; provides medium for chemical reactions; transports chemicals; regulates temperature; removes waste products	Fruits, vegetables, liquids

Tracking Your Junk Food Intake

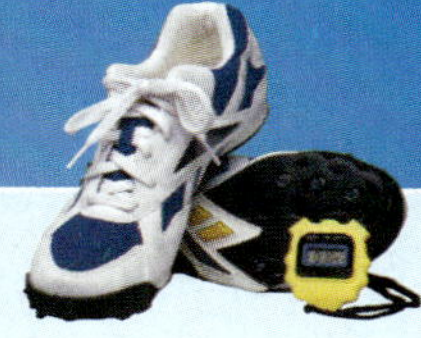

PERSONAL CHALLENGE

How much junk food do you eat on any given day? Let's find out. Write down all the different kinds of junk food you eat during the day today:

____

____

____

____

____

____

Now, write down your reason for eating each of those items:

____

____

____

____

____

____

Whether you eat junk for pleasure or to help cope with stress, it pays to be mindful of your eating habits. Consider your reasons for eating junk food, and try to catch yourself the next time you're tempted to reach for some. If you're able to stop yourself, you can make healthier choices.

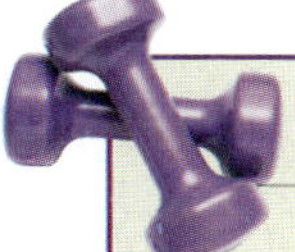

Fitness Tip

A pound of body fat is equal to 3500 calories. If you eat 100 calories more than you expend every day, you will gain more than 10 pounds in a year.

Just meeting energy needs is not enough. Our bodies need enough of the essential nutrients to grow and function properly. Practically all foods contain combinations of nutrients, although foods are commonly classified according to their predominant nutrients. For example, spaghetti is considered a carbohydrate food, although it contains small amounts of other nutrients. The following sections discuss the functions and sources of each class of nutrients.

Proteins—The Basis of Body Structure

Proteins form important parts of the body's main structural components: muscles and bones. Proteins also form

KEY TERMS

nutrition The science of food and how the body uses it in health and disease.

essential nutrients Substances the body must get from foods because it cannot manufacture them at all or fast enough to meet its needs. These nutrients include proteins, fats, carbohydrates, vitamins, minerals, and water.

macronutrient An essential nutrient required by the body in relatively large amounts.

micronutrient An essential nutrient required by the body in minute amounts.

digestion The process of breaking down foods into compounds the gastrointestinal tract can absorb and the body can use.

kilocalorie A measure of energy content in food; 1 kilocalorie represents the amount of heat needed to raise the temperature of 1 liter of water 1°C; commonly referred to as *calorie*.

protein An essential nutrient that forms important parts of the body's main structures (muscles and bones) as well as blood, enzymes, hormones, and cell membranes; also provides energy.

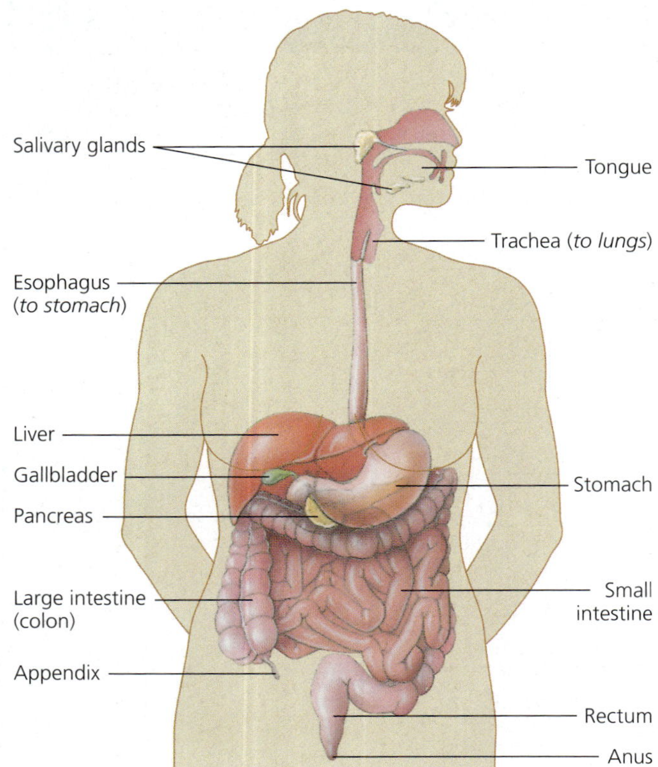

FIGURE 3.1 The digestive system.
Food is partially broken down by being chewed and mixed with saliva in the mouth. After traveling to the stomach via the esophagus, food is broken down further by stomach acids and other secretions. As food moves through the digestive tract, it is mixed by muscular contractions and broken down by chemicals. Most absorption of nutrients occurs in the small intestine, aided by secretions from the pancreas, gallbladder, and intestinal lining. The large intestine reabsorbs excess water; the remaining solid wastes are collected in the rectum and excreted through the anus.

important parts of blood, enzymes, cell membranes, and some hormones. As mentioned earlier, proteins also provide energy (4 calories per gram) for the body.

Amino Acids The building blocks of proteins are called **amino acids.** Twenty common amino acids are found in food. Nine of these are essential (or indispensable). The other 11 amino acids can be produced by the body as long as the necessary components are supplied by foods.

Complete and Incomplete Proteins Individual protein sources are considered "complete" if they supply all the essential amino acids in adequate amounts and "incomplete" if they do not. Meat, fish, poultry, eggs, milk, cheese, and soy provide complete proteins. Incomplete proteins, which come from plant sources such as nuts and **legumes** (dried beans and peas), are good sources of most essential amino acids but are usually low in one or two.

Certain combinations of vegetable proteins, such as wheat and peanuts in a peanut butter sandwich, allow each vegetable protein to make up for the amino acids missing in the other protein. The combination yields a complete protein. It was once believed that vegetarians had to "complement" their proteins at each meal in order to receive the benefit of a complete protein. It is now known, however, that proteins consumed throughout the course of the day can complement each other to form a pool of amino acids the body can draw from to produce proteins. Vegetarians should include a variety of vegetable protein sources in their diets to make sure they get all the essential amino acids in adequate amounts. (Healthy vegetarian diets are discussed later in the chapter.)

Table 3.2 Protein Content of Common Food Items

ITEM	PROTEIN (GRAMS)
3 ounces lean meat, poultry, or fish	20–25
⅓ cup tofu	20–25
1 cup dried beans	15–20
1 cup milk, yogurt	8–12
1½ ounces cheese	8–12
1 serving of cereals, grains, nuts, vegetables	2–4

Recommended Protein Intake Adequate daily intake of protein for adults is 0.8 gram per kilogram (0.36 gram per pound) of body weight, corresponding to 50 grams of protein per day for someone who weighs 140 pounds and 65 grams of protein for someone who weighs 180 pounds. Table 3.2 lists some popular food items and the amount of protein each provides.

Most Americans meet or exceed the protein intake needed for adequate nutrition. If you consume more protein than your body needs, the extra protein is synthesized into fat for energy storage or burned for energy requirements. A little extra protein is not harmful, but it can contribute fat to the diet because protein-rich foods are often fat-rich, as well.

A fairly broad range of protein intakes is associated with good health, and the Food and Nutrition Board of the Institute of Medicine recommends that the amount of protein adults eat should fall within the range of 10–35% of total daily calories, depending on the individual's age. The average American diet includes about 15–16% of total daily calories as protein.

Wellness Tip

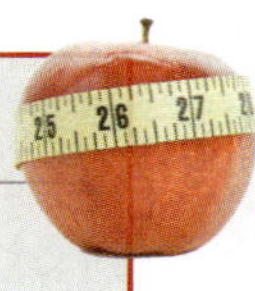

Research shows that some protein-rich foods can give you a quick mental boost, which can be helpful before an exam.

Fats—Essential in Small Amounts

Fats, also known as *lipids*, are the most concentrated source of energy, at 9 calories per gram. The fats stored in your body represent usable energy, help insulate your body, and support and cushion your organs. Fats in the diet help your body absorb fat-soluble vitamins, and they add flavor and texture to foods. Fats are the major fuel for the body during rest and light activity.

Two fats—linoleic acid and alpha-linolenic acid—are essential components of the diet. They are used to make compounds that are key regulators of such body functions as the maintenance of blood pressure and the progress of a healthy pregnancy.

Types and Sources of Fats Most of the fats in foods are fairly similar in composition, generally including a molecule of glycerol (an alcohol) with three fatty acid chains attached to it. The resulting structure is called a *triglyceride*. Animal fat, for example, is primarily made of triglycerides. Within a triglyceride, differences in the fatty acid structure result in different types of fats. Depending on this structure, a fat may be unsaturated, monounsaturated, polyunsaturated, or saturated. (The essential fatty acids—linoleic and alpha-linolenic acids—are both polyunsaturated.) The different types of fatty acids have different characteristics and different effects on your health.

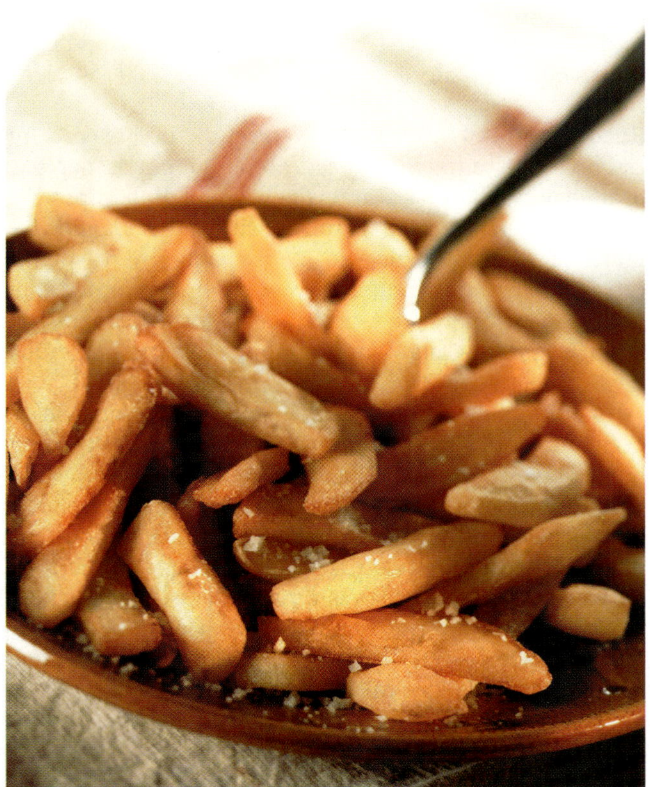

Food fats are often composed of both saturated and unsaturated fatty acids; the dominant type of fatty acid determines the fat's characteristics. Food fats containing large amounts of saturated fatty acids are usually solid at room temperature; they are generally found naturally in animal products. The leading sources of saturated fat in the American diet are red meats (hamburger, steak, roasts), whole milk, cheese, hot dogs, and lunch meats. Food fats containing large amounts of monounsaturated and polyunsaturated fatty acids usually come from plant sources and are liquid at room temperature. Olive, canola, safflower, and peanut oils contain mostly monounsaturated fatty acids. Corn, soybean, and cottonseed oils contain mostly polyunsaturated fatty acids.

Hydrogenation There are notable exceptions to these generalizations. When unsaturated vegetable oils undergo the process of **hydrogenation**, a mixture of saturated and unsaturated fatty acids is produced, creating a more solid fat from a liquid oil. Hydrogenation also changes some unsaturated fatty acids into **trans fatty acids (trans fats)**, unsaturated fatty acids with an atypical shape that affects their behavior in the body. Food manufacturers use hydrogenation to increase the stability of an oil so it can be reused for deep frying, to improve the texture of certain foods (to make pastries and pie crusts flakier, for example), and to extend the shelf life of foods made with oil. Hydrogenation is also used to transform liquid vegetable oils into margarine or shortening.

Many baked and fried foods are prepared with hydrogenated vegetable oils, which means they can be relatively high in saturated and trans fatty acids. Leading sources of trans fats in the American diet are deep-fried fast foods such as french fries and fried chicken (typically fried in vegetable shortening rather than oil), baked and snack foods, and stick margarine.

In general, the more solid a hydrogenated oil is, the more saturated and trans fats it contains. For example, stick margarines typically contain more saturated and trans fats than do tub or squeeze margarines. Small amounts of trans fatty acids are also found naturally in meat and milk.

Hydrogenated vegetable oils are not the only plant fats that contain saturated fats. Palm and coconut oils,

KEY TERMS

amino acids The building blocks of proteins.

legumes Vegetables such as dried beans and peas that are high in fiber and are also important sources of protein.

hydrogenation A process by which hydrogens are added to unsaturated fats, increasing the degree of saturation and turning liquid oils into solid fats. Hydrogenation produces a mixture of saturated fatty acids and standard and trans forms of unsaturated fatty acids.

trans fatty acid (trans fat) A type of unsaturated fatty acid produced during the process of hydrogenation; trans fats have an atypical shape that affects their chemical activity.

although derived from plants, are also highly saturated. Yet fish oils, derived from an animal source, are rich in polyunsaturated fats.

Fats and Health Different types of fats have very different effects on health. Many studies have examined the effects of dietary fat intake on blood **cholesterol** levels and the risk of heart disease. However, the results of a recent analysis concluded that dietary saturated fat is not associated with an increased risk of certain forms of heart disease, and that the benefits of diets low in saturated fat may come from the higher amounts of polyunsaturated fats that these diets provide.

Saturated and trans fatty acids raise blood levels of **low-density lipoprotein (LDL)**, or "bad" cholesterol, thereby increasing a person's risk of heart disease. Unsaturated fatty acids lower LDL. Monounsaturated fatty acids, such as those found in olive and canola oils, may also increase levels of **high-density lipoprotein (HDL)**, or "good" cholesterol, providing even greater benefits for heart health. In large amounts, trans fatty acids may lower HDL. Saturated fats impair the ability of HDLs to prevent inflammation of the blood vessels, a key factor in vascular disease. Saturated fats also reduce the blood vessels' ability to react normally to stress. Thus, to reduce the risk of heart disease, it is important to choose unsaturated fats instead of saturated and trans fats. (See Chapter 5 for more on cholesterol.)

Most Americans consume 4–5 times as much saturated fat as trans fat (8–10% versus 2% of total daily calories). However, health experts are particularly concerned about trans fats because of their double-negative effect on heart health—they not only raise LDL but also lower HDL—and because there is less public awareness of trans fats, although awareness is growing. Since 2006, federal law has required food labels to include trans fat content, and numerous states and cities have banned the use of trans fats in restaurant food. Consumers can also check for the presence of trans fats by examining a food's ingredient list for partially hydrogenated oil or vegetable shortening.

For heart health, it's important to limit your consumption of both saturated and trans fats. The best way to reduce saturated fat in your diet is to eat less meat and full-fat dairy products (whole milk, cream, butter, cheese, ice cream). To lower trans fats, eat fewer deep-fried foods and baked goods made with hydrogenated vegetable oils (such as many kinds of crackers and cookies), use liquid oils for cooking, and favor tub or squeeze margarines over stick margarines. Remember: The softer or more liquid a fat is, the less saturated and trans fat it is likely to contain.

Although saturated and trans fats pose health hazards, other fats can be beneficial. When used in place of saturated fats, monounsaturated fatty acids—as found in avocados, most nuts, and olive, canola, peanut, and safflower oils—improve cholesterol levels and may help protect against some cancers.

Omega-3 fatty acids, a form of polyunsaturated fat found primarily in fish, may be even more healthful. Omega-3s and the compounds the body makes from them have a number of heart-healthy effects: They reduce the tendency of blood to clot, inhibit inflammation and abnormal heart rhythms, and reduce blood pressure and the risk of heart attack and stroke in some people. Because of these benefits, nutritionists recommend that Americans increase the proportion of omega-3s in their diet by eating fish two or more times a week. Salmon, tuna, trout, mackerel, herring, sardines, and anchovies are all good sources of omega-3s. Lesser amounts are found in plant foods, including dark green leafy vegetables; walnuts; flaxseeds; and canola, walnut, and flaxseed oils.

Most of the polyunsaturated fats currently consumed by Americans are *omega-6* fatty acids, primarily from corn oil and soybean oil. The American Heart Association (AHA) recommends consuming at least 5–10% of energy from omega-6 fatty acids as part of a low-saturated-fat and low-cholesterol diet to reduce the risk of coronary heart disease.

In addition to its effects on heart disease risk, dietary fat can affect health in other ways. Diets high in fatty red meat are associated with an increased risk of certain forms of cancer, especially colon cancer. A high-fat diet can also make weight management more difficult. Because fat is a concentrated source of calories, a high-fat diet is often a high-calorie diet that can lead to weight gain.

Although more research is needed on the precise effects of different types and amounts of fat on overall health, a great deal of evidence points to the fact that most people benefit from lowering their overall fat intake to recommended levels and choosing unsaturated fats instead of saturated and trans fats. The types of fatty acids and their effects on health are summarized in Table 3.3.

Recommended Fat Intake To meet the body's need for essential fats, adult men need about 17 grams per day of linoleic acid and 1.6 grams per day of alpha-linolenic acid. Women need 12 grams of linoleic acid and 1.1 grams of alpha-linolenic acid. It takes only 3–4 teaspoons (15–20 grams) of vegetable oil per day incorporated into your diet to supply the essential fats. Most Americans get enough essential fats. Limiting unhealthy fats is a much greater health concern.

Limits for total fat, saturated fat, and trans fat intake have been set by a number of government and research organizations. The Institute of Medicine's Food and Nutrition Board has released recommendations for the balance of energy sources in a healthful diet. These recommendations—called Acceptable Macronutrient Distribution Ranges (AMDRs)—are based on ensuring adequate intake of essential nutrients while reducing the risk of chronic diseases. As with protein, a range of levels of fat intake is associated with good health. The AMDR for total fat is 20–35% of total calories. Although more difficult for consumers to monitor, AMDRs have also been set for omega-6 fatty acids (5–10%) and omega-3 fatty acids (0.6–1.2%) as part of total fat intake.

Table 3.3 Types of Fatty Acids and Their Possible Effects on Health

	TYPE OF FATTY ACID	FOUND IN[a]	POSSIBLE EFFECTS ON HEALTH
Keep Intake Low	SATURATED	• Animal fats (especially fatty meats and poultry fat and skin) • Butter, cheese, and other high-fat dairy products • Palm and coconut oils	• Raises total cholesterol and LDL cholesterol • May increase risk of heart disease • May increase risk of colon and prostate cancers
Keep Intake Low	TRANS	• Deep-fried fast foods • Stick margarines, shortening • Packaged cookies and crackers • Processed snacks and sweets	• Raises total cholesterol and LDL cholesterol • Lowers HDL cholesterol • May increase risk of heart disease and breast cancer
Choose Moderate Amounts	MONOUNSATURATED	• Olive, canola, and safflower oils • Avocados, olives • Peanut butter (without added fat) • Many nuts, including almonds, cashews, pecans, and pistachios	• Lowers total cholesterol and LDL cholesterol • May reduce blood pressure and lower triglycerides (a risk factor for heart disease) • May reduce risk of heart disease, stroke, and some cancers
Choose Moderate Amounts	POLYUNSATURATED (two groups)[b]		
Choose Moderate Amounts	Omega-3	• Fatty fish, including salmon, white albacore tuna, mackerel, anchovies, and sardines • Lesser amounts in walnut, flaxseed, canola, and soybean oils; tofu, walnuts; flaxseeds; and dark green leafy vegetables	• Reduces blood clotting and inflammation and inhibits abnormal heart rhythms • Lowers triglycerides • May lower blood pressure in some people • May reduce the risk of fatal heart attack, stroke, and some cancers
Choose Moderate Amounts	Omega-6	• Corn, soybean, and cottonseed oils (often used in margarine, mayonnaise, and salad dressings)	• Lowers total cholesterol and LDL cholesterol • May lower HDL cholesterol • May reduce risk of heart disease • May slightly increase risk of cancer if omega-6 intake is high and omega-3 is low

[a] Food fats contain a combination of types of fatty acids in various proportions. For example, canola oil is composed mainly of monounsaturated fatty acids (62%) but also contains polyunsaturated (32%) and saturated (6%) fatty acids. Food fats are categorized here according to their predominant fatty acid.

[b] The essential fatty acids are polyunsaturated: Linoleic acid is an omega-6 fatty acid and alpha-linolenic acid is an omega-3 fatty acid.

Because any amount of saturated and trans fat increases the risk of heart disease, the Food and Nutrition Board recommends that saturated and trans fat intake be kept as low as possible; most fat in a healthy diet should be unsaturated.

For advice on setting individual intake goals, see the box "Setting Intake Goals for Protein, Fat, and Carbohydrate." To determine how close you are to meeting your personal intake goals for fat, keep a running total over the course of the day. For prepared foods, food labels list the number of grams of fat, protein, and carbohydrate. Nutrition information is also available in many grocery stores, in published nutrition guides, and online (see For Further Exploration at the end of the chapter). By checking these resources, you can keep track of the total grams of fat, protein, and carbohydrate you eat and assess your current diet.

In reducing fat intake to recommended levels, the emphasis should be on lowering saturated and trans fats (see Table 3.3). You can still eat high-fat foods, but it makes sense to limit the size of your portions and to balance your intake with low-fat foods. For example, peanut butter is high in fat, with 8 grams (72 calories) of fat in each 90-calorie tablespoon. Two tablespoons of peanut butter eaten on whole-wheat bread and served with a banana, carrot sticks, and a glass of nonfat milk make a nutritious lunch—high in protein and carbohydrate, relatively low in total and saturated fat (500 calories, 18 grams of total fat, 4 grams of saturated fat). By comparison, four tablespoons of peanut butter on high-fat crackers with potato chips, cookies, and whole milk is a less healthy combination (1000 calories, 62 grams of total fat, 15 grams of saturated fat). So although it's important to evaluate individual food items for their fat content, it is more important to look at them in the context of your overall diet.

KEY TERMS

cholesterol A waxy substance found in the blood and cells and needed for synthesis of cell membranes, vitamin D, and hormones.

low-density lipoprotein (LDL) Blood fat that transports cholesterol to organs and tissues; excess amounts result in the accumulation of fatty deposits on artery walls.

high-density lipoprotein (HDL) Blood fat that helps transport cholesterol out of the arteries, thereby protecting against heart disease.

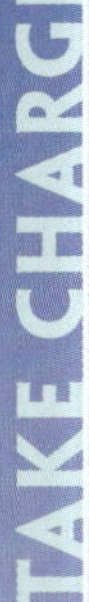

Setting Intake Goals for Protein, Fat, and Carbohydrate

The Food and Nutrition Board has established goals to help ensure adequate intake of the essential amino acids, fatty acids, and carbohydrate. The daily goals for adequate intake for adults follow:

	MEN	WOMEN
Protein	56 grams	46 grams
Fat: Linoleic acid	17 grams	12 grams
Alpha-linoleic acid	1.6 grams	1.1 grams
Carbohydrate	130 grams	130 grams

Protein intake goals can be calculated more specifically by multiplying your body weight in kilograms by 0.8 or your body weight in pounds by 0.36. (Refer to the Nutrition Resources section at the end of the chapter for information for specific age groups and life stages.)

To meet your daily energy needs, you need to consume more than the minimally adequate amounts of the energy-providing nutrients listed above, which alone supply only about 800–900 calories.

The Food and Nutrition Board provides additional guidance in the form of Acceptable Macronutrient Distribution Ranges (AMDRs). These ranges can help you balance your intake of energy-providing nutrients in ways that ensure adequate intake and reduce the risk of chronic disease.

The AMDRs for protein, total fat, and carbohydrate are as follows:

Protein	10–35% of total daily calories
Total fat	20–35% of total daily calories
Carbohydrate	45–65% of total daily calories

To set individual goals, begin by estimating your total daily energy (calorie) needs. If your weight is stable, your current energy intake is the number of calories you need to maintain your weight at your current activity level. Next, select percentage goals for protein, fat, and carbohydrate. You can allocate your total daily calories among the three classes of macronutrients to suit your preferences; just make sure that the three percentages you select total 100% and that you meet the minimum intake goals listed. Two samples reflecting different total energy intake and nutrient intake goals are shown in the table below.

To translate your percentage goals into daily intake goals expressed in calories and grams, multiply the appropriate percentages by total calorie intake, and then divide the results by the corresponding calories per gram. For example, a fat limit of 35% applied to a 2200-calorie diet would be calculated as follows: 0.35 x 2200 = 770 calories of total fat; 770 ÷ 9 calories per gram = 86 grams of total fat. (Remember that fat has 9 calories per gram and that protein and carbohydrate have 4 calories per gram.)

Two Sample Macronutrient Distributions

		SAMPLE 1		SAMPLE 2	
NUTRIENT	AMDR	INDIVIDUAL GOALS	AMOUNTS FOR A 1600-CALORIE DIET	INDIVIDUAL GOALS	AMOUNTS FOR A 2800-CALORIE DIET
PROTEIN	10–35%	15%	240 calories = 60 grams	30%	840 calories = 210 grams
FAT	20–35%	30%	480 calories = 53 grams	25%	700 calories = 78 grams
CARBOHYDRATE	45–65%	55%	880 calories = 220 grams	45%	1260 calories = 315 grams

SOURCE: Food and Nutrition Board, Institute of Medicine, National Academies. 2002. *Dietary Reference Intakes: Applications in Dietary Planning.* Washington, D.C.: National Academies Press.

Carbohydrates—An Ideal Source of Energy

Carbohydrates ("carbs") are needed in the diet primarily to supply energy to body cells. Some cells, such as those in the brain and other parts of the nervous system and in the blood, use only carbohydrates for fuel. During high-intensity exercise, muscles also get most of their energy from carbohydrates.

Simple and Complex Carbohydrates Carbohydrates are classified into two groups: simple and complex. *Simple carbohydrates* include sucrose (table sugar), fructose (fruit sugar, honey), maltose (malt sugar), and lactose (milk sugar). Simple carbohydrates provide much of the sweetness in foods. They are found naturally in fruits and milk and are added to soft drinks, fruit drinks, candy, and sweet desserts. There is no evidence that any type of simple carbohydrate is more nutritious than others.

Complex carbohydrates include starches and most types of dietary fiber. Starches are found in a variety of plants, especially grains (wheat, rye, rice, oats, barley, and millet), legumes (dried beans, peas, and lentils), and tubers (potatoes and yams). Most other vegetables contain a mix of complex and simple carbohydrates. Fiber, which is discussed later in this chapter, is found in fruits, vegetables, and grains.

During digestion, your body breaks down carbohydrates into simple sugar molecules, such as **glucose**, for absorption. Once glucose is in the bloodstream, the

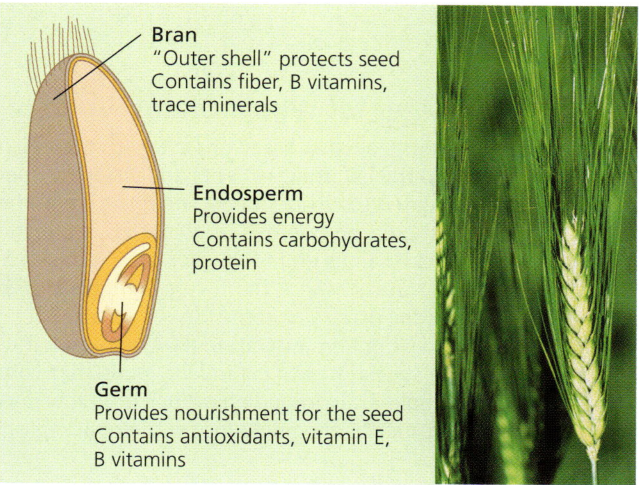

FIGURE 3.2 The parts of a whole grain kernel.

pancreas releases the hormone insulin, which allows cells to take up glucose and use it for energy. The liver and muscles also take up glucose and store it in the form of a starch called **glycogen.** The muscles use glucose from glycogen as fuel during endurance events or long workouts.

Refined Carbohydrates Versus Whole Grains Complex carbohydrates can be further divided between refined, or processed, carbohydrates and unrefined carbohydrates, or whole grains. Before they are processed, all grains are **whole grains,** consisting of an inner layer of germ, a middle layer called the endosperm, and an outer layer of bran (Figure 3.2). During processing, the germ and bran are often removed, leaving just the starchy endosperm. The refinement of whole grains transforms whole-wheat flour into white flour, brown rice into white rice, and so on.

Refined carbohydrates usually retain all the calories of their unrefined counterparts, but they tend to be much lower in fiber, vitamins, minerals, and other beneficial compounds. Refined grain products are often enriched or fortified with vitamins and minerals, but many of the nutrients lost in processing are not replaced.

Unrefined carbohydrates tend to take longer to chew and digest than refined ones; they also enter the bloodstream more slowly. This slower digestive pace tends to make people feel full sooner and for a longer period. Also, a slower rise in blood glucose levels following consumption of complex carbohydrates may help in the management of diabetes. Whole grains are also high in dietary fiber (discussed later).

Consumption of whole grains has been linked to a reduced risk of heart disease, diabetes, high blood pressure, stroke, and certain forms of cancer. For all these reasons, whole grains are recommended over those that have been refined. This does not mean you should never eat refined carbohydrates such as white bread or white rice; it simply means that whole-wheat bread, brown rice, and other whole grains are healthier choices. See the box "Choosing More Whole-Grain Foods" for tips on increasing your intake of whole grains.

Glycemic Index and Glycemic Response Insulin and glucose levels rise following a meal or snack containing any type of carbohydrate. Some foods cause a quick and dramatic rise in glucose and insulin levels, while others have a slower, more moderate effect. A food that has a rapid effect on blood glucose levels is said to have a high **glycemic index.** The glycemic index of a food indicates the type of carbohydrate in that food. High-glycemic-index foods do not, as some popular diets claim, directly cause weight gain beyond the calories they contain.

Attempting to base food choices on glycemic index is a difficult task. Unrefined complex carbohydrates and high-fiber foods generally tend to have a lower glycemic index, but patterns are less clear for other types of foods. The fat content of a food also affects its glycemic index; the higher in fat a food is, the lower its effect on glucose levels. Ripeness, storage time, processing, and food preparation are other factors that can affect a food's glycemic index. The body's response to carbohydrates also depends on other factors, such as what other foods are consumed at the same time, as well as the individual's fitness status.

For people with particular health concerns, such as diabetes, glycemic index may be an important consideration in choosing foods. Still, it should not be the sole criterion for food choices. Carbohydrate choices (low versus high glycemic index) that replace dietary saturated fat may also be an important factor in determining the effects of diet on the risk of cardiovascular disease. Some unrefined grains, fruits, vegetables, and legumes are rich in nutrients, have a relatively low energy density, and have a

Wellness Tip

Certain carbohydrate-rich foods, such as a bagel or a plain baked potato, can have a temporary calming effect on some people during stressful situations.

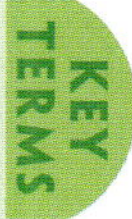

KEY TERMS

carbohydrate An essential nutrient; sugars, starches, and dietary fiber are all carbohydrates.

glucose A simple sugar that is the body's basic fuel.

glycogen A starch stored in the liver and muscles.

whole grain The entire edible portion of a grain (such as wheat, rice, or oats), including the germ, endosperm, and bran; processing removes parts of the grain, often leaving just the endosperm.

glycemic index A measure of how a particular food affects blood glucose levels.

TAKE CHARGE

Choosing More Whole-Grain Foods

What Are Whole Grains?

The first step in increasing your intake of whole grains is to correctly identify them. The following are whole grains:

- whole wheat
- whole rye
- whole oats
- oatmeal
- whole-grain corn
- popcorn
- brown rice
- whole-grain barley

Other choices include bulgur (cracked wheat), millet, kasha (roasted buckwheat kernels), quinoa, wheat and rye berries, amaranth, wild rice, graham flour, whole-grain kamut, whole-grain spelt, and whole-grain triticale.

Wheat flour, unbleached flour, enriched flour, and degerminated corn meal are not whole grains. Wheat germ and wheat bran are also not whole grains, but they are the constituents of wheat typically left out when wheat is processed and so are healthier choices than regular wheat flour, which typically contains just the grain's endosperm.

Checking Packages for Whole Grains

To find packaged foods—such as bread or pasta—that are rich in whole grains, read the list of ingredients and check for special health claims related to whole grains. The *first* item in the list of ingredients should be one of the whole grains in the preceding list. Product names and food color can be misleading. *When in doubt, always check the list of ingredients and make sure "whole" is the first word in the list.*

The U.S. Food and Drug Administration (FDA) allows manufacturers to include special health claims for foods that contain 51% or more whole-grain ingredients. Such products may contain a statement such as the following on their packaging:

- "Rich in whole grain"
- "Made with 100% whole grain"
- "Diets rich in whole-grain foods may help reduce the risk of heart disease and certain cancers."

However, many whole-grain products will not carry such claims. This is one more reason to check the ingredient list to make sure you're buying a product made from one or more whole grains.

low to moderate glycemic index. Your best bet, therefore, is to choose a variety of vegetables daily and limit refined grains as well as foods that are high in added sugars but low in other nutrients.

Recommended Carbohydrate Intake On average, Americans consume 200–300 grams of carbohydrate per day, well above the 130 grams needed to meet the body's requirement for essential carbohydrate. A range of intakes is associated with good health, and experts recommend that adults consume 45–65% of total daily calories as carbohydrate. (That's about 225–325 grams of carbohydrate for someone who consumes 2000 calories per day.) The focus should be on consuming a variety of foods rich in complex carbohydrates, especially whole grains.

Athletes in training can especially benefit from high-carbohydrate diets (60–70% of total daily calories), which enhance the amount of carbohydrates stored in their muscles as glycogen and therefore provide more carbohydrate fuel for use during endurance events or long workouts. Carbohydrates consumed during prolonged athletic events (often in the form of sports beverages) can help fuel muscles and extend the availability of the glycogen stored in muscles. Caution is in order, however, because overconsumption of carbohydrates can lead to feelings of fatigue and underconsumption of other nutrients.

Although the Food and Nutrition Board set an AMDR for added sugars of 25% or less of total daily calories, many health experts recommend an even lower intake. (Recall that sugars are a form of carbohydrate.) World Health Organization guidelines suggest a limit of 10% of total daily calories from added sugars. Limits set by the U.S. Department of Agriculture (USDA) are even lower, with a maximum of about 8 teaspoons (32 grams) suggested for someone consuming 2000 calories per day. Foods high in added sugar are generally high in calories and low in nutrients and fiber, thus providing "empty" calories.

To reduce your intake of added sugars, limit soft drinks, candy, desserts, and sweetened fruit drinks. The simple carbohydrates in your diet shoulde come mainly from fruits, which are excellent sources of vitamins and minerals, and from low-fat or fat-free milk and other dairy products, which are high in protein and calcium.

Fiber—A Closer Look

Fiber is the term given to nondigestible carbohydrates provided by plants. Instead of being digested, like starch, fiber moves through the intestinal tract and provides bulk for feces in the large intestine, which in turn facilitates elimination. In the large intestine, some types of fiber are broken down by bacteria into acids and gases, which explains why eating too much fiber-rich food can lead to intestinal gas. Even though humans don't digest fiber, it is necessary for good health.

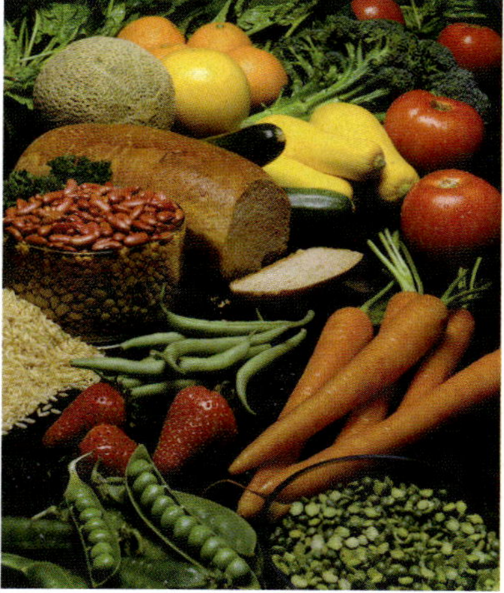

Fruits, vegetables, and whole grains are excellent sources of carbohydrates and fiber.

Types of Dietary Fiber The Food and Nutrition Board has defined two types of fiber:

- **Dietary fiber** is the nondigestible carbohydrates (and the noncarbohydrate substance lignin) that are present naturally in plants such as grains, legumes, and vegetables.
- **Functional fiber** is any nondigestible carbohydrate that has been either isolated from natural sources or synthesized in a lab and then added to a food product or supplement.
- **Total fiber** is the sum of dietary and functional fiber in a person's diet.

Fibers have different properties that lead to different physiological effects in the body. **Soluble (viscous) fiber** such as that found in oat bran or legumes can delay stomach emptying, slow the movement of glucose into the blood after eating, and reduce absorption of cholesterol. **Insoluble fiber**, such as that found in wheat bran or psyllium seed, increases fecal bulk and helps prevent constipation, hemorrhoids, and other digestive disorders.

A high-fiber diet can help reduce the risk of type 2 diabetes, heart disease, and pulmonary disease, as well as improve gastrointestinal health and aid in weight management. Some studies have linked high-fiber diets with a reduced risk of colon and rectal cancer. Other studies have suggested that other characteristics of diets rich in fruits, vegetables, and whole grains may be responsible for this reduction in risk.

Sources of Fiber All plant foods contain some dietary fiber. Fruits, legumes, oats (especially oat bran), and barley all contain the viscous types of fiber that help lower blood glucose and cholesterol levels. Wheat (especially wheat bran), cereals, grains, and vegetables are all good sources of cellulose and other fibers that help prevent constipation. Psyllium, which is often added to cereals or used in fiber supplements and laxatives, improves intestinal health and also helps control glucose and cholesterol levels. The processing of packaged foods can remove fiber, so it's important to depend on fresh fruits and vegetables and foods made from whole grains as your main sources of fiber.

> **Wellness Tip**
>
> To avoid intestinal discomfort, add fiber to your diet slowly so you can build a tolerance to it.

Recommended Fiber Intake To reduce the risk of chronic disease and maintain intestinal health, the Food and Nutrition Board recommends a daily fiber intake of 38 grams for adult men and 25 grams for adult women. Americans currently consume about half this amount. Fiber should come from foods, not supplements, which should be used only under medical supervision.

Vitamins—Organic Micronutrients

Vitamins are organic (carbon-containing) substances required in small amounts to regulate various processes within living cells (Table 3.4). Humans need 13 vitamins; of these, four are fat-soluble (A, D, E, and K), and nine are water-soluble (C and the B-complex vitamins thiamin, riboflavin, niacin, vitamin B-6, folate, vitamin B-12, biotin, and pantothenic acid).

Solubility affects how a vitamin is absorbed, transported, and stored in the body. The water-soluble vitamins are absorbed directly into the bloodstream, where they travel freely. Excess water-soluble vitamins are removed by the kidneys and excreted in urine. Fat-soluble vitamins require a more complex absorptive process. They are usually carried in the blood by special proteins and are stored in the liver and in fat tissues rather than excreted.

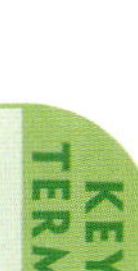

dietary fiber Nondigestible carbohydrates and lignin that are intact in plants.

functional fiber Nondigestible carbohydrates either isolated from natural sources or synthesized; these may be added to foods and dietary supplements.

total fiber The total amount of dietary fiber and functional fiber in the diet.

soluble (viscous) fiber Fiber that dissolves in water or is broken down by bacteria in the large intestine.

insoluble fiber Fiber that does not dissolve in water and is not broken down by bacteria in the large intestine.

vitamins Carbon-containing substances needed in small amounts to help promote and regulate chemical reactions and processes in the body.

Table 3.4 Facts About Vitamins

VITAMIN	IMPORTANT DIETARY SOURCES	MAJOR FUNCTIONS	SIGNS OF PROLONGED DEFICIENCY	TOXIC EFFECTS OF MEGADOSES
FAT-SOLUBLE				
Vitamin A	Liver, milk, butter, cheese, fortified margarine; carrots, spinach, and other orange and deep green vegetables and fruits	Maintenance of vision, skin, linings of the nose, mouth, digestive and urinary tracts, immune function	Night blindness; dry, scaling skin; increased susceptibility to infection; loss of appetite; anemia; kidney stones	Liver damage, miscarriage and birth defects, headache, vomiting and diarrhea, vertigo, double vision, bone abnormalities
Vitamin D	Fortified milk and margarine, fish oils, butter, egg yolks (sunlight on skin also produces vitamin D)	Development and maintenance of bones and teeth; promotion of calcium absorption	Rickets (bone deformities) in children; bone softening, loss, fractures in adults	Kidney damage, calcium deposits in soft tissues, depression, death
Vitamin E	Vegetable oils, whole grains, nuts and seeds, green leafy vegetables, asparagus, peaches	Protection and maintenance of cellular membranes	Red blood cell breakage and anemia, weakness, neurological problems, muscle cramps	Relatively nontoxic, but may cause excess bleeding or formation of blood clots
Vitamin K	Green leafy vegetables; smaller amounts widespread in other foods	Production of factors essential for blood clotting and bone metabolism	Hemorrhaging	None reported
WATER-SOLUBLE				
Biotin	Cereals, yeast, egg yolks, soy flour, liver; widespread in foods	Synthesis of fat, glycogen, and amino acids	Rash, nausea, vomiting, weight loss, depression, fatigue, hair loss	None reported
Folate	Green leafy vegetables, yeast, oranges, whole grains, legumes, liver	Amino acid metabolism, synthesis of RNA and DNA, new cell synthesis	Anemia, weakness, fatigue, irritability, shortness of breath, swollen tongue	Masking of vitamin B-12 deficiency
Niacin	Eggs, poultry, fish, milk, whole grains, nuts, enriched breads and cereals, meats, legumes	Conversion of carbohydrates, fats, and proteins into usable forms of energy	Pellagra (symptoms include diarrhea, dermatitis, inflammation of mucous membranes, dementia)	Flushing of skin, nausea, vomiting, diarrhea, liver dysfunction, glucose intolerance
Pantothenic acid	Animal foods, whole grains, broccoli, potatoes; widespread in foods	Metabolism of fats, carbohydrates, and proteins	Fatigue, numbness and tingling of hands and feet, gastrointestinal disturbances	None reported
Riboflavin	Dairy products, enriched breads and cereals, lean meats, poultry, fish, green vegetables	Energy metabolism; maintenance of skin, mucous membranes, nervous system structures	Cracks at corners of mouth, sore throat, skin rash, hypersensitivity to light, purple tongue	None reported
Thiamin	Whole-grain and enriched breads and cereals, organ meats, lean pork, nuts, legumes	Conversion of carbohydrates into usable forms of energy; maintenance of appetite and nervous system function	Beriberi (symptoms include muscle wasting, mental confusion, anorexia, enlarged heart, nerve changes)	None reported
Vitamin B-6	Eggs, poultry, fish, whole grains, nuts, soybeans, liver, kidney, pork	Metabolism of amino acids and glycogen	Anemia, convulsions, cracks at corners of mouth, dermatitis, nausea, confusion	Neurological abnormalities and damage
Vitamin B-12	Meat, fish, poultry, fortified cereals	Synthesis of blood cells; other metabolic reactions	Anemia, fatigue, nervous system damage, sore tongue	None reported
Vitamin C	Peppers, broccoli, brussels sprouts, spinach, citrus fruits, strawberries, tomatoes, potatoes, cabbage, other fruits and vegetables	Maintenance and repair , of connective tissue, bones, teeth, cartilage; promotion of healing; aid in iron absorption	Scurvy, anemia, reduced resistance to infection, loosened teeth, joint pain, poor wound healing, hair loss, poor iron absorption	Urinary stones in some people, acid stomach from ingesting supplements in pill form, nausea, diarrhea, headache, fatigue

SOURCES: Food and Nutrition Board, Institute of Medicine. 2006. *Dietary Reference Intakes: The Essential Guide to Nutrient Requirements.* Washington, D.C.: National Academies Press. The complete Dietary Reference Intake reports are available from the National Academies Press (http://www.nap.edu). Shils, M. E., et al., eds. 2005. *Modern Nutrition in Health and Disease,* 10th ed. Baltimore: Lippincott Williams and Wilkins.

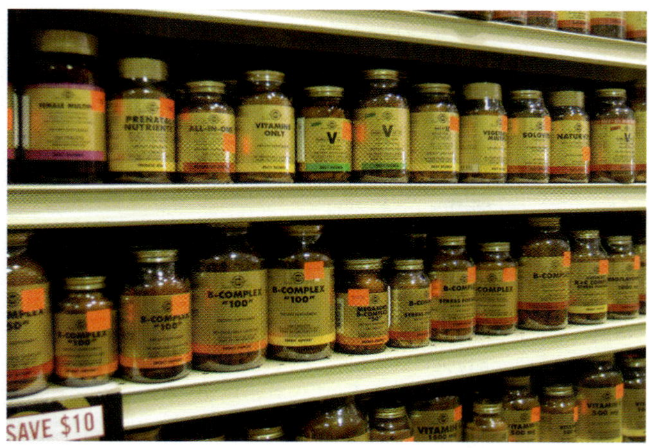

Vitamin and mineral supplements are popular, but they are not usually necessary for healthy people who eat a balanced diet.

Functions of Vitamins Many vitamins help chemical reactions take place. They provide no energy to the body directly but help unleash the energy stored in carbohydrates, proteins, and fats. Other vitamins are critical in the production of red blood cells and the maintenance of the nervous, skeletal, and immune systems. Some vitamins act as **antioxidants**, which help preserve the health of cells. Key vitamin antioxidants include vitamin E, vitamin C, and the vitamin A precursor beta-carotene. (Antioxidants are described later in the chapter.)

Sources of Vitamins The human body does not manufacture most of the vitamins it requires and must obtain them from foods. Vitamins are abundant in fruits, vegetables, and grains. In addition, many processed foods, such as flour and breakfast cereals, contain added vitamins. A few vitamins are made in certain parts of the body: The skin makes vitamin D when it is exposed to sunlight, and intestinal bacteria make vitamin K. Nonetheless, you still need to get vitamin D and vitamin K from foods (see Table 3.4).

Vitamin Deficiencies and Excesses If your diet lacks a particular vitamin, characteristic symptoms of deficiency can develop (see Table 3.4). For example, vitamin A deficiency can cause blindness, and vitamin B-12 deficiency can cause anemia. Vitamin deficiency diseases are most often seen in developing countries; they are relatively rare in the United States because vitamins are readily available from our food supply. However, intakes below recommended levels can have adverse effects on health even if they are not low enough to cause a deficiency disease. For example, low intake of folate increases a woman's chance of giving birth to a baby with a neural tube defect (a congenital malformation of the central nervous system). Low intake of folate and vitamins B-6 and B-12 has been linked to increased heart disease risk. A great deal of recent research has focused on vitamin D, suggesting that vitamin D supplementation can reduce the risk of cardiovascular disease and linking low vitamin D levels to an increased risk of several cancers. As important as vitamins are, however, many Americans consume less-than-recommended amounts of some vitamins.

Extra vitamins in the diet can be harmful, especially when taken as supplements. Megadoses of fat-soluble vitamins are particularly dangerous because the excess is stored in the body rather than excreted, increasing the risk of toxicity. Even when supplements are not taken in excess, relying on them for an adequate intake of vitamins can be problematic. There are many substances in foods other than vitamins and minerals, and some of these compounds may have important health effects. Later, this chapter discusses specific recommendations for vitamin intake and when a supplement is advisable. For now, keep in mind that it's best to get most of your vitamins from foods rather than supplements.

The vitamins and minerals in foods can be easily lost or destroyed during storage or cooking. To retain their value, eat or process vegetables immediately after buying them. If you can't do this, store them in a cool place, covered to retain moisture—either in the refrigerator (for a few days) or in the freezer (for a longer term). To reduce nutrient losses during food preparation, minimize the amount of water used and the total cooking time. Develop a taste for a crunchier texture in cooked vegetables. Baking, steaming, broiling, grilling, and microwaving are all good methods of preparing vegetables.

Minerals—Inorganic Micronutrients

Minerals are inorganic (non-carbon-containing) elements you need in relatively small amounts to help regulate body functions, aid in the growth and maintenance of body tissues, and help release energy (Table 3.5). There are about 17 essential minerals. The major minerals, those that the body needs in amounts exceeding 100 milligrams per day, include calcium, phosphorus, magnesium, sodium, potassium, and chloride. The essential trace minerals, which you need in minute amounts, include copper, fluoride, iodine, iron, selenium, and zinc.

Characteristic symptoms develop if an essential mineral is consumed in a quantity too small or too large for good health. The minerals commonly lacking in the American diet are iron, calcium, magnesium, and potassium. Iron-deficiency **anemia** is a problem in some

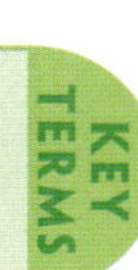

antioxidant A substance that protects against the breakdown of food or body constituents by free radicals; antioxidants' actions include binding oxygen, donating electrons to free radicals, and repairing damage to molecules.

minerals Inorganic compounds needed in relatively small amounts for the regulation, growth, and maintenance of body tissues and functions.

anemia A deficiency in the oxygen-carrying material in the red blood cells.

Table 3.5 Facts About Selected Minerals

MINERAL	IMPORTANT DIETARY SOURCES	MAJOR FUNCTIONS	SIGNS OF PROLONGED DEFICIENCY	TOXIC EFFECTS OF MEGADOSES
Calcium	Milk and milk products, tofu, fortified orange juice and bread, green leafy vegetables, bones in fish	Formation of bones and teeth; control of nerve impulses, muscle contraction, blood clotting	Stunted growth in children, bone mineral loss in adults; urinary stones	Kidney stones, calcium deposits in soft tissues, inhibition of mineral absorption, constipation
Fluoride	Fluoridated water, tea, marine fish eaten with bones	Maintenance of tooth and bone structure	Higher frequency of tooth decay	Increased bone density, mottling of teeth, impaired kidney function
Iodine	Iodized salt, seafood, processed foods	Essential part of thyroid hormones, regulation of body metabolism	Goiter (enlarged thyroid), cretinism (birth defect)	Depression of thyroid activity, hyperthyroidism in susceptible people
Iron	Meat and poultry, fortified grain products, dark green vegetables, dried fruit	Component of hemoglobin, myoglobin, and enzymes	Iron-deficiency anemia, weakness, impaired immune function, gastrointestinal distress	Nausea, diarrhea, liver and kidney damage, joint pains, sterility, disruption of cardiac function, death
Magnesium	Widespread in foods and water (except soft water); especially found in grains, legumes, nuts, seeds, green vegetables, milk	Transmission of nerve impulses, energy transfer, activation of many enzymes	Neurological disturbances, cardiovascular problems, kidney disorders, nausea, growth failure in children	Nausea, vomiting, diarrhea, central nervous system depression, coma; death in people with impaired kidney function
Phosphorus	Present in nearly all foods, especially milk, cereal, peas, eggs, meat	Bone growth and maintenance, energy transfer in cells	Impaired growth, weakness, kidney disorders, cardiorespiratory and nervous system dysfunction	Drop in blood calcium levels, calcium deposits in soft tissues, bone loss
Potassium	Meats, milk, fruits, vegetables, grains, legumes	Nerve function and body water balance	Muscular weakness, nausea, drowsiness, paralysis, confusion, disruption of cardiac rhythm	Cardiac arrest
Selenium	Seafood, meat, eggs, whole grains	Defense against oxidative stress; regulation of thyroid hormone action	Muscle pain and weakness, heart disorders	Hair and nail loss, nausea and vomiting, weakness, irritability
Sodium	Salt, soy sauce, fast food, processed foods, especially lunch meats, canned soups and vegetables, salty snacks, processed cheese	Body water balance, acid-base balance, nerve function	Muscle weakness, loss of appetite, nausea, vomiting; deficiency rarely seen	Edema, hypertension in sensitive people
Zinc	Whole grains, meat, eggs, liver, seafood (especially oysters)	Synthesis of proteins, RNA, and DNA; wound healing; immune response; ability to taste	Growth failure, loss of appetite, impaired taste acuity, skin rash, impaired immune function, poor wound healing	Vomiting, impaired immune function, decline in blood HDL levels, impaired copper absorption

SOURCES: Food and Nutrition Board, Institute of Medicine. 2006. *Dietary Reference Intakes: The Essential Guide to Nutrient Requirements.* Washington, D.C.: National Academies Press. The complete Dietary Reference Intake reports are available from the National Academies Press (http://www.nap.edu). Shils, M. E., et al., eds. 2005. *Modern Nutrition in Health and Disease,* 10th ed. Baltimore: Lippincott Williams and Wilkins.

age groups, and researchers fear poor calcium intakes in childhood are sowing the seeds for future **osteoporosis**, especially in women. See the box "Eating for Healthy Bones" to learn more.

Water—Vital but Often Ignored

Water is the major component in both foods and the human body: You are composed of about 50–60% water. Your need for other nutrients, in terms of weight, is much less than your need for water. You can live up to 50 days without food but only a few days without water.

Water is distributed all over the body, among lean and other tissues and in blood and other body fluids. Water is used in the digestion and absorption of food and is the medium in which most chemical reactions take place within the body. Some water-based fluids, such as blood, transport substances around the body; other fluids serve as lubricants or cushions. Water also helps regulate body temperature.

Eating for Healthy Bones

TAKE CHARGE

Osteoporosis is a condition in which the bones become dangerously thin and fragile over time. An estimated 10 million Americans over age 50 have osteoporosis, and another 34 million are at risk. Women account for about 80% of osteoporosis cases.

Most bone mass is built by age 18. After bone density peaks between ages 25 and 35, bone mass is lost over time. To prevent osteoporosis, the best strategy is to build as much bone as possible during your youth and do everything you can to maintain it as you age. Up to 50% of bone loss is determined by controllable lifestyle factors such as diet and exercise. Key nutrients for bone health include the following:

- ***Calcium.*** Getting enough calcium is important throughout life to build and maintain bone mass. Milk, yogurt, and calcium-fortified orange juice, bread, and cereals are all good sources.
- ***Vitamin D.*** Vitamin D is necessary for bones to absorb calcium; a daily intake of 600 IU is recommended for individuals age 1–70. Vitamin D can be obtained from foods and is manufactured by the skin when exposed to sunlight. Candidates for vitamin D supplements include people who don't eat many foods rich in vitamin D; those who don't expose their face, arms, and hands to the sun (without sunscreen) for 5–15 minutes a few times each week; and people who live north of an imaginary line drawn across the United States from Boston to the Oregon-California border (where the sun is weaker).
- ***Vitamin K.*** Vitamin K promotes the synthesis of proteins that help keep bones strong. Broccoli and leafy green vegetables are rich in vitamin K.
- ***Other nutrients.*** Other nutrients that may play an important role in bone health include vitamin C, magnesium, potassium, phosphorus, fluoride, manganese, zinc, copper, and boron.

Several dietary substances may have a *negative* effect on bone health, especially if consumed in excess. These include alcohol, sodium, caffeine, and retinol (a form of vitamin A). Drinking lots of soda, which often replaces milk in the diet, has been shown to increase the risk of bone fracture in teenage girls.

The effect of protein intake on bone mass depends on other nutrients: Protein helps build bone as long as calcium and vitamin D intake are adequate. But if intake of calcium and vitamin D is low, high protein intake can lead to bone loss.

Weight-bearing aerobic exercise helps maintain bone mass throughout life, and strength training improves bone density, muscle mass, strength, and balance. Drinking alcohol only in moderation, refraining from smoking, and managing depression and stress are also important for maintaining strong bones. For people who develop osteoporosis, a variety of medications are available to treat the condition.

Water is contained in almost all foods, particularly in liquids, fruits, and vegetables. The foods and fluids you consume provide 80–90% of your daily water intake; the remainder is generated through metabolism. You lose water each day in urine, feces, and sweat and through evaporation from your lungs.

Most people can maintain a healthy water balance by consuming beverages at meals and drinking fluids in response to thirst. The Food and Nutrition Board has set levels of adequate water intake to maintain hydration. All fluids, including those containing caffeine, can count toward your total daily fluid intake. Under these guidelines, men need to consume about 3.7 total liters of water, with 3.0 liters (about 13 cups) coming from beverages; women need 2.7 total liters, with 2.2 liters (about 9 cups) coming from beverages. About 20% of daily water intake comes from food. (See Table 1 in the Nutrition Resources section at the end of the chapter for recommendations for specific age groups.) If you exercise vigorously or live in a hot climate, you need to consume additional fluids to maintain a balance between water consumed and water lost. Severe dehydration causes weakness and can lead to death.

Other Substances in Food

Many substances in food are not essential nutrients but may influence health.

Antioxidants When the body uses oxygen or breaks down certain fats or proteins as a normal part of metabolism, it gives rise to substances called **free radicals.** Environmental factors such as cigarette smoke, exhaust fumes, radiation, excessive sunlight, certain drugs, and stress can increase free radical production. A free radical is a

Fitness Tip

Drink plenty of water before, during, and after workouts, especially when the weather is warm. Proper hydration helps you avoid cramps and heat-related problems such as heat stroke.

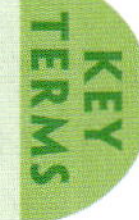

KEY TERMS

osteoporosis A condition in which the bones become extremely thin and brittle and break easily; due largely to insufficient calcium intake.

free radical An electron-seeking compound that can react with fats, proteins, and DNA, damaging cell membranes and mutating genes in its search for electrons; produced through chemical reactions in the body and by exposure to environmental factors such as sunlight and tobacco smoke.

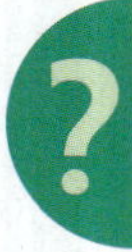

Ask Yourself

QUESTIONS FOR CRITICAL THINKING AND REFLECTION

Experts say that two of the most important factors in a healthy diet are eating the "right" kinds of carbohydrates and eating the "right" kinds of fats. Based on what you've read so far in this chapter, which are the "right" carbohydrates and the "right" fats? How would you say your own diet stacks up when it comes to carbs and fats?

chemically unstable molecule that reacts with fats, proteins, and DNA, damaging cell membranes and mutating genes. Free radicals have been implicated in aging, cancer, cardiovascular disease, and other degenerative diseases like arthritis.

Antioxidants found in foods can help protect the body by blocking the formation and action of free radicals and repairing the damage they cause. Some antioxidants, such as vitamin C, vitamin E, and selenium, are also essential nutrients. Others—such as carotenoids, found in yellow, orange, and dark green leafy vegetables—are not. Researchers recently identified the top antioxidant-containing foods and beverages as blackberries, walnuts, strawberries, artichokes, cranberries, brewed coffee, raspberries, pecans, blueberries, cloves, grape juice, unsweetened baking chocolate, sour cherries, and red wine. Also high in antioxidants are brussels sprouts, kale, cauliflower, and pomegranates.

Phytochemicals Antioxidants fall into the broader category of **phytochemicals**, substances found in plant foods that may help prevent chronic disease. In the past 30 years, researchers have identified and studied hundreds of different compounds found in foods, and many findings are promising. For example, certain substances found in soy foods may help lower cholesterol levels. Sulforaphane, a compound isolated from broccoli and other **cruciferous vegetables**, may render some carcinogenic compounds harmless. Allyl sulfides, a group of chemicals found in garlic and onions, appear to boost the activity of cancer-fighting immune cells. Carotenoids found in green vegetables may help preserve eyesight with age. Further research on phytochemicals may extend the role of nutrition to the prevention and treatment of many chronic diseases.

To increase your intake of phytochemicals, eat a variety of fruits, vegetables, and grains rather than relying on supplements. Like many vitamins and minerals, isolated phytochemicals may be harmful if taken in high doses. In many cases, their health benefits may be the result of chemical substances working in combination. The role of phytochemicals in disease prevention is discussed further in Chapter 5.

NUTRITIONAL GUIDELINES: PLANNING YOUR DIET

Various tools have been created by scientific and government groups to help people design healthy diets:

- The **Dietary Reference Intakes (DRIs)** are standards for nutrient intake designed to prevent nutritional deficiencies and reduce the risk of chronic diseases.
- The **Dietary Guidelines for Americans** were established to promote health and reduce the risk of major chronic diseases through diet and physical activity.
- **MyPlate** (formerly MyPyramid) provides daily food intake patterns that meet the DRIs and are consistent with the Dietary Guidelines for Americans.

Dietary Reference Intakes (DRIs)

The Food and Nutrition Board establishes dietary standards, or recommended intake levels, for Americans of all ages. The current set of standards, called Dietary Reference Intakes (DRIs), was introduced in 1997. The DRIs are frequently reviewed and are updated as substantial new nutrition-related information becomes available. The DRIs present different categories of nutrients in easy-to-read table format. The DRIs have a broad focus, being based on research that looks not just at the prevention of nutrient deficiencies but also at the role of nutrients in promoting health and preventing chronic diseases such as cancer, osteoporosis, and heart disease.

The DRIs include standards for both recommended intakes and maximum safe intakes. The recommended intake of each nutrient is expressed as either a *Recommended Dietary Allowance (RDA)* or as *Adequate Intake (AI)*. An AI is set when there is not enough information available to set an RDA value; regardless of the type of standard used, however, the DRI represents the best available estimate of intake for optimal health. The Estimated Average Requirement (EAR) is the average daily nutrient intake level estimated to meet the requirement of half the healthy individuals in a particular life stage and gender group. The *Tolerable Upper Intake Level (UL)* is the maximum daily intake that is unlikely to cause health problems in a healthy person. For example, the RDA for calcium for an 18-year-old female is 1300 milligrams (mg) per day; the UL is 3000 milligrams per day.

Because of a lack of data, ULs have not been set for all nutrients. This does not mean that people can tolerate long-term intakes of these vitamins and minerals above recommended levels. Like all chemical agents, nutrients can produce adverse effects if intakes are excessive. There is no established benefit from consuming nutrients at levels above the RDA or AI. The DRIs can be found in the Nutrition Resources section at the end of the chapter.

Daily Values Because the DRIs are too cumbersome to use as a basis for food labels, the FDA developed another set of dietary standards, the **Daily Values.** The Daily Values are based on several different sets of guidelines and include standards for fat, cholesterol, carbohydrate, dietary fiber, and selected vitamins and minerals. The Daily Values represent appropriate intake levels for a 2000-calorie diet. The percent Daily Value shown on a food label shows how well that food contributes to your recommended daily intake. Food labels are described in detail later in the chapter.

Should You Take Supplements? The aim of the DRIs is to guide you in meeting your nutritional needs primarily with food, rather than with vitamin and mineral supplements. Supplements lack potentially beneficial phytochemicals and fiber that are found only in whole foods. Most Americans can get the vitamins and minerals they need by eating a varied, nutritionally balanced diet.

The question of whether to take supplements is a serious one. Some vitamins and minerals are dangerous when ingested in excess, as described previously in Tables 3.4 and 3.5. Large doses of particular nutrients can also cause health problems by affecting the absorption of other vitamins and minerals. For all these reasons, you should think carefully about whether to take high-dose supplements; consider consulting a physician or registered dietitian.

Over the past two decades, high-dose supplement use has been promoted as a way to prevent or delay the onset of many diseases, including heart disease and several forms of cancer. These claims remain controversial, however, and a growing body of research shows that vitamin or mineral supplements have no significant impact on the risk of developing such illnesses. For example, a 2008 study conducted as part of the Women's Health Initiative showed no differences in the levels of heart disease, cancer, or overall mortality between postmenopausal women who took multivitamin supplements and those who did not. A similar study of adult men indicated that taking vitamins C and E did not reduce the risk of heart disease or certain cancers. According to the experts behind these and other studies, the research provides further proof that a balanced diet of whole foods—not high-dose supplementation—is the best way to promote health and prevent disease.

In setting the DRIs, the Food and Nutrition Board recommended supplements of particular nutrients for the following groups:

- Women who are capable of becoming pregnant should take 400 micrograms (μg) per day of folic acid (the synthetic form of the vitamin folate) from fortified foods and/or supplements in addition to folate from a varied diet. Research indicates that this level of folate intake will reduce the risk of neural tube defects. Enriched breads, flours, corn meals, rice, noodles, and other grain products are fortified with folic acid. Folate is found naturally in green leafy vegetables, legumes, oranges, and strawberries.
- People over age 50 should eat foods fortified with vitamin B-12, take B-12 supplements, or both to meet the majority of the DRI of 2.4 micrograms of B-12 daily. Up to 30% of people over 50 may have problems absorbing protein-bound B-12 in foods.
- Because of the oxidative stress caused by smoking, smokers should get 35 milligrams *more* vitamin C per day than the RDA set for their age and sex. However, supplements are not usually needed because this extra vitamin C can easily be found in foods. For example, an 8-ounce glass of orange juice has about 100 mg of vitamin C.

Supplements may also be recommended in other cases. Women with heavy menstrual flows may need extra iron. Older people, people with dark skin, and people exposed to little sunlight may need extra vitamin D. Some vegetarians may need supplemental calcium, iron, zinc, and vitamin B-12, depending on their food choices. Other people may benefit from supplementation based on their lifestyle physical condition, medicines, or dietary habits.

Before deciding whether to take a vitamin or mineral supplement, consider whether you already eat a fortified breakfast cereal every day. Many breakfast cereals contain almost as many nutrients as a multivitamin pill. If you

Wellness Tip

If you take a supplement, *never* take more than the recommended dosage unless your doctor tells you to.

KEY TERMS

phytochemical A naturally occurring substance found in plant foods that may help prevent and treat chronic diseases such as heart disease and cancer; *phyto* means "plant."

cruciferous vegetables Vegetables of the cabbage family, including cabbage, broccoli, brussels sprouts, kale, and cauliflower; the flower petals of these plants form the shape of a cross, hence the name.

Dietary Reference Intakes (DRIs) An umbrella term for four types of nutrient standards: Adequate Intake (AI), Estimated Average Requirement (EAR), and Recommended Dietary Allowance (RDA) are levels of intake considered adequate to prevent nutrient deficiencies and reduce the risk of chronic disease; Tolerable Upper Intake Level (UL) is the maximum daily intake that is unlikely to cause health problems.

Dietary Guidelines for Americans General principles of good nutrition intended to help prevent certain diet-related diseases.

MyPlate A food-group plan that provides practical advice to ensure a balanced intake of the essential nutrients.

Daily Values A simplified version of the RDAs used on food labels; also included are values for nutrients with no established RDA.

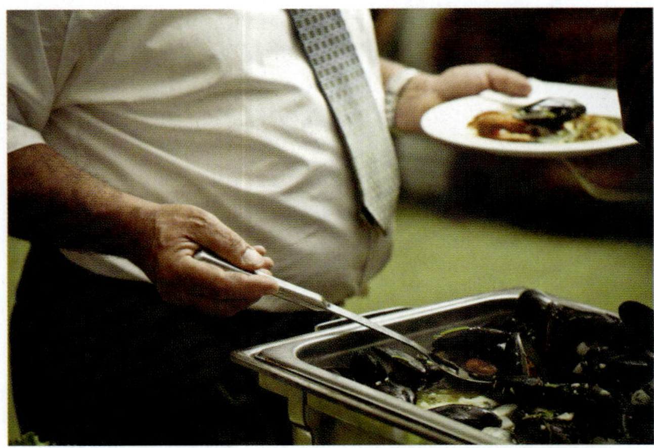

Food choices and portion control are key factors in weight management.

elect to take a supplement, choose one that contains 50–100% of the Daily Value for vitamins and minerals. Avoid supplements containing large doses of nutrients that may be harmful.

Dietary Guidelines for Americans

To provide general guidance for choosing a healthy diet, the USDA and the U.S. Department of Health and Human Services (DHHS) jointly issue the Dietary Guidelines for Americans, updating and revising the guidelines every 5 years. The guidelines are intended for all Americans aged 2 and older. Following these guidelines promotes health and reduces the risk of chronic diseases, including heart disease, cancer, diabetes, stroke, osteoporosis, and obesity. Each of the recommendations is supported by an extensive review of scientific and medical evidence.

The 2010 Dietary Guidelines highlight four areas. First, because the majority of Americans are overweight or obese, the guidelines focus on ways to balance calorie consumption and calorie expenditure to manage weight. Second, because Americans also tend to consume too many calories without getting enough of certain nutrients, the guidelines focus on foods to reduce in the diet (the second highlighted area) and foods to increase in the diet (the third highlighted area). Finally, the guidelines focus on ways to incorporate the recommendations into overall healthy eating patterns. Specific recommendations for putting the Dietary Guidelines into practice are provided in MyPlate (discussed in the next section).

Balancing Calories to Manage Weight Calorie balance—the balance between calories consumed and calories expended—is the key to weight management. Current high rates of overweight and obesity can be attributed at least in part to people consuming more calories in foods and beverages than they expend in physical activity.

The guidelines recognize that many aspects of American life promote obesity, leading to an "obesogenic food environment." Factors contributing to this environment include an increase in the number of fast-food restaurants in communities, an increase in meals eaten outside the home, increased portion sizes, sedentary work and home environments, limited availability of safe outdoor walking and recreational spaces, and increased dependence on transportation and technological advances that lead to lower calorie expenditure on everyday tasks.

Still, managing body weight means that individuals need to control total calorie intake, and for people who are overweight or obese, this means consuming fewer calories from foods and beverages. The guidelines encourage people to become more conscious of what, when, why, and how much they eat; to deliberately make better choices; and to seek ways to be more physically active. Several specific behaviors and practices can help people manage their calorie balance and maintain a healthy weight. Recommendations include:

- Know what calorie level is appropriate for you at your current level of activity, and be aware of how many calories you are consuming.
- Cook at home more and eat out less, and when you do eat out, eat smaller portions and lower-calorie options.
- Limit screen time, whether watching television, playing games, or using a computer, and don't eat when watching TV.

Foods and Food Components to Reduce In addition to overall calories, Americans tend to consume certain foods and food components in excess—in particular, sodium, solid fats, added sugars, and refined grains. These foods often replace needed nutrients in the diet. Key recommendations include:

- Reduce daily sodium intake to less than 2300 mg, and further reduce intake to 1500 mg if you are 51 or older, are African American, or have hypertension, diabetes, or chronic kidney disease. The 1500 mg recommendation applies to about half the U.S. population, including children, and the majority of adults. The average intake of sodium for all Americans is estimated at 3400 mg; for boys and men between the ages of 12 and 50, it is estimated at more than 4000 mg. High sodium intake is associated with high blood pressure. Most salt in the diet comes from salt added during food processing.
- Limit intake of saturated fat, trans fat, and dietary cholesterol. Consume less than 10% of calories from saturated fats by replacing them with monounsaturated and polyunsaturated fats. Keep trans fatty acid consumption as low as possible, especially by limiting foods that contain synthetic sources of trans fats, such as partially hydrogenated oils. (See the

Nutrient	Recommended Daily Intake* 2000 calories	Orange Juice 168 calories % Daily	Orange Juice Nutrient value	Low-Fat (1%) Milk 150 calories % Daily	Low-Fat (1%) Milk Nutrient value	Regular Cola 152 calories % Daily	Regular Cola Nutrient value	Bottled Iced Tea 150 calories % Daily	Bottled Iced Tea Nutrient value
Carbohydrate	300 g	14%	40.5 g	6%	18 g	13%	38 g	13%	37.5 g
Added sugars	32 g					119%	38 g +	108%	34.5 g +
Fat	65 g			6%	3.9 g				
Protein	55 g			22%	12 g				
Calcium	1000 mg	3%	33 mg	45%	450 mg	1%	11 mg		
Potassium	4700 mg	15%	710 mg	12%	570 mg	<1%	4 mg		
Vitamin A	700 µg	4%	30 µg	31%	216 µg				
Vitamin C	75 mg	193%	145.5 mg +	5%	3.6 mg				
Vitamin D	5 µg			74%	3.7 µg				
Folate	400 µg	40%	160 µg	5%	20 µg				

Bars show percentage of recommended daily intake or limit

+ = Greater than 100% of recommended

*Recommended intakes and limits appropriate for a 20-year-old woman consuming 2000 calories per day.

FIGURE 3.3 Nutrient density of 12-ounce portions of selected beverages.
Color bars represent percentage of recommended daily intake or limit for each nutrient.

box "Reducing the Saturated and Trans Fats in Your Diet" for more information.) Consume less than 300 mg per day of dietary cholesterol.

- Reduce the intake of calories from solid fats and added sugars. Together, solid fats and added sugars contribute about 35% of the calories consumed by Americans, without contributing many nutrients. Most people should consume no more than 5–15% of daily calories from foods in these categories. Suggestions include limiting the amount of solid fats and added sugars when cooking and eating; consuming smaller and fewer portions of foods and beverages with these components, such as desserts and sodas; and eating the most nutrient-dense forms of foods in all food groups. Sodas, energy drinks, and sports drinks are the biggest source of added sugars in the American diet. The differences in nutrients between soda and other beverages are shown in Figure 3.3.
- Limit the consumption of foods that contain refined grains, especially refined grain foods that contain solid fats, added sugars, and sodium.

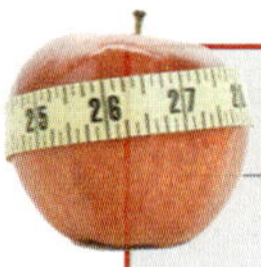

Wellness Tip

About a dozen major American cities, and the entire state of California, have enacted laws restricting the use of trans fats in commercially prepared foods.

- If alcohol is consumed, it should be consumed in moderation.

Foods and Nutrients to Increase In general, Americans don't eat a wide enough variety of nutrient-dense foods to obtain all the nutrients they need for optimal health. Recommendations include:

- Eat more fruits and vegetables, and eat a variety of vegetables, especially dark green, red, and orange vegetables and beans and peas. These foods are major sources of many nutrients that are underconsumed by many Americans, and they are relatively low in calories (unless prepared with added fats and sugars).
- Consume at least half of all grains as whole grains, which are a source of important nutrients such as iron, B vitamins, and dietary fiber.
- Increase intake of fat-free and low-fat milk and milk products, such as milk, yogurt, cheese, and fortified soy beverages. These foods are important sources of calcium, potassium, magnesium, vitamin D, and vitamin A. Milk and yogurt are preferable to cheese, which has more solid fat and more calories.
- Choose a variety of protein foods, including seafood, lean meat and poultry, eggs, beans and peas, soy products, and unsalted nuts and seeds. Increase the amount and variety of seafood, and reduce protein foods that are high in solid fats and calories. In addition to protein, these foods provide B vitamins,

TAKE CHARGE

Reducing the Saturated and Trans Fats in Your Diet

Your overall goal is to limit total fat intake to no more than 35% of total calories. Favor unsaturated fats over saturated and trans fats. Here are some steps that can help reduce these types of fat in your diet:

- Be moderate in your consumption of foods high in fat, including fast foods, commercially prepared baked goods and desserts, deep-fried food, meat, poultry, nuts and seeds, and regular dairy products.
- When you eat high-fat foods, limit your portion sizes, and balance your intake with other foods that are low in fat.
- Choose lean cuts of meat, and trim any visible fat from meat before and after cooking. Remove skin from poultry before or after cooking.
- Drink fat-free or low-fat milk instead of whole milk, and use lower-fat milk when cooking or baking. Substitute plain low-fat yogurt, low-fat cottage cheese, or buttermilk for sour cream.
- Use vegetable oil instead of butter or margarine. Use tub or squeeze margarine instead of stick margarine. Look for margarines that are free of trans fats. Minimize intake of coconut or palm oil.
- Season vegetables, seafood, and meats with herbs and spices rather than with creamy sauces, butter, or margarine.
- Use olive oil and lemon juice on salad, or use a yogurt-based salad dressing instead of mayonnaise or sour cream dressings.
- Steam, boil, bake, or microwave vegetables, or stir-fry them in a small amount of vegetable oil.
- Roast, bake, or broil meat, poultry, or fish so that fat drains away as the food cooks.
- Use a nonstick pan for cooking so that added fat will be unnecessary; use a vegetable spray for frying.
- Substitute egg whites for whole eggs when baking; limit the number of egg yolks when scrambling eggs.
- Choose fruits as desserts most often.
- Eat a low-fat vegetarian main dish at least once a week.

vitamin E, zinc, and magnesium. Seafood provides a range of nutrients, notably omega-3 fatty acids, which are associated with reduced risk of heart disease. (Seafood consumption is discussed in more detail later in the chapter.)

- Replace solid fats with oils where possible. Oils should not be added to the diet in addition to solid fats; instead, they should replace them.
- Because most Americans do not get enough potassium, dietary fiber, calcium, or vitamin D in their diet, they should consume more foods that contain these nutrients.
  - Potassium, which can help lower blood pressure, is found in many fruits, vegetables, and milk products. Recommended intake is 4700 mg per day.
  - Dietary fiber is found in beans and peas, other vegetables, fruits, nuts, and whole grains. Recommended daily intake for fiber is 25 g for women and 38 g for men; the current average daily intake is only about 15 g.
  - Calcium plays several important roles in health, including bone health. Low intake of calcium is a concern in children 9 and older, adolescent girls, adult women, and all adults age 51 and older. The chief sources of calcium in the diet are milk and milk products.
  - Vitamin D also has an important role in bone health. Chief sources are fortified foods, especially milk and yogurt.
- Other nutrients are a concern for certain special population groups, such as folic acid for women who may become pregnant.

Building Healthy Eating Patterns There are many different ways to incorporate the recommendations of the 2010 Dietary Guidelines into healthy eating patterns that (1) meet nutrient needs; (2) stay within calorie limits; (3) accommodate cultural, ethnic, traditional, and personal preferences; and (4) consider food cost and availability. In other words, people can eat healthfully in many different ways. Currently, howevere, there is a large discrepancy between the guidelines and the actual American diet.

Three eating plans that show how to put the Dietary Guidelines recommendations into action are the USDA Food Pattern (MyPlate), vegetarian adaptations of the USDA Food Pattern, and the DASH Eating Plan. (MyPlate and vegetarian diets are discussed later in the chapter, and the DASH Eating Plan is explained in the Nutrition Resources section at the end of this chapter.) A general principle in all these diets is that people should eat nutrient-dense foods—foods with little or no solid fats and added sugars. Another principle is that people should get their nutrients from foods rather than from supplements, although dietary supplements or fortification may be helpful in certain situations.

Helping Americans Make Healthy Choices A final area covered by the 2010 Dietary Guidelines for Americans is the environment in which people make their food choices.

To make healthy choices, individuals need *opportunities* to obtain healthy foods and engage in physical activity. Significant numbers of Americans—notably, members of racial and ethnic minorities, people with disabilities, and people with lower incomes—lack access to affordable, nutritious foods and/or opportunities for safe physical activity in their neighborhoods. The guidelines recognize the problem of *food security* in the United States—the ability to acquire adequate food to meet nutritional needs. Nearly 15% of the population is not able to obtain sufficient food to meet basic nutritional needs, and as noted above, many more Americans have diets that provide adequate calories but are deficient in essential nutrients.

The Dietary Guidelines propose the Social Ecological Model as a way to understand and address these complex problems. This model considers the interaction among individual factors (such as gender, income, and race/ethnicity), environmental settings (such as schools, workplaces, and restaurants), various sectors of influence (such as health care systems, agriculture, and media), and social and cultural norms and values (such as assumptions regarding body weight, types of foods consumed, and amount of physical activity incorporated into one's free time). All these factors play a role in a person's food and physical activity choices—and ultimately, in the person's health risks and outcomes.

The guidelines call on all elements of society, ranging from educators to communities to government policy makers, to implement strategies aimed at improving the food and activity environment in the United States. Examples of such strategies are expanding access to grocery stores, farmers markets, and other sources of healthy food; ensuring that meals and snacks served in schools are consistent with the Dietary Guidelines; encouraging physical activity in schools; developing policies to limit food and beverage marketing to children; supporting sustainable agricultural practices; and providing nutrition assistance programs. Such measures have the potential to improve the health of current and future generations by making healthy physical activity and eating choices the norm.

USDA's MyPlate

To help consumers put the Dietary Guidelines for Americans into practice, the USDA also issues the food guidance system known as MyPlate (called MyPyramid until 2011). MyPlate is designed for individuals to take advantage of the customization made possible by the Internet (Figure 3.4).

Key Messages of MyPlate MyPlate was developed to remind consumers to make healthy food choices and to be active every day. Key messages include the following:

- *Personalization* is an important element of the MyPlate program and the ChooseMyPlate.gov site, which includes individualized recommendations, interactive assessments of food intake and physical activity, weight-management tools, and tips for success.
- *Daily physical activity* is important for maintaining a healthy weight and reducing the risk of chronic disease.
- *Moderation* of food intake is represented by advice to use smaller plates and to carefully watch portion sizes.
- *Proportionality* is represented by the different sizes of the food groups on the plate. The serving sizes provide a general guide for how much food a person should choose from each group.
- *Variety* is represented by the five food groups. Foods from all groups are needed daily for good health.
- *Gradual improvement* is a good strategy; people can benefit from taking small steps to improve their diet and activity habits each day.

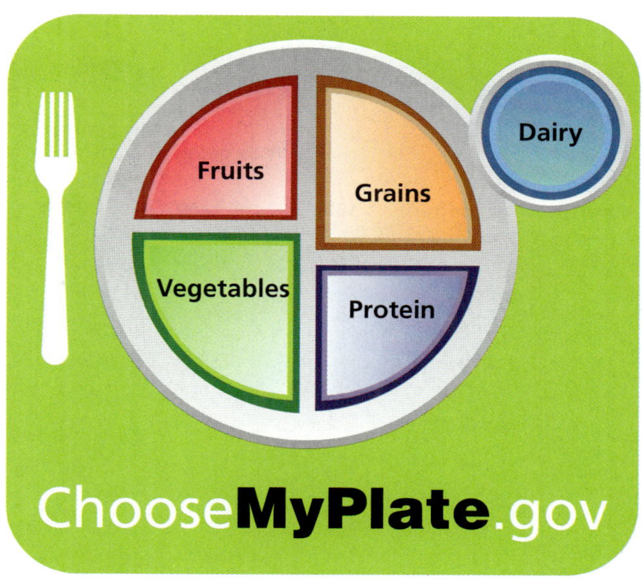

FIGURE 3.4 USDA's MyPlate.
The USDA food guidance system, called MyPlate, can be personalized based on an individual's sex, age, and activity level; visit www.ChooseMyPlate.gov to obtain a food plan appropriate for you.
SOURCE: U.S. Department of Agriculture. 2011. *MyPlate* (http://www.choosemyplate.gov; retrieved August 6, 2011).

The MyPlate chart in Figure 3.5 shows the food intake patterns recommended for different levels of calorie intake. Table 3.6 provides guidance for determining an appropriate calorie intake for weight maintenance. Use the table to identify an energy intake that is about right for you, and then refer to the appropriate column in Figure 3.5. You can also get a personalized version of MyPlate recommendations by visiting ChooseMyPlate.gov. Each food group is described briefly in the following sections. Many Americans have trouble identifying serving sizes, so recommended daily intakes from each group are given in terms of cups and ounces; see the box "Judging Portion Sizes" for additional advice.

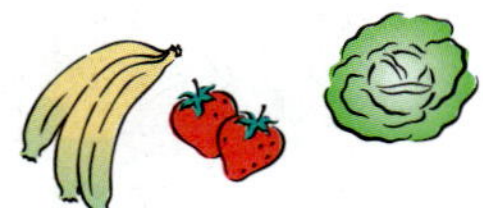
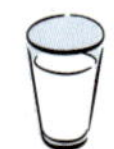
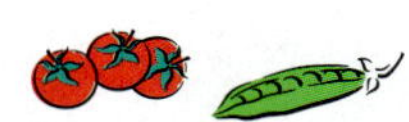
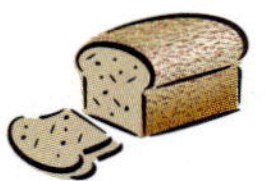
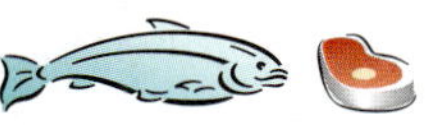
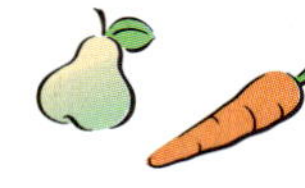
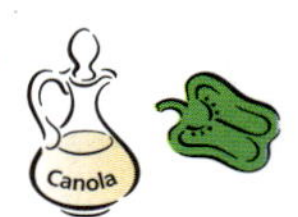

Daily Amount of Food from Each Group
Food group amounts shown in cups (c) or ounce-equivalents (oz-eq)

Calorie level of pattern	1600	1800	2000	2200	2400	2600	2800	3000
Fruits	1.5 c	1.5 c	2 c	2 c	2 c	2 c	2.5 c	2.5 c
Vegetables	2 c	2.5 c	2.5 c	3 c	3 c	3.5 c	3.5 c	4 c
Dark-green	1.5 c/wk	1.5 c/wk	1.5 c/wk	2 c/wk	2 c/wk	2.5 c/wk	2.5 c/wk	2.5 c/wk
Red and orange	4 c/wk	5.5 c/wk	5.5 c/wk	6 c/wk	6 c/wk	7 c/wk	7 c/wk	7.5 c/wk
Beans and peas (legumes)	1 c/wk	1.5 c/wk	1.5 c/wk	2 c/wk	2 c/wk	2.5 c/wk	2.5 c/wk	3 c/wk
Starchy	4 c/wk	5 c/wk	5 c/wk	6 c/wk	6 c/wk	7 c/wk	7 c/wk	8 c/wk
Other	3.5 c/wk	4 c/wk	4 c/wk	5 c/wk	5 c/wk	5.5 c/wk	5.5 c/wk	7 c/wk
Grains	5 oz-eq	6 oz-eq	6 oz-eq	7 oz-eq	8 oz-eq	9 oz-eq	10 oz-eq	10 oz-eq
Whole grains	3 oz-eq	3 oz-eq	3 oz-eq	3.5 oz-eq	4 oz-eq	4.5 oz-eq	5 oz-eq	5 oz-eq
Enriched grains	2 oz-eq	3 oz-eq	3 oz-eq	3.5 oz-eq	4 oz-eq	4.5 oz-eq	5 oz-eq	5 oz-eq
Protein foods	5 oz-eq	5 oz-eq	5.5 oz-eq	6 oz-eq	6.5 oz-eq	6.5 oz-eq	7 oz-eq	7 oz-eq
Seafood	8 oz/wk	8 oz/wk	8 oz/wk	9 oz/wk	10 oz/wk	10 oz/wk	11 oz/wk	11 oz/wk
Meat poultry, eggs	24 oz/wk	24 oz/wk	26 oz/wk	29 oz/wk	31 oz/wk	31 oz/wk	34 oz/wk	34 oz/wk
Nuts, seeds, soy products	4 oz/wk	4 oz/wk	4 oz/wk	4 oz/wk	5 oz/wk	5 oz/wk	5 oz/wk	5 oz/wk
Dairy	3 c	3 c	3 c	3 c	3 c	3 c	3 c	3 c
Oils	22 g	24 g	27 g	29 g	31 g	34 g	36 g	44 g
Maximum SoFAS limit, calories (% of calories)	121 (8%)	161 (9%)	258 (13%)	266 (12%)	330 (14%)	362 (14%)	395 (14%)	459 (15%)

FIGURE 3.5 MyPlate food intake patterns.
To determine an appropriate amount of food from each group, find the column with your approximate daily energy intake. That column lists the daily recommended intake from each food group. Visit ChooseMyPlate.gov for a personalized intake plan and for intakes for other calorie levels.
SOURCE: U.S. Department of Health and Human Services and U.S. Department of Agriculture. 2011. *Dietary Guidelines for Americans, 2010, Appendix 7. USDA Food Patterns* (http://www.cnpp.usda.gov/Publications/DietaryGuidelines/2010/PolicyDoc/PolicyDoc.pdf; retrieved August 7, 2011).

Whole and Refined Grains Foods from this group are usually low in fat and rich in complex carbohydrates, dietary fiber (if grains are unrefined), and many vitamins and minerals. A 2000-calorie diet should include 6 ounce-equivalents each day. The following count as 1 ounce-equivalent:

- 1 slice of bread
- 1 small (2½-inch diameter) muffin
- 1 cup ready-to-eat cereal flakes
- ½ cup cooked cereal, rice, grains, or pasta
- 1 6-inch tortilla

Choose foods that are typically made with little fat or added sugar (bread, rice, pasta) over those that are high in fat and added sugar (croissants, chips, cookies, doughnuts). The key message is to make at least half your grains whole grains.

Vegetables Vegetables contain carbohydrates, dietary fiber, and many other nutrients, and they are naturally low in fat. A 2000-calorie diet should include 2½ cups of

Judging Portion Sizes

TAKE CHARGE

Studies have shown that most people underestimate the size of their food portions, in many cases by as much as 50%. If you need to retrain your eye, try using measuring cups and spoons and an inexpensive kitchen scale when you eat at home. With a little practice, you'll learn the difference between 3 and 8 ounces of chicken or meat, and what a half-cup of rice really looks like. For quick estimates, use the following equivalents:

- 1 teaspoon of margarine = one dice
- 1 ½ ounce of cheese = your thumb, four dice stacked together
- 3 ounces of chicken or meat = a deck of cards
- ½ cup of cooked rice, pasta, or potato = ½ baseball
- 1 cup of cereal flakes = a fist
- 2 tablespoons of peanut butter = a ping-pong ball
- 1 medium potato = a computer mouse
- 1–2-ounce muffin or roll = a plum or large egg
- 2-ounce bagel = a hockey puck or yo-yo
- 1 medium fruit (apple or orange) = a baseball
- ¼ cup nuts = a golf ball
- Small cookie or cracker = a poker chip

vegetables daily. Each of the following counts as 1/2 cup or equivalent of vegetables:

- ½ cup raw or cooked vegetables
- 1 cup raw leafy salad greens
- ½ cup vegetable juice

Because vegetables vary in the nutrients they provide, MyPlate recommends servings from five different subgroups within the vegetables group. Choose vegetables from several subgroups each day. (For clarity, Figure 3.5 shows servings from the subgroups in terms of weekly consumption.) The key message is to fill half your plate with fruits and vegetables.

Fruits Fruits are rich in carbohydrates, dietary fiber, and many vitamins, especially vitamin C. A 2000-calorie diet should include 2 cups of fruits daily. Each of the following counts as ½ cup or equivalent of fruit:

- ½ cup fresh, canned, or frozen fruit
- ½ cup fruit juice (100% juice)
- ½ large (3½" diameter) whole fruit
- ¼ cup dried fruit

Choose whole fruits often; they are higher in fiber and often lower in calories than fruit juices. Fruit *juices* typically contain more nutrients and less added sugar than fruit *drinks*. Choose canned fruits packed in 100% fruit juice or water rather than in syrup. Again, MyPlate's key message for consumers is to fill half your plate with fruits and vegetables.

Dairy This group includes all milk and milk products, as well as lactose-free and lactose-reduced products. Those consuming 2000 calories per day should include 3 cups of milk or the equivalent daily. Each of the following counts as the equivalent of 1 cup:

- 1 cup milk or yogurt
- ½ cup ricotta cheese
- 1½ ounces natural cheese
- 2 ounces processed cheese

Cottage cheese is lower in calcium than most other cheeses; ½ cup is equivalent to ¼ cup milk. Ice cream is also lower in calcium and higher in sugar and fat than many other dairy products; one scoop counts as ⅓ cup milk. MyPlate's key message for consumers is to switch to fat-free or low-fat (1%) milk and dairy products.

Protein Foods (Meat and Beans) This group includes meat, poultry, fish, dried beans and peas, eggs, nuts, and seeds. A 2000-calorie diet should include 5½ ounce-equivalents daily. Each of the following counts as equivalent to 1 ounce:

- 1 ounce cooked lean meat, poultry, or fish
- ¼ cup cooked dry beans (legumes) or tofu
- 1 egg
- 1 tablespoon peanut butter
- ½ ounce nuts or seeds

Choose lean meats and skinless poultry, and watch your serving sizes carefully. Choose at least one serving of plant proteins, such as black beans, lentils, or tofu, every day.

Oils Oils and soft margarines include vegetable oils and soft vegetable oil table spreads that have no trans fats. These are major sources of vitamin E and unsaturated fatty

Table 3.6 USDA Daily Calorie Intake Levels

AGE (YEARS)	SEDENTARY*	MODERATELY ACTIVE**	ACTIVE+
FEMALE			
2–3	1000	1000–1200	1000–1400
4–8	1200–1400	1400–1600	1400–1800
9–13	1400–1600	1600–2000	1800–2200
14–18	1800	2000	2400
19–25	2000	2200	2400
26–30	1800	2000	2400
31–50	1800	2000	2200
51 +	1600	1800	2000–2200
MALE			
2–3	1000–1200	1000–1400	1000–1400
4–8	1200–1400	1400–1600	1600–2000
9–13	1600–2000	1800–2200	2000–2600
14–18	2000–2400	2400–2800	2800–3200
19–20	2600	2800	3000
21–25	2400	2800	3000
26–30	2400	2600	3000
31–35	2400	2600	3000
36–40	2400	2600	2800
41–45	2200	2600	2800
46–50	2200	2400	2800
51–55	2200	2400	2800
56 +	2000–2200	2200–2400	2400–2600

*A lifestyle that includes only the light physical activity associated with typical day-to-day life.

**A lifestyle that includes physical activity equivalent to walking about 1.5–3 miles per day at 3–4 miles per hour (30–60 minutes a day of moderate physical activity), in addition to the light physical activity associated with typical day-to-day life.

+A lifestyle that includes physical activity equivalent to walking more than 3 miles per day at 3–4 miles per hour (60 or more minutes a day of moderate physical activity), in addition to the light physical activity associated with typical day-to-day life.

SOURCE: U.S. Department of Health and Human Services and U.S. Department of Agriculture. 2011. *Dietary Guidelines for Americans, 2010, Appendix 6. Estimated Calorie Needs per Day by Age, Gender, and Physical Activity Level* (http://www.cnpp.usda.gov/Publications/DietaryGuidelines/2010/PolicyDoc/PolicyDoc.pdf; retrieved August 7, 2011).

acids, including the essential fatty acids. A 2000-calorie diet should include 6 teaspoons of oils per day. One teaspoon is the equivalent of the following:

- 1 teaspoon vegetable oil or soft margarine
- 1 tablespoon salad dressing or light mayonnaise

Foods that are mostly oils include nuts, olives, avocados, and some fish. The following portions include about 1 teaspoon of oil: 4 large olives, ½ medium avocado, 2 tablespoons peanut butter, and 1 ounce roasted nuts. Food labels can help you identify the type and amount of fat in various foods.

Solid Fats and Added Sugars If you consistently choose nutrient-dense foods that are fat-free or low-fat and that contain no added sugars, you can also have a small amount of additional calories in the form of solid fats and added sugars (SoFAS). Figure 3.5 shows the maximum number of SoFAS calories allowed at each calorie level in MyPlate.

People who are trying to lose weight may choose not to use SoFAS calories. For those wanting to maintain weight, these calories may be used to increase the amount of food from a food group; to consume foods that are not in the lowest-fat form or that contain added sugars; to add oil, fat, or sugars to foods; or to consume alcohol.

The current American diet includes higher levels of sugar intake and more calories per day from sugar than recommended. For teenagers age 14–18, sodas and energy and sports drinks are the top source of calories in the diet, accounting for 226 calories per beverage; teens typically drink more than one such beverage daily. In particular, experts advise consumers to be wary of products containing high-fructose corn syrup. Although this sweetener is not harmful in itself, it is high in calories and very low in nutritional value. High-fructose corn syrup is found in many products, especially soft drinks and processed foods. Research has linked high consumption of high-fructose corn syrup with obesity, diabetes, and other health problems.

Physical Activity Like the Dietary Guidelines and other plans, MyPlate encourages physical activity for improving health, preventing chronic diseases, and managing weight. The physical activity recommendations in MyPlate are very similar to those found in the Dietary Guidelines (described earlier in this chapter); if you meet the Department of Health and Human Services' guidelines of 150 minutes per week of moderate physical activity, you will meet the recommendations found in MyPlate.

Other Food-Group Plans

A variety of experts have proposed other food-group plans. Some of these address perceived shortcomings in the USDA plans, and some have adapted the old MyPyramid plans to special populations. Two alternative food plans appear in the Nutrition Resources section at the end

Fitness Tip

Consumption of red meats, sweets, eggs, and butter is greatly reduced or eliminated entirely in most forms of the Mediterranean diet.

of the chapter: the DASH eating plan and the Harvard Healthy Eating Pyramid. The USDA Center for Nutrition Policy and Promotion (www.usda.gov/cnpp) has more on alternative food plans for special populations such as young children, older adults, and people choosing particular ethnic diets. MyPlate is available in Spanish, and there are special adaptations of MyPlate for children and for women who are pregnant or breastfeeding.

Another food plan that has received attention in recent years is the Mediterranean diet, which emphasizes vegetables, fruits, and whole grains; daily servings of beans, legumes, and nuts; moderate consumption of fish, poultry, and dairy products; and the use of olive oil over other types of fat, especially saturated fat. The Mediterranean diet has been associated with lower rates of heart disease and cancer, and recent studies have found a link between the diet and a greatly reduced risk of Parkinson's disease and Alzheimer's disease.

The Vegetarian Alternative

Vegetarians choose a diet with one essential difference from the diets described previously—they eliminate or restrict foods of animal origin (meat, poultry, fish, eggs, milk). Many people choose such diets for health reasons; vegetarian diets tend to be lower in saturated fat, cholesterol, and animal protein and higher in complex carbohydrates, dietary fiber, folate, vitamins C and E, carotenoids, and phytochemicals. Some people adopt a vegetarian diet out of concern for the environment, for financial considerations, or for reasons related to ethics or religion.

Types of Vegetarian Diets There are various vegetarian styles. The wider the variety of the diet eaten, the easier it is to meet nutritional needs.

- *Vegans* eat only plant foods.
- *Lacto-vegetarians* eat plant foods and dairy products.
- *Lacto-ovo-vegetarians* eat plant foods, dairy products, and eggs.

Others can be categorized as partial vegetarians, semivegetarians, or pescovegetarians. These people eat plant foods, dairy products, eggs, and usually a small selection of poultry, fish, and other seafood. Many other people choose vegetarian meals frequently but are not strictly vegetarian. Including some animal protein (such as dairy products) in a mostly vegetarian diet makes meal planning easier, but it is not necessary.

A Food Plan for Vegetarians MyPlate can be adapted for use by vegetarians with only a few key modifications. For the meat and beans group, vegetarians can focus on the nonmeat choices of dry beans and peas, nuts, seeds, eggs, and soy foods like tofu. Vegans and other vegetarians who do not eat or drink any dairy products must find other rich sources of calcium (see the following list). Fruits, vegetables, and whole grains are healthy choices for people following all types of vegetarian diets.

A healthy vegetarian diet emphasizes a wide variety of plant foods. Although plant proteins are generally of a lower quality than animal proteins, choosing a variety of plant foods will supply all of the essential amino acids. Choosing minimally processed and unrefined foods will maximize nutrient value and provide ample dietary fiber. Daily consumption of a variety of plant foods in amounts that meet total energy needs can provide all needed nutrients except vitamin B-12 and possibly vitamin D. Strategies for getting these and other nutrients include the following:

- *Vitamin B-12* is found naturally only in animal foods. If dairy products and eggs are limited or avoided, B-12

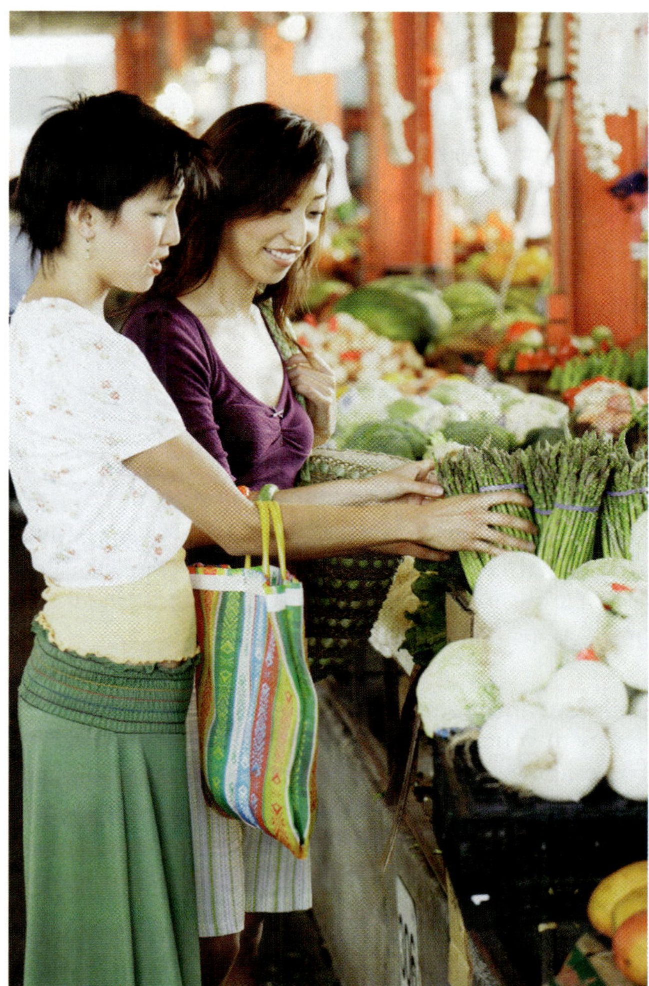

Variety is the key to maintaining a healthy, balanced vegetarian diet.

vegetarian Someone who follows a diet that restricts or eliminates foods of animal origin.

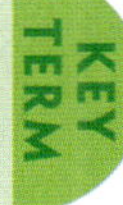

can be found in fortified foods such as ready-to-eat cereals, soy beverages, meat substitutes, special yeast products, and supplements.

- *Vitamin D* can be obtained by spending 5–15 minutes a day in the sun, by consuming vitamin D–fortified products like ready-to-eat cereals and soy or rice milk, or by taking a supplement.
- *Calcium* is found in legumes, tofu processed with calcium, dark-green leafy vegetables, nuts, tortillas made from lime-processed corn, fortified orange juice, soy milk, bread, and other foods.
- *Iron* is found in whole grains, fortified bread and breakfast cereals, dried fruits, leafy green vegetables, nuts and seeds, legumes, and soy foods. The iron in plant foods is more difficult for the body to absorb than the iron from animal sources. Eating or drinking a good source of vitamin C with most meals is helpful because vitamin C improves iron absorption.
- *Zinc* is found in whole grains, nuts, legumes, and soy foods.

If you are a vegetarian, remember that it's especially important to eat as wide a variety of foods as possible to ensure that all your nutritional needs are satisfied. Consulting with a registered dietitian will make your planning easier. Vegetarian diets for children, teens, and pregnant and lactating women warrant professional guidance.

Dietary Challenges for Various Population Groups

MyPlate and the Dietary Guidelines for Americans provide a basis that nearly everyone can use to create a healthy diet. However, different population groups should be aware of special dietary challenges.

Children and Teenagers The best approach for parents with young children is to provide a variety of foods. For example, parents can add vegetables to casseroles and fruit to cereal, or they can offer fruit and vegetable juices or homemade yogurt or fruit shakes instead of sugary drinks. Allowing children to help prepare meals is another good way to encourage good eating habits.

Women Women tend to need fewer calories than men, so they may need to focus more on nutrient-dense foods to make sure they are getting enough of all the essential nutrients. Two nutrients of special concern to women are calcium and iron. Low calcium intake may be linked to the development of osteoporosis in later life. Nonfat and low-fat dairy products and fortified cereal, bread, and orange juice are good sources of calcium.

Ask Yourself ?

QUESTIONS FOR CRITICAL THINKING AND REFLECTION

What factors influence your food choices—convenience, cost, availability, habit? Do you ever consider nutritional content or nutritional recommendations like those found in MyPlate? If not, how big a change would it be for you to think of nutritional content first when choosing food? Is it something you could do easily?

Menstruating women have higher iron requirements than other groups, and a lack of iron in the diet can lead to iron-deficiency anemia. Lean red meat, leafy green vegetables, and fortified breakfast cereals are good sources of iron. As discussed earlier, all women capable of becoming pregnant should also get enough folate or folic acid from fortified foods and/or supplements.

Good nutrition is essential to a healthy pregnancy. Nutritional counseling can help a woman create a plan for healthy eating before and during pregnancy. Diet is especially important for any woman with special nutritional needs or an eating disorder, or who is overweight or obese. Physicians commonly prescribe prenatal vitamin supplements to pregnant women. The U.S. Public Health Service recommends that all women of childbearing age get 400 μg of folic acid from fortified foods and/or supplements each day to reduce the risk of neural tube defects that can arise in the fetus.

College Students Foods that are convenient for college students are not always the healthiest choices. However, it is possible to make healthy eating both convenient and affordable. See the tips in the box "Eating Strategies for College Students."

Older Adults As people age, they tend to become less active, so they require fewer calories to maintain their weight. At the same time, the absorption of nutrients tends to be lower in older adults because of age-related changes in the digestive tract. As discussed earlier, foods fortified with vitamin B-12 and/or B-12 supplements are recommended for people over age 50. Because constipation is a common problem, consuming foods high in dietary fiber and drinking enough fluids are important goals.

Athletes Key dietary concerns for athletes are meeting increased energy and fluid requirements for training and making healthy food choices throughout the day. For more on this topic, see the box "Do Athletes Need a Different Diet?"

People with Special Health Concerns Many Americans have special health concerns that affect their dietary needs. For example, women who are pregnant or breastfeeding

Eating Strategies for College Students

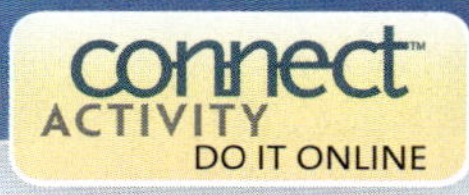

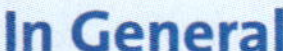

In General

- Eat a colorful, varied diet. The more colorful your diet is, the more varied and rich in fruits and vegetables it will be. Fruits and vegetables are typically inexpensive, delicious, nutritious, and low in fat and calories.
- Eat breakfast. You'll have more energy in the morning and be less likely to grab an unhealthy snack later on.
- Choose healthy snacks—fruits, vegetables, whole grains, and cereals.
- Drink nonfat milk, water, mineral water, or 100% fruit juice more often than soft drinks or sweetened beverages.
- Pay attention to portion sizes.
- Combine physical activity with healthy eating.

Eating in the Dining Hall

- Choose a meal plan that includes breakfast.
- Decide what you want to eat before you get in line, and stick to your choices.
- Build your meals around whole grains and vegetables. Ask for small servings of meat and high-fat main dishes.
- Choose leaner poultry, fish, or bean dishes rather than high-fat meats and fried entrees.
- Ask that gravies and sauces be served on the side; limit your intake.
- Choose broth-based or vegetable soups rather than cream soups.
- At the salad bar, load up on leafy greens, beans, and fresh vegetables. Avoid mayonnaise-coated salads, bacon, croutons, and high-fat dressings. Put dressing on the side; dip your fork into it rather than pouring it over the salad.
- Choose fruit for dessert rather than cookies or cakes.

Eating in Fast-Food Restaurants

- Most fast-food chains can provide a brochure with the nutritional content of their menu items. Ask for it, or check the restaurant's Web site for nutritional information. Order small single burgers with no cheese instead of double burgers with many toppings. If possible, get them broiled instead of fried.
- Ask for items to be prepared without mayonnaise, tartar sauce, sour cream, or other high-fat sauces. Ketchup, mustard, and fat-free mayonnaise or sour cream are better choices and are available at many fast-food restaurants.
- Choose whole-grain buns or bread for sandwiches.
- Choose chicken items made from chicken breast, not processed chicken.
- Order vegetable pizzas without extra cheese.
- If you order french fries or onion rings, get the smallest size and/or share them with a friend. Better yet, get a salad or a fruit cup instead.

Eating on the Run

- When you need to eat in a hurry, remember that you can carry healthy foods in your backpack or a small insulated lunch sack (with a frozen gel pack to keep fresh food from spoiling).
- Carry items that are small and convenient but nutritious, such as fresh fruits or vegetables, whole-wheat buns or muffins, snack-size cereal boxes, and water.

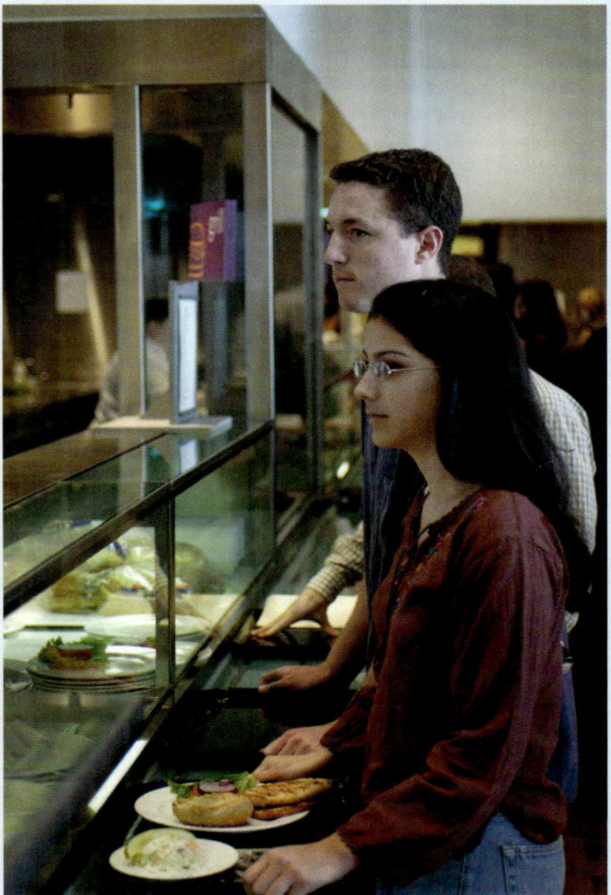

THE EVIDENCE FOR EXERCISE

Do Athletes Need a Different Diet?

If you exercise vigorously and frequently, or if you are an athlete in training, you likely have increased energy and fluid requirements. Research supports the following recommendations for athletes:

- **Energy intake:** Someone engaged in a vigorous training program may have energy needs as high as 6000 calories per day—far greater than the energy needs of a moderately active person. For athletes, the Academy of Nutrition and Dietetics (formerly the American Dietetic Association) recommends a diet with 60–65% of calories coming from carbohydrates, 10–15% from protein, and no more than 30% from fat.

  Athletes who need to maintain low body weight and fat (such as gymnasts, skaters, and wrestlers) need to get enough calories and nutrients while avoiding unhealthy eating patterns such as bulimia. The combination of low body fat, high physical activity, disordered eating habits—and, in women, amenorrhea—is associated with osteoporosis, stress fractures, and other injuries. If keeping your weight and body fat low for athletic reasons is important to you, seek dietary advice from a qualified dietician and make sure your physician is aware of your eating habits.

- **Carbohydrates:** Endurance athletes involved in competitive events lasting longer than 90 minutes may benefit from increasing carbohydrate intake to 65–70% of their total calories. Specifically, the American College of Sports Medicine (ACSM) recommends that athletes consume 2.7–4.5 grams per pound of body weight daily, depending on their weight, sport, and other nutritional needs. This increase should come in the form of complex carbohydrates.

  High carbohydrate intake builds and maintains glycogen stores in the muscles, resulting in greater endurance and delayed fatigue during competitive events. The ACSM recommends that before exercise an active adult or athlete eat a meal or snack that is relatively high in carbohydrates, moderate in protein, and low in fat and fiber. Eating carbohydrates 30 minutes, 2 hours, and 4 hours after exercise can help replenish glycogen stores in the liver and muscles.

- **Fat:** The ACSM recommends that all athletes get 20–35% of calories from fat in their diets. This is in line with the daily intake suggested by the Food and Nutrition Board. Reducing fat intake to less than 20% of daily calories can negatively affect performance and be harmful to health.

- **Protein:** For endurance and strength-trained athletes, the ACSM recommends eating 0.5–0.8 gram of protein per pound of body weight each day, which is considerably higher than the standard DRI of 0.36 gram per pound. This level of protein is easily obtainable from foods; in fact, most Americans eat more protein than they need every day. A balanced, moderate-protein diet can provide the protein most athletes need.

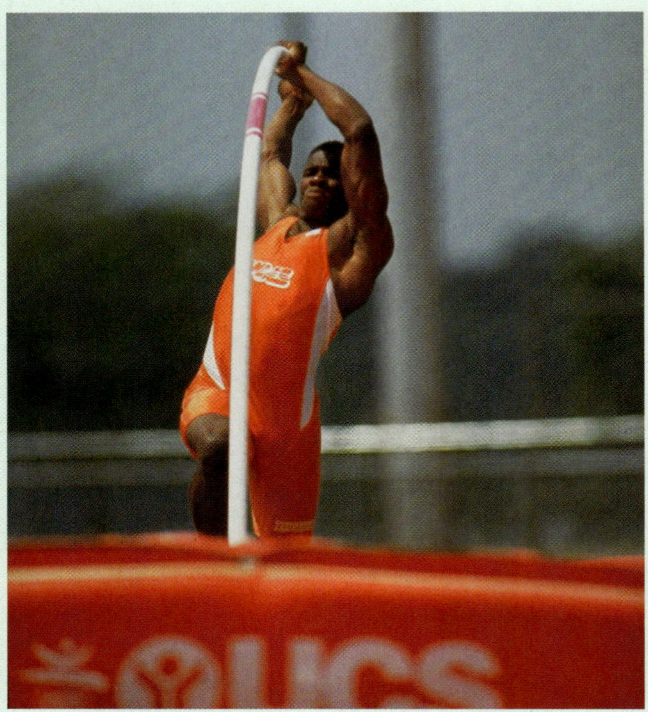

  There is no evidence that consuming supplements containing vitamins, minerals, protein, or specific amino acids builds muscle or improves sports performance. Strength and muscle are built with exercise, not extra protein, and carbohydrates provide the fuel needed for muscle-building exercise.

- **Fluids:** If you exercise heavily or live in a hot climate, you should drink extra fluids to maximize performance and prevent heat illness. For a strenuous endurance event, prepare yourself the day before by drinking plenty of fluids. The ACSM recommends drinking 2–3 milliliters of fluid per pound of body weight about 4 hours before the event. During the event, take in enough fluids to compensate for fluid loss due to sweating; the amount required depends on the individual and his or her sweat rate. Afterward, drink enough to replace lost fluids—about 16–24 ounces for every pound of weight lost.

  Water is a good choice for fluid replacement for events lasting 60–90 minutes. For longer workouts or events, a sports drink can be a good choice. These contain water, electrolytes, and carbohydrates and can provide some extra energy as well as replace electrolytes like sodium lost in sweat.

SOURCE: American College of Sports Medicine. 2009. *American College of Sports Medicine Position Stand: Nutrition and Athletic Performance* (http://www.acsm-msse.org/pt/pt-core/template-journal/msse/media/0309nutrition.pdf; retrived April 23, 2011).

require extra calories, vitamins, and minerals. People with diabetes benefit from a well-balanced diet that is low in simple sugars, high in complex carbohydrates, and relatively rich in monounsaturated fats. People with high blood pressure need to limit their sodium consumption and control their weight. If you have a health problem or concern that may require a special diet, discuss your situation with a physician or registered dietitian.

Using Food Labels

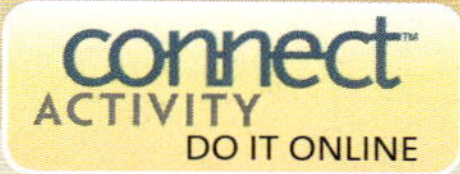

The "Nutrition Facts" section of a food label designed to help consumers make food choices based on the nutrients that are most important to good health. In addition to listing nutrient content by weight, the label puts the information in the context of a daily diet of 2000 calories that includes no more than 65 grams of fat (approximately 30% of total calories). For example, if a serving of a particular product has 13 grams of fat, the label will show that the serving represents 20% of the daily fat allowance. If your daily diet contains fewer or more than 2000 calories, you need to adjust these calculations accordingly.

Food labels contain uniform serving sizes. This means that if you look at different brands of salad dressing, for example, you can compare calories and fat content based on the serving amount. (Food label serving sizes may be larger or smaller than USDA serving size equivalents, however.) Regulations also require that foods meet strict definitions if their packaging includes the terms *light, low-fat,* or *high-fiber* (see below). Health claims such as "good source of dietary fiber" or "low in saturated fat" on packages are signals that those products can wisely be included in your diet. Overall, the food label is an important tool to help you choose a diet that conforms to MyPlate and the Dietary Guidelines.

Selected Nutrient Claims and What They Mean

- ***Healthy*** A food that is low in fat, is low in saturated fat, has no more than 360–480 mg of sodium and 60 mg of cholesterol, *and* provides 10% or more of the Daily Value for vitamin A, vitamin C, protein, calcium, iron, or dietary fiber.
- ***Light or lite*** 33% fewer calories or 50% less fat than a similar product.
- ***Reduced or fewer*** At least 25% less of a nutrient than a similar product; can be applied to fat ("reduced fat"), saturated fat, cholesterol, sodium, and calories.
- ***Extra or added*** 10% or more of the Daily Value per serving when compared to what a similar product has.
- ***Good source*** 10–19% of the Daily Value for a particular nutrient per serving.
- ***High, rich in, or excellent source of*** 20% or more of the Daily Value for a particular nutrient per serving.
- ***Low calorie*** 40 calories or less per serving.
- ***High fiber*** 5 g or more of fiber per serving.
- ***Good source of fiber*** 2.5–4.9 g of fiber per serving.
- ***Fat-free*** Less than 0.5 g of fat per serving.
- ***Low-fat*** 3 g of fat or less per serving.
- ***Saturated fat-free*** Less than 0.5 g of saturated fat and 0.5 g of trans fatty acids per serving.
- ***Low saturated fat*** 1 g or less of saturated fat per serving and no more than 15% of total calories.
- ***Cholesterol-free*** Less than 2 mg of cholesterol and 2 g or less of saturated fat per serving.
- ***Low cholesterol*** 20 mg or less of cholesterol and 2 g or less of saturated fat per serving.
- ***Low sodium*** 140 mg or less of sodium per serving.
- ***Very low sodium*** 35 mg or less of sodium per serving.
- ***Lean*** Cooked seafood, meat, or poultry with less than 10 g of fat, 4.5 g or less of saturated fat, and less than 95 mg of cholesterol per serving.
- ***Extra lean*** Cooked seafood, meat, or poultry with less than 5 g of fat, 2 g of saturated fat, and 95 mg of cholesterol per serving.

NOTE: The FDA has not yet defined nutrient claims relating to carbohydrates, so foods labeled low- or reduced-carbohydrate do not conform to any approved standard.

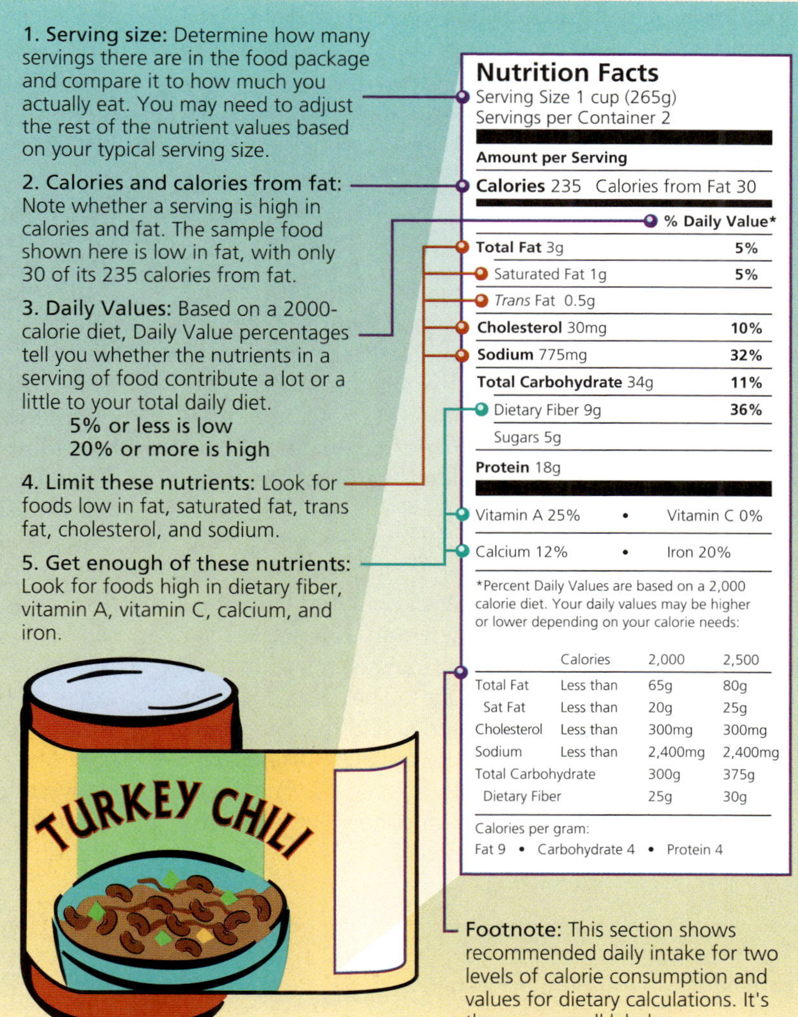

NUTRITIONAL PLANNING: MAKING INFORMED CHOICES ABOUT FOOD

Knowing about nutrition is a good start to making sound choices about food. It also helps if you can interpret food labels, understand food additives, and avoid foodborne illnesses.

Food Labels

All processed foods regulated by either the FDA or the USDA include standardized nutrition information on their labels. Every food label shows serving sizes and the amount of fat, saturated fat, trans fat, cholesterol, protein, dietary fiber, sugars, total carbohydrate, and sodium in each serving. To make intelligent choices about food, learn to read and understand food labels (see the box "Using Food Labels").

Food labels are not required on fresh meat, poultry, fish, fruits, and vegetables (many of these products are not packaged). You can get information on the nutrient content of these items from basic nutrition books, registered dietitians, nutrient analysis computer software, the Web, and the companies that produce or distribute these foods. Also, supermarkets often have posters or pamphlets listing the nutrient contents of these foods. In Lab 3.3, you compare foods using the information on their labels.

Dietary Supplements

Dietary supplements include vitamins, minerals, amino acids, herbs, enzymes, and other compounds. Although dietary supplements are often thought of as safe and natural, they contain powerful bioactive chemicals that have the potential for harm. About one-quarter of all pharmaceutical drugs are derived from botanical sources, and even essential vitamins and minerals can have toxic effects if consumed in excess.

In the United States, supplements are not legally considered drugs and are not regulated the way drugs are. Before they are approved by the FDA and put on the market, drugs undergo clinical studies to determine safety, effectiveness, side effects and risks, possible interactions with other substances, and appropriate dosages. The FDA does not authorize or test dietary supplements, and manufacturers are not required to demonstrate either safety or effectiveness before they are marketed. Although dosage guidelines exist for some of the compounds in dietary supplements, dosages for many are not well established.

KEY TERM

pathogen A microorganism that causes disease.

Many ingredients in dietary supplements are classified by the FDA as "generally recognized as safe," but some have been found to be dangerous on their own or to interact with prescription or over-the-counter drugs in dangerous ways. Garlic supplements, for example, can cause bleeding if taken with anticoagulant (blood-thinning) medications. Some supplements can have side effects. St. John's wort, for example, increases the skin's sensitivity to sunlight and may decrease the effectiveness of oral contraceptives, drugs used to treat HIV infection, and many other medications.

There are also key differences in the way drugs and supplements are manufactured: FDA-approved medications are standardized for potency, and quality control and proof of purity are required. Dietary supplement manufacture is not as closely regulated, and there is no guarantee that a product contains a given ingredient at all, let alone in the appropriate amount. The potency of herbal supplements can vary widely due to differences in growing and harvesting conditions, preparation methods, and storage. Contamination and misidentification of plant compounds are also potential problems.

In an effort to provide consumers with more reliable and consistent information about supplements, the FDA has developed labeling regulations. Labels similar to those found on foods are now required for dietary supplements; for more information, see the box "Using Dietary Supplement Labels."

Food Additives

Today, some 2800 substances are intentionally added to foods to maintain or improve nutritional quality, to maintain freshness, to help in processing or preparation, or to alter taste or appearance. Additives make up less than 1% of our food. The most widely used are sugar, salt, and corn syrup; these three, plus citric acid, baking soda, vegetable colors, mustard, and pepper, account for 98% by weight of all food additives used in the United States.

Food additives pose no significant health hazard to most people because the levels used are well below any that could produce toxic effects. Two additives of potential concern for some people are sulfites, used to keep vegetables from turning brown, and monosodium glutamate (MSG), used as a flavor enhancer. Sulfites can cause severe reactions in some people, and the FDA strictly limits their use and requires clear labeling on any food containing sulfites. MSG may cause some people to experience episodes of sweating and increased blood pressure. If you have any sensitivity to an additive, check food labels when you shop and ask questions when you eat out.

Foodborne Illness

Many people worry about additives or pesticide residues in their food, but a greater threat comes from microorganisms that cause foodborne illnesses. Raw or

Using Dietary Supplement Labels

Since 1999, specific types of information have been required on the labels of dietary supplements. In addition to basic information about the product, labels include a "Supplement Facts" panel, modeled after the "Nutrition Facts" panel used on food labels (see the figure). Under the Dietary Supplement Health and Education Act (DSHEA) and food labeling laws, supplement labels can make three types of health-related claims:

- *Nutrient-content claims,* such as "high in calcium," "excellent source of vitamin C," or "high potency." The claims "high in" and "excellent source of" mean the same as they do on food labels. A "high potency" single-ingredient supplement must contain 100% of its Daily Value; a "high potency" multi-ingredient product must contain 100% or more of the Daily Value of at least two-thirds of the nutrients present for which Daily Values have been established.
- *Health claims,* if they have been authorized by the FDA or another authoritative scientific body. The association between adequate calcium intake and lower risk of osteoporosis is an example of an approved health claim. The FDA also allows so-called *qualified health claims* for situations in which there is emerging but as yet inconclusive evidence for a particular claim. Such claims must include qualifying language such as "scientific evidence suggests but does not prove" the claim.
- *Structure-function claims,* such as "antioxidants maintain cellular integrity" or "this product enhances energy levels." Because these claims are not reviewed by the FDA, they must carry a disclaimer (see the sample label).

Tips for Choosing and Using Dietary Supplements

- Check with your physician before taking a supplement. Many are not meant for children, older people, women who are pregnant or breastfeeding, people with chronic illnesses or upcoming surgery, or people taking prescription or over-the-counter medications.
- Follow the cautions, instructions for use, and dosage given on the label.
- Look for the USP verification mark on the label, indicating that the product meets minimum safety and purity standards developed under the Dietary Supplement Verification Program by the United States Pharmacopeia (USP). The USP mark means that the product (1) contains the ingredients stated on the label, (2) has the declared amount and strength of ingredients, (3) will dissolve effectively, (4) has been screened for harmful contaminants, and (5) has been manufactured using safe, sanitary, and well-controlled procedures. The National Nutritional Foods Association has a self-regulatory testing program for its members; other, smaller associations and labs, including ConsumerLab.com, also test and rate dietary supplements.
- Choose brands made by nationally known food and drug manufacturers or " house brands" from large retail chains. Due to their size and visibility, such sources are likely to have high manufacturing standards.
- If you experience side effects, stop using the product and contact your physician. Report any serious reactions to the FDA's MedWatch monitoring program (1-800-FDA-1088 or online at http://www.fda.gov/Safety/MedWatch/default.htm).

For More Information About Dietary Supplements

ConsumerLab.Com: http://www.consumerlab.com

Food and Drug Administration: http://www.fda.gov/Food/DietarySupplements/default.htm

National Institutes of Health, Office of Dietary Supplements: http://ods.od.nih.gov

Natural Products Association: http://www.npainfo.org

U.S. Department of Agriculture: http://fnic.nal.usda.gov/nal_display/index.php?info_center=4&tax_level=1&tax_subject=274

U.S. Pharmacopeia: http://www.usp.org/USPVerified/DietarySupplements

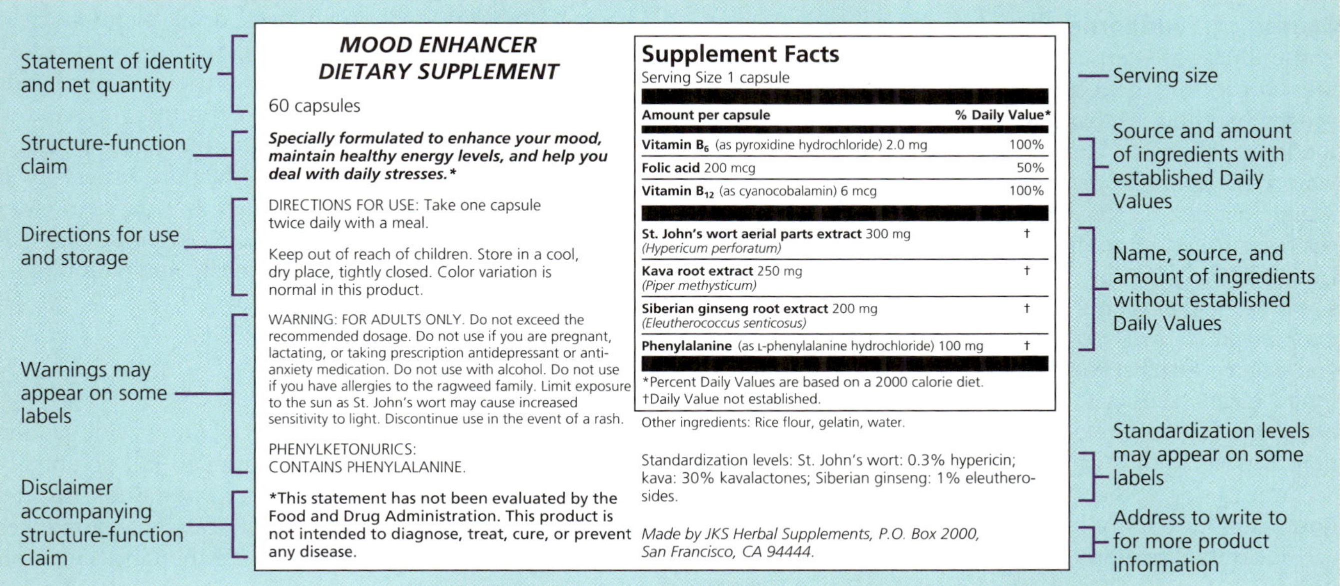

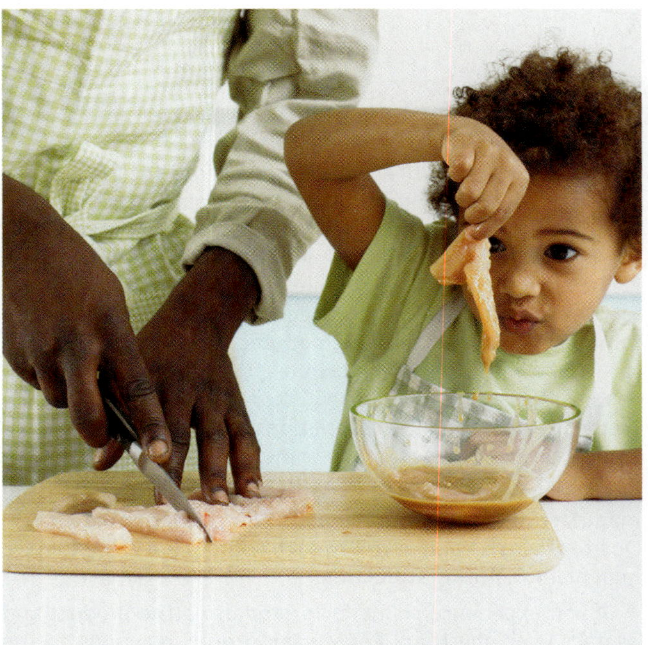

Careful food handling greatly reduces the risk of foodborne illness.

undercooked animal products, such as chicken, hamburger, and oysters, pose the greatest risk, although in recent years contaminated fruits and vegetables have been catching up.

The CDC estimates that 48 million illnesses, 128,000 hospitalizations, and 3000 deaths occur each year in the United States due to foodborne contaminants. Symptoms include diarrhea, vomiting, fever, pain, headache, and weakness. Although the effects of foodborne illness are usually not serious, some groups, such as children, pregnant women, and elderly people, are more at risk for severe complications such as rheumatic diseases, seizures, blood poisoning, and death.

Causes of Foodborne Illnesses Most cases of foodborne illness are caused by **pathogens**, disease-causing microorganisms that contaminate food, usually from improper handling. According to the CDC, about 90% of foodborne illnesses, hospitalizations, and deaths in 2010 were due to seven pathogens: *Salmonella* (most often found in eggs, on vegetables, and on poultry); norovirus (most often found in salad ingredients and shellfish); *Campylobacter jejuni* (most often found in meat and poultry); *Toxoplasma* (most often found in meat); *Escherichia coli (E. coli)* O157:H7 (most often found in meat and water); *Listeria monocytogenes* (most often found in lunch meats, sausages, and hot dogs); and *Clostridium perfringens* (most often found in meat and gravy). Salmonella was the leading cause of hospitalizations and deaths, accounting for 28% of deaths and 35% of hospitalizations. About 60% of illness, but a much smaller percentage of severe illness, was caused by norovirus.

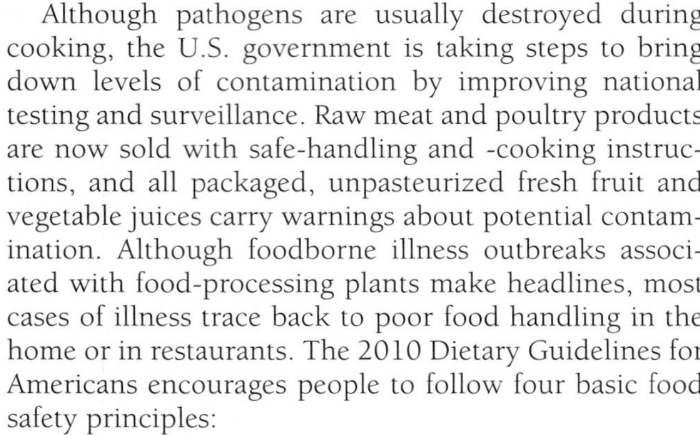

Wellness Tip

To get produce as clean as possible, rub it with a soft brush while holding it under running water.

Although pathogens are usually destroyed during cooking, the U.S. government is taking steps to bring down levels of contamination by improving national testing and surveillance. Raw meat and poultry products are now sold with safe-handling and -cooking instructions, and all packaged, unpasteurized fresh fruit and vegetable juices carry warnings about potential contamination. Although foodborne illness outbreaks associated with food-processing plants make headlines, most cases of illness trace back to poor food handling in the home or in restaurants. The 2010 Dietary Guidelines for Americans encourages people to follow four basic food safety principles:

- **Clean** hands, food contact surfaces, and vegetables and fruits.
- **Separate** raw, cooked, and read-to-eat foods while shopping, storing, and preparing foods.
- **Cook** foods to a safe temperature.
- **Chill** (refrigerate) perishable foods promptly.

The Dietary Guidelines also advise people to avoid certain high-risk foods, including raw (unpasteurized) milk, cheeses, and juices; raw or undercooked animal foods, such as seafood, meat, poultry, and eggs; and raw sprouts. These precautions are especially important for pregnant women, young children, older adults, and people with weakened immune systems or certain chronic diseases. For more information on food safety, see the box "Safe Food Handling."

Treating Foodborne Illness If you think you may be having a bout of foodborne illness, drink plenty of clear fluids to prevent dehydration, and rest to speed recovery. To prevent further contamination, wash your hands often and always before handling food until you recover. A fever higher than 102°F, blood in the stool, or dehydration deserves a physician's evaluation, especially if the symptoms persist for more than 2–3 days. In cases of suspected botulism—characterized by symptoms such as double vision, paralysis, dizziness, and vomiting—consult a physician immediately.

Irradiated Foods

Food irradiation is the treatment of foods with gamma rays, X-rays, or high-voltage electrons to kill potentially harmful pathogens, including bacteria, parasites, insects, and fungi that cause foodborne illness. It also reduces spoilage and extends shelf life. Even though irradiation

Safe Food Handling

TAKE CHARGE

Shopping

- Don't buy food in containers that leak, bulge, or are severely dented. Refrigerated foods should be cold, and frozen foods should be solid.
- Check the food label for an expiration date and for safe-handling instructions.
- Place meat, poultry, and seafood in plastic bags, and separate foods in your grocery cart.
- Select cold and frozen food last to ensure that they stay refrigerated until just before checkout.

Storing Food

- Store raw meat, poultry, fish, and shellfish in containers in the refrigerator so that the juices don't drip onto other foods. Keep these items away from other foods, surfaces, utensils, and serving dishes to prevent cross-contamination.
- Store eggs in the coldest part of the refrigerator, not in the door, and use them within 3–5 weeks.
- Keep hot foods hot (140°F or above) and cold foods cold (40°F or below); harmful bacteria can grow rapidly between these two temperatures. Refrigerate foods within 2 hours of purchase or preparation and within 1 hour if the air temperature is above 90°F. Freeze foods at or below 0°F. Use or freeze fresh meats within 3–5 days and fresh poultry, fish, and ground meat within 1–2 days. Use refrigerated leftovers within 3–4 days.

Preparing Food

- Thoroughly wash your hands with warm soapy water for 20 seconds before and after handling food, especially raw meat, fish, shellfish, poultry, or eggs.
- Make sure counters, cutting boards, dishes, utensils, and other equipment are thoroughly cleaned with hot soapy water before and after use. Wash dishcloths and kitchen towels frequently.
- Use separate cutting boards for meat, poultry, and seafood and for foods that will be eaten raw, such as fruits and vegetables. Replace cutting boards once they become worn or develop hard-to-clean grooves.
- Thoroughly rinse and scrub fruits and vegetables with a brush (but not with soap or detergent), or peel off the skin.
- Don't eat raw animal products, including raw eggs in homemade hollandaise sauce, eggnog, or cookie dough.
- Thaw frozen food in the refrigerator, in cold water, or in the microwave, not on the kitchen counter. Cook foods immediately after thawing.

Cooking

- Cook foods thoroughly, especially beef, poultry, fish, pork, and eggs; cooking kills most microorganisms. Use a food thermometer to ensure that foods are cooked to a safe temperature. Hamburgers should be cooked to 160°F. Turn or stir microwaved food to make sure it is heated evenly throughout.

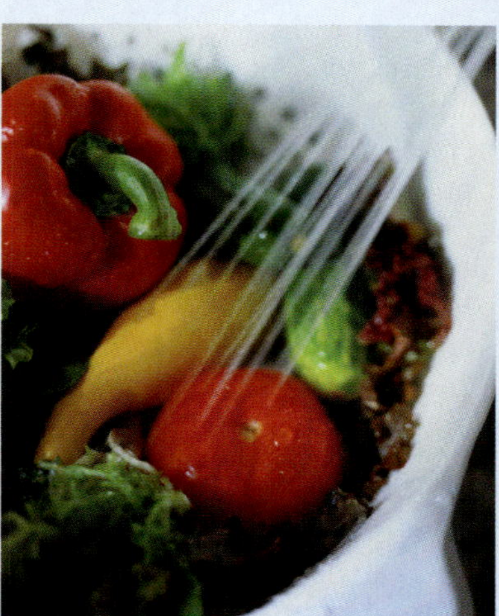

- Cook stuffing separately from poultry; or wash poultry thoroughly, stuff immediately before cooking, and transfer the stuffing to a clean bowl immediately after cooking. The temperature of cooked stuffing should reach 165°F.
- Cook eggs until they're firm, and fully cook foods containing eggs.
- To protect against *Listeria*, reheat ready-to-eat foods like hot dogs and cold cuts until steaming hot.
- Because of possible contamination with *E. coli* 0157:H7 and *Salmonella,* avoid raw sprouts.

According to the USDA, "When in doubt, throw it out." Even if a food looks and smells fine, it may not be safe. If you aren't sure that a food has been prepared, served, and stored safely, don't eat it. For more information, see the USDA's *Kitchen Companion: Your Safe Food Handbook* at http://www.fsis.usda.gov/PDF/Kitchen_Companion.pdf.

has been generally endorsed by agencies such as the World Health Organization, the CDC, and the American Medical Association, few irradiated foods are currently on the market due to consumer resistance and skepticism. Studies haven't conclusively identified any harmful effects of food irradiation, and newer methods of irradiation involving electricity and X-rays do not require the use of any radioactive materials. Studies indicate that when consumers are given information about the process of irradiation and the benefits of irradiated foods, most want to purchase them.

food irradiation The treatment of foods with gamma rays, X-rays, or high-voltage electrons to kill potentially harmful pathogens and increase shelf life.

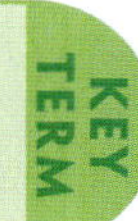

All primary irradiated foods (meat, vegetables, and so on) are labeled with the flowerlike radura symbol and a brief information label; spices and foods that are merely ingredients do not have to be labeled. It is important to remember that although irradiation kills most pathogens, it does not completely sterilize foods. Proper handling of irradiated foods is still critical for preventing foodborne illness.

Environmental Contaminants and Organic Foods

Contaminants are present in the food-growing environment. Environmental contaminants include various minerals, antibiotics, hormones, pesticides, and industrial chemicals. Safety regulations attempt to keep our exposure to contaminants at safe levels, but monitoring is difficult, and many substances (such as pesticides) persist in the environment long after being banned from use.

Organic Foods Some people who are concerned about pesticides and other environmental contaminants choose to buy foods that are **organic.** To be certified as organic, foods must meet strict production, processing, handling, and labeling criteria. Organic crops must meet limits on pesticide residues. For meat, milk, eggs, and other animal products to be certified organic, animals must be given organic feed and access to the outdoors and may not be given antibiotics or growth hormones. The use of genetic engineering, ionizing radiation, and sewage sludge is prohibited. Products can be labeled "100% organic" if they contain all organic ingredients and "organic" if they contain at least 95% organic ingredients; all such products may carry the USDA organic seal. A product with at least 70% organic ingredients can be labeled "made with organic ingredients" but cannot use the USDA seal.

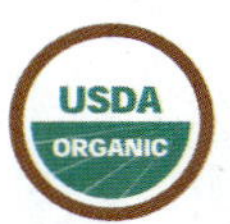

Organic foods, however, are not necessarily free of chemicals. They may be contaminated with pesticides used on neighboring lands or on foods transported in the same train or truck. However, they tend to have lower levels of pesticide residues than conventionally grown crops. Some experts recommend that consumers who want to buy organic fruits and vegetables spend their money on those that carry lower pesticide residues than their conventional counterparts (the "dirty dozen"): apples, bell peppers, celery, cherries, imported grapes, nectarines, peaches, pears, potatoes, red raspberries, spinach, and strawberries. Experts also recommend buying organic beef, poultry, eggs, dairy products, and baby food. Fruits and vegetables that carry little pesticide residue whether grown conventionally or organically include asparagus, avocadoes, bananas, broccoli, cauliflower, corn, kiwi, mangoes, onions, papaya, pineapples, and peas. All foods are subject to strict pesticide limits; the debate about the health effects of small amounts of residue is ongoing.

Whether organic foods are better for your health cannot be said for certain, but organic farming is better for the environment. It helps maintain biodiversity of crops and replenish the Earth's resources. It is less likely to degrade soil, contaminate water, or expose farm workers to toxic chemicals. As multinational food companies get into the organic food business, however, consumers who want to support environmentally friendly farming methods should look for foods that are not only organic but also locally grown.

Guidelines for Fish Consumption A specific area of concern has been possible mercury contamination in fish. Overall, fish and shellfish are healthy sources of protein, omega-3 fats, and other nutrients. Prudent choices can minimize the risk of any possible negative health effects. High mercury concentrations are most likely to be found in predator fish—large fish that eat smaller fish. Mercury can cause brain damage to fetuses and young children. According to FDA and Environmental Protection Agency (EPA) guidelines, women who are or who may become pregnant and nursing mothers should follow these guidelines to minimize their exposure to mercury:

- Do not eat shark, swordfish, king mackerel, or tilefish.
- Eat up to 12 ounces a week of a variety of fish and shellfish that are lower in mercury, such as shrimp, canned light tuna, salmon, pollock, and catfish. Limit consumption of albacore tuna to 6 ounces per week.
- Check advisories about the safety of recreationally caught fish from local lakes, rivers, and coastal areas. If no information is available, limit consumption to 6 ounces per week.

The same FDA/EPA guidelines apply to children, although they should consume smaller servings.

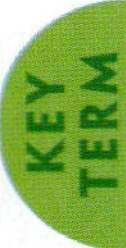

organic A designation applied to foods grown and produced according to strict guidelines limiting the use of pesticides, nonorganic ingredients, hormones, antibiotics, genetic engineering, irradiation, and other practices.

Ask Yourself ?

QUESTIONS FOR CRITICAL THINKING AND REFLECTION

Have you ever taken a dietary supplement, such as St. John's wort for mild depression or echinacea or zinc for a cold? If so, who or what influenced your decision to use this product? Did you do any research before taking it? Did you read the label on the package? Do you think the product had the desired effect?

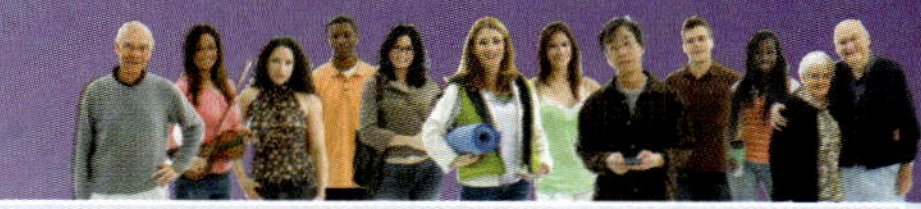

Ethnic Foods

There is no one ethnic diet that clearly surpasses all others in providing people with healthful foods. Every diet has its advantages and disadvantages, and within each cuisine, some foods are better choices. The dietary guidelines described in this chapter can be applied to any ethnic cuisine. For additional guidance, refer to the table below.

	Choose More Often	Choose Less Often
CHINESE	Dishes that are steamed, poached (jum), boiled (chu), roasted (kow), barbecued (shu), or lightly stir-fried Hoisin sauce, oyster sauce, wine sauce, plum sauce, velvet sauce, or hot mustard Fresh fish and seafood, skinless chicken, tofu Mixed vegetables, Chinese greens Steamed rice, steamed spring rolls, soft noodles	Fried wontons or egg rolls Crab rangoon Crispy (Peking) duck or chicken Sweet-and-sour dishes made with breaded and deep-fried meat, poultry, or fish Fried or crispy noodles Fried rice
FRENCH	Dishes prepared au vapeur (steamed), en brochette (skewered and broiled), or grillé (grilled) Fresh fish, shrimp, scallops, mussels, or skinless chicken, without sauces Clear soups	Dishes prepared á la créme (in cream sauce), au gratin or gratinée (baked with cream and cheese), or en croûte (in pastry crust) Drawn butter, hollandaise sauce, and remoulade (mayonnaise-based sauce)
GREEK	Dishes that are stewed, broiled, or grilled, including shish kabobs (souvlaki) Dolmas (grape leaves) stuffed with rice Tzatziki (yogurt, cucumbers, and garlic) Tabouli (bulgur-based salad) Pita bread, especially whole wheat	Moussaka, saganaki (fried cheese) Vegetable pies such as spanakopita and tyropita Baba ghanoush (eggplant and olive oil) Deep-fried falafel (chickpea patties) Gyros stuffed with ground meat Baklava
INDIAN	Dishes prepared masala (curry), tandoori (roasted in a clay oven), or tikke (pan roasted); kabobs Raita (yogurt and cucumber salad) and other yogurt-based dishes and sauces Dal (lentils), pullao or pilau (basmati rice) Chapati (baked bread)	Ghee (clarified butter) Korma (meat in cream sauce) Samosas, pakoras (fried dishes) Molee and other coconut milk-based dishes Poori, bhatura, or paratha (fried breads)
ITALIAN	Pasta primavera or pasta, polenta, risotto, or gnocchi withmarinara, red or white wine, white or red clam, or light mushroom sauce Dishes that are grilled or prepared cacciatore (tomato-based sauce), marsala (broth and wine sauce), or piccata (lemon sauce) Cioppino (seafood stew) Vegetable soup, minestrone or fagioli (beans)	Antipasto (cheese, smoked meats) Dishes that are prepared alfredo, frito (fried), crema (creamed), alla panna (with cream), or carbonara Veal scaloppini Chicken, veal, or eggplant parmigiana Italian sausage, salami, and prosciutto Buttered garlic bread Cannoli
JAPANESE	Dishes prepared nabemono (boiled), shabu-shabu (in boiling broth), mushimono (steamed), nimono (simmered), yaki (broiled), or yakimono (grilled) Sushi or domburi (mixed rice dish) Steamed rice or soba (buckwheat), udon (wheat), or rice noodles	Tempura (battered and fried) Agemono (deep fried) Katsu (fried pork cutlet) Sukiyaki Fried tofu
MEXICAN	Soft corn or wheat tortillas Burritos, fajitas, enchiladas, soft tacos, and tamales filled with beans, vegetables, or lean meats Refried beans, nonfat or low-fat; rice and beans Ceviche (fish marinated in lime juice) Salsa, enchilada sauce, and picante sauce Gazpacho, menudo, or black bean soup Fruit or flan for dessert	Crispy, fried tortillas Dishes that are fried, such as chile rellenos, chimichangas, flautas, and tostadas Nachos and cheese, chili con queso, and other dishes made with cheese or cheese sauce Guacamole, sour cream, and extra cheese Refried beans made with lard Fried ice cream
THAI	Dishes that are barbecued, sauteed, broiled, boiled, steamed, braised, or marinated Sáte (skewered and grilled meats) Fish sauce, basil sauce, chili or hot sauces Bean thread noodles, Thai salad	Coconut milk soup Peanut sauce or dishes topped with nuts Mee-krob (crispy noodles) Red, green, and yellow curries, which typically contain coconut milk

Some experts have also expressed concern about the presence of toxins in farmed fish, especially farmed salmon. Although no federal guidelines have been set, some researchers suggest that consumers limit themselves to 8 ounces of farmed salmon per month. Fish should be labeled with its country of origin and whether it is wild or farmed; most canned salmon is wild.

A PERSONAL PLAN: APPLYING NUTRITIONAL PRINCIPLES

Based on your particular nutrition and health status, there probably is an ideal diet for you, but no single type of diet provides optimal health for everyone. Many cultural dietary patterns can meet people's nutritional requirements (see the box "Ethnic Foods"). Customize your food plan based on your age, gender, weight, activity level, medical risk factors, and personal tastes.

Assessing and Changing Your Diet

The first step in planning a healthy diet is to examine what you currently eat. Labs 3.1 and 3.2 help you analyze your current diet and compare it with optimal dietary goals. (This analysis can be completed using a nutritional analysis software program or one of several Web sites.)

To put your plan into action, use the behavioral self-management techniques and tips described in Chapter 1. If you identify several changes you want to make, focus on one at a time. You might start, for example, by substituting nonfat or low-fat milk for whole milk. When you become used to that, you can try substituting whole-wheat bread for white bread. The information on eating behavior in Lab 3.1 will help you identify and change unhealthy patterns of eating.

Staying Committed to a Healthy Diet

Beyond knowledge and information, you also need support in difficult situations. Keeping to your plan is easiest when you choose and prepare your own food at home. Advance planning is the key: mapping out meals and shopping appropriately, cooking in advance when possible, and preparing enough food for leftovers. A tight budget does not necessarily make it more difficult to eat healthy meals. It makes good health sense and good budget sense to use only small amounts of meat and to have a few meatless meals each week.

In restaurants, sticking to food plan goals becomes somewhat more difficult. Portion sizes in restaurants tend to be larger than MyPlate serving size equivalents, but by remaining focused on your goals, you can eat only part of your meal and take the rest home for a meal later in the week. Don't hesitate to ask questions when you're eating in a restaurant. Most restaurant personnel are glad to explain how menu selections are prepared and to make small adjustments, such as serving salad dressings and sauces on the side so they can be avoided or used sparingly.

Strategies like these are helpful, but small changes cannot change a fundamentally high-fat, high-calorie meal into a moderate, healthful one. Often, the best advice is to bypass a large steak with potatoes au gratin for a flavorful but low-fat entree. Many of the selections offered in ethnic restaurants are healthy choices (refer to the box on ethnic foods for suggestions).

TIPS FOR TODAY AND THE FUTURE

Opportunities to improve your diet present themselves every day, and small changes add up.

RIGHT NOW YOU CAN

- Substitute a healthy snack for an unhealthy one.
- Drink a glass of water and put a bottle of water in your backpack for tomorrow.
- Plan to make healthy selections when you eat out, such as steamed vegetables instead of french fries or salmon instead of steak.

IN THE FUTURE YOU CAN

- Visit the MyPlate Web site at www.choosemyplate.gov and use the online tools to create a personalized nutrition plan and begin tracking your eating habits.
- Learn to cook healthier meals. There are hundreds of free Web sites and low-cost cookbooks that provide recipes for healthy dishes.

Ask yourself

QUESTIONS FOR CRITICAL THINKING AND REFLECTION

What is the least healthy food you eat every day (either during meals or as a snack)? Identify at least one substitute that would be healthier but just as satisfying.

SUMMARY

- The six classes of nutrients are carbohydrates, proteins, fats, vitamins, minerals, and water.
- The nutrients essential to humans are released into the body through digestion. Nutrients in foods provide energy, measured in kilocalories (commonly called calories), build and maintain body tissues, and regulate body functions.
- Protein, an important component of body tissue, is composed of amino acids; nine are essential to good health. Foods

from animal sources provide complete proteins. Plants provide incomplete proteins.

- Fats, a major source of energy, also insulate the body and cushion the organs. Just 3–4 teaspoons of vegetable oil per day supply the essential fats. For most people, dietary fat intake should be 20–35% of total calories, and unsaturated fats should be favored over saturated and trans fats.

- Carbohydrates provide energy to the brain, nervous system, and blood and to muscles during high-intensity exercise. Naturally occurring simple carbohydrates and unrefined complex carbohydrates should be favored over added sugars and refined carbohydrates.

- Fiber includes plant substances that are impossible for the human body to digest. It helps reduce cholesterol levels and promotes the passage of wastes through the intestines.

- The 13 essential vitamins are organic substances that promote specific chemical and cell processes and act as antioxidants. The 17 known essential minerals are inorganic substances that regulate body functions, aid in growth and tissue maintenance, and help in the release of energy from food. Deficiencies in vitamins and minerals can cause severe symptoms over time, but excess doses are also dangerous.

- Water aids in digestion and food absorption, allows chemical reactions to take place, serves as a lubricant or cushion, and helps regulate body temperature.

- Foods contain other substances, such as phytochemicals, that may not be essential nutrients but that may protect against chronic diseases.

- The Dietary Reference Intakes, Dietary Guidelines for Americans, and MyPlate food guidance system provide standards and recommendations for getting all essential nutrients from a varied, balanced diet and for eating in ways that protect against chronic disease.

- The Dietary Guidelines for Americans advise us to balance calorie intake and calorie expenditure to manage weight; reduce consumption of sodium, solid fats, added sugars, and refined grains; increase consumption of fruits, vegetables, and whole grains; and follow a healthy eating pattern.

- Choosing foods from each group in MyPlate every day helps ensure the appropriate amounts of necessary nutrients.

- A vegetarian diet requires special planning but can meet all human nutritional needs.

- Different population groups, such as college students and athletes, face special dietary challenges and should plan their diets to meet their particular needs.

- Consumers can get help applying nutritional principles by reading the standardized labels that appear on all packaged foods and on dietary supplements.

- Although nutritional basics are well established, no single diet provides wellness for everyone. Individuals should focus on their particular needs and adapt general dietary principles to meet them.

FOR FURTHER EXPLORATION

BOOKS

Byrd-Bredbenner, C., et al. 2009. *Wardlaw's Perspectives in Nutrition,* 8th ed. New York: McGraw-Hill. *An easy-to-understand review of major concepts in nutrition.*

Duyff, R. L. 2006. *ADA Complete Food and Nutrition Guide,* 3rd ed. Hoboken, N.J.: Wiley. *An excellent review of current nutrition information.*

Insel, P., D. Ross, K. McMahon, and M. Bernstein. 2011. *Nutrition,* 4th ed. Sudbury, Mass.: Jones & Bartlett. *An introductory nutrition textbook covering a variety of key topics.*

Nestle, M. 2007. *What to Eat.* New York: North Point Press. *A nutritionist examines the marketing of food and explains how to interpret food-related information while shopping.*

Selkowitz, A. 2005. *The College Student's Guide to Eating Well on Campus,* revised ed. Bethesda, Md.: Tulip Hill Press. *Provides practical advice for students, including how to make healthy choices when eating in a dorm or restaurant and how to stock a first pantry.*

Warshaw, H. 2008. *Eat Out Eat Right: The Guide to Healthier Restaurant Eating.* 3rd ed. Agate Surrey. *A registered dietitian provides realistic, informative guidelines for restaurant eating to enable diners to make healthy menu choices from a wide variety of foods and cuisines.*

NEWSLETTERS

Environmental Nutrition (800-424-7887;
http://www.environmentalnutrition.com)
Nutrition Action Health Letter (202-332-9110;
http://www.cspinet.org/nah/index.htm)
Tufts University Health & Nutrition Letter (800-274-7581;
http://www.tuftshealthletter.com)

ORGANIZATIONS, HOTLINES, AND WEB SITES

Academy of Nutrition and Dietetics. Provides a wide variety of educational materials on nutrition.
http://www.eatright.org

American Heart Association: Delicious Decisions. Provides basic information about nutrition, tips for shopping and eating out, and heart-healthy recipes.
http://www.deliciousdecisions.org

FDA: Food. Offers information and interactive tools about topics such as food labeling, food additives, dietary supplements, and foodborne illness.
http://www.fda.gov/food/default.htm

Food Safety Hotlines. Provide information on the safe purchase, handling, cooking, and storage of food.
800-535-4555 (USDA)
888-SAFEFOOD (FDA)

Q Which should I eat—butter or margarine?

A Both butter and margarine are concentrated sources of fat, containing about 11 grams of fat and 100 calories per tablespoon. Butter is higher in saturated fat, which raises levels of artery-clogging LDL ("bad" cholesterol). Each tablespoon of butter has about 8 grams of saturated fat; margarine has about 2. Butter also contains cholesterol, which margarine does not.

Margarine, on the other hand, contains trans fat, which not only raises LDL but lowers HDL ("good" cholesterol). A tablespoon of stick margarine contains about 2 grams of trans fat. Butter contains a small amount of trans fat as well. Although butter has a combined total of saturated and trans fats that is twice that of stick margarine, the trans fat in stick margarine may be worse for you. Clearly, you should avoid both butter and stick margarine. To solve this dilemma, remember that softer is better. The softer or more liquid a margarine or spread is, the less hydrogenated it is and the less trans fat it contains. Tub and squeeze margarines contain less trans fat than stick margarines; some margarines are modified to be low-trans or trans-fat-free and are labeled as such. Vegetable oils are an even better choice for cooking and for table use (such as olive oil for dipping bread) because most are low in saturated fat and completely free of trans fats.

Q MyPlate recommends such large amounts of vegetables and fruit. How can I possibly eat that many servings without gaining weight?

A First, consider your typical portion sizes; you may be closer to meeting the recommendations than you think. Many people consume large servings of foods and underestimate the size of their portions. For example, a large banana may contain the equivalent of a cup of fruit, or half the recommended daily total for someone consuming 2000–2600 calories per day. Likewise, a medium baked potato (3-inch diameter) or an ear of corn (8-inch length) counts as a cup of vegetables. Use a measuring cup or a food scale for a few days to train your eye to accurately estimate food portion sizes. The ChooseMyPlate .gov Web site includes charts of portion-size equivalents for each food group.

If an analysis of your diet indicates that you need to increase your overall intake of fruits and vegetables, look for healthy substitutions. If you are like most Americans, you are consuming more than the recommended number of calories from added sugars and solid fats; trim some of these calories to make room for additional servings of fruits and vegetables. Your beverage choices may be a good place to start. Do you routinely consume regular sodas, sweetened energy or fruit drinks, or whole milk? One regular 12-ounce soda contains the equivalent of about 150 calories of added sugars; an 8-ounce glass of whole milk provides about 75 calories as discretionary fats. Substituting water or low-fat milk would free up calories for additional servings of fruits and vegetables. A half-cup of carrots, tomatoes, apples, or melon has only about 25 calories; you could consume 6 cups of these foods for the calories in one can of regular soda. Substituting lower-fat condiments for such full-fat items as butter, mayonnaise, and salad dressing is another good way to trim calories to make room for additional servings of nutrient-rich fruits and vegetables.

Also consider your portion sizes and/or the frequency with which you consume foods high in discretionary calories: You may not need to eliminate a favorite food—instead, just cut back. For example, cut your consumption of fast-food fries from four times a week to once a week, or reduce the size of your ice cream dessert from a cup to half a cup. Treats should be consumed infrequently, and in small amounts.

For additional help on improving food choices to meet dietary recommendations, visit the ChooseMyPlate.gov Web site and the family-friendly chart of "Go, Slow, and Whoa" foods at the site for the National Heart, Lung, and Blood Institute (www.nhlbi.nih.gov/health /public/heart/ obesity/wecan/downloads /gswtips.pdf).

Q What exactly are genetically modified foods? Are they safe? How can I recognize them on the shelf, and how can I know when I'm eating them?

A Genetic engineering involves altering the characteristics of a plant, animal, or microorganism by adding, rearranging, or replacing genes in its

Fruits and Veggies Matter. Hosted by a partnership of the CDC, DHHS, and National Cancer Institute; promotes the consumption of fruits and vegetables every day.

http://www.fruitsandveggiesmatter.gov

Gateways to Government Nutrition Information. Provides access to government resources relating to food safety, including consumer advice and information on specific pathogens.

http://www.foodsafety.gov

http://www.nutrition.gov

Harvard School of Public Health: Nutrition Source. Provides advice on interpreting news on nutrition; an overview of the Healthy Eating Pyramid, an alternative to the basic USDA pyramid; and suggestions for building a healthy diet.

http://www.hsph.harvard.edu/nutritionsource

International Food Information Council. Provides information on food safety and nutrition for consumers, journalists, and educators.

http://www.ific.org

DNA; the result is a genetically modified (GM) organism. New DNA may come from related species of organisms or from entirely different types of organisms. Many GM crops are already grown in the United States: About 75% of the current U.S. soybean crop has been genetically modified to be resistant to an herbicide used to kill weeds, and about a third of the U.S. corn crop carries genes for herbicide resistance or to produce a protein lethal to a destructive type of caterpillar. Products made with GM organisms include juice, soda, nuts, tuna, frozen pizza, spaghetti sauce, canola oil, chips, salad dressing, and soup.

The potential benefits of GM foods cited by supporters include improved yields overall and in difficult growing conditions, increased disease resistance, improved nutritional content, lower prices, and less use of pesticides. Critics of biotechnology argue that unexpected effects may occur: Gene manipulation could elevate levels of naturally occurring toxins or allergens, permanently change the gene pool and reduce biodiversity, and produce pesticide-resistant insects through the transfer of genes. In 2000, a form of GM corn approved for use only in animal feed was found to have commingled with other varieties of corn and to have been used in human foods; this mistake sparked fears of allergic reactions and led to recalls. Opposition to GM foods is particularly strong in Europe; in many developing nations that face food shortages, responses to GM crops have tended to be more positive.

In April 2000, the National Academy of Sciences released a report stating that there is no proof that GM food on the market is unsafe but that changes are needed to better coordinate regulation of GM foods and to assess potential problems.

Labeling has been another major concern. Surveys indicate that the majority of Americans want to know if their foods contain GM organisms. However, under current rules, the FDA requires special labeling only when a food's composition is changed significantly or when a known allergen is introduced. For example, soybeans that contain a gene from a peanut would have to be labeled because peanuts are a common allergen. The only foods guaranteed not to contain GM ingredients are those certified as organic.

Q How can I tell if I'm allergic to a food?

A A true food allergy is a reaction of the body's immune system to a food or food ingredient, usually a protein. This immune reaction can occur within minutes of ingesting the food, resulting in symptoms such as hives, diarrhea, difficulty breathing, or swelling of the lips or tongue. The most severe response is a systemic reaction called anaphylaxis, which involves a potentially life-threatening drop in blood pressure. Food allergies affect only about 1.5% of the adult population and 4% of children. Between 1997 and 2007, the food allergy rate among American children increased 18%. People with food allergies, especially children, are more likely to have asthma or other allergic conditions.

Just eight foods account for more than 90% of the food allergies in the United States: cow's milk, eggs, peanuts, tree nuts (walnuts, cashews, and so on), soy, wheat, fish, and shellfish. Food manufacturers are now required to state the presence of these eight allergens in plain language in the list of ingredients on food labels.

Many people who believe they have food allergies may actually suffer from a food intolerance, a much more common source of adverse food reactions that typically involves problems with metabolism rather than with the immune system. The body may not be able to adequately digest a food or the body may react to a particular food compound. Food intolerances have been attributed to lactose (milk sugar), gluten (a protein in some grains), tartrazine (yellow food coloring), sulfite (a food additive), MSG, and the sweetener aspartame. Although symptoms of a food intolerance may be similar to those of a food allergy, they are typically more localized and not life-threatening. Many people with food intolerance can safely and comfortably consume small amounts of the food that affects them.

If you suspect you have a food allergy or intolerance, a good first step is to keep a food diary. Note everything you eat or drink, any symptoms you develop, and how long after eating the symptoms appear. Then make an appointment with your physician to go over your diary and determine if any additional tests are needed. People at risk for severe allergic reactions must diligently avoid trigger foods and carry medications to treat anaphylaxis.

For more Common Questions Answered about nutrition, visit the Online Learning Center at www.mhhe.com/fahey.

MedlinePlus: Nutrition. Provides links to information from government agencies and major medical associations on a variety of nutrition topics.

http://www.nlm.nih.gov/medlineplus/nutrition.html

MyPlate. Provides personalized dietary plans and interactive food and activity tracking tools.

http://www.choosemyplate.gov

National Academies' Food and Nutrition Board. Provides information about the Dietary Reference Intakes and related guidelines.

http://www.iom.edu/CMS/3788.aspx

National Institutes of Health: Osteoporosis and Related Bone Diseases' National Resource Center. Provides information about osteoporosis prevention and treatment; includes a special section on men and osteoporosis.

http://www.osteo.org

National Osteoporosis Foundation. Provides information on the causes, prevention, detection, and treatment of osteoporosis.

http://www.nof.org

USDA Center for Nutrition Policy and Promotion. Includes information on the Dietary Guidelines and the Food Guide Pyramid.

http://www.cnpp.usda.gov

USDA Food and Nutrition Information Center. Provides a variety of materials relating to the Dietary Guidelines, food labels, Food Guide Pyramid, MyPlate, and many other topics.

http://www.nal.usda.gov/fnic

Vegetarian Resource Group. Provides information and links for vegetarians and people interested in learning more about vegetarian diets.

http://www.vrg.org

You can find nutrient breakdowns of individual food items at the following sites:

Nutrition Analysis Tool, University of Illinois, Urbana/Champaign

http://www.nat.uiuc.edu

USDA Nutrient Data Laboratory

http://www.ars.usda.gov/ba/bhnrc/ndl

See also the resources listed in Chapters 5 and 7.

SELECTED BIBLIOGRAPHY

A guide to the best and worst drinks. 2006. *Consumer Reports on Health*, July, 8–9.

American Heart Association. 2010. *Diet and Lifestyle Recommendations* (http://www.americanheart.org/presenter.jhtml?identifier=851; retrieved September 15, 2010).

American Heart Association. 2010. *Fish, Levels of Mercury and Omega-3 Fatty Acids* (http://www.americanheart.org/presenter.jhtml?identifier=3013797; retrieved September 15, 2010).

American Heart Association. 2010. Trans Fats (http://www.americanheart.org/presenter.jhtml?identifier=3045792; retrieved September 15, 2010).

Bleich, S. N., et al. 2009. Increasing consumption of sugar-sweetened beverages among U.S. adults: 1988–1994 to 1999–2004. *American Journal of Clinical Nutrition* 89(1): 372–381.

Centers for Disease Control and Prevention. 2009. Application of lower sodium intake recommendations to adults—United States, 1999–2006. *Morbidity and Mortality Weekly Report* 58(11): 281–283.

Centers for Disease Control and Prevention. 2009. *Listeriosis* (http://www.cdc.gov/nczved/divisions/dfbmd/diseases/listeriosis; retrieved September 15, 2010).

Centers for Disease Control and Prevention. 2010. *Foodborne Illness* (http://www.cdc.gov/ncidod/dbmd/diseaseinfo/foodborneinfections_g.htm; retrieved September 15, 2010).

Council for Responsible Nutrition. 2009. *Dietary Supplements: Safe, Regulated and Beneficial* (http://www.crnusa.org/pdfs/CRN_FACT_DSSafeRegulatedBeneficial_09.pdf; retrieved September 15, 2010).

Food and Agriculture Organization of the United Nations. 2009. 1.02 billion people hungry (http://www.fao.org/news/story/en/item/20568/icode: retrieved September 15, 2010).

Food and Nutrition Board, Institute of Medicine. 2005. *Dietary Reference Intakes for Energy, Carbohydrate, Fiber, Fat, Fatty Acids, Cholesterol, Protein, and Amino Acids.* Washington, D.C.: National Academy Press.

Food and Nutrition Board, Institute of Medicine. 2005. *Dietary Reference Intakes for Water, Potassium, Sodium, Chloride, and Sulfate.* Washington, D.C.: National Academy Press.

Grisenbeck, J. S., et al. 2010. Maternal characteristics associated with the dietary intake of nitrates, nitrites, and nitrosamines in women of child-bearing age: A cross-sectional study. *Environmental Health* 9(1): 10.

Harris, W. S., et al. 2009. Omega-6 fatty acids and risk for cardiovascular disease: A science advisory from the American Heart Association Nutrition Subcommittee of the Council on Nutrition, Physical Activity, and Metabolism; Council on Cardiovascular Nursing; and Council on Epidemiology and Prevention. *Circulation* 119(6): 902–907

Harvard School of Public Health, Department of Nutrition. 2010. *The Nutrition Source: Knowledge for Healthy Eating* (http://www.hsph.harvard.edu/nutritionsource; retrieved September 15, 2010).

Hasler, C. M., et al. 2009. Position of the American Dietetic Association: Functional foods. *Journal of the American Dietetic Association* 109(4): 735–736.

Johnson, R. K., et al. 2009. Dietary sugars intake and cardiovascular health: A scientific statement from the American Heart Association. *Circulation* 120(11): 1011–1020.

Lichtenstein, A. H., et al. 2006. Diet and Lifestyle Recommendations, Revision 2006. A Scientific Statement from the American Heart Association Nutrition Committee. *Circulation* 114(1): 82–96.

Liebman, B. 2006. Whole Grains: The Inside Story. *Nutrition Action Health Letter* 33(4): 1–5.

Maki, K. C., et al. 2010. Whole-grain ready-to-eat oat cereal, as part of a dietary program for weight loss, reduces low-density lipoprotein cholesterol in adults with overweight and obesity more than a dietary program including low-fiber control foods. *Journal of the American Dietetic Association* 110(2): 205–214.

Mayo Clinic. 2010. *Food Pyramids: Explore These Healthy Diet Options* (http://www.mayoclinic.com/health/healthy-diet/NU00190; retrieved September 15, 2010).

Mosaffarian, D., et al. 2006. Trans fatty acids and cardiovascular disease. *New England Journal of Medicine* 354(15): 1601–1613.

Nicholls, S. J., et al. 2006. Consumption of saturated fat impairs the anti-inflammatory properties of high-density lipoproteins and endothelial function. *Journal of the American College of Cardiology* 48(4): 715–720.

Siri-Tarino, P. W., et al. 2010. Meta-analysis of prospective cohort studies evaluating the association of saturated fat with cardiovascular disease. *American Journal of Clinical Nutrition* 91(3): 535–546.

Trump, D. L., et al. 2010. Vitamin D: Considerations in the continued development as an agent for cancer prevention and therapy. *Cancer Journal* 16(1): 1–9.

Tucker, K. L. 2009. Osteoporosis prevention and nutrition. *Current Osteoporosis Reports* 7(4): 111–117.

U.S. Department of Agriculture and Centers for Disease Control and Prevention. 2010. *What We Eat in America* (http://www.ars.usda.gov/Services/docs.htm?docid=15044; retrieved September 15, 2010).

U.S. Department of Health and Human Services and U.S. Department of Agriculture. 2010. *Dietary Guidelines for Americans 2010* (http://www.cnpp.usda.gov/DGAs2010-PolicyDocument.htm; retrieved April 1, 2011).

U.S. Food and Drug Administration. 2009. *Food Allergies* (http://www.fda.gov/Food/FoodSafety/FoodAllergens/default.htm; retrieved September 15, 2010).

Varraso R, et al. 2010. Prospective study of dietary fiber and risk of chronic obstructive pulmonary disease among U.S. women and men. *American Journal of Epidemiology* (Published online Feb. 19).

Wang, Y. C., et al. 2008. Increasing caloric contribution from sugar-sweetened beverages and 100% fruit juices among U.S. children and adolescents, 1988–2004. *Pediatrics* 121(6): e1604–e1614.

Nutrition Resources

Table 1 Dietary Reference Intakes (DRIs): Recommended Levels for Individual Intake

Life Stage	Group	BIOTIN (µg/day)	CHOLINE (mg/day)[a]	FOLATE (µg/day)[b]	NIACIN (mg/day)[c]	PANTOTHENIC ACID (mg/day)	RIBOFLAVIN (mg/day)	THIAMIN (mg/day)	VITAMIN A (µg/day)[d]	VITAMIN B-6 (mg/day)	VITAMIN B-12 (µg/day)	VITAMIN C (mg/day)[e]	VITAMIN D (IU/day)[f]	VITAMIN E (mg/day)[g]
Infants	0–6 months	5	125	65	**2**	1.7	0.3	0.2	400	0.1	0.4	40	400	4
	7–12 months	6	150	**80**	**4**	1.8	0.4	0.3	500	0.3	0.5	50	400	5
Children	1–3 years	8	200	**150**	**6**	2	**0.5**	**0.5**	**300**	**0.5**	**0.9**	**15**	600	**6**
	4–8 years	12	250	**200**	**8**	3	**0.6**	**0.6**	**400**	**0.6**	**1.2**	**25**	600	**7**
Males	9–13 years	20	375	**300**	**12**	4	**0.9**	**0.9**	**600**	**1.0**	**1.8**	**45**	600	**11**
	14–18 years	25	550	**400**	**16**	5	**1.3**	**1.2**	**900**	**1.3**	**2.4**	**75**	600	**15**
	19–30 years	30	550	**400**	**16**	5	**1.3**	**1.2**	**900**	**1.3**	**2.4**	**90**	600	**15**
	31–50 years	30	550	**400**	**16**	5	**1.3**	**1.2**	**900**	**1.3**	**2.4**	**90**	600	**15**
	51–70 years	30	550	**400**	**16**	5	**1.3**	**1.2**	**900**	**1.7**	**2.4**[h]	**90**	600	**15**
	>70 years	30	550	**400**	**16**	5	**1.3**	**1.2**	**900**	**1.7**	**2.4**[h]	**90**	600	**15**
Females	9–13 years	20	375	**300**	**12**	4	**0.9**	**0.9**	**600**	**1.0**	**1.8**	**45**	800	**11**
	14–18 years	25	400	**400**[i]	**14**	5	**1.0**	**1.0**	**700**	**1.2**	**2.4**	**65**	600	**15**
	19–30 years	30	425	**400**[i]	**14**	5	**1.1**	**1.1**	**700**	**1.3**	**2.4**	**75**	600	**15**
	31–50 years	30	425	**400**[i]	**14**	5	**1.1**	**1.1**	**700**	**1.3**	**2.4**	**75**	600	**15**
	51–70 years	30	425	**400**[i]	**14**	5	**1.1**	**1.1**	**700**	**1.5**	**2.4**[h]	**75**	600	**15**
	>70 years	30	425	**400**	**14**	5	**1.1**	**1.1**	**700**	**1.5**	**2.4**[h]	**75**	600	**15**
Pregnancy	≤18 years	30	450	**600**[i]	**18**	6	**1.4**	**1.4**	**750**	**1.9**	**2.6**	**80**	800	**15**
	19–30 years	30	450	**600**[j]	**18**	6	**1.4**	**1.4**	**770**	**1.9**	**2.6**	**85**	600	**15**
	31–50 years	30	450	**600**[j]	**18**	6	**1.4**	**1.4**	**770**	**1.9**	**2.6**	**85**	600	**15**
Lactation	≤18 years	35	550	**500**	**17**	7	**1.6**	**1.4**	**1200**	**2.0**	**2.8**	**115**	600	**19**
	19–30 years	35	550	**500**	**17**	7	**1.6**	**1.4**	**1300**	**2.0**	**2.8**	**120**	600	**19**
	31–50 years	35	550	**500**	**17**	7	**1.6**	**1.4**	**1300**	**2.0**	**2.8**	**120**	600	**19**
Tolerable Upper Intake Levels for Adults (19–70)		*3500*	*1000*[k]	*35*[k]				*3000*	*100*		*2000*	*50*	*4000*[k]	

NOTE: The table includes values for the type of DRI standard—Adequate Intake (AI) or Recommended Dietary Allowance (RDA)—that has been established for that particular nutrient and life stage; RDAs are shown in **bold type.** The final row of the table shows the Tolerable Upper Intake Levels (ULs) for adults; refer to the full DRI report for information on other ages and life stages. A UL is the maximum level of daily nutrient intake that is likely to pose no risk of adverse effects. There is insufficient data to set ULs for all nutrients, but this does not mean that there is no potential for adverse effects; source of intake should be from food only to prevent high levels of intake of nutrients without established ULs. In healthy individuals, there is no established benefit from nutrient intakes above the RDA or AI.

[a]Although AIs have been set for choline, there are few data to assess whether a dietary supply of choline is needed at all stages of the life cycle, and it may be that the choline requirement can be met by endogenous synthesis at some of these stages.

[b]As dietary folate equivalents (DFE): 1 DFE = 1 µg food folate = 0.6 µg folate from fortified food or as a supplement consumed with food = 0.5 µg of a supplement taken on an empty stomach.

[c]As niacin equivalents (NE): 1 mg niacin = 60 mg tryptophan.

Table 1 Dietary Reference Intakes (DRIs): Recommended Levels for Individual Intake *(continued)*

Life Stage	Group	VITAMIN K (μg/day)	CALCIUM (mg/day)	CHROMIUM (μg/day)	COPPER (μg/day)	FLUORIDE (mg/day)	IODINE (mg/day)	IRON (mg/day)[l]	MAGNESIUM (mg/day)	MANGANESE (mg/day)	MOLYBDENUM (μg/day)	PHOSPHORUS (mg/day)	SELENIUM (μg/day)	ZINC (mg/day)[m]
Infants	0–6 months	2.0	200	0.2	200	0.01	110	0.27	30	0.003	2	100	15	2
	7–12 months	2.5	260	5.5	220	0.5	130	11	75	0.6	3	275	20	3
Children	1–3 years	30	700	11	340	0.7	90	7	80	1.2	17	460	20	3
	4–8 years	55	1000	15	440	1	90	10	130	1.5	22	500	30	5
Males	9–13 years	60	1300	25	700	2	120	8	240	1.9	34	1250	40	8
	14–18 years	75	1300	35	890	3	150	11	410	2.2	43	1250	55	11
	19–30 years	120	1000	35	900	4	150	8	400	2.3	45	700	55	11
	31–50 years	120	1000	35	900	4	150	8	420	2.3	45	700	55	11
	51–70 years	120	1000	30	900	4	150	8	420	2.3	45	700	55	11
	>70 years	120	1200	30	900	4	150	8	420	2.3	45	700	55	11
Females	9–13 years	60	1300	21	700	2	120	8	240	1.6	34	1250	40	8
	14–18 years	75	1300	24	890	3	150	15	360	1.6	43	1250	55	9
	19–30 years	90	1000	25	900	3	150	18	310	1.8	45	700	55	8
	31–50 years	90	1000	25	900	3	150	18	320	1.8	45	700	55	8
	51–70 years	90	1200	20	900	3	150	8	320	1.8	45	700	55	8
	>70 years	90	1200	20	900	3	150	8	320	1.8	45	700	55	8
Pregnancy	≤18 years	75	3000	29	1000	3	220	27	400	2.0	50	1250	60	13
	19–30 years	90	2500	30	1000	3	220	27	350	2.0	50	700	60	11
	31–50 years	90	2500	30	1000	3	220	27	360	2.0	50	700	60	11
Lactation	≤18 years	75	3000	44	1300	3	290	10	360	2.6	50	1250	70	14
	19–30 years	90	2500	45	1300	3	290	9	310	2.6	50	700	70	12
	31–50 years	90	2500	45	1300	3	290	9	320	2.6	50	700	70	12
Tolerable Upper Intake Levels for Adults (19–70)			*2500*		*10,000*	*10*	*1100*	*45*	*350*[k]	*11*	*2000*	*4000*	*400*	*40*

[d]As retinol activity equivalents (RAEs): 1 RAE = 1 μg retinol, 12 μg β-carotene, or 24 μg α-carotene or β-cryptoxanthin. Preformed vitamin A (retinol) is abundant in animal-derived foods; provitamin A carotenoids are abundant in some dark yellow, orange, red, and deep-green fruits and vegetables. For preformed vitamin A and for provitamin A carotenoids in supplements, IRE = 1 RAE; for provitamin A carotenoids in foods, divide the REs by 2 to obtain RAEs. The UL applies only to preformed vitamin A.

[e]Individuals who smoke require an additional 35 mg/day of vitamin C over that needed by nonsmokers; nonsmokers regularly exposed to tobacco smoke should ensure they meet the RDA for vitamin C.

[f]IU = International Unit.

[g]As α-tocopherol. Includes naturally occurring RRR-α-tocopherol and the 2R-stereoisomeric forms from supplements; does not include the 2S-stereoisomeric forms from supplements.

[h]Because 10–30% of older people may malabsorb food-bound B-12, those over age 50 should meet their RDA mainly with supplements or foods fortified with B-12.

[i]In view of evidence linking folate intake with neural tube defects in the fetus it is recommended that all women capable of becoming pregnant consume 400 μg from supplements or fortified foods in addition to consuming folate from a varied diet.

[j]It is assumed that women will continue consuming 400 μg from supplements or fortified food until their pregnancy is confirmed and they enter prenatal care, which ordinarily occurs after the end of the periconceptional period—the critical time for formation of the neural tube.

[k]The UL applies only to intake from supplements, fortified foods, and/or pharmacological agents and not to intake from foods.

[l]Because the absorption of iron from plant foods is low compared to that from animal foods, the RDA for strict vegetarians is approximately 1.8 times higher than the values established for omnivores (14 mg/day for adult male vegetarians; 33 mg/day for premenopausal female vegetarians). Oral contraceptives (OCs) reduce menstrual blood losses, so women taking them need less daily iron; the RDA for premenopausal women taking OCs is 10.9 mg/day. For more on iron requirements for other special situations, refer to *Dietary Reference Intakes for Vitamin A, Vitamin K, Arsenic, Boron, Chromium, Copper, Iodine, Iron, Manganese, Molybdenum, Nickel, Silicon, Vanadium, and Zinc* (visit http://www.nap.edu for the complete report).

[m]Zinc absorption is lower for those consuming vegetarian diets, so the zinc requirement for vegetarians is approximately twofold greater than for those consuming a nonvegetarian diet.

Table 1 Dietary Reference Intakes (DRIs): Recommended Levels for Individual Intake *(continued)*

Life Stage	Group	POTASSIUM (g/day)	SODIUM (g/day)	CHLORIDE (g/day)	CARBOHYDRATE RDA/AI (g/day)	CARBOHYDRATE AMDR[n] (%)	TOTAL FIBER RDA/AI (g/day)	TOTAL FAT AMDR[o] (%)	LINOLEIC ACID RDA/AI (g/day)	LINOLEIC ACID AMDR[o] (%)	ALPHA-LINOLENIC ACID RDA/AI (g/day)	ALPHA-LINOLENIC ACID AMDR[o] (%)	PROTEIN[n] RDA/AI (g/day)	PROTEIN[n] AMDR[o] (%)	WATER[p] (L/day)
Infants	0–6 months	0.4	0.12	0.18	60	ND[q]	ND	r	4.4	ND[q]	0.5	ND[q]	9.1	ND[q]	0.7
	7–12 months	0.7	0.37	0.57	95	ND[q]	ND	r	4.6	ND[q]	0.5	ND[q]	**13.5**	ND[q]	0.8
Children	1–3 years	3.0	1.0	1.5	**130**	45–65	19	30–40	7	5–10	0.7	0.6–1.2	**13**	5–20	1.3
	4–8 years	3.8	1.2	1.9	**130**	45–65	25	25–35	10	5–10	0.9	0.6–1.2	**19**	10–30	1.7
Males	9–13 years	4.5	1.5	2.3	**130**	45–65	31	25–35	12	5–10	1.2	0.6–1.2	**34**	10–30	2.4
	14–18 years	4.7	1.5	2.3	**130**	45–65	38	25–35	16	5–10	1.6	0.6–1.2	**52**	10–30	3.3
	19–30 years	4.7	1.5	2.3	**130**	45–65	38	20–35	17	5–10	1.6	0.6–1.2	**56**	10–35	3.7
	31–50 years	4.7	1.5	2.3	**130**	45–65	38	20–35	17	5–10	1.6	0.6–1.2	**56**	10–35	3.7
	51–70 years	4.7	1.3	2.0	**130**	45–65	30	20–35	14	5–10	1.6	0.6–1.2	**56**	10–35	3.7
	>70 years	4.7	1.2	1.8	**130**	45–65	30	20–35	14	5–10	1.6	0.6–1.2	**56**	10–35	3.7
Females	9–13 years	4.5	1.5	2.3	**130**	45–65	26	25–35	10	5–10	1.0	0.6–1.2	**34**	10–30	2.1
	14–18 years	4.7	1.5	2.3	**130**	45–65	26	25–35	11	5–10	1.1	0.6–1.2	**46**	10–30	2.3
	19–30 years	4.7	1.5	2.3	**130**	45–65	25	20–35	12	5–10	1.1	0.6–1.2	**46**	10–35	2.7
	31–50 years	4.7	1.5	2.3	**130**	45–65	25	20–35	12	5–10	1.1	0.6–1.2	**46**	10–35	2.7
	51–70 years	4.7	1.3	2.0	**130**	45–65	21	20–35	11	5–10	1.1	0.6–1.2	**46**	10–35	2.7
	>70 years	4.7	1.2	1.8	**130**	45–65	21	20–35	11	5–10	1.1	0.6–1.2	**46**	10–35	2.7
Pregnancy	≤18 years	4.7	1.5	2.3	**175**	45–65	28	20–35	13	5–10	1.4	0.6–1.2	**71**	10–35	3.0
	19–30 years	4.7	1.5	2.3	**175**	45–65	28	20–35	13	5–10	1.4	0.6–1.2	**71**	10–35	3.0
	31–50 years	4.7	1.5	2.3	**175**	45–65	28	20–35	13	5–10	1.4	0.6–1.2	**71**	10–35	3.0
Lactation	≤18 years	5.1	1.5	2.3	**210**	45–65	29	20–35	13	5–10	1.3	0.6–1.2	**71**	10–35	3.8
	19–30 years	5.1	1.5	2.3	**210**	45–65	29	20–35	13	5–10	1.3	0.6–1.2	**71**	10–35	3.8
	31–50 years	5.1	1.5	2.3	**210**	45–65	29	20–35	13	5–10	1.3	0.6–1.2	**71**	10–35	3.8
Tolerable Upper Intake Level for Adults (19–70)			2.3	3.6											

[n]Daily protein recommendations are based on body weight for reference body weights. To calculate for a specific body weight, use the following values: 1.5 g/kg for infants, 1.1 g/kg for 1–3 years, 0.95 g/kg for 4–13 years, 0.85 g/kg for 14–18 years, 0.8 g/kg for adults, and 1.1 g/kg for pregnant (using prepregnancy weight) and lactating women.

[o]Acceptable Macronutrient Distribution Range (AMDR), expressed as a percent of total daily calories, is the range of intake for a particular energy source that is associated with reduced risk of chronic disease while providing intakes of essential nutrients. If an individual consumes in excess of the AMDR, there is a potential for increasing the risk of chronic diseases and/or insufficient intakes of essential nutrients.

[p]Total water intake from fluids and food.

[q]Not determinable due to lack of data of adverse effects in this age group and concern with regard to lack of ability to handle excess amounts. Source of intake should be from food only to prevent high levels of intake.

[r]For infants, Adequate Intake of total fat is 31 grams/day (0–6 months) and 30 grams per day (7–12 months) from breast milk and, for infants 7–12 months, complementary food and beverages.

SOURCE: Food and Nutrition Board, Institute of Medicine, National Academies. 2004. *Dietary Reference Intakes Tables.* Washington, D.C.: National Academics Press. The complete Dietary Reference Intake reports are available from the National Academy Press (http://www.nap.edu).

*Reprinted with permission from *Dietary Reference Intakes Applications in Dietary Planning.* Copyright © 2004 by the National Academy of Sciences. Reprinted with permission from the National Academies Press, Washington, D.C.

Nutrition Resources

Food groups	Number of servings per day (or per week, as noted) 1600 calories	2000 calories	2600 calories	3100 calories	Serving sizes and notes
Grains	6	6–8	10–11	12–13	1 slice bread, 1 oz dry cereal, 1/2 cup cooked rice, pasta, or cereal; choose whole grains
Vegetables	3–4	4–5	5–6	6	1 cup raw leafy vegetables, 1/2 cup cooked vegetables, 1/2 cup vegetable juice
Fruits	4	4–5	5–6	6	1/2 cup fruit juice, 1 medium fruit, 1/4 cup dried fruit, 1/2 cup fresh, frozen, or canned fruit
Low-fat or fat-free dairy foods	2–3	2–3	3	3–4	1 cup milk; 1 cup yogurt, 1 1/2 oz cheese; choose fat-free or low-fat types
Meat, poultry, fish	3–6	6 or less	6	6–9	1 oz cooked meats, poultry, or fish: select only lean; trim away visible fats; broil, roast, or boil instead of frying; remove skin from poultry
Nuts, seeds, legumes	3 servings per week	4–5 servings per week	1	1	1/3 cup or 1 1/2 oz nuts, 2 Tbsp or 1/2 oz seeds, 1/2 cup cooked dry beans/peas, 2 Tbsp peanut butter
Fats and oils	2	2–3	3	4	1 tsp soft margarine, 1 Tbsp low-fat mayonnaise, 2 Tbsp light salad dressing, 1 tsp vegetable oil; DASH has 27% of calories as fat (low in saturated fat)
Sweets	0	5 servings/ week or less	2	2	1 Tbsp sugar, 1 Tbsp jelly or jam, 1/2 cup sorbet, 1 cup lemonade; sweets should be low in fat

FIGURE 1 The DASH Eating Plan.

SOURCE: National Institutes of Health, National Heart, Lung, and Blood Institute. 2006. *Your Guide to Lowering Your Blood Pressure with DASH: How Do I Make the Dash?* (http://www.nhlbi.nih.gov/health/public/heart/hbp/dash/how_make_dash html; retrieved April 30, 2009).

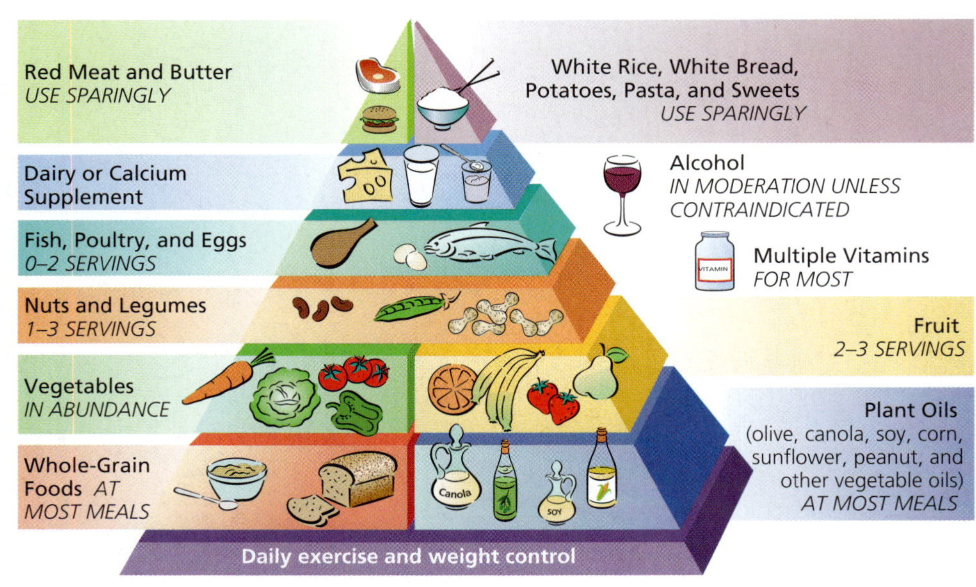

FIGURE 2 Healthy Eating Pyramid. The Healthy Eating Pyramid is an alternative food-group plan developed by researchers at the Harvard School of Public Health. This pyramid reflects many major research studies that have looked at the relationship between diet and long-term health. The Healthy Eating Pyramid differentiates between the various dietary sources of fat, protein, and carbohydrates, and it emphasizes whole grains, vegetable oils, fruits and vegetables, nuts, and dried peas and beans.

SOURCE: Reprinted by permission of Simon & Schuster Inc., from *Eat, Drink, and Be Healthy: The Harvard Medical School Guide to Healthy Eating* by Walter C. Willett, M.D. Copyright © 2001, 2005 by President and Fellows of Harvard College. All rights reserved.

Name ______________________________ Section ______________ Date ____________

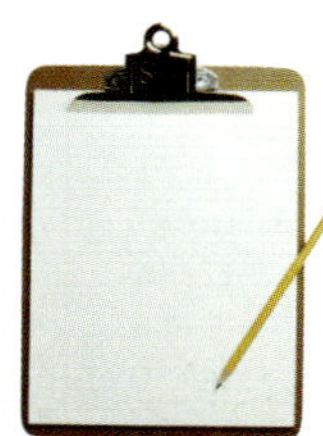

LAB 3.1 Your Daily Diet Versus MyPlate

Make three photocopies of the worksheet in this lab and use them to keep track of everything you eat for 3 consecutive days. Break down each food item into its component parts, and list them separately in the column labeled "Food." Then enter the portion size you consumed in the correct food-group column. For example, a turkey sandwich might be listed as follows: whole-wheat bread, 2 oz-equiv of whole grains; turkey, 2 oz-equiv of meat/beans; tomato, $\frac{1}{3}$ cup other vegetables; romaine lettuce, $\frac{1}{4}$ cup dark green vegetables; 1 tablespoon mayonnaise dressing, 1 teaspoon oils. It can be challenging to track values for added sugars and oils and fats, but use food labels to be as accurate as you can. ChooseMyPlate.gov has additional guidelines for counting discretionary calories.

For vegetables, enter your portion sizes in both the "Total" column and the column corresponding to the correct subgroup; for example, the spinach in a spinach salad would be entered under "Dark Green" and carrots would be entered under "Orange." For the purpose of this 3-day activity, you will compare only your total vegetable consumption against MyPlate guidelines; as described in the chapter, vegetable subgroup recommendations are based on weekly consumption. However, it is important to note which vegetable subgroups are represented in your diet; over a 3-day period, you should consume several servings from each of the subgroups.

Date: ______________________

	Grains (oz-eq)		Vegetable (cups)										Discretionary Calories	
Food	**Whole**	**Other**	**Total**	*Dark Green*	*Orange*	*Legume*	*Starchy*	*Other*	**Fruits (cups)**	**Milk (cups)**	**Meat/ Beans (oz-eq)**	**Oils (tsp)**	**Solid Fats (g)**	**Added Sugars (g/tsp)**
Daily Total														

Next, average your daily intake totals for the 3 days and enter them in the chart below. For example, if your three daily totals for the fruit group were 1 cup, 1½ cups, and 2 cups, your average daily intake would be 1½ cups. Fill in the recommended intake totals that apply to you from Figure 3.5 and Table 3.6.

MyPlate Food Group	Recommended Daily Amounts or Limits	Your Actual Average Daily Intake
Grains (total)	oz-eq	oz-eq
Whole grains	oz-eq	oz-eq
Other grains	oz-eq	oz-eq
Vegetables (total)	cups	cups
Fruits	cups	cups
Milk	cups	cups
Meat and beans	oz-eq	oz-eq
Oils	tsp	tsp
Solid fats	g	g
Added sugars	g/tsp	g/tsp

Using Your Results

How did you score? How close is your diet to that recommended by MyPlate? Are you surprised by the amount of food you are consuming from each food group or from added sugars and solid fats?

What should you do next? If the results of the assessment indicate that you could boost your level of wellness by improving your diet, set realistic goals for change. Do you need to increase or decrease your consumption of any food groups? List any areas of concern below, along with a goal for change and strategies for achieving the goal you've set. If you see that you are falling short in one food group, such as fruits or vegetables, but have many foods that are rich in discretionary calories from solid fats and added sugars, you might try decreasing those items in favor of an apple, a bunch of grapes, or some baby carrots. Think carefully about the reasons behind your food choices. For example, if you eat doughnuts for breakfast every morning because you feel rushed, make a list of ways to save time to allow for a healthier breakfast.

Problem: ____________________

Goal: ____________________

Strategies for change: ____________________

____

____

Problem: ____________________

Goal: ____________________

Strategies for change: ____________________

____

____

Problem: ____________________

Goal: ____________________

Strategies for change: ____________________

____

____

Enter the results of this lab in the Preprogram Assessment column in Appendix C. If you've set goals and identified strategies for change, begin putting your plan into action. After several weeks of your program, complete this lab again and enter the results in the Postprogram Assessment column of Appendix C. How do the results compare?

Name ______________________ **Section** ____________ **Date** __________

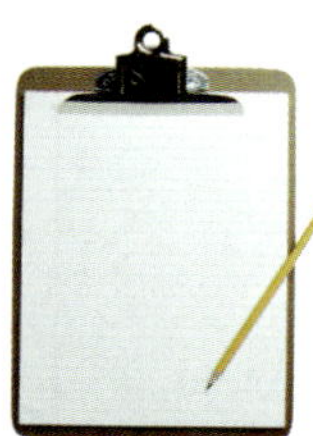

LAB 3.2 Dietary Analysis

You can complete this activity using either a nutrition analysis software program or information about the nutrient content of foods available online; see the For Further Exploration section and page A–1 for recommended Web sites. (This lab asks you to analyze 1 day's diet. For a more complete and accurate assessment of your diet, analyze the results from several different days, including a weekday and a weekend day.)

DATE ______________________ **DAY: M Tu W Th F Sa Su**

Food	Amount	Calories	Protein (g)	Carbohydrate (g)	Dietary fiber (g)	Fat, total (g)	Saturated fat (g)	Cholesterol (mg)	Sodium (mg)	Vitamin A (RE)	Vitamin C (mg)	Calcium (mg)	Iron (mg)
Recommended totals*			10–35%	45–65%	25–38 g	20–35%	<10%	≤300 mg	≤2300 mg	RE	mg	mg	mg
Actual totals**		cal	g / %	g / %	g	g / %	g / %	mg	mg	RE	mg	mg	mg

*Fill in the appropriate DRI values for vitamin A, vitamin C, calcium, and iron from Table 1 in the Nutrition Resources section.

**Total the values in each column. Protein and carbohydrate provide 4 calories per gram; fat provides 9 calories per gram. For example, if you consume a total of 270 grams of carbohydrates and 2000 calories, your percentage of total calories from carbohydrates would be (270 g × 4 cal/g) ÷ 2000 cal = 54%. Do not include data for alcoholic beverages in your calculations. Percentages may not total 100% due to rounding.

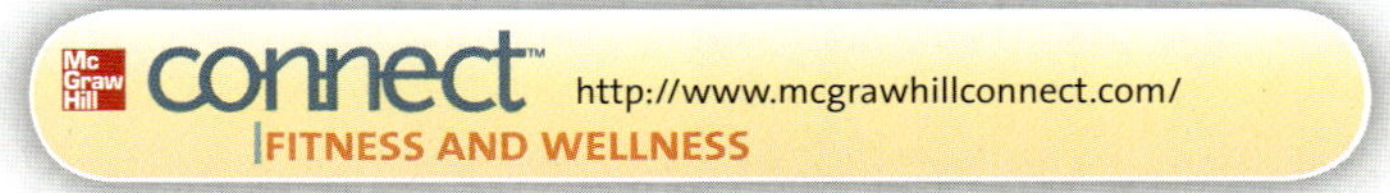

Using Your Results

How did you score? How close is your diet to that recommended in this chapter? Are you surprised by any of the results of this assessment?

What should you do next? Enter the results of this lab in the Preprogram Assessment column in Appendix C. If your daily diet meets all the recommended intakes, congratulations—and keep up the good work. If the results of the assessment pinpoint areas of concern, then work with your food record on the previous page to determine what changes you could make to meet all the guidelines. Make changes, additions, and deletions until it conforms to all or most of the guidelines. Or, if you prefer, start from scratch to create a day's diet that meets the guidelines. Use the chart below to experiment and record your final, healthy sample diet for 1 day. Then put what you learned from this exercise into practice in your daily life. After several weeks of your program, complete this lab again and enter the results in the Postprogram Assessment column of Appendix C. How do the results compare?

DATE ______________ **DAY: M Tu W Th F Sa Su**

Food	Amount	Calories	Protein (g)	Carbohydrate (g)	Dietary fiber (g)	Fat, total (g)	Saturated fat (g)	Cholesterol (mg)	Sodium (mg)	Vitamin A (RE)	Vitamin C (mg)	Calcium (mg)	Iron (mg)
Recommended totals			10–35%	45–65%	25–38 g	20–38%	< 10%	≤300 mg	≤2300 mg	RE	mg	mg	mg
Actual totals		cal	g / %	g / %	g	g / %	g / %	mg	mg	RE	mg	mg	mg

Name ______________________ Section ____________ Date __________

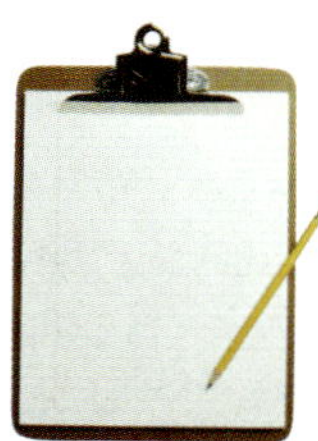

LAB 3.3 Informed Food Choices

Part I Using Food Labels

Choose three food items to evaluate. You might want to select three similar items, such as regular, low-fat, and nonfat salad dressing, or three very different items. Record the information from their food labels in the table below.

Food Items			
Serving size			
Total calories	cal	cal	cal
Total fat—grams	g	g	g
—% Daily Value	%	%	%
Saturated fat—grams	g	g	g
—% Daily Value	%	%	%
Trans fat—grams	g	g	g
Cholesterol—milligrams	mg	mg	mg
—% Daily Value	%	%	%
Sodium—milligrams	mg	mg	mg
—% Daily Value	%	%	%
Carbohydrates (total)—gram	g	g	g
—% Daily Value	%	%	%
Dietary fiber—grams	g	g	g
—% Daily Value	%	%	%
Sugars—grams	g	g	g
Protein—grams	g	g	g
Vitamin A—% Daily Value	%	%	%
Vitamin C—% Daily Value	%	%	%
Calcium—% Daily Value	%	%	%
Iron—% Daily Value	%	%	%

How do the items you chose compare? You can do a quick nutrient check by totaling the Daily Value percentages for nutrients you should limit (total fat, cholesterol, sodium) and the nutrients you should favor (dietary fiber, vitamin A, vitamin C, calcium, iron) for each food. Which food has the largest percent Daily Value sum for nutrients to limit? For nutrients to favor?

Food Items			
Calories	cal	cal	cal
% Daily Value total for nutrients to limit (total fat, cholesterol, sodium)	%	%	%
% Daily Value total for nutrients to favor (fiber, vitamin A, vitamin C, calcium, iron)	%	%	%

Part II Evaluating Fast Food

Use the nutritional information available from fast-food restaurants to complete the chart on this page for the last fast-food meal you ate. Add up your totals for the meal. Compare the values for fat, protein, carbohydrate, cholesterol, and sodium content for each food item and for the meal as a whole with the levels suggested by the Dietary Guidelines for Americans. Calculate the percent of total calories derived from fat, saturated fat, protein, and carbohydrate using the formulas given.

To get fast-food nutritional information, ask for a nutrition information brochure when you visit the restaurant, or visit restaurant Web sites: Arby's (http://www.arbysrestaurant.com), Burger King (http://www.burgerking.com), Domino's Pizza (http://www.dominos.com), Jack in the Box (http://www.jackinthebox.com), KFC (http://www.kfc.com), McDonald's (http://www.mcdonalds.com), Subway (http://www.subway.com), Taco Bell (http://www.tacobell.com), Wendy's (http://www.wendys.com).

If you haven't recently been to a fast-food restaurant, fill in the chart for any sample meal you might eat.

FOOD ITEMS

	Dietary Guidelines							Total**
Serving size (g)		g	g	g	g	g	g	g
Calories		cal	cal	cal	cal	cal	cal	cal
Total fat—grams		g	g	g	g	g	g	g
—% calories*	20–35%	%	%	%	%	%	%	%
Saturated fat—grams		g	g	g	g	g	g	g
—% calories*	<10%	%	%	%	%	%	%	%
Protein—grams		g	g	g	g	g	g	g
—% calories*	10–35%	%	%	%	%	%	%	%
Carbohydrate—grams		g	g	g	g	g	g	g
—% calories*	45–65%	%	%	%	%	%	%	%
Cholesterol[†]	100 mg	mg	mg	mg	mg	mg	mg	mg
Sodium[†]	800 mg	mg	mg	mg	mg	mg	mg	mg

*To calculate the percent of total calories from each food energy source (fat, carbohydrate, protein), use the following formula:

$$\frac{\text{(number of grams of energy source)} \times \text{(number of calories per gram of energy source)}}{\text{(total calories in serving of food item)}}$$

(*Note:* Fat and saturated fat provide 9 calories per gram; protein and carbohydrate provide 4 calories per gram.) For example, the percent of total calories from protein in a 150-calorie dish containing 10 grams of protein is

$$\frac{\text{(10 grams of protein)} \times \text{(4 calories per gram)}}{\text{(150 calories)}} = \frac{40}{150} - 0.27\text{, or 27\% of total calories from protein}$$

**For the Total column, add up the total grams of fat, carbohydrate, and protein contained in your sample meal and calculate the percentages based on the total calories in the meal. (Percentages may not total 100% due to rounding.) For cholesterol and sodium values, add up the total number of milligrams.

[†]Recommended daily limits of cholesterol and sodium are divided by 3 here to give an approximate recommended limit for a single meal.

CHAPTER 4

Cardiorespiratory Endurance

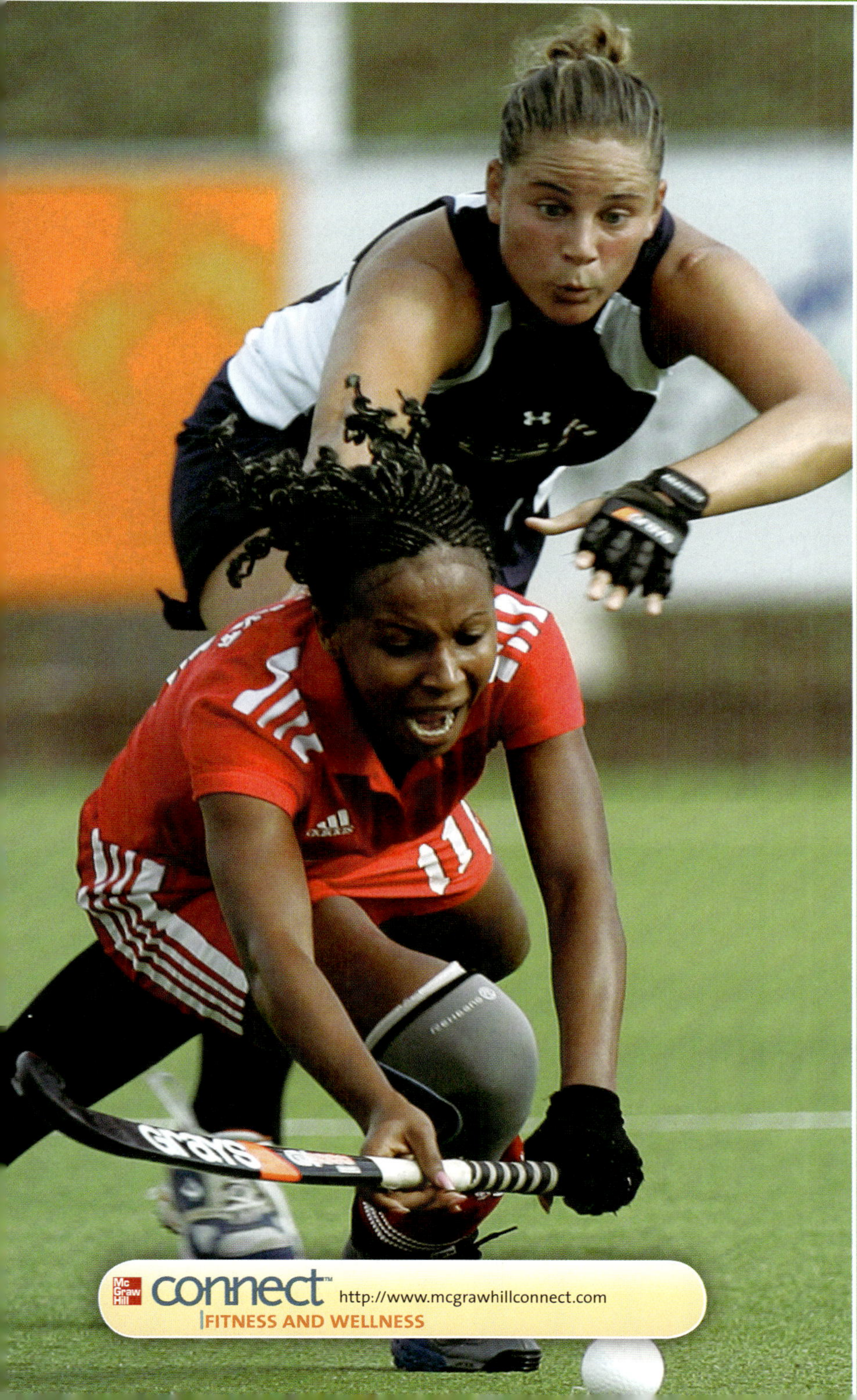

LOOKING AHEAD...

After reading this chapter, you should be able to:

- Describe how the body produces the energy it needs for exercise
- List the major effects and benefits of cardiorespiratory endurance exercise
- Explain how cardiorespiratory endurance is measured and assessed
- Describe how frequency, intensity, time (duration), and type of exercise affect the development of cardiorespiratory endurance
- Explain the best ways to prevent and treat common exercise injuries

TEST YOUR KNOWLEDGE

1. Compared to sedentary people, those who engage in regular moderate endurance exercise are likely to
   a. have fewer colds.
   b. be less anxious and depressed.
   c. fall asleep more quickly and sleep better.
   d. be more alert and creative.
2. About how much blood does the heart pump each minute during aerobic exercise?
   a. 5 quarts
   b. 10 quarts
   c. 20 quarts
3. During an effective 30-minute cardiorespiratory endurance workout, you should lose 1–2 pounds. True or false?

Answers

1. **All four.** Endurance exercise has many immediate benefits that affect all the dimensions of wellness and improve overall quality of life.
2. **c.** During exercise, cardiac output increases to 20 or more quarts per minute, compared to about 5 quarts per minute at rest.
3. **False.** Any weight loss during an exercise session is due to fluid loss that needs to be replaced to prevent dehydration and enhance performance. It is best to drink enough during exercise to match fluid lost as sweat; weigh yourself before and after a workout to make sure you are drinking enough.

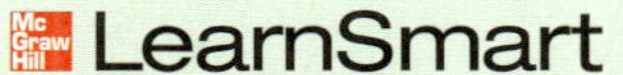

Cardiorespiratory endurance—the ability of the body to perform prolonged, large-muscle, dynamic exercise at moderate to high levels of intensity—is a key health-related component of fitness. As explained in Chapter 2, a healthy cardiorespiratory system is essential to high levels of fitness and wellness.

This chapter reviews the short- and long-term effects and benefits of cardiorespiratory endurance exercise. It then describes several tests that are commonly used to assess cardiorespiratory fitness. Finally, it provides guidelines for creating your own cardiorespiratory endurance training program—one that is geared to your current level of fitness and built around activities you enjoy.

BASIC PHYSIOLOGY OF CARDIORESPIRATORY ENDURANCE EXERCISE

A basic understanding of the body processes involved in cardiorespiratory endurance exercise can help you design a safe and effective fitness program.

The Cardiorespiratory System

The **cardiorespiratory system** consists of the heart, the blood vessels, and the respiratory system. (See page T3-2 of the color transparency insert "Touring the Cardiorespiratory System" in this chapter.) The cardiorespiratory system circulates blood through the body, transporting oxygen, nutrients, and other key substances to the organs and tissues that need them. It also carries away waste products so they can be used or expelled.

The Heart The heart is a four-chambered, fist-sized muscle located just beneath the sternum (breastbone) (Figure 4.1). It pumps deoxygenated (oxygen-poor) blood to the lungs and delivers oxygenated (oxygen-rich) blood to the rest of the body. Blood actually travels through two separate circulatory systems: The right side of the heart pumps blood to the lungs in what is called **pulmonary circulation**, and the left side pumps blood through the rest of the body in **systemic circulation.**

The path of blood flow through the heart and cardiorespiratory system is illustrated on page T3-3 of the color transparency insert "Touring the Cardiorespiratory System" in this chapter. Refer to that illustration as you trace these steps:

1. Waste-laden, oxygen-poor blood travels through large vessels, called **venae cavae**, into the heart's right upper chamber, or **atrium.**
2. After the right atrium fills, it contracts and pumps blood into the heart's right lower chamber, or **ventricle.**
3. When the right ventricle is full, it contracts and pumps blood through the pulmonary artery into the lungs.
4. In the lungs, blood picks up oxygen and discards carbon dioxide.
5. The cleaned, oxygenated blood flows from the lungs through the pulmonary veins into the heart's left atrium.
6. After the left atrium fills, it contracts and pumps blood into the left ventricle.
7. When the left ventricle is full, it pumps blood through the **aorta**—the body's largest artery—for distribution to the rest of the body's blood vessels.

The period of the heart's contraction is called **systole;** the period of relaxation is called **diastole.** During systole, the atria contract first, pumping blood into the ventricles. A fraction of a second later, the ventricles contract, pumping blood to the lungs and the body. During diastole, blood flows into the heart.

Blood pressure, the force exerted by blood on the walls of the blood vessels, is created by the pumping action of the heart. Blood pressure is greater during systole than during diastole. A person weighing 150 pounds has about 5 quarts of blood, which are circulated about once every minute.

The heartbeat—the split-second sequence of contractions of the heart's four chambers—is controlled by nerve impulses. These signals originate in a bundle of specialized cells in the right atrium called the *pacemaker,* or *sinoatrial (SA) node*. Unless it is speeded up or slowed down by the brain in response to such stimuli as danger or the tissues' need for more oxygen, the heart produces nerve impulses at a steady rate.

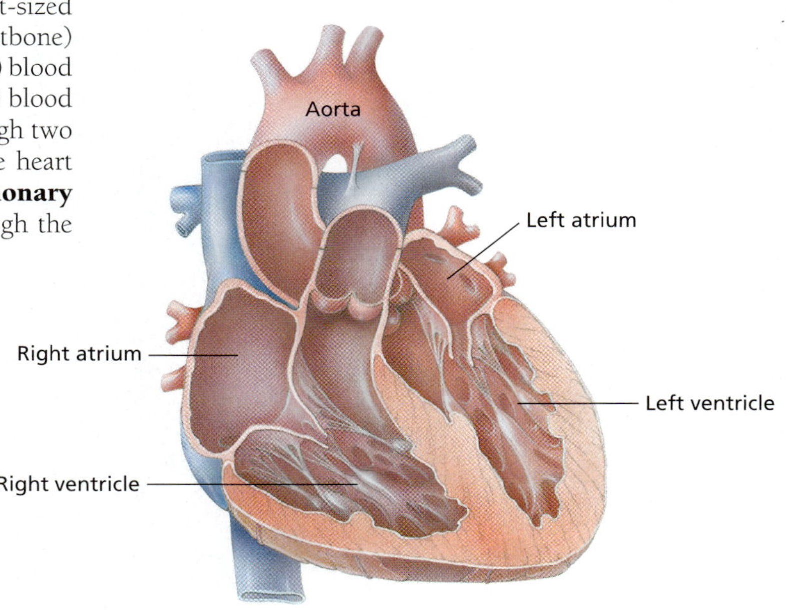

FIGURE 4.1 Chambers of the heart.

Wellness Tip

Aerobic exercise reduces blood pressure. Regular physical activity, regardless of intensity, helps you maintain a healthy blood pressure.

The Blood Vessels Blood vessels are classified by size and function. **Veins** carry blood to the heart. **Arteries** carry it away from the heart. Veins have thin walls, but arteries have thick elastic walls that enable them to expand and relax with the volume of blood being pumped through them.

After leaving the heart, the aorta branches into smaller and smaller vessels. The smallest arteries branch still further into **capillaries,** tiny vessels only one cell thick. The capillaries deliver oxygen and nutrient-rich blood to the tissues and pick up oxygen-poor, waste-laden blood. From the capillaries, this blood empties into small veins (*venules*) and then into larger veins that return it to the heart to repeat the cycle.

Blood pumped through the heart doesn't reach the heart's own cells, so the organ has its own network of blood vessels. Two large vessels, the right and left **coronary arteries,** branch off the aorta and supply the heart muscle with oxygenated blood. The coronary arteries are shown on page T3-3 of the color transparency insert "Touring the Cardiorespiratory System" in this chapter.

The Respiratory System The **respiratory system** supplies oxygen to the body, carries off carbon dioxide—a waste product of body processes—and helps regulate acid produced during metabolism. Air passes in and out of the lungs as a result of pressure changes brought about by the contraction and relaxation of the diaphragm and rib muscles. As air is inhaled, it passes through the nasal passages, throat, larynx, trachea (windpipe), and bronchi into the lungs. The lungs consist of many branching tubes that end in tiny, thin-walled air sacs called **alveoli.**

Carbon dioxide and oxygen are exchanged between alveoli and capillaries in the lungs. Carbon dioxide passes from blood cells into the alveoli, where it is carried up and out of the lungs (exhaled). Oxygen from inhaled air is passed from the alveoli into blood cells; these oxygen-rich blood cells then return to the heart and are pumped throughout the body. Oxygen is an important component of the body's energy-producing system, so the cardiorespiratory system's ability to pick up and deliver oxygen is critical for the functioning of the body.

The Cardiorespiratory System at Rest and During Exercise At rest and during light activity, the cardiorespiratory system functions at a fairly steady pace. Your heart beats at a rate of about 50–90 beats per minute, and you take about 12–20 breaths per minute. A typical resting blood pressure in a healthy adult, measured in millimeters of mercury, is 120 systolic and 80 diastolic (120/80).

During exercise, the demands on the cardiorespiratory system increase. Body cells, particularly working muscles, need to obtain more oxygen and fuel and to eliminate more waste products. To meet these demands, your body makes the following changes:

- Heart rate increases, up to 170–210 beats per minute during intense exercise.
- The heart's **stroke volume** increases, meaning that the heart pumps out more blood with each beat.
- The heart pumps and circulates more blood per minute as a result of the faster heart rate and greater

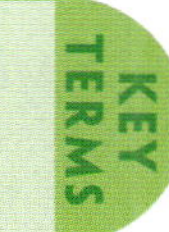

cardiorespiratory system The system that circulates blood through the body; consists of the heart, blood vessels, and respiratory system.

pulmonary circulation The part of the circulatory system that moves blood between the heart and lungs; controlled by the right side of the heart.

systemic circulation The part of the circulatory system that moves blood between the heart and the rest of the body; controlled by the left side of the heart.

venae cavae The large veins through which blood is returned to the right atrium of the heart.

atrium One of the two upper chambers of the heart in which blood collects before passing to the ventricles (pl. *atria*).

ventricle One of the two lower chambers of the heart, from which blood flows through arteries to the lungs and other parts of the body.

aorta The body's largest artery; receives blood from the left ventricle and distributes it to the body.

systole Contraction of the heart.

diastole Relaxation of the heart.

blood pressure The force exerted by the blood on the walls of the blood vessels; created by the pumping action of the heart.

veins Vessels that carry blood to the heart.

arteries Vessels that carry blood away from the heart.

capillaries Very small blood vessels that distribute blood to all parts of the body.

coronary arteries A pair of large blood vessels that branch off the aorta and supply the heart muscle with oxygenated blood.

respiratory system The lungs, air passages, and breathing muscles; supplies oxygen to the body and removes carbon dioxide.

alveoli Tiny air sacs in the lungs that allow the exchange of oxygen and carbon dioxide between the lungs and blood.

stroke volume The amount of blood the heart pumps with each beat.

stroke volume. During exercise, this **cardiac output** increases to 20 or more quarts per minute, compared to about 5 quarts per minute at rest.

- Blood flow changes, so as much as 85–90% of the blood may be delivered to working muscles. At rest, about 15–20% of blood is distributed to the skeletal muscles.
- Systolic blood pressure increases, while diastolic blood pressure holds steady or declines slightly. A typical exercise blood pressure might be 175/65.
- To oxygenate this increased blood flow, you take deeper breaths and breathe faster, up to 40–60 breaths per minute.

All of these changes are controlled and coordinated by special centers in the brain, which use the nervous system and chemical messengers to control the process.

Energy Production

Metabolism is the sum of all the chemical processes necessary to maintain the body. Energy is required to fuel vital body functions—to build and break down tissue, contract muscles, conduct nerve impulses, regulate body temperature, and so on.

The rate at which your body uses energy—its **metabolic rate**—depends on your level of activity. At rest, you have a low metabolic rate; if you begin to walk, your metabolic rate increases. If you jog, your metabolic rate may increase more than 800% above its resting level. Olympic-caliber distance runners can increase their metabolic rate by 2000% or more.

Energy from Food The body converts chemical energy from food into substances that cells can use as fuel. These fuels can be used immediately or stored for later use. The body's ability to store fuel is critical, because if all the energy from food were released immediately, much of it would be wasted.

The three classes of energy-containing nutrients in food are carbohydrates, fats, and proteins. During digestion, most carbohydrates are broken down into the simple sugar **glucose.** Some glucose remains circulating in the blood ("blood sugar"), where it can be used as a quick source of fuel to produce energy. Glucose may also be converted to **glycogen** and stored in the liver, muscles, and kidneys. If glycogen stores are full and the body's immediate need for energy is met, the remaining glucose is converted to fat and stored in the body's fatty tissues. Excess energy from dietary fat is also stored as body fat. Protein in the diet is used primarily to build new tissue, but it can be broken down for energy or incorporated into fat stores. Glucose, glycogen, and fat are important fuels for the production of energy in the cells; protein is a significant energy source only when other fuels are lacking. (See Chapter 3 for more on the roles of carbohydrate, fat, and protein in the body.)

ATP: The Energy "Currency" of Cells The basic form of energy used by cells is **adenosine triphosphate**, or ATP. When a cell needs energy, it breaks down ATP, a process that releases energy in the only form the cell can use directly. Cells store a small amount of ATP; when they need more, they create it through chemical reactions that utilize the body's stored fuels—glucose, glycogen, and fat. When you exercise, your cells need to produce more energy. Consequently, your body mobilizes its stores of fuel to increase ATP production.

Exercise and the Three Energy Systems

The muscles in your body use three energy systems to create ATP and fuel cellular activity. These systems use different fuels and chemical processes and perform different, specific functions during exercise (Table 4.1).

Table 4.1 Characteristics of the Body's Energy Systems

	ENERGY SYSTEM*		
	IMMEDIATE	NONOXIDATIVE	OXIDATIVE
DURATION OF ACTIVITY FOR WHICH SYSTEM PREDOMINATES	0–10 seconds	10 seconds–2 minutes	>2 minutes
INTENSITY OF ACTIVITY FOR WHICH SYSTEM PREDOMINATES	High	High	Low to moderately high
RATE OF ATP PRODUCTION	Immediate, very rapid	Rapid	Slower, but prolonged
FUEL	Adenosine triphosphate (ATP), creatine phosphate (CP)	Muscle stores of glucose and glycogen	Body stores of glycogen, glucose, fat, and protein
OXYGEN USED?	No	No	Yes
SAMPLE ACTIVITIES	Weight lifting, picking up a bag of groceries	400-meter run, running up several flights of stairs	1500-meter run, 30-minute walk, standing in line for a long time

*For most activities, all three systems contribute to energy production; the duration and intensity of the activity determine which system predominates.

SOURCE: Adapted from Brooks, G. A., et al. 2005. *Exercise Physiology: Human Bioenergetics and Its Applications,* 4th ed. New York: McGraw-Hill. Copyright © 2005 The McGraw-Hill Companies. Reproduced with permission of The McGraw-Hill Companies.

The Immediate Energy System The **immediate ("explosive") energy system** provides energy rapidly but for only a short period of time. It is used to fuel activities that last for about 10 or fewer seconds—examples in sports include weight lifting and shot-putting; examples in daily life include rising from a chair or picking up a bag of groceries. The components of this energy system include existing cellular ATP stores and creatine phosphate (CP), a chemical that cells can use to make ATP. CP levels are depleted rapidly during exercise, so the maximum capacity of this energy system is reached within a few seconds. Cells must then switch to the other energy systems to restore levels of ATP and CP. (Without adequate ATP, muscles will stiffen and become unusable.)

The Nonoxidative Energy System The **nonoxidative (anaerobic) energy system** is used at the start of an exercise session and for high-intensity activities lasting for about 10 seconds to 2 minutes, such as the 400-meter run. During daily activities, this system may be called on to help you run to catch a bus or dash up several flights of stairs. The nonoxidative energy system creates ATP by breaking down glucose and glycogen. This system doesn't require oxygen, which is why it is sometimes referred to as the **anaerobic** system. This system's capacity to produce energy is limited, but it can generate a great deal of ATP in a short period of time. For this reason, it is the most important energy system for very intense exercise.

There are two key limitations to the nonoxidative energy system. First, the body's supply of glucose and glycogen is limited. If these are depleted, a person may experience fatigue and dizziness, and judgment may be impaired. (The brain and nervous system rely on carbohydrates as fuel.) Second, increases in hydrogen and potassium ions (which are thought to interfere with metabolism and muscle contraction) cause fatigue. During heavy exercise, such as sprinting, large increases in hydrogen and potassium ions cause muscles to fatigue rapidly.

The anaerobic energy system also creates metabolic acids. Fortunately, exercise training increases the body's ability to cope with metabolic acid. Improved fitness allows you to exercise at higher intensities before the abrupt buildup of metabolic acids—a point that scientists call the *lactate threshold*. One metabolic acid, called **lactic acid** (lactate), is often linked to fatigue during intense exercise. However, lactic acid is an important fuel at rest and during exercise.

The Oxidative Energy System The **oxidative (aerobic) energy system** is used during any physical activity that lasts longer than about 2 minutes, such as distance running, swimming, hiking, or even standing in line. The oxidative system requires oxygen to generate ATP, which is why it is considered an **aerobic** system. The oxidative system cannot produce energy as quickly as the other two systems, but it can supply energy for much longer periods of time. It provides energy during most daily activities.

In the oxidative energy system, ATP production takes place in cellular structures called **mitochondria.** Because mitochondria can use carbohydrates (glucose and glycogen) or fats to produce ATP, the body's stores of fuel for this system are much greater than those for the other two energy systems. The actual fuel used depends on the intensity and duration of exercise and on the fitness status of the individual. Carbohydrates are favored during more intense exercise (over 65% of maximum capacity); fats are used for mild, low-intensity activities. During a prolonged exercise session, carbohydrates are the predominant fuel at the start of the workout, but fat utilization increases over time. Fit individuals use a greater proportion of fat as fuel because increased fitness allows people to do activities at lower intensities. This is an important adaptation because glycogen depletion is one of the limiting factors for the oxidative energy system. Thus, by being able to use more fat as fuel, a fit individual can exercise for a longer time before glycogen is depleted and muscles become fatigued.

Oxygen is another limiting factor. The oxygen requirement of this energy system is proportional to the intensity of exercise. As intensity increases, so does oxygen

KEY TERMS

cardiac output The amount of blood pumped by the heart each minute; a function of heart rate and stroke volume.

metabolic rate The rate at which the body uses energy.

glucose A simple sugar that circulates in the blood and can be used by cells to fuel adenosine triphosphate (ATP) production.

glycogen A complex carbohydrate stored principally in the liver and skeletal muscles; the major fuel source during most forms of intense exercise. Glycogen is the storage form of glucose.

adenosine triphosphate (ATP) The energy source for cellular processes.

immediate ("explosive") energy system The system that supplies energy to muscle cells through the breakdown of cellular stores of ATP and creatine phosphate (CP).

nonoxidative (anaerobic) energy system The system that supplies energy to muscle cells through the breakdown of muscle stores of glucose and glycogen; also called the *anaerobic system* or the *lactic acid system* because chemical reactions take place without oxygen and produce lactic acid.

anaerobic Occurring in the absence of oxygen.

lactic acid A metabolic acid resulting from the metabolism of glucose and glycogen.

oxidative (aerobic) energy system The system that supplies energy to cells through the breakdown of glucose, glycogen, and fats; also called the *aerobic system* because its chemical reactions require oxygen.

aerobic Dependent on the presence of oxygen.

mitochondria Cell structures that convert the energy in food to a form the body can use.

consumption. The body's ability to increase oxygen use is limited; this limit is referred to as **maximal oxygen consumption**, or $\dot{V}O_{2max}$. $\dot{V}O_{2max}$ determines how intensely a person can perform endurance exercise and for how long, and it is considered the best overall measure of the capacity of the cardiorespiratory system. (The assessment tests described later in the chapter are designed to help you evaluate your $\dot{V}O_{2max}$.)

The Energy Systems in Combination Your body typically uses all three energy systems when you exercise. The intensity and duration of the activity determine which system predominates. For example, when you play tennis, you use the immediate energy system when hitting the ball, but you replenish cellular energy stores by using the nonoxidative and oxidative systems. When cycling, the oxidative system predominates. However, if you must suddenly exercise intensely—by riding up a steep hill, for example—the other systems become important because the oxidative system is unable to supply ATP fast enough to sustain high-intensity effort.

Physical Fitness and Energy Production Physically fit people can increase their metabolic rate substantially, generating the energy needed for powerful or sustained exercise. People who are not fit cannot respond to exercise in the same way. Their bodies are less capable of delivering oxygen and fuel to exercising muscles, they can't burn as many calories during or after exercise, and they are less able to cope with lactic acid and other substances produced during intense physical activity that contribute to fatigue. Because of this, they become fatigued more rapidly; their legs hurt and they breathe heavily walking up a flight of stairs, for example. Regular physical training can substantially improve the body's ability to produce energy and meet the challenges of increased physical activity.

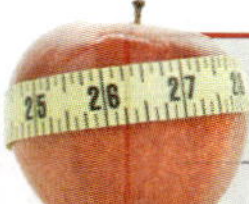

Wellness Tip

Feeling tired? Try taking a brisk walk instead of a nap. The more physically active you are, the more energetic you'll feel over the long run.

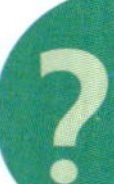

Ask Yourself

QUESTIONS FOR CRITICAL THINKING AND REFLECTION

When you think about the types of physical activity you engage in during your typical day or week, which ones use the immediate energy system? The nonoxidative energy system? The oxidative energy system? How can you increase activities that use the oxidative energy system?

In designing an exercise program, focus on the energy system most important to your goals. Because improving the functioning of the cardiorespiratory system is critical to overall wellness, endurance exercise that utilizes the oxidative energy system—activities performed at moderate to high intensities for a prolonged duration—is a key component of any health-related fitness program.

BENEFITS OF CARDIORESPIRATORY ENDURANCE EXERCISE

Cardiorespiratory endurance exercise helps the body become more efficient and better able to cope with physical challenges. It also lowers risk for many chronic diseases.

Improved Cardiorespiratory Functioning

Earlier, this chapter described some of the major changes that occur in the cardiorespiratory system when you exercise, such as increases in cardiac output and blood

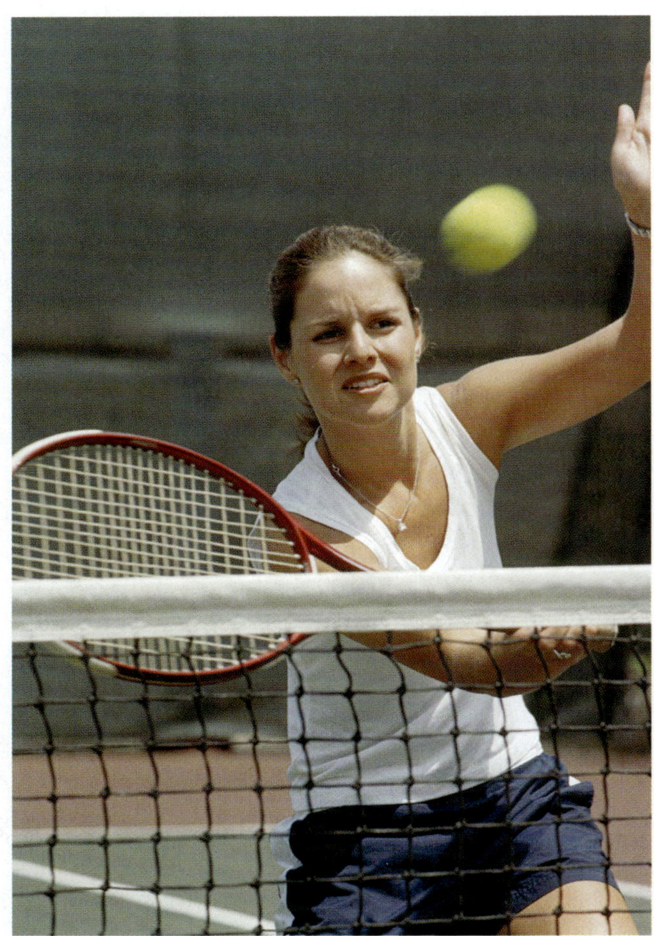

Exercise offers both long-term health benefits and immediate pleasures. Many popular sports and activities develop cardiorespiratory endurance.

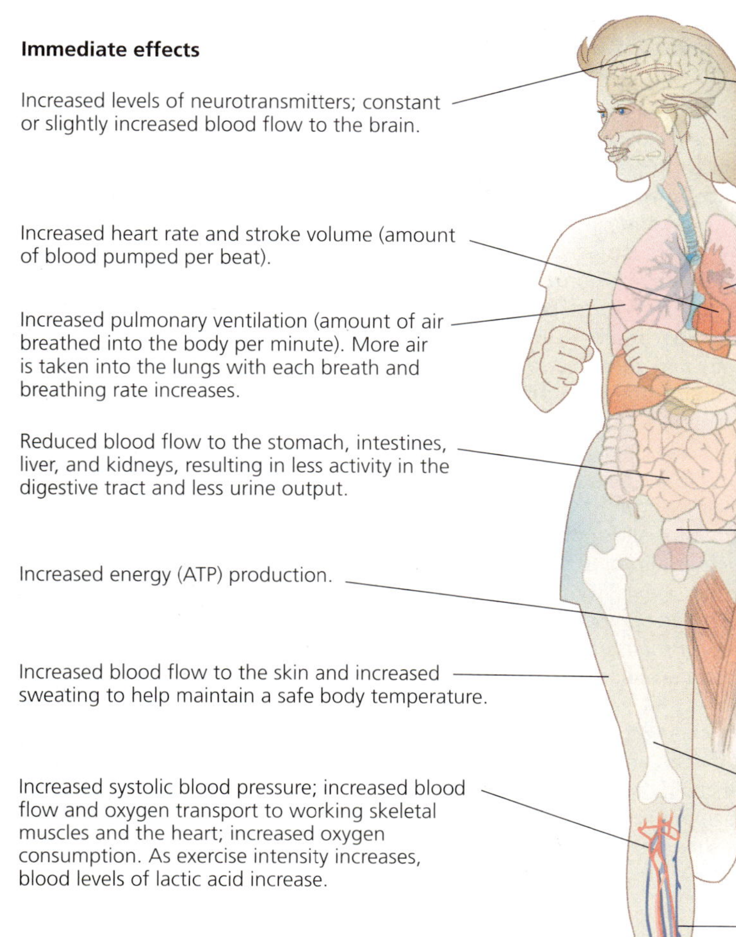

FIGURE 4.2 Immediate and long-term effects of regular cardiorespiratory endurance exercise. When endurance exercise is performed regularly, short-term changes in the body develop into more permanent adaptations; these include improved ability to exercise, reduced risk of many chronic diseases, and improved psychological and emotional well-being.

pressure, breathing rate, and blood flow to the skeletal muscles. In the short term, all these changes help the body respond to the challenge of exercise. When performed regularly, endurance exercise also leads to permanent adaptations in the cardiorespiratory system (Figure 4.2). These improvements reduce the effort required to perform everyday tasks and make the body better able to respond to physical challenges. This, in a nutshell, is what it means to be physically fit.

Endurance exercise enhances the heart's health by:

- Maintaining or increasing the heart's own blood and oxygen supply.
- Improving the heart muscle's function, so it pumps more blood per beat. This improved function keeps the heart rate lower both at rest and during exercise. The resting heart rate of a fit person is often 10–20 beats per minute lower than that of an unfit person. This translates into as many as 10 million fewer beats in the course of a year.
- Strengthening the heart's contractions.
- Increasing the heart's cavity size (in young adults).
- Increasing blood volume so the heart pushes more blood into the circulatory system during each contraction (larger stroke volume).
- Reducing blood pressure.

KEY TERM

maximal oxygen consumption ($\dot{V}O_{2max}$) The highest rate of oxygen consumption an individual is capable of during maximum physical effort, reflecting the body's ability to transport and use oxygen; measured in milliliters of oxygen used per minute per kilogram of body weight.

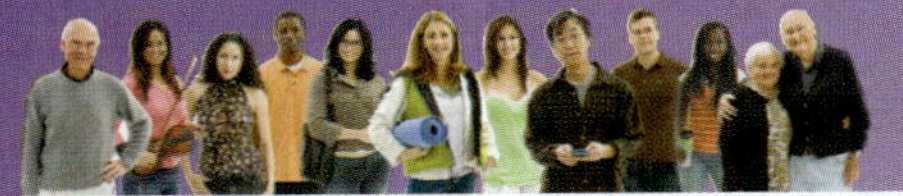

DIMENSIONS OF DIVERSITY

Benefits of Exercise for Older Adults

Research has shown that most aspects of physiological functioning peak when people are about 30 years old, then decline at a rate of about 0.5–1.0% per year. This decline in physical capacity is characterized by a decrease in maximal oxygen consumption, cardiac output, muscular strength, fat-free mass, joint mobility, and other factors. However, regular exercise can substantially alter the rate of decline in functional status, and it is associated with both longevity and improved quality of life.

Regular endurance exercise can improve maximal oxygen consumption in older adults by up to 15–30%—the same degree of improvement seen in younger adults. In fact, studies have shown that Masters athletes in their seventies have $\dot{V}O_{2max}$ values equivalent to those of sedentary 20-year-olds. At any age, endurance training can improve cardiorespiratory functioning, cellular metabolism, body composition, and psychological and emotional well-being. Older adults who exercise regularly have better balance and greater bone density and are less likely than their sedentary peers to suffer injuries as a result of falls. Regular endurance training also substantially reduces the risk of many chronic and disabling diseases, including heart disease, cancer, diabetes, osteoporosis, and dementia.

Other forms of exercise training are also beneficial for older adults. Resistance training is a safe and effective way to build strength and fat-free mass and can help people remain independent as they age. Lifting weights has also been shown to boost spirits in older people, perhaps because improvements in strength appear quickly and are easily applied to everyday tasks such as climbing stairs and carrying groceries. Flexibility exercises can improve the range of motion in joints and also help people maintain functional independence as they age.

It's never too late to start exercising. Even in people over 80, beginning an exercise program can improve physical functioning and quality of life. Most older adults can participate in moderate walking and strengthening and stretching exercises, and modified programs can be created for people with chronic conditions and other special health concerns. The wellness benefits of exercise are available to people of all ages and levels of ability.

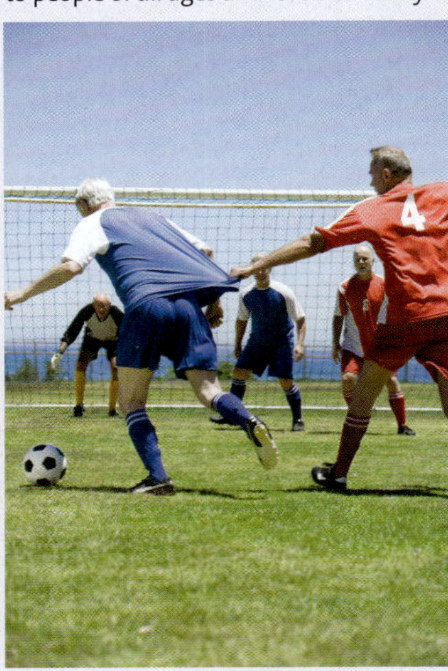

Improved Cellular Metabolism

Regular endurance exercise improves the body's metabolism, down to the cellular level, enhancing your ability to produce and use energy efficiently. Cardiorespiratory training improves metabolism by doing the following:

- Increasing the number of capillaries in the muscles. Additional capillaries supply the muscles with more fuel and oxygen and more quickly eliminate waste products. Greater capillary density also helps heal injuries and reduce muscle aches.
- Training muscles to make the most of oxygen and fuel so they work more efficiently.
- Increasing the size of and number of mitochondria in muscle cells, increasing cells' energy capacity.
- Preventing glycogen depletion and increasing the muscles' ability to use lactate and fat as fuels.

Regular exercise may also help protect cells from chemical damage caused by agents called *free radicals*. (See Chapter 3 for details on free radicals and special enzymes the body uses to fight them.)

Fitness programs that best develop metabolic efficiency include both long-duration, moderately intense endurance exercise and brief periods of more intense effort. For example, climbing a small hill while jogging or cycling introduces the kind of intense exercise that leads to more efficient use of lactate and fats.

Reduced Risk of Chronic Disease

Regular endurance exercise lowers your risk of many chronic, disabling diseases. It can also help people with those diseases improve their health (see the box "Benefits of Exercise for Older Adults"). The most significant health benefits occur when someone who is sedentary becomes moderately active.

Cardiovascular Diseases Sedentary living is a key contributor to cardiovascular disease (CVD). CVD is a general category that encompasses several diseases of the heart and blood vessels, including coronary heart disease (which can cause heart attacks), stroke, and high blood pressure (see the box "Why Is It Important to Combine Aerobic Exercise with Strength Training?"). Sedentary people are significantly more likely to die of CVD than are fit individuals.

Cardiorespiratory endurance exercise lowers your risk of CVD by doing the following:

- Promoting a healthy balance of fats in the blood. High concentrations of blood fats such as cholesterol and triglycerides are linked to CVD. Exercise raises levels

Why Is It Important to Combine Aerobic Exercise with Strength Training?

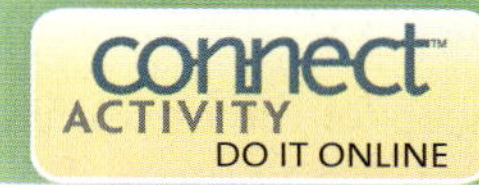

THE EVIDENCE FOR EXERCISE

For a variety of reasons, many people choose to focus on only one aspect of physical wellness or fitness. For example, many women concentrate on cardiorespiratory and flexibility exercises but ignore weight training for fear of developing bulky muscles. Many men, conversely, focus exclusively on resistance training in the hope of developing large, strong muscles. They often avoid cardio or flexibility workouts, fearing such exercises will result in loss of hard-earned muscle mass. The fact remains, however, that it is best to include activities that develop all components of health-related fitness.

Emphasizing one aspect of fitness at the expense of others may be a special concern for weight trainers who don't do enough cardiorespiratory conditioning. Although exercise experts universally agree that resistance training is beneficial for a variety of reasons (as detailed in Chapter 8), it also has a downside.

A number of studies conducted around the world have tracked the impact of weight-training exercises on the cardiovascular system, to determine whether resistance training is helpful or harmful to the heart and blood vessels. These studies have shown that strength training poses short- and long-term risks to cardiovascular health and especially to arterial health. Aside from the risk of injury, lifting weights has been shown to have the following adverse effects on the cardiovascular system:

- Weight training promotes short-term stiffness of the blood vessels, which could promote hypertension (high blood pressure) over time and increase the load on the heart.
- Lifting weights (especially heavy weights) causes extreme short-term boosts in blood pressure; a Canadian study revealed that blood pressure can reach 480/350 mm Hg during heavy lifting. Over the long term, sharp elevations in blood pressure can damage arteries, even if each pressure increase lasts only a few seconds.
- Weight training places stress on the endothelial cells that line blood vessels. Because these cells secrete nitric oxide (a chemical messenger involved in a variety of bodily functions), this stress can contribute to a wide range of negative effects, from erectile dysfunction to heart disease.

A variety of studies have shown that the best way to offset cardiovascular stress caused by strength training is to do cardiorespiratory endurance exercise (such as brisk walking or using an elliptical machine) immediately after a weight-training session. Ground-breaking Japanese research showed that following resistance training with aerobic exercise prevents the stiffening of blood vessels and its associated damage. In this 8-week study, participants did aerobics before lifting weights, after lifting weights, or not at all. The group that did aerobics after weight training saw the greatest positive impact on arterial health; participants who did aerobics before lifting weights did not see any improvement in the health of their blood vessels.

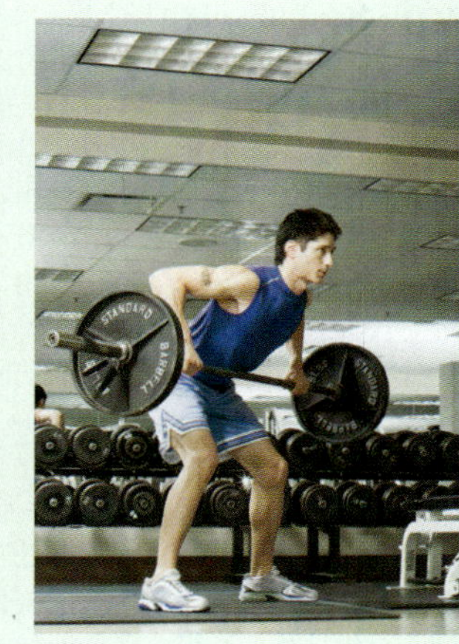

Strength training also promotes endurance fitness by improving nervous control of the muscles, increasing type IIa motor units (muscle fibers have a blend of strength and endurance capacity), and increasing tendon stiffness. These changes increase muscle strength and the rate of force development, enhance the economy of movement, and increase the speed that blood cells travel through the muscles.

The bottom line of all this research? Resistance training and cardiorespiratory exercise are both good for you, if you do them in the right order. So, when you plan your workouts, be sure to do 15–60 minutes of aerobic exercise after each weight-training session.

SOURCES: Aagaard, P., and J. L. Andersen. 2010. Effects of strength training on endurance capacity in top-level endurance athletes. *Scandinavian Journal Medicine Science Sports.* 20(supplement 2): 39–47; Okamoto, T., M. Masuhara, and K. Ikuta. 2006. Effects of eccentric and concentric resistance training on arterial stiffness. *Journal of Human Hypertension* 20(5): 348–354; Okamoto, T., M. Masuhara, and K. Ikuta. 2007. Combined aerobic and resistance training and vascular function: Effect of aerobic exercise before and after resistance training. *Journal of Applied Physiology* 103(5): 1655–1661; Physical Activity Guidelines Advisory Committee. 2008. *Physical Activity Guidelines Advisory Committee Report, 2008.* Washington, D.C.: U.S. Department of Health and Human Services.

of "good cholesterol" (high-density lipoproteins, or HDL) and may lower levels of "bad cholesterol" (low-density lipoproteins, or LDL).

- Reducing high blood pressure, which is a contributing factor to several kinds of CVD.
- Enhancing the function of the cells that line the arteries (endothelial cells).
- Reducing inflammation.
- Preventing obesity and type 2 diabetes, both of which contribute to CVD.

Details on various types of CVD, their associated risk factors, and lifestyle factors that can reduce your risk for developing CVD are discussed in Chapter 5. To learn more about atherosclerosis, the underlying disease process in CVD, see page T3-4 of the color transparency insert "Touring the Cardiorespiratory System" in this chapter.

Cancer Although the findings are not conclusive, some studies have shown a relationship between increased physical activity and a reduction in a person's risk of cancer. Exercise reduces the risk of colon cancer, and it may reduce the risk of cancers of the breast and reproductive organs. Physical activity during the high school and college years may be particularly important for preventing breast cancer later in life. Exercise may also reduce the risk of lung cancer, endometrial cancer, pancreatic cancer, and prostate cancer.

Type 2 Diabetes Regular exercise helps prevent the development of type 2 diabetes, the most common form of diabetes. Exercise metabolizes (burns) excess sugar and makes cells more sensitive to the hormone insulin, which is involved in the regulation of blood sugar levels. Obesity is a key risk factor for diabetes, and exercise helps keep body fat at healthy levels. But even without fat loss, exercise improves control of blood sugar levels in many people with diabetes, and physical activity is an important part of treatment. (See Chapter 6 for more on diabetes and insulin resistance.)

Osteoporosis A special benefit of exercise, especially for women, is protection against osteoporosis, a disease that results in loss of bone density and strength. Weight-bearing exercise—particularly weight training—helps build bone during the teens and twenties. People with denser bones can better endure the bone loss that occurs with aging. With stronger bones and muscles and better balance, fit people are less likely to experience debilitating falls and bone fractures. (See Chapter 3 for more on osteoporosis.)

Deaths from All Causes Physically active people have a reduced risk of dying prematurely from all causes, with the greatest benefits found for people with the highest levels of physical activity (Figure 4.3). Physical inactivity is a predictor of premature death and is as important a risk factor as smoking, high blood pressure, obesity, and diabetes.

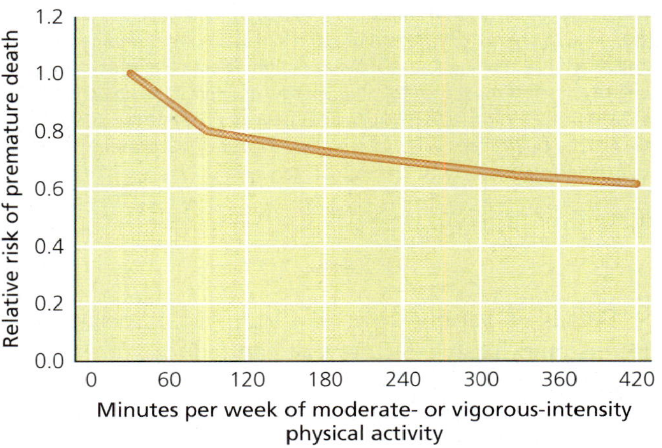

FIGURE 4.3 Doing only 150 minutes of moderate-intensity physical activity per week provides significant health benefits. As you exercise longer or more intensely, you reduce your risk of dying prematurely from a variety of causes.

SOURCE: Physical Activity Guidelines Advisory Committee. 2008. *Physical Activity Guidelines Advisory Committee Report, 2008*. Washington, D.C.: U. S. Department of Health and Human Services.

Fitness Tip

To prevent weight gain, you should exercise 150 to 250 minutes per week, which equals an energy expenditure of 1200 to 2000 calories per week. To lose weight, you should exercise at least 150 minutes per week and up to 420 minutes per week for significant weight loss.

Better Control of Body Fat

Too much body fat is linked to a variety of health problems, including CVD, cancer, and type 2 diabetes. Healthy body composition can be difficult to achieve and maintain—especially for someone who is sedentary—because a diet that contains all essential nutrients can be relatively high in calories. Excess calories are stored in the body as fat. Regular exercise increases daily calorie expenditure so that a healthy diet is less likely to lead to weight gain. Endurance exercise burns calories directly and, if intense enough, continues to do so by raising resting metabolic rate for several hours following an exercise session. A higher metabolic rate makes it easier for a person to maintain a healthy weight or to lose weight. However, exercise alone cannot ensure a healthy body composition. As described in Chapters 6 and 7, you will lose more weight more rapidly and keep it off longer if you decrease your calorie intake and boost your calorie expenditure through exercise.

Improved Immune Function

Exercise can have either positive or negative effects on the immune system, the physiological processes that protect us from diseases such as colds, bacterial infections, and even cancer. Moderate endurance exercise boosts immune function, whereas overtraining (excessive training) depresses it, at least temporarily. Physically fit people get fewer colds and upper respiratory tract infections than people who are not fit. Exercise affects immune function by influencing levels of specialized cells and chemicals involved in the immune response. In addition to getting regular moderate exercise, you can further strengthen your immune system by eating a well-balanced diet, managing stress, and getting 7–8 hours of sleep every night.

Improved Psychological and Emotional Well-Being

Most people who participate in regular endurance exercise experience social, psychological, and emotional benefits. Performing physical activities provides proof of skill mastery and self-control, thus enhancing self-image. Recreational sports provide an opportunity to socialize, have fun, and strive to excel. Endurance exercise lessens

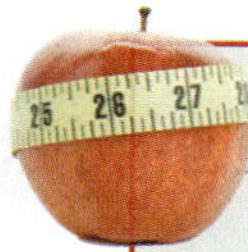

Wellness Tip

If you have trouble sleeping, exercise could be the cure. Regular physical activity helps people fall asleep more easily; it also improves the quality of sleep.

Ask Yourself

QUESTIONS FOR CRITICAL THINKING AND REFLECTION

If you already follow an exercise program, how could you modify it to help improve your cellular metabolism? What specific activities (or changes to existing ones) could you incorporate into your program for this purpose?

anxiety, depression, stress, anger, and hostility, thereby improving mood and boosting cardiovascular health. Regular exercise also improves sleep.

ASSESSING CARDIORESPIRATORY FITNESS

The body's ability to maintain a level of exertion (exercise) for an extended time is a direct reflection of cardiorespiratory fitness. One's level of fitness is determined by the body's ability to take up, distribute, and use oxygen during physical activity. As explained earlier, the best quantitative measure of cardiorespiratory endurance is maximal oxygen consumption, expressed as $\dot{V}O_{2max}$, the amount of oxygen the body uses when a person reaches his or her maximum ability to supply oxygen during exercise (measured in milliliters of oxygen used per minute for each kilogram of body weight). Maximal oxygen consumption can be measured pecisely in an exercise physiology laboratory through analysis of the air a person inhales and exhales when exercising to a level of exhaustion (maximum intensity). This procedure can be expensive and time-consuming, however, making it impractical for the average person.

Choosing an Assessment Test

Fortunately, several simple assessment tests provide reasonably good estimates of maximal oxygen consumption (within 10–15% of the results of a laboratory test). Three commonly used assessments are the following:

- ***The 1-mile walk test.*** This estimates your level of cardiorespiratory fitness (maximal oxygen consumption) based on the amount of time it takes you to complete 1 mile of brisk walking and your heart rate at the end of your walk. A fast time and a low heart rate indicate a high level of cardiorespiratory endurance.
- ***The 3-minute step test.*** The rate at which the pulse returns to normal after exercise is also a good measure of cardiorespiratory capacity; heart rate remains lower and recovers faster in people who are more physically fit. For the step test, you step continually at a steady rate and then monitor your heart rate during recovery.
- ***The 1.5-mile run-walk test.*** Oxygen consumption increases with speed in distance running, so a fast time on this test indicates high maximal oxygen consumption.

Lab 4.1 provides detailed instructions for each of these tests. An additional assessment, the 12-minute swim test, is also provided. To assess yourself, choose one of these methods based on your access to equipment, your current physical condition, and your own preference. Don't take any of these tests without checking with your physician if you are ill or have any of the risk factors for exercise discussed in Chapter 2 and Lab 2.1. Table 4.2 lists the fitness prerequisites and cautions recommended for each test.

Table 4.2 Fitness Prerequisites and Cautions for the Cardiorespiratory Endurance Assessment Tests

TEST	FITNESS PREREQUISITES/CAUTIONS
1-mile walk test	Recommended for anyone who meets the criteria for safe exercise. This test can be used by individuals who cannot perform other tests because of low fitness level or injury.
3-minute step test	If you suffer from joint problems in your ankles, knees, or hips or are significantly overweight, check with your physician before taking this test. People with balance problems or for whom a fall would be particularly dangerous, including older adults and pregnant women, should use special caution or avoid this test.
1.5-mile run-walk test	Recommended for people who are healthy and at least moderately active. If you have been sedentary, you should participate in a 4- to 8-week walk-run program before taking the test. Don't take this test in extremely hot or cold weather if you aren't used to exercising under those conditions.

NOTE: The conditions for exercise safety given in Chapter 2 apply to all fitness assessment tests. If you answered yes to any question on the PAR-Q in Lab 2.1, see your physician before taking any assessment test. If you experience any unusual symptoms while taking a test, stop exercising and discuss your condition with your instructor.

Monitoring Your Heart Rate

Each time your heart beats, it pumps blood into your arteries; this surge of blood causes a pulse that you can feel by holding your fingers against an artery. Counting your pulse to determine your exercise heart rate is a key part of most assessment tests for maximal oxygen consumption. Heart rate can also be used to monitor exercise intensity during a workout. (Intensity is described in more detail in the next section.)

The two most common sites for monitoring heart rate are the carotid artery in the neck and the radial artery in the wrist (Figure 4.4). To take your pulse, press your index and middle fingers gently on the correct site. You may have to shift position several times to find the best place to feel your pulse. Don't use your thumb to check your pulse; it has a pulse of its own that can confuse your count. (Use your middle and ring finger if you have a strong pulse in your index finger.) Be careful not to push too hard, particularly when taking your pulse in the carotid artery (strong pressure on this artery may cause a reflex that slows the heart rate).

> **Ask Yourself**
>
> **QUESTIONS FOR CRITICAL THINKING AND REFLECTION**
>
> Why do you think a relatively slow resting pulse rate is a sign of good cardiorespiratory fitness? What physical conditions or attributes are reflected in your pulse rate?

Heart rates are usually assessed in beats per minute (bpm). But counting your pulse for an entire minute isn't practical when you're exercising. And because heart rate slows rapidly when you stop exercising, a full minute's worth of counting can give inaccurate results. It's best to do a shorter count—10 seconds—and then multiply the result by 6 to get your heart rate in beats per minute. (You can also use a heart rate monitor to check your pulse. See the box "Heart Rate Monitors and GPS Devices" for more information.)

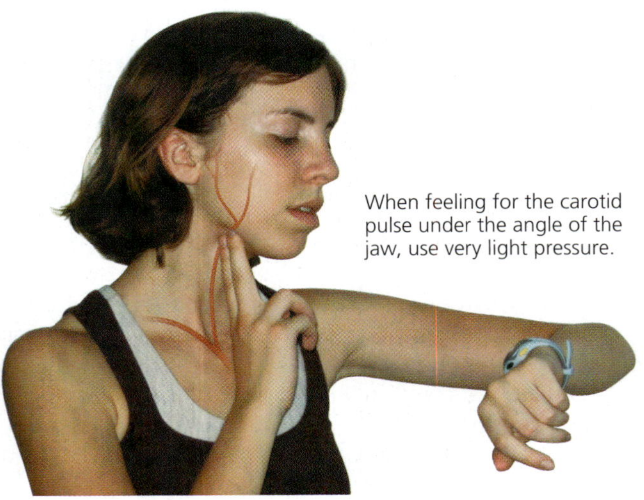

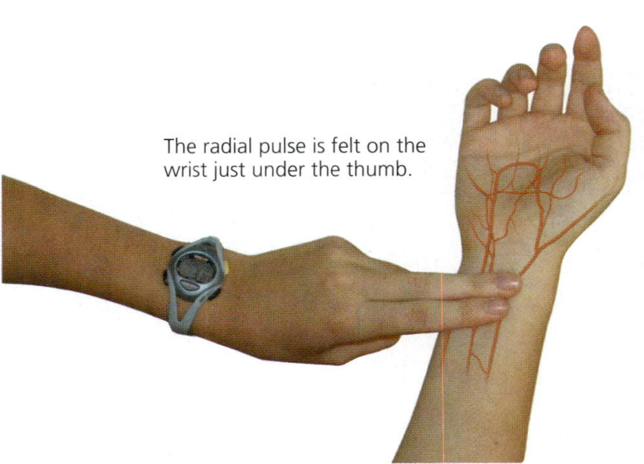

FIGURE 4.4 Checking your pulse.
The pulse can be taken at the carotid artery in the neck (top) or at the radial artery in the wrist (bottom).

Interpreting Your Score

Once you've completed one or more of the assessment tests, use the table under "Rating Your Cardiovascular Fitness" in Lab 4.1 to determine your current level of cardiorespiratory fitness. As you interpret your score, remember that field tests of cardiorespiratory fitness are not precise scientific measurements and have up to a 10–15% margin of error.

You can use the assessment tests to monitor the progress of your fitness program by retesting yourself from time to time. Always compare scores for the *same* test: Your scores on different tests may vary considerably because of differences in skill and motivation and weaknesses in the tests themselves.

DEVELOPING A CARDIORESPIRATORY ENDURANCE PROGRAM

Cardiorespiratory endurance exercises are best for developing the type of fitness associated with good health, so they should serve as the focus of your exercise program. To create a successful endurance exercise program, follow these guidelines:

- Set realistic goals.
- Set your starting frequency, intensity, and duration of exercise at appropriate levels.
- Choose suitable activities.
- Warm up and cool down.
- Adjust your program as your fitness improves.

Heart Rate Monitors and GPS Devices

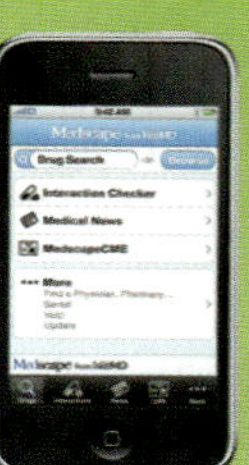

A heart rate monitor is an electronic device that checks the user's pulse, either continuously or on demand. These devices make it easy to monitor your heart rate before, during, and after exercise. Some include global positioning system (GPS) receivers that help you track the distance you walk, run, or bike.

Wearable Monitors

Most consumer-grade monitors have two pieces—a strap that wraps around the user's chest and a wrist strap. The chest strap contains one or more small electrodes, which detect changes in the heart's electrical voltage. A transmitter in the chest strap sends this data to a receiver in the wrist strap. A small computer in the wrist strap calculates the wearer's heart rate and displays it on a small screen.

In a few low-cost monitors, the chest and wrist straps are connected together by a wire, but the most popular monitors use wireless technology to transmit data between the straps. In advanced wireless monitors, data is encoded so that it cannot be read by other monitors that may be nearby, as is often the case in a crowded gym. A one-piece (or "strapless") heart rate monitor does not include a chest strap; the wrist-worn device contains sensors that detect a pulse in the wearer's hand.

Monitors in Gym Equipment

Many pieces of workout equipment—including newer-model treadmills, stationary bikes, and elliptical trainers—feature built-in heart rate monitors. The monitor is usually mounted into the device's handles. To check your heart rate at any time while working out, simply grip the handles in the appropriate place; within a few seconds, your current heart rate will appear on the device's console.

Other Features

Heart rate monitors can do more than just check your pulse. For example, most monitors can tell you the following kinds of information:

- Highest and lowest heart rate during a session
- Average heart rate
- Target heart range, based on your age, weight, and other factors
- Time spent within the target range
- Number of calories burned during a session

Some monitors can upload their data to a computer, so information can be stored and analyzed. The analytical software can help you track your progress over a period of time or a number of workouts. Monitors with GPS provide an accurate estimate of distance traveled during a workout or over an entire day.

Advantages

Heart rate monitors are useful if very close tracking of heart rate is important in your program. They offer several advantages:

- They are accurate, and they reduce the risk of mistakes when checking your own pulse. (Note: Chest-strap monitors are considered more accurate than strapless models. If you use a monitor built into gym equipment, its accuracy will depend on how well the device is maintained.)
- They are easy to use, although a sophisticated, multifunction monitor may take some time to master.
- They do the monitoring for you, so you don't have to worry about checking your own pulse.

When shopping for a heart rate or exercise GPS monitor, do your homework. Quality, reliability, and warranties vary. Ask personal trainers in your area for their recommendations, and look for product reviews in consumer magazines or online.

Setting Goals

You can use the results of cardiorespiratory fitness assessment tests to set a specific oxygen consumption goal for your cardiorespiratory endurance program. Your goal should be high enough to ensure a healthy cardiorespiratory system, but not so high that it will be impossible to achieve. Scores in the fair and good ranges for maximal oxygen consumption suggest good fitness; scores in the excellent and superior ranges indicate a high standard of physical performance.

Through endurance training, an individual may be able to improve maximal oxygen consumption ($\dot{V}O_{2max}$) by about 10–30%. The amount of improvement possible depends on genetics, age, health status, and initial fitness level. People who start at a very low fitness level can improve by a greater percentage than elite athletes because the latter are already at a much higher fitness level, one that may approach their genetic physical limits. If you are tracking $\dot{V}O_{2max}$ by using the field tests described in this chapter, you may be able to increase your score by more than 30% due to improvements in other physical factors, such as muscle power, which can affect your performance on the tests.

Another physical factor you can track to monitor progress is resting heart rate—your heart rate at complete rest, measured in the morning before you get out of bed and move around. Resting heart rate may decrease by as much as 10–15 beats per minute in response to endurance training. Changes in resting heart rate may be noticeable after only about 4–6 weeks of training.

You may want to set other types of goals for your fitness program. For example, if you walk, jog, or cycle as part of your fitness program, you may want to set a time or distance goal—working up to walking 5 miles in one session, completing a 4-mile run in 28 minutes, or cycling a total of 35 miles per week. A more modest goal might be to achieve the U.S. Department of Health and Human Services and ACSM's recommendation of 150 minutes per week of moderate-intensity physical activity. Although it's best to base your program on "SMART" goals, you may also want to set more qualitative goals, such as becoming more energetic, sleeping better, and improving the fit of your clothes.

Applying the FITT Equation

As described in Chapter 2, you can use the acronym FITT to remember key parameters of your fitness program: Frequency, Intensity, Time (duration), and Type of activity.

Frequency of Training Accumulating at least 150 minutes per week of moderate-intensity physical activity (or at least 75 minutes per week of vigorous physical activity) is enough to promote health. Most experts recommend that people exercise 3 to 5 days per week to build cardiorespiratory endurance. Training more than 5 days per week can lead to injury and isn't necessary for the typical person on an exercise program designed to promote wellness. It is safe to do moderate-intensity activity such as walking and gardening every day. Training fewer than 3 days per week makes it difficult to improve your fitness (unless exercise intensity is very high) or to use exercise to lose weight. Remember, however, that some exercise is better than none.

Intensity of Training Intensity is the most important factor for increasing aerobic fitness. You must exercise intensely enough to stress your body so that fitness improves. Four methods of monitoring exercise intensity are described in the following sections; choose the method that works best for you. Be sure to make adjustments in your intensity levels for environmental or individual factors. For example, on a hot and humid day or on your first day back to your program after an illness, you should decrease your intensity level.

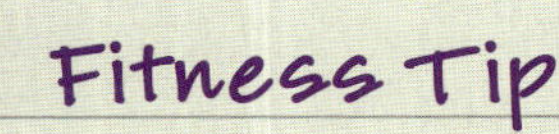

Listen to fast-paced music for a better workout! In a British study, students rode a stationary bike while listening to music at different tempos. The subjects rode harder when listening to faster music and performed less exercise in response to slower music.

TARGET HEART RATE ZONE One of the best ways to monitor the intensity of cardiorespiratory endurance exercise is to measure your heart rate. It isn't necessary to exercise at your maximum heart rate to improve maximal oxygen consumption. Fitness adaptations occur at lower heart rates with a much lower risk of injury.

According to the American College of Sports Medicine, your **target heart rate zone**—rates at which you should exercise to experience cardiorespiratory benefits—is between 65% and 90% of your maximum heart rate. To calculate your target heart rate zone, follow these steps:

1. Estimate your maximum heart rate (MHR) by subtracting your age from 220, or have it measured precisely by undergoing an exercise stress test in a doctor's office, hospital, or sports medicine lab. (*Note:* The formula to estimate MHR carries an error of about ±10–15 beats per minute and can be very inaccurate for some people, particularly older adults and young children. If your exercise heart rate seems inaccurate—that is, exercise within your target zone seems either too easy or too difficult—then use the perceived exertion method described in the next section, or have your maximum heart rate measured precisely.)
2. Multiply your MHR by 65% and 90% to calculate your target heart rate zone. (*Note:* Very unfit people should use 55% of MHR for their training threshold.)

For example, a 19-year-old would calculate her target heart rate zone as follows:

MHR = 220 − 19 = 201

65% training intensity = 0.65 × 201 = 131 bpm

90% training intensity = 0.90 × 201 = 181 bpm

To gain fitness benefits, the young woman in our example would have to exercise at an intensity that raises her heart rate to between 131 and 181 bpm.

An alternative method for calculating target heart rate range uses **heart rate reserve,** the difference between maximum heart rate and resting heart rate. Using this method, target heart rate is equal to resting heart rate plus between 50% (40% for very unfit people) and 85% of heart rate reserve. Although some people (particularly those with very low levels of fitness) will obtain more accurate results using this more complex method, both methods provide reasonable estimates of an appropriate target heart rate zone. Formulas for both methods of calculating target heart rate are given in Lab 4.2.

If you have been sedentary, start by exercising at the lower end of your target heart rate range (65% of maximum heart rate or 50% of heart rate reserve) for at least 4–6 weeks. Fast and significant gains in maximal oxygen consumption can be made by exercising closer to the top of the range, but you may increase your risk of injury and overtraining. You *can* achieve significant health benefits by exercising at the bottom of your target range, so don't feel pressure to exercise at an unnecessarily intense level. If you exercise at a lower intensity, you can increase the duration or frequency of training to obtain as much benefit to your health, as long as you are above the 65% training threshold. For people with a very low initial level of fitness, a lower training intensity of 55–64% of maximum heart rate or 40–49% of heart rate reserve may be sufficient to achieve improvements in maximal oxygen consumption, especially at the start of an exercise program. Intensities of 70–85% of maximum heart rate are appropriate for average individuals.

By monitoring your heart rate, you will always know if you are working hard enough to improve, not hard enough, or too hard. As your program progresses and your fitness improves, you will need to jog, cycle, or walk faster in order to reach your target heart rate zone. To monitor your heart rate during exercise, count your pulse while you're still moving or immediately after you stop exercising. Count beats for 10 seconds, then multiply that number by 6 to see if your heart rate is in your target zone. Table 4.3 shows target heart rate ranges and 10-second counts based on the maximum heart rate formula.

METS One way scientists describe fitness is in terms of the capacity to increase metabolism (energy usage level) above rest. Scientists use METs to measure the metabolic cost of an exercise. One **MET** represents the body's resting metabolic rate—that is, the energy or calorie requirement of the body at rest. Exercise intensity is expressed in multiples of resting metabolic rate. For example, an exercise intensity of 2 METs is twice the resting metabolic rate.

METs are used to describe exercise intensities for occupational activities and exercise programs. Exercise intensities of less than 3–4 METs are considered low. Household chores and most industrial jobs fall into this category. Exercise at these intensities does not improve fitness for most people, but it will improve fitness for people with low physical capacities. Activities that increase metabolism by 6–8 METs are classified as moderate-intensity exercises and are suitable for most people beginning an exercise program. Vigorous exercise increases metabolic rate by more than 10 METs. Fast running or cycling, as well as intense play in sports like racquetball, can place people in this category. Table 4.4 lists the MET ratings for various activities.

METs are intended to be only an approximation of exercise intensity. Skill, body weight, body fat, and environment affect the accuracy of METs. As a practical matter, however, these limitations can be disregarded. METs are

Table 4.3 Target Heart Rate Range and 10-Second Counts

AGE (years)	TARGET HEART RATE RANGE (bpm)*	10-SECOND COUNT (beats)
20–24	127–180	21–30
25–29	124–176	20–29
30–34	121–171	20–28
35–39	118–167	19–27
40–44	114–162	19–27
45–49	111–158	18–26
50–54	108–153	18–25
55–59	105–149	17–24
60–64	101–144	16–24
65+	97–140	16–23

*Target heart rates lower than those shown here are appropriate for individuals with a very low initial level of fitness. Ranges are based on the following formula: target heart rate = 0.65 to 0.90 of maximum heart rate, assuming maximum heart rate = 220 − age. The heart rate range values shown here correspond to ratings of perceived exertion (rpe) values of about 12–18.

Table 4.4 Approximate MET and Caloric Costs of Selected Activities for a 154-Pound Person

ACTIVITY	METS	CALORIC EXPENDITURE (kilocalories/min)
Rest	1	1.2
Light housework	2–4	2.4–4.8
Bowling	2–4	2.5–5
Walking	2–7	2.5–8.5
Archery	3–4	3.7–5
Dancing	3–7	3.7–8.5
Hiking	3–7	3.7–8.5
Horseback riding	3–8	3.7–10
Cycling	3–8	3.7–10
Basketball (recreational)	3–9	3.7–11
Swimming	4–8	5–10
Tennis	4–9	5–11
Fishing (fly, stream)	5–6	6–7.5
In-line skating	5–8	6–10
Skiing (downhill)	5–8	6–10
Rock climbing	5–10	6–12
Scuba diving	5–10	6–12
Skiing (cross-country)	6–12	7.5–15
Jogging	8–12	10–15

NOTE: Intensity varies greatly with effort, skill, and motivation.

SOURCE: Adapted from American College of Sports Medicine. 2009. *ACSM's Guidelines for Excercise Testing and Prescription*, 8th ed. Philadelphia: Lippincott Williams and Wilkins.

KEY TERMS

target heart rate zone The range of heart rates that should be reached and maintained during cardiorespiratory endurance exercise to obtain training effects.

heart rate reserve The difference between maximum heart rate and resting heart rate; used in one method for calculating target heart rate range.

MET A unit of measure that represents the body's resting metabolic rate—that is, the energy requirement of the body at rest.

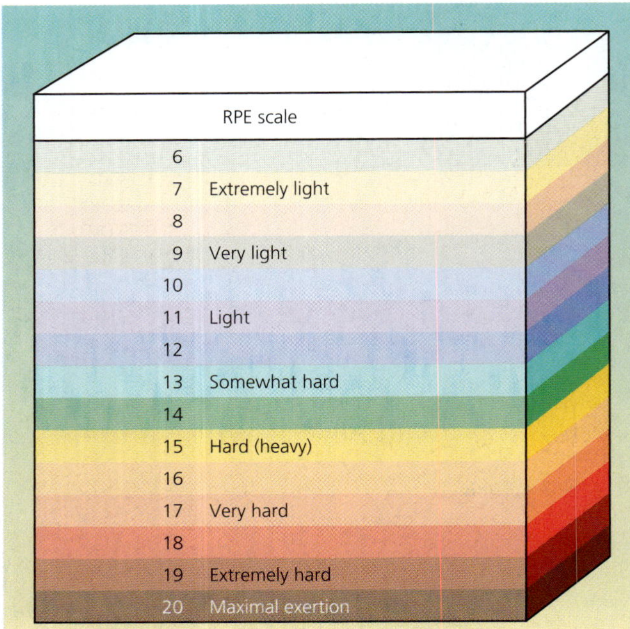

FIGURE 4.5 Ratings of perceived exertion (RPE). Experienced exercisers may use this subjective scale to estimate how near they are to their target heart rate zone.

SOURCE: *Psychology from Research to Practice* (1978), ed. H. L. Pick. Kluwer Academic/Plenum Publishing Corporation. With kind permission of Springer Science and Business Media and the author.

a good way to express exercise intensity because this system is easy for people to remember and apply.

RATINGS OF PERCEIVED EXERTION Another way to monitor intensity is to monitor your perceived level of exertion. Repeated pulse counting during exercise can become a nuisance if it interferes with the activity. As your exercise program progresses, you will probably become familiar with the amount of exertion required to raise your heart rate to target levels. In other words, you will know how you feel when you have exercised intensely enough. If this is the case, you can use the scale of **ratings of perceived exertion (RPE)** shown in Figure 4.5 to monitor the intensity of your exercise session without checking your pulse.

To use the RPE scale, select a rating that corresponds to your subjective perception of how hard you are exercising when you are training in your target heart rate zone. If your target zone is about 135–155 bpm, exercise intensely enough to raise your heart rate to that level, and then associate a rating—for example, "somewhat hard" or "hard" (14 or 15)—with how hard you feel you are working. To reach and maintain a similar intensity in future workouts, exercise hard enough to reach what you feel is the same level of exertion. You should periodically check your RPE against your target heart rate zone to make sure it's correct. RPE is an accurate means of monitoring exercise intensity, and you may find it easier and more convenient than pulse counting.

KEY TERM

ratings of perceived exertion (RPE) A system of monitoring exercise intensity by assigning a number to the subjective perception of target intensity.

Table 4.5 Estimating Exercise Intensity

METHOD	MODERATE INTENSITY	VIGOROUS INTENSITY
Percentage of maximum heart rate	55–69%	70–90%
Heart rate reserve	40–59%	60–85%
Rating of perceived exertion	12–13 (somewhat hard)	14–16 (hard)
Talk test	Speech with some difficulty	Speech limited to short phrases

TALK TEST Another easy method of monitoring exercise exertion—in particular, to prevent overly intense exercise—is the talk test. Although your breathing rate will increase during moderate-intensity cardiorespiratory endurance exercise, you should not work out so intensely that you cannot speak comfortably. Speech is limited to short phrases during vigorous-intensity exercise. The talk test is an effective gauge of intensity for many types of activities.

Table 4.5 provides a quick reference to each of the four methods of estimating exercise intensity discussed here.

Time (Duration) of Training

A total duration of 20–60 minutes per day is recommended; exercise can take place in a single session or in multiple sessions lasting 10 or more minutes. The total duration of exercise depends on its intensity. To improve cardiorespiratory endurance during a low- to moderate-intensity activity such as walking or slow swimming, you should exercise for 30–60 minutes. For high-intensity exercise performed at the top of your target heart rate zone, a duration of 20 minutes is sufficient.

Some studies have shown that 5–10 minutes of extremely intense exercise (greater than 90% of maximal oxygen consumption) improves cardiorespiratory endurance. However, training at high intensity, particularly during high-impact activities, increases the risk of injury. Also, because of the discomfort of high-intensity exercise, you are more likely to discontinue your exercise program. Longer-duration, low- to moderate-intensity activities generally result in more gradual gains in maximal oxygen consumption. In planning your program, start with less vigorous activities and gradually increase intensity.

Type of Activity

Cardiorespiratory endurance exercises include activities that involve the rhythmic use of large-muscle groups for an extended period of time, such as jogging, walking, cycling, aerobic dancing and other forms of group exercise, cross-country skiing, and swimming. Start-and-stop sports, such as tennis and racquetball, also qualify if you have enough skill to play continuously and intensely enough to raise your heart rate to target levels.

Other important considerations are access to facilities, expense, equipment, and the time required to achieve an adequate skill level and workout.

Warming Up and Cooling Down

It's important to warm up before every session of cardiorespiratory endurance exercise and to cool down afterward. Because the body's muscles work better when their temperature is slightly above resting level, warming up enhances performance and decreases the chance of injury. It gives the body time to redirect blood to active muscles and the heart time to adapt to increased demands. Warming up also helps spread protective fluid throughout the joints, preventing injury to their surfaces.

A warm-up session should include low-intensity, whole-body movements similar to those in the activity that will follow, such as walking slowly before beginning a brisk walk. An active warm-up of 5–10 minutes is adequate for most types of exercise. However, warm-up time will depend on your level of fitness, experience, and individual preferences.

Do not use stretching as part of your preexercise warm-up. Warm-up stretches do not prevent injury and have little or no effect on postexercise muscle soreness. Stretching before exercise can increase the energy cost of your workout and adversely affect strength, power, balance, reaction time, and movement time. Stretching interferes with muscle and joint receptors that are vital to performance of sport and movement skills. For these reasons, it is best to stretch at the end of your workout, while your muscles are still warm and your joints are lubricated. (See Chapter 9 for a detailed discussion of stretching and flexibility exercises.)

Cooling down after exercise is important for returning the body to a nonexercising state. A cool-down helps maintain blood flow to the heart and brain and redirects blood from working muscles to other areas of the body. This helps prevent a large drop in blood pressure, dizziness, and other potential cardiovascular complications. A cool-down, consisting of 5–10 minutes of reduced activity, should follow every workout to allow heart rate, breathing, and circulation to return to normal. Decrease the intensity of exercise gradually during your cool-down. For example, following a running workout, begin your cool-down by jogging at half speed for 30 seconds to a minute; then do several minutes of walking, reducing your speed slowly. A good rule of thumb is to cool down at least until your heart rate drops below 100 beats per minute.

Fitness Tip

Always make warming up and cooling down a part of your exercise routine! Doing so helps the body adapt to being more active, protects from certain injuries, and may make the health benefits of exercise last longer.

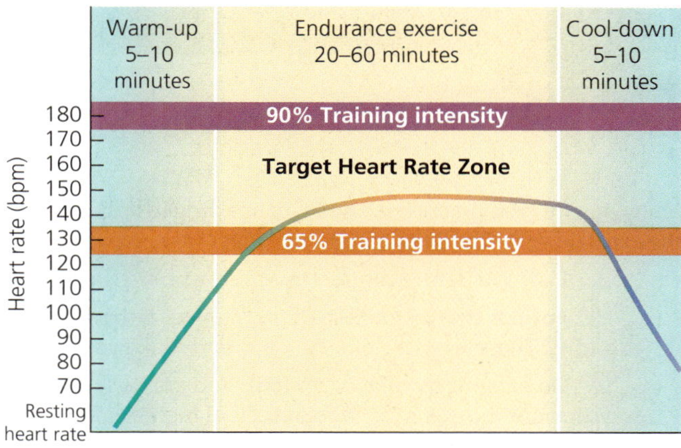

Frequency: 3–5 days per week

Intensity: 55/65–90% of maximum heart rate, 40/50–85% of heart rate reserve plus resting heart rate, or an RPE rating of about 12–18 (lower intensities—55–64% of maximum heart rate and 40–49% of heart rate reserve—are applicable to people who are quite unfit; for average individuals, intensities of 70–85% of maximum heart rate are appropriate)

Time (duration): 20–60 minutes (one session or multiple sessions lasting 10 or more minutes)

Type of activity: Cardiorespiratory endurance exercises, such as walking, jogging, biking, swimming, cross-country skiing, and rope skipping

FIGURE 4.6 The FITT principle for a cardiorespiratory endurance workout.
Longer-duration exercise at lower intensities can often be as beneficial for promoting health as shorter-duration, high-intensity exercise.

The general pattern of a safe and successful workout for cardiorespiratory fitness is illustrated in Figure 4.6.

Building Cardiorespiratory Fitness

Building fitness is as much an art as a science. Your fitness improves when you overload your body. However, you must increase the intensity, frequency, and duration of exercise carefully to avoid injury and overtraining.

For the initial stage of your program, which may last anywhere from 3 to 6 weeks, exercise at the low end of your target heart rate zone. Begin with a frequency of 3–4 days per week, and choose a duration appropriate for your fitness level: 12–15 minutes if you are very unfit, 20 minutes if you are sedentary but otherwise healthy, and 30–40 minutes if you are an experienced exerciser. Use this stage of your program to allow both your body and your schedule to adjust to your new exercise routine. Once you can exercise at the upper levels of frequency (4–5 days per week) and duration (30–40 minutes) without excessive fatigue or muscle soreness, you are ready to progress.

The next phase of your program is the improvement stage, lasting from 4 to 6 months. During this phase, slowly and gradually increase the amount of overload until you reach your target level of fitness (see the sample

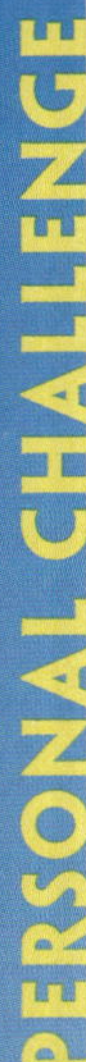

Staying Active between Workouts

Many people who practice formal exercise programs do less activity during the rest of the day, which partially defeats the purpose of the exercise program. Below are some ideas for becoming more active during the day. Check which one you can work into your lifestyle:

1. ______ **Exercise before dinner:** Pre-meal exercise decreases appetite and promotes a feeling of fullness.
2. ______ **Enter a charity walk-a-thon:** Many charities make money by getting people to sign up as sponsors in walk-a-thons and fun runs. These events help charities and make you look better in a bikini.
3. ______ **Do errands by bike or on foot:** You are not chained to your car. Buy a grocery cart and walk to the store. Carts are small, so you won't buy as much food and will increase fitness at the same time.
4. ______ **Take the dog for a walk:** Do your dog and yourself a favor and go for a walk together.
5. ______ **Hit softballs or baseballs at the batting cage:** Hitting balls is a great way to get ready for springtime softball games and is a terrific total body exercise.
6. ______ **Hit a bucket of balls at the golf course:** Many people think golf is a wimpy sport. Hit a couple of hundred balls at the driving range and see how you feel the next day. This is a great way to burn calories and improve your game.
7. ______ **Do aerobics 30 to 90 minutes a day:** People who walk only 30 minutes, 5 times per week will lose an average of 5 pounds in 6 to 12 months—without dieting, watching what they eat, or exercising intensely.
8. ______ **Do calisthenics first thing in the morning**: Calisthenics are resistive exercises that use body weight as resistance. These are excellent for a person who wants to develop muscle strength but is unwilling to join a health club or devote too much time to the activity. Examples include push-ups, squats, curl-ups, chair dips, crunches, and jumping jacks.
9. ______ **Exercise in the housework gym:** A vacuum cleaner is actually a lunge machine. Use a little creativity and you can turn simple household chores into a weight and aerobics workout. Try wearing a weighted vest while you sweep or mop the floor. Don't walk up the stairs— run. Jog in place as you wash the dishes. Stretch while putting away the dishes.
10. ______ **Active shopping:** Go on a window-shopping hike. Walk through the mall and check out every single shop. If you live in a small town, check out each store twice. If you live near the Mall of America, cover the stores in four days.
11. ______**Trim the hedge**: Go to the hardware store and purchase hand hedge trimmers. This garden chore burns calories and builds chest, shoulder, leg, and core muscles.
12. ______ **Sweep the walkway**: Try interval sweeping: Pick a 10-yard strip of cement and sweep as fast and as hard as you can. Also, try lunge sweeping: Do a lunge every time you sweep the broom—first your left leg, then your right.

By themselves, few of these methods will make you physically fit. But combining two or three of these techniques gives you powerful tools that will help you build fitness and keep the fat off.

training progression in Table 4.6). Take care not to increase overload too quickly. It is usually best to avoid increasing intensity and duration during the same session or all three training variables in one week. Increasing duration in increments of 5–10 minutes every 2–3 weeks is usually appropriate. Signs that you are increasing overload too quickly include muscle aches and pains, lack of usual interest in exercise, extreme fatigue, and inability to complete a workout. Keep an exercise log or training diary to monitor your workouts and progress.

Maintaining Cardiorespiratory Fitness

You will not improve your fitness indefinitely. The more fit you become, the harder you must work to improve (see the box "Interval Training: Pros and Cons"). There are limits to the level of fitness you can achieve, and if you increase intensity and duration indefinitely, you are likely to become injured or overtrained. After an improvement stage of 4–6 months, you may reach your goal of an acceptable level of fitness. You can then maintain fitness by continuing to exercise at the same intensity at least 3 nonconsecutive days every week. If you stop exercising, you lose your gains in fitness fairly rapidly. If you take time off for any reason, start your program again at a lower level and rebuild your fitness in a slow and systematic way.

Fitness Tip

A 40-meter running track, found in almost any high school or college, is a great place to do interval training. Start by striding the straight-a-ways and walking the turns. Begin with just one lap and increase the number of laps until you can do 4 to 8 (1 to 2 miles).

Table 4.6 Sample Progression for an Endurance Program

STAGE/WEEK	FREQUENCY (days/week)	INTENSITY* (beats/minute)	TIME (duration in minutes)
Initial stage			
1	3	120–130	15–20
2	3	120–130	20–25
3	4	130–145	20–25
4	4	130–145	25–30
Improvement stage			
5–7	3–4	145–160	25–30
8–10	3–4	145–160	30–35
11–13	3–4	150–165	30–35
14–16	4–5	150–165	30–35
17–20	4–5	160–180	35–40
21–24	4–5	160–180	35–40
Maintenance stage			
25+	3–5	160–180	20–60

*The target heart rates shown here are based on calculations for a healthy 20-year-old with a resting heart rate of 60 beats per minute; the program progresses from an initial target heart rate of 50% to a maintenance range of 70–85% of heart rate reserve.

SOURCE: Adapted from American College of Sports Medicine. 2009. *ACSM's Guidelines for Exercise Testing and Prescription*, 8th ed. Philadelphia: Lippincott Williams and Wilkins. Reprinted with permission from the publisher.

When you reach the maintenance stage, you may want to set new goals for your program and make some adjustments to maintain your motivation. Adding variety to your program can be a helpful strategy. Engaging in multiple types of endurance activities, an approach known as **cross-training**, can help boost enjoyment and prevent some types of injuries. For example, someone who has been jogging 5 days a week may change her program so that she jogs 3 days a week, plays tennis 1 day a week, and goes for a bike ride 1 day a week.

? **Ask Yourself**

QUESTIONS FOR CRITICAL THINKING AND REFLECTION

Suppose you want to start a new cardiorespiratory exercise program. How do your age, health status, and current level of fitness affect the kind of program you design for yourself? For the first few weeks, how often would you exercise, at what intensity (heart rate), and for how long?

EXERCISE SAFETY AND INJURY PREVENTION

Exercising safely and preventing injuries are two important challenges for people who engage in cardiorespiratory endurance exercise. This section provides basic safety guidelines that can be applied to a variety of fitness activities. Chapters 8 and 9 include additional advice specific to strength training and flexibility training.

Hot Weather and Heat Stress

Human beings require a relatively constant body temperature to survive. A change of just a few degrees in body temperature can quickly lead to distress and even death. If you lose too much water or if your body temperature gets too high, you may suffer from heat stress. Problems associated with heat stress include dehydration, heat cramps, heat exhaustion, and heatstroke.

In a high-temperature environment, exercise safety depends on the body's ability to dissipate heat and maintain blood flow to active muscles. The body releases heat from exercise through the evaporation of sweat. This process cools the skin and the blood circulating near the body's surface. Sweating is an efficient process as long as the air is relatively dry. As humidity increases, however, the sweating mechanism becomes less efficient because extra moisture in the air inhibits the evaporation of sweat from the skin. This is why it takes longer to cool down in humid weather than in dry weather.

You can avoid significant heat stress by staying fit, avoiding overly intense or prolonged exercise for which you are not prepared, drinking adequate fluids before and during exercise, and wearing clothes that allow heat to dissipate.

Dehydration Your body needs water to carry out many chemical reactions and to regulate body temperature. Sweating during exercise depletes your body's water supply and can lead to **dehydration** if fluids aren't replaced. Although dehydration is most common in hot weather, it can occur even in comfortable temperatures if fluid intake is insufficient.

Dehydration increases body temperature and decreases sweat rate, plasma volume, cardiac output, maximal oxygen consumption, exercise capacity, muscular strength, and stores of liver glycogen. You may begin to feel thirsty when you have a fluid deficit of about 1% of total body weight.

Drinking fluids before and during exercise is important to prevent dehydration and enhance performance. Thirst receptors in the brain make you want to drink fluids, but during heavy or prolonged exercise or exercise

cross-training Alternating two or more activities to improve a single component of fitness.

dehydration Excessive loss of body fluid.

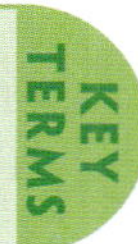

IN FOCUS

Interval Training: Pros and Cons

Few exercise techniques are more effective at improving fitness rapidly than *high-intensity interval training (HIT)*—a series of very brief, high-intensity exercise sessions interspersed with short rest periods. The four components of interval training are distance, repetition, intensity, and rest, defined as follows:

- *Distance* refers to either the distance or the time of the exercise interval.
- *Repetition* is the number of times the exercise is repeated.
- *Intensity* is the speed at which the exercise is performed.
- *Rest* is the time spent recovering between exercises.

Canadian researchers found that 6 sessions of high-intensity interval training on a stationary bike increased muscle oxidative capacity by almost 50%, muscle glycogen by 20%, and cycle endurance capacity by 100%. The subjects made these amazing improvements by exercising only 15 minutes in 2 weeks. Each workout consisted of 4–7 repetitions of high-intensity exercise (each repetition consisted of 30 seconds at near maximum effort) on a stationary bike. A follow-up study of moderately active women using the same training method showed that interval training increased the body's capacity for burning fat during exercise. These studies (and more than 20 others) showed the value of high-intensity training for building aerobic capacity and endurance.

You can use interval training in your favorite aerobic exercises. In fact, the type of exercise you select is not important as long as you exercise at a high intensity. HIT training can even be used to help develop sports skills. For example, a runner might do 4 to 8 repetitions of 200-meter sprints at near-maximum effort. A tennis player might practice volleys against a wall as fast as possible for 4 to 8 repetitions lasting 30 seconds each. A swimmer might swim 4 to 8 repetitions of 50 meters at 100% effort. It is important to rest from 3 to 5 minutes between repetitions, regardless of the type of exercise being performed.

If you add HIT to your exercise program, do not practice interval training more than 3 days per week. Intervals are exhausting and easily lead to injury. Let your body tell you how many days you can tolerate. If you become overly tired after doing interval training 3 days per week, cut back to 2 days. If you feel good, try increasing the intensity or volume of intervals (but not the number of days per week) and see what happens. As with any kind of exercise program, begin HIT training slowly and progress conservatively. Although the Canadian studies showed that HIT training produced substantial fitness improvements by themselves, it is best to integrate HIT into your total exercise program.

High-intensity interval training appears to be safe and effective in the short term, but there are concerns about the long-term safety and effectiveness of this type of training, so consider the following issues:

- Maximal-intensity training could be dangerous for some people. A physician might be reluctant to give certain patients the green light for this type of exercise.
- Always warm up with several minutes of low-intensity exercise before practicing HIT. Maximal-intensity exercise without a warm-up can cause cardiac arrhythmias (abnormal heart rhythms) even in healthy people.
- HIT might trigger overuse injuries in unfit people. For this reason, it is essential to start gradually, especially for someone at a low level of fitness. Exercise at sub-maximal intensities for at least 4 to 6 weeks before starting high-intensity interval training. Cut back on interval training or rest if you feel overly fatigued or develop overly sore joints or muscles.

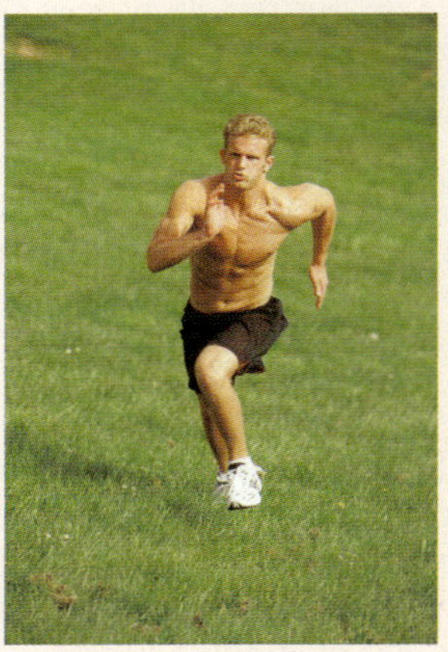

in hot weather, thirst alone isn't a good indicator of how much you need to drink. As a rule of thumb, drink at least 2 cups (16 ounces) of fluid 2 hours before exercise, and then drink enough during exercise to match fluid loss in sweat. Drink at least 1 cup of fluid every 20–30 minutes during exercise, more in hot weather or if you sweat heavily. To determine if you're drinking enough fluid, weigh yourself before and after an exercise session; any weight loss is due to fluid loss that needs to be replaced.

Very rarely, active people consume too much water and develop ***hyponatremia***, a condition characterized by lung congestion, muscle weakness, and nervous system problems. Following the guidelines presented here can help prevent this condition.

Bring a water bottle when you exercise so you can replace your fluids when they're being depleted. For exercise sessions lasting less than 60–90 minutes, cool water is an excellent fluid replacement. For longer workouts, choose a sports drink that contains water and small amounts of electrolytes (sodium, potassium, and magnesium) and simple carbohydrates ("sugar," usually in the form of sucrose, glucose, lactate, or glucose polymers). Electrolytes, which are lost from the body in sweat, are important because they help regulate the balance of fluids in body cells and the bloodstream. The carbohydrates in typical sports drinks are rapidly digestible and can thus help maintain blood glucose levels. Choose a beverage with no more than 8 grams of simple carbohydrate per 100 milliliters. Nonfat milk or chocolate milk, for those who can tolerate dairy products, are excellent fluid replacement beverages because they promote long-term hydration. See Chapter 3 for more on diet and fluid recommendations for active people.

Heat Cramps Involuntary cramping and spasms in the muscle groups used during exercise are sometimes called **heat cramps.** Although depletion of sodium and potassium from the muscles is involved with the problem, the primary cause of cramps is muscle fatigue. Children are particularly susceptible to heat cramps, but the condition can also occur in adults, even those who are fit. The best treatment for heat cramps is a combination of gentle stretching, replacement of fluid and electrolytes, and rest.

Heat Exhaustion Symptoms of **heat exhaustion** include the following:

- Rapid, weak pulse
- Low blood pressure
- Headache
- Faintness, weakness, dizziness
- Profuse sweating
- Pale face
- Psychological disorientation (in some cases)
- Normal or slightly elevated core body temperature

Heat exhaustion occurs when an insufficient amount of blood returns to the heart because so much of the body's blood volume is being directed to working muscles (for exercise) and to the skin (for cooling). Treatment for heat exhaustion includes resting in a cool area, removing excess clothing, applying cool or damp towels to the body, and drinking fluids. An affected individual should rest for the remainder of the day and drink plenty of fluids for the next 24 hours.

Heatstroke **Heatstroke** is a major medical emergency involving the failure of the brain's temperature regulatory center. The body does not sweat enough, and body temperature rises dramatically to extremely dangerous levels. In addition to high body temperature, symptoms can include the following:

- Hot, flushed skin (dry or sweaty), red face
- Chills, shivering
- Very high or very low blood pressure
- Confusion, erratic behavior
- Convulsions, loss of consciousness

A heatstroke victim should be cooled as rapidly as possible and immediately transported to a hospital. To lower body temperature, get out of the heat, remove excess clothing, drink cold fluids, and apply cool or damp towels to the body or immerse the body in cold water. People experiencing heatstroke during exercise may still be sweating.

Cold Weather

In extremely cold conditions, problems can occur if a person's body temperature drops or if particular parts of the body are exposed. If the body's ability to warm itself through shivering or exercise can't keep pace with heat loss, the core body temperature begins to drop. This condition, known as **hypothermia**, depresses the central nervous system, resulting in sleepiness and a lower metabolic rate. As metabolic rate drops, body temperature declines even further, and coma and death can result. The risk of hypothermia is particularly great in cold water.

Frostbite—the freezing of body tissues—is another potential danger of exercise in extremely cold conditions. Frostbite most commonly occurs in exposed body parts like earlobes, fingers, and the nose, and it can cause permanent circulatory damage. Hypothermia and frostbite both require immediate medical treatment.

To exercise safely in cold conditions, don't stay out in very cold temperatures for too long. Take both the temperature and the wind into account when planning your exercise session. Frostbite is possible within 30 minutes in calm conditions when the temperature is colder than −5°F, or in windy conditions (30 mph) if the temperature is below 10°F. **Wind chill** values that reflect both the temperature and the wind speed are available as part of a local weather forecast and from the National Weather Service (http://www.weather.gov).

Appropriate clothing provides insulation and helps trap warm air next to the skin. Dress in layers so you can remove them as you warm up and can put them back on if you get cold. A substantial amount of heat loss comes from the head and neck, so keep these areas covered. In subfreezing temperatures, protect the areas of your body most susceptible to frostbite—fingers, toes, ears, nose, and cheeks—with warm socks, mittens or gloves, and a cap, hood, or ski mask. Wear clothing that breathes and will wick moisture away from your skin to avoid being cooled or overheated by trapped perspiration. Many types of comfortable, lightweight clothing that provide good insulation are available. It's also important to warm up thoroughly and to drink plenty of fluids.

KEY TERMS

heat cramps Sudden muscle spasms and pain associated with intense exercise in hot weather.

heat exhaustion Heat illness resulting from exertion in hot weather.

heatstroke A severe and often fatal heat illness characterized by significantly elevated core body temperature.

hypothermia Low body temperature due to exposure to cold conditions.

frostbite Freezing of body tissues characterized by pallor, numbness, and a loss of cold sensation.

wind chill A measure of how cold it feels based on the rate of heat loss from exposed skin caused by cold and wind; the temperature that would have the same cooling effect on a person as a given combination of temperature and wind speed.

Table 4.7 Care of Common Exercise Injuries and Discomforts

INJURY	SYMPTOMS	TREATMENT
Blister	Accumulation of fluid in one spot under the skin	Don't pop or drain it unless it interferes too much with your daily activities. If it does pop, clean the area with antiseptic and cover with a bandage. Do not remove the skin covering the blister.
Bruise (contusion)	Pain, swelling, and discoloration	R-I-C-E: rest, ice, compression, elevation.
Fracture and/or dislocation	Pain, swelling, tenderness, loss of function, and deformity	Seek medical attention, immobilize the affected area, and apply cold.
Joint sprain	Pain, tenderness, swelling, discoloration, and loss of function	R-I-C-E; apply heat when swelling has disappeared. Stretch and strengthen affected area.
Muscle cramp	Painful, spasmodic muscle contractions	Gently stretch for 15–30 seconds at a time and/or massage the cramped area. Drink fluids and increase dietary salt intake if exercising in hot weather.
Muscle soreness or stiffness	Pain and tenderness in the affected muscle	Stretch the affected muscle gently; exercise at a low intensity; apply heat. Nonsteroidal anti-inflammatory drugs, such as ibuprofen, help some people.
Muscle strain	Pain, tenderness, swelling, and loss of strength in the affected muscle	R-I-C-E; apply heat when swelling has disappeared. Stretch and strengthen the affected area.
Plantar fascitis	Pain and tenderness in the connective tissue on the bottom of the foot	Apply ice, take nonsteroidal anti-inflammatory drugs, and stretch. Wear night splints when sleeping.
Shin splint	Pain and tenderness on the front of the lower leg; sometimes also pain in the calf muscle	Rest; apply ice to the affected area several times a day and before exercise; wrap with tape for support. Stretch and strengthen muscles in the lower legs. Purchase good-quality footwear and run on soft surfaces.
Side stitch	Pain on the side of the abdomen	Stretch the arm on the affected side as high as possible; if that doesn't help, try bending forward while tightening the abdominal muscles.
Tendinitis	Pain, swelling, and tenderness of the affected area	R-I-C-E; apply heat when swelling has disappeared. Stretch and strengthen the affected area.

Poor Air Quality

Air pollution can decrease exercise performance and negatively affect health, particularly if you smoke or have respiratory problems such as asthma, bronchitis, or emphysema. The effects of smog are worse during exercise than at rest because air enters the lungs faster. Polluted air may also contain carbon monoxide, which displaces oxygen in the blood and reduces the amount of oxygen available to working muscles. In a 2007 study, scientists from the ACSM found that exercise in polluted air could decrease lung function to the same extent as heavy smoking. Symptoms of poor air quality include eye and throat irritations, difficulty breathing, and possibly headache and malaise.

Do not exercise outdoors during a smog alert or if air quality is very poor. If you have any type of cardiorespiratory difficulty, you should also avoid exertion outdoors when air quality is poor. You can avoid some smog and air pollution by exercising in indoor facilities, in parks, near water (riverbanks, lakeshores, and ocean beaches), or in residential areas with less traffic (areas with stop-and-go traffic will have lower air quality than areas where traffic moves quickly). Air quality is also usually better in the early morning and late evening, before and after the commute hours.

Exercise Injuries

Most injuries are annoying rather than serious or permanent. However, an injury that isn't cared for properly can escalate into a chronic problem, sometimes serious enough to permanently curtail the activity. It's important to learn how to deal with injuries so they don't derail your fitness program. Strategies for the care of common exercise injuries and discomforts appear in Table 4.7; some general guidelines are given in the following sections.

When to Call a Physician Some injuries require medical attention. Consult a physician for the following:

- Head and eye injuries
- Possible ligament injuries
- Broken bones
- Internal disorders: chest pain, fainting, elevated body temperature, intolerance to hot weather

Also seek medical attention for ostensibly minor injuries that do not get better within a reasonable amount of time. You may need to modify your exercise program for a few weeks to allow an injury to heal.

Wellness Tip

It may be easy to nurse some injuries yourself, but if you aren't sure what to do, call your doctor.

Rehabilitation Following a Minor Athletic Injury

connect ACTIVITY DO IT ONLINE

TAKE CHARGE

- Reduce the initial inflammation using the R-I-C-E principle (see text).
- After 36–48 hours, apply heat *if the swelling has disappeared completely.* Immerse the affected area in warm water or apply warm compresses, a hot water bottle, or a heating pad. As soon as it's comfortable, begin moving the affected joints slowly. If you feel pain, or if the injured area begins to swell again, reduce the amount of movement. Continue gently stretching and moving the affected area until you have regained normal range of motion.
- Gradually begin exercising the injured area to build strength and endurance. Depending on the type of injury, weight training, walking, and resistance training can all be effective.
- Gradually reintroduce the stress of an activity until you can return to full intensity. Don't progress too rapidly or you'll re-injure yourself. Before returning to full exercise participation, you should have a full range of motion in your joints, normal strength and balance among your muscles, normal coordinated patterns of movement (with no injury compensation movements, such as limping), and little or no pain.

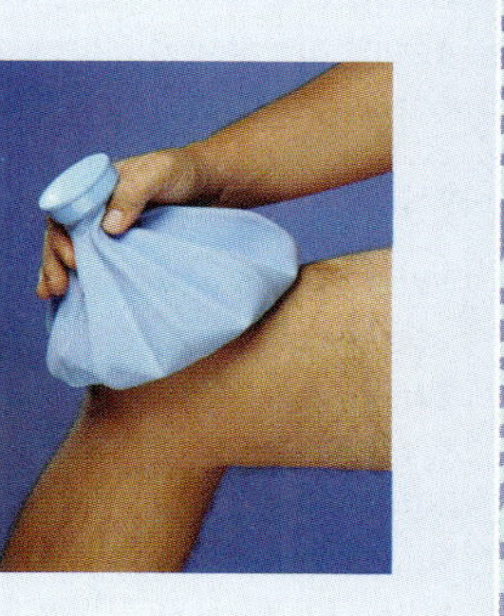

Managing Minor Exercise Injuries For minor cuts and scrapes, stop the bleeding and clean the wound. Treat injuries to soft tissue (muscles and joints) with the R-I-C-E principle: rest, ice, compression, and elevation.

- ***Rest:*** Stop using the injured area as soon as you experience pain. Avoid any activity that causes pain.
- ***Ice:*** Apply ice to the injured area to reduce swelling and alleviate pain. Apply ice immediately for 10–20 minutes, and repeat every few hours until the swelling disappears. Let the injured part return to normal temperature between icings, and do not apply ice to one area for more than 20 minutes. An easy method for applying ice is to freeze water in a paper cup, peel some of the paper away, and rub the exposed ice on the injured area. If the injured area is large, you can surround it with several bags of crushed ice or ice cubes, or bags of frozen vegetables. Place a thin towel between the bag and your skin. If you use a cold gel pack, limit application time to 10 minutes. Apply ice regularly for 36–48 hours or until the swelling is gone; it may be necessary to apply ice for a week or more if swelling persists.
- ***Compression:*** Wrap the injured area firmly with an elastic or compression bandage between icings. If the area starts throbbing or begins to change color, the bandage may be wrapped too tightly. Do not sleep with the wrap on.
- ***Elevation:*** Raise the injured area above heart level to decrease the blood supply and reduce swelling. Use pillows, books, or a low chair or stool to raise the injured area.

The day after the injury, some experts recommend also taking an over-the-counter medication, such as aspirin, ibuprofen, or naproxen, to decrease inflammation. To rehabilitate your body, follow the steps listed in the box "Rehabilitation Following a Minor Athletic Injury."

Preventing Injuries The best method for dealing with exercise injuries is to prevent them. If you choose activities for your program carefully and follow the training guidelines described here and in Chapter 2, you should be able to avoid most types of injuries. Important guidelines for preventing athletic injuries include the following:

- Train regularly and stay in condition.
- Gradually increase the intensity, duration, or frequency of your workouts.
- Avoid or minimize high-impact activities; alternate them with low-impact activities.
- Get proper rest between exercise sessions.
- Drink plenty of fluids.
- Warm up thoroughly before you exercise and cool down afterward.
- Achieve and maintain a normal range of motion in your joints.
- Use proper body mechanics when lifting objects or executing sports skills.
- Don't exercise when you are ill or overtrained.
- Use proper equipment, particularly shoes, and choose an appropriate exercise surface. If you exercise on a grass field, soft track, or wooden floor, you are less likely to be injured than on concrete or a hard track. (For information on athletic shoes, see the box "Choosing Exercise Footwear.")
- Don't return to your normal exercise program until any athletic injuries have healed. Restart your program at a lower intensity and gradually increase the amount of overload.

CRITICAL CONSUMER

Choosing Exercise Footwear

Footwear is perhaps the most important item of equipment for almost any activity. Shoes protect and support your feet and improve your traction. When you jump or run, you place as much as six times more force on your feet than when you stand still. Shoes can help cushion against the stress that this additional force places on your lower legs, thereby preventing injuries. Some athletic shoes are also designed to help prevent ankle rollover, another common source of injury.

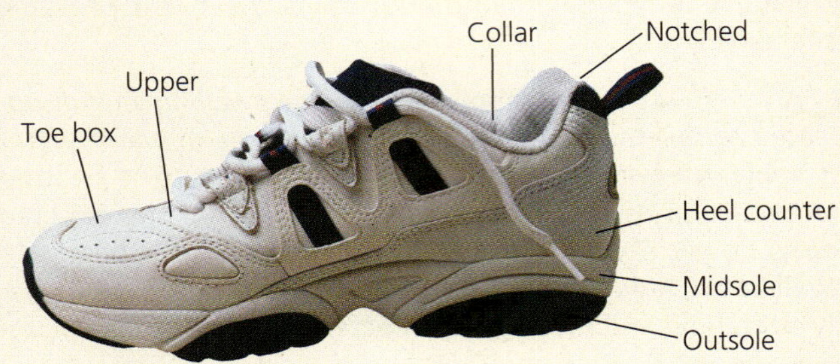

General Guidelines

When choosing athletic shoes, first consider the activity you've chosen for your exercise program. Shoes appropriate for different activities have very different characteristics.

Foot type is another important consideration. If your feet tend to roll inward excessively, you may need shoes with additional stability features on the inner side of the shoe to counteract this movement. If your feet tend to roll outward excessively, you may need highly flexible and cushioned shoes that promote foot motion. Most women will get a better fit if they choose shoes specifically designed for women's feet rather than downsized versions of men's shoes.

Successful Shopping For successful shoe shopping, keep the following strategies in mind:

- Shop late in the day or, ideally, following a workout. Your foot size increases over the course of the day and after exercise.
- Wear socks like those you plan to wear during exercise.
- Try on both shoes and wear them around for 10 or more minutes. Try walking on a noncarpeted surface. Approximate the movements of your activity: walk, jog, run, jump, and so on.
- Check the fit and style carefully:
  - Is the toe box roomy enough? Your toes will spread out when your foot hits the ground or you push off. There should be at least one thumb's width of space from the longest toe to the end of the toe box.
  - Do the shoes have enough cushioning? Do your feet feel supported when you bounce up and down? Try bouncing on your toes and on your heels.
  - Do your heels fit snugly into the shoe? Do they stay put when you walk, or do they slide up?
  - Are the arches of your feet right on top of the shoes' arch supports?
  - Do the shoes feel stable when you twist and turn on the balls of your feet? Try twisting from side to side while standing on one foot.
  - Do you feel any pressure points?
- If you exercise at dawn or dusk, choose shoes with reflective sections for added visibility and safety.
- Replace athletic shoes about every 3 months or 300–500 miles of jogging or walking.

Ask Yourself

QUESTIONS FOR CRITICAL THINKING AND REFLECTION

Have you ever suffered an injury while exercising? If so, how did you treat the injury? Compare your treatment with the guidelines given in this chapter. Did you do the right things? What can you do to avoid such injuries in the future?

TIPS FOR TODAY AND THE FUTURE

Regular, moderate exercise, even in short bouts spread through the day, can improve cardiorespiratory fitness.

RIGHT NOW YOU CAN

- Assess your cardiorespiratory fitness by using one of the methods discussed in this chapter and in Lab 4.1.
- Do a short bout of endurance exercise, such as 10–15 minutes of walking, jogging, or cycling.
- If you have physical activity planned for later in the day, drink some fluids now to make sure you are fully hydrated for your workout.
- Consider the exercise equipment, including shoes, you currently have on hand. If you need new equipment, start researching your options to get the best equipment you can afford.

IN THE FUTURE YOU CAN

- Graduate to a different, more challenging fitness assessment as your cardiorespiratory fitness improves.
- Incorporate different types of exercises into your cardiorespiratory endurance training to keep yourself challenged and motivated.

COMMON QUESTIONS ANSWERED

Q Do I need a special diet for my endurance exercise program?

A No. For most people, a nutritionally balanced diet contains all the energy and nutrients needed to sustain an exercise program. Don't waste your money on unnecessary supplements. (Chapter 3 provides detailed information about putting together a healthy diet.)

Q How can I measure how far I walk or run?

A The simplest and cheapest way to measure distance is with a pedometer, which counts your steps. Although stride length varies among individuals, 2000 steps typically equals about 1 mile, and 10,000 steps equals about 5 miles. To track your distance and your progress using a pedometer, follow the guidelines in Lab 2.3.

Q How can I avoid being so sore when I start an exercise program?

A Postexercise muscle soreness is caused by muscle injury followed by muscle inflammation. Muscles get stronger and larger in response to muscle tension and injury. However, excessive injury can delay progress. The best approach is to begin conservatively with low-volume, low-intensity workouts, and gradually increase the severity of the exercise sessions. If you are currently sedentary, begin with 5 to 10 minutes of exercise and gradually increase the distance and speed you walk, run, cycle, or swim.

Q Is it OK to do cardiorespiratory endurance exercise while menstruating?

A Yes. There is no evidence that exercise during menstruation is unhealthy or that it has negative effects on performance. If you have headaches, backaches, and abdominal pain during menstruation, you may not feel like exercising. For some women, exercise helps relieve these symptoms. Listen to your body and exercise at whatever intensity is comfortable for you.

Q Will high altitude affect my ability to exercise?

A At high altitudes (above 1500 meters, or about 4900 feet), there is less oxygen available in the air than at lower altitudes. High altitude doesn't affect anaerobic exercise, such as stretching and weight lifting, but it does affect aerobic activities—that is, any type of cardiovascular endurance exercise—because the heart and lungs have to work harder, even when the body is at rest, to deliver enough oxygen to body cells. The increased cardiovascular strain of exercise reduces endurance. To play it safe when at high altitudes, avoid heavy exercise—at least for the first few days—and drink plenty of water. And don't expect to reach your normal lower-altitude exercise capacity.

For more Common Questions Answered about endurance training, visit the Online Learning Center at www.mhhe.com/fahey.

SUMMARY

- The cardiorespiratory system consists of the heart, blood vessels, and respiratory system; it picks up and transports oxygen, nutrients, and waste products.
- The body takes chemical energy from food and uses it to produce ATP and fuel cellular activities. ATP is stored in the body's cells as the basic form of energy.
- During exercise, the body supplies ATP and fuels cellular activities by combining three energy systems: immediate, for short periods of activity; nonoxidative (anaerobic), for intense activity; and oxidative (aerobic), for prolonged activity. Which energy system predominates depends on the duration and intensity of the activity.
- Cardiorespiratory endurance exercise improves cardiorespiratory functioning and cellular metabolism; it reduces the risk of chronic diseases such as heart disease, cancer, type 2 diabetes, obesity, and osteoporosis; and it improves immune function and psychological and emotional well-being.
- Cardiorespiratory fitness is measured by determining how well the cardiorespiratory system transports and uses oxygen. The upper limit of this measure, called maximal oxygen consumption, or $\dot{V}O_{2max}$, can be measured precisely in a laboratory, or it can be estimated reasonably well through self-assessment tests.
- To create a successful exercise program, set realistic goals, choose suitable activities, begin slowly, and always warm up and cool down. As fitness improves, exercise more often, longer, and/or harder.
- Intensity of training can be measured through target heart rate zone, METs, ratings of perceived exertion, or the talk test.
- With careful attention to fluid intake, clothing, duration of exercise, and exercise intensity, endurance training can be safe in hot and cold weather conditions.

• Serious injuries require medical attention. Application of the R-I-C-E principle (rest, ice, compression, elevation) is appropriate for treating many types of muscle or joint injuries.

FOR FURTHER EXPLORATION

BOOKS

American College of Sports Medicine. 2003. *ACSM Fitness Book.* 3rd ed. Champaign, Ill.: Human Kinetics. *Includes fitness assessment tests and advice on creating a complete fitness program.*

Centers for Disease Control and Prevention. 2010. *Promoting Physical Activity: A Guide for Community Action*, 2nd ed. Champaign, Ill.: Human Kinetics. *Presents a guide for community action that offers the tools and information you need to help people become more active.*

Coffman, S. 2007. *Successful Programs for Fitness and Health Clubs.* Champaign, Ill.: Human Kinetics. *Presents more than 100 ready-to-use programs for fitness centers, group exercise studios, pools, gyms, and classrooms.*

Edwards, S., and S. Reed. 2006. *Heart Zones Cycling: The Avid Cyclist's Guide to Riding Faster and Farther.* Boulder, Colo: VeloPress. *An excellent guide to using heart rate in endurance training written by a top athlete and scientist.*

Fenton, M. 2008. *The Complete Guide to Walking, New and Revised: For Health, Weight Loss, and Fitness.* Guilford, Conn.: Lyons Press. *Discusses walking as a fitness method and a way to avoid diseases such as diabetes.*

Gotlin, R. 2007. *Sports Injuries Guidebook.* Champaign, Ill.: Human Kinetics. *Provides information and care instructions on many types of sports-related injuries.*

Howley, E. T., and B. D Franks. 2007. *Fitness Professional's Handbook,* 5th ed. Champaign, Ill.: Human Kinetics. *A comprehensive manual on physical training for professionals and people interested in exercise and sports.*

Maffetone, P. 2010. *The Big Book of Endurance Training and Racing*. New York: Skyhorse Publishing. *An excellent book for people of all levels interested in running, swimming, cycling, and triathlon.*

Marcus, B. H., and L A. Forsyth. 2009. *Motivating People to be Physically Active,* 2nd ed. Champaign, Ill.: Human Kinetics. *Describes methods for helping people increase their level of physical activity.*

Nieman, D. C. 2010. *Exercise Testing and Prescription: A Health-Related Approach,* 7th ed. New York: McGraw-Hill. *A comprehensive discussion of the effect of exercise and exercise testing and prescription.*

Richmond, M. 2011. *The Physiology Storybook: An Owner's Manual for the Human Body*. Monterey, Calif.: Healthy Learning. *A discussion of human physiology and wellness written for the average person.*

Rothman, J., and T. LaFontaine. 2011. *The Exercise Professional's Guide to Optimizing Health: Strategies for Preventing and Reducing Chronic Disease.* Baltimore: Lippincott Williams & Wilkins. *Written for professionals in association with the American College of Sports Medicine, the book describes how exercise can help prevent and treat chronic disease.*

ORGANIZATIONS AND WEB SITES

American Academy of Orthopaedic Surgeons: Sports and Exercise. Provides fact sheets on many fitness and sports topics, including how to begin a program, how to choose equipment, and how to prevent and treat many types of injuries.
http://orthoinfo.aaos.org/menus/sports.cfm

American Cancer Society: Staying Active. Provides tools for managing an exercise program and discusses the links between cancer and lifestyle, including the importance of physical activity in preventing some cancers.
http://www.cancer.org/docroot/PED/ped_6.asp?sitearea-PED

American Heart Association: Exercise and Fitness. Provides information on cardiovascular health and disease, including the role of exercise in maintaining heart health and exercise tips for people of all ages.
http://www.americanheart.org/presenter.jhtml?identifier_1200013

Centers for Disease Control and Prevention: Physical Activity for Everyone. Explains the latest government recommendations on exercise and physical activity and provides strategies for getting the appropriate type and amount of exercise.
http://www.cdc.gov/physicalactivity/everyone/guidelines/adults.html

Dr. Pribut's Running Injuries Page. Provides information about running and many types of running injuries.
http://www.drpribut.com/sports/spsport.html

The Human Heart. An online museum exhibit with information on the structure and function of the heart, blood vessels, and respiratory system.
http://www.fi.edu/learn/heart/index.html

President's Challenge Adult Fitness Test: Aerobics. Provides step-by-step instructions for taking and interpreting standard tests of aerobic fitness.
http://www.adultfitnesstest.org/testInstructions/aerobicFitness/default.aspx

Runner's World Online. Contains a wide variety of information about running, including tips for beginning runners, advice about training, and a shoe buyer's guide.
http://www.runnersworld.com

Weight Control Information Network: Walking. An online fact sheet that explains the benefits of walking for exercise, tips for starting a walking program, and techniques for getting the most from walking workouts.
http://win.niddk.nih.gov/publications/walking.htm

Women's Sports Foundation. Provides information and links about training and about many specific sports activities.
http://www.womenssportsfoundation.org

SELECTED BIBLIOGRAPHY

Adler, P. A., and B. L. Roberts. 2009. The use of Tai Chi to improve health in older adults. *Orthopedic Nursing* 25(2): 122–126.

American College of Sports Medicine. 2009. *ACSM's Resource Manual for Guidelines for Exercise Testing and Prescription,* 6th ed. Philadelphia: Lippincott Williams and Wilkins.

American College of Sports Medicine. 2009. *ACSM's Guidelines for Exercise Testing and Prescription,* 8th ed. Philadelphia: Lippincott Williams and Wilkins.

American Heart Association. 2010. *Heart Disease and Stroke Statistics—2010 Update.* Dallas: American Heart Association.

Brooks, G. A., et al. 2005. *Exercise Physiology: Human Bioenergetics and Its Applications,* 4th ed. New York: McGraw-Hill.

Budde H., et al. 2008. Acute coordinative exercise improves attentional performance in adolescents. *Neuroscience Letters* 441(2): 219–223.

Cadore, E. L., et al. 2011. Effects of strength, endurance, and concurrent training on aerobic power and dynamic neuromuscular economy in elderly men. *J Strength Conditioning Research* 25(3): 758–766.

Courneya, K. S., and C. M. Friedenreich. 2011. Physical activity and cancer: an introduction. *Recent Results Cancer Research.* 186: 1–10.

Denadai, B. S., et al. 2006. Interval training at 95% and 100% of the velocity at $\dot{V}O_{2max}$: Effects on aerobic physiological indexes and running performance. *Applied Physiology, Nutrition, and Metabolism* 31(6): 737–743.

Erickson, K. I., et al. 2011. Exercise training increases size of hippocampus and improves memory. *Proceedings of the National Academy of Sciences.* 108(7): 3017–3022.

Garber, C. E., et al. 2011. Quantity and quality of exercise for developing and maintaining cardiorespiratory, musculoskeletal, and neuromotor fitness in apparently healthy adults: Guidance for prescribing exercise. *Medicine and Science in Sport and Exercise* 43(7):1334–1359.

Haskell, W. L., et al. 2007. Physical activity and public health: Updated recommendation for adults from the American College of Sports Medicine and the American Heart Association. *Medicine and Science in Sport and Exercise* 39(8): 1423–1434.

Hautala, A. J., et al. 2009. Individual responses to aerobic exercise: The role of the autonomic nervous system. *Neuroscience and Biobehavioral Reviews* 33(2): 107–115.

Keller, P., et al. 2011. A transcriptional map of the impact of endurance exercise training on skeletal muscle phenotype. *Journal of Applied Physiology* 110(1): 46–59.

Moien-Afshari, F., et al. 2009. Exercise restores endothelial function independently of weight loss or hyperglycaemic status in db/db mice. *Diabetologia* 51(7): 1327–1337.

Morikawa, M., et al. 2011. Physical fitness and indices of lifestyle-related diseases before and after interval walking training in middle-aged and older males and females. *British Journal Sports Medicine* 45(3): 216–224.

Murphy, M. H., et al. 2009. Accumulated versus continuous exercise for health benefit: A review of empirical studies. *Sports Medicine* 39(1): 29–43.

Netz, Y. T., et al. 2011. Aerobic fitness and multi-domain cognitive function in advanced age. *International Psychogeriatrics.* 23(1): 114–124.

Okura, T., et al. 2006. Effect of regular exercise on homocysteine concentrations: The HERITAGE Family Study. *European Journal of Applied Physiology* 98(4): 394–401.

Physical Activity Guidelines Advisory Committee. 2008. *Physical Activity Guidelines Advisory Committee Report, 2008.* Washington, D.C.: U.S. Department of Health and Human Services.

Ploughman, M. 2008. Exercise is brain food: The effects of physical activity on cognitive function. *Developmental Neurorehabilitation* 11(3): 236–240.

Reigle, B. S., and K. Wonders. 2009. Breast cancer and the role of exercise in women. *Methods in Molecular Biology* 472(1): 169–189.

Ruiz, J. R., et al. 2011. Strenuous endurance exercise improves life expectancy: It's in our genes. *British Journal of Sports Medicine* 45(3): 159–161.

Sui, X., et al. 2008. A prospective study of cardiorespiratory fitness and risk of type 2 diabetes in women. *Diabetes Care* 31(3): 550–555.

Suominen, H. 2006. Muscle training for bone strength. *Aging Clinical and Experimental Research* 18(2): 85–93.

U.S. Department of Health and Human Services. 2008. *Physical Activity Guidelines for Americans.* Washington, D.C.: U.S. Department of Health and Human Services.

Waterhouse, J., et al. 2010. Effects of music tempo upon submaximal cycling performance. *Scandinavian Journal of Medicine and Science in Sports* 20(4): 662–669.

Yeo, W. K., et al. 2011. Fat adaptation in well-trained athletes: effects on cell metabolism. *Applied Physiology Nutrition Metabolism* 36(1): 12–22.

Yung, L. M., et al. 2009. Exercise, vascular wall and cardiovascular diseases: An update (part 2). *Sports Medicine* 39(1): 45–63.

Name ______________________ Section ______________ Date ____________

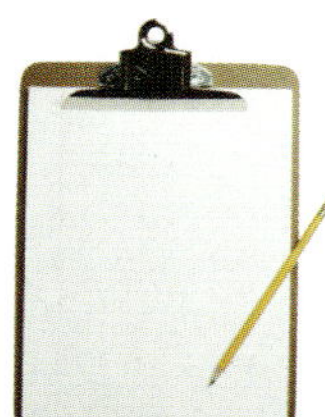

LAB 4.1 Assessing Your Current Level of Cardiorespiratory Endurance

Before taking any of the cardiorespiratory endurance assessment tests, refer to the fitness prerequisites and cautions given in Table 4.2. Choose one of the following four tests presented in this lab:

- 1-mile walk test
- 3-minute step test
- 1.5-mile run-walk test
- 12-minute swim test

For best results, don't exercise strenuously or consume caffeine the day of the test, and don't smoke or eat a heavy meal within about 3 hours of the test.

The 1-Mile Walk Test

Equipment

1. A track or course that provides a measurement of 1 mile
2. A stopwatch, clock, or watch with a second hand
3. A weight scale

Preparation

Measure your body weight (in pounds) before taking the test.
Body weight: ____________ lb

Instructions

1. Warm up before taking the test. Do some walking, easy jogging, or calisthenics.
2. Cover the 1-mile course as quickly as possible. Walk at a pace that is brisk but comfortable. You must raise your heart rate above 120 beats per minute (bpm).
3. As soon as you complete the distance, note your time and take your pulse for 10 seconds.
   Walking time: ____________ min ____________ sec
   10-second pulse count: ____________ beats
4. Cool down after the test by walking slowly for several minutes.

Determining Maximal Oxygen Consumption

1. Convert your 10-second pulse count into a value for exercise heart rate by multiplying it by 6.
   Exercise heart rate: ____________ × 6 = ____________ bpm
2. Convert your walking time from minutes and seconds to a decimal figure. For example, a time of 14 minutes and 45 seconds would be 14 + (45/60), or 14.75 minutes.
   Walking time: ____________ min + (____________ sec ÷ 60 sec/min) = ____________ min
3. Insert values for your age, gender, weight, walking time, and exercise heart rate in the following equation, where
   W = your weight (in pounds)
   A = your age (in years)
   G = your gender (male = 1; female = 0)
   T = your time to complete the 1-mile course (in minutes)
   H = your exercise heart rate (in beats per minute)
   $\dot{V}O_{2max} = 132.853 - (0.0769 \times W) - (0.3877 \times A) + (6.315 \times G) - (3.2649 \times T) - (0.1565 \times H)$

For example, a 20-year-old, 190-pound male with a time of 14.75 minutes and an exercise heart rate of 152 bpm would calculate maximal oxygen consumption as follows:

$\dot{V}O_{2max} = 132.853 - (0.0769 \times 190) - (0.3877 \times 20) + (6.315 \times 1) - (3.2649 \times 14.75) - (0.1565 \times 152) = 45$ *ml/kg/min*

$\dot{V}O_{2max}$ = 132.853 − (0.0769 × ____________ [weight (lb)]) − (0.3877 × ____________ [age (years)]) + (6.315 × ____________ [gender])

− (3.2649 × ____________ [walking time (min)]) − (0.1565 × ____________ [exercise heart rate (bpm)]) = ____________ ml/kg/min

4. Copy this value for $\dot{V}O_{2max}$ into the appropriate place in the chart on page 142.

The 3-Minute Step Test

Equipment

1. A step, bench, or bleacher step that is 16.25 inches from ground level
2. A stopwatch, clock, or watch with a second hand
3. A metronome

Preparation

Practice stepping up onto and down from the step before you begin the test. Each step has four beats: up-up-down-down. Males should perform the test with the metronome set for a rate of 96 beats per minute, or 24 steps per minute. Females should set the metronome at 88 beats per minute, or 22 steps per minute.

Instructions

1. Warm up before taking the test. Do some walking or easy jogging.
2. Set the metronome at the proper rate. Your instructor or a partner can call out starting and stopping times; otherwise, have a clock or watch within easy viewing during the test.
3. Begin the test and continue to step at the correct pace for 3 minutes.
4. Stop after 3 minutes. Remain standing and count your pulse for the 15-second period from 5 to 20 seconds into recovery.
   15-second pulse count: ____________ beats
5. Cool down after the test by walking slowly for several minutes.

Determining Maximal Oxygen Consumption

1. Convert your 15-second pulse count to a value for recovery heart rate by multiplying by 4.
   Recovery heart rate: ____________ [bpm 15-sec pulse count] × 4 = ____________
2. Insert your recovery heart rate in the equation below, where
   H = recovery heart rate (in beats per minute)
   Males: $\dot{V}O_{2max} = 111.33 - (0.42 \times H)$
   Females: $\dot{V}O_{2max} = 65.81 - (0.1847 \times H)$
   For example, a man with a recovery heart rate of 162 bpm would calculate maximal oxygen consumption as follows:
   $\dot{V}O_{2max} = 111.33 - (0.42 \times 162) = 43$ *ml/kg/min*
   Males: $\dot{V}O_{2max}$ = 111.33 − (0.42 × ____________ [recovery heart rate (bpm)]) = ____________ ml/kg/min
   Females: $\dot{V}O_{2max}$ = 65.81 − (0.1847 × ____________ [recovery heart rate (bpm)]) = ____________ ml/kg/min
3. Copy this value for $\dot{V}O_{2max}$ into the appropriate place in the chart on page 142.

LABORATORY ACTIVITIES

The 1.5-Mile Run-Walk Test

Equipment

1. A running track or course that is flat and provides exact measurements of up to 1.5 miles
2. A stopwatch, clock, or watch with a second hand

Preparation

You may want to practice pacing yourself prior to taking the test to avoid going too fast at the start and becoming prematurely fatigued. Allow yourself a day or two to recover from your practice run before taking the test.

Instructions

1. Warm up before taking the test. Do some walking or easy jogging.
2. Try to cover the distance as fast as possible without overexerting yourself. If possible, monitor your own time, or have someone call out your time at various intervals of the test to determine whether your pace is correct.
3. Record the amount of time, in minutes and seconds, it takes you to complete the 1.5-mile distance.

   Running-walking time: ________________ min ________________ sec
4. Cool down after the test by walking or jogging slowly for about 5 minutes.

Determining Maximal Oxygen Consumption

1. Convert your running time from minutes and seconds to a decimal figure. For example, a time of 14 minutes and 25 seconds would be 14 + (25/60), or 14.4 minutes.

   Running-walking time: ________________ min + (________________ sec ÷ 60 sec/min) = ________________ min
2. Insert your running time into the equation below, where

   T = running time (in minutes)

   $\dot{V}O_{2max} = (483 \div T) + 3.5$

   For example, a person who completes 1.5 miles in 14.4 minutes would calculate maximal oxygen consumption as follows:

   $\dot{V}O_{2max} = (483 \div 14.4) + 3.5 = 37$ *ml/kg/min*

   $\dot{V}O_{2max}$ = (483 ÷ ________________) + 3.5 = ________________ ml/kg/min

   run-walk time (min)
3. Copy this value for $\dot{V}O_{2max}$ into the appropriate place in the chart on page 142.

Rating Your Cardiovascular Fitness

Record your $\dot{V}O_{2max}$ score(s) and the corresponding fitness rating from the table below.

Women	*Very Poor*	*Poor*	*Fair*	*Good*	*Excellent*	*Superior*
Age: 18–29	Below 31.6	31.6–35.4	35.5–39.4	39.5–43.9	44.0–50.1	Above 50.1
30–39	Below 29.9	29.9–33.7	33.8–36.7	36.8–40.9	41.0–46.8	Above 46.8
40–49	Below 28.0	28.0–31.5	31.6–35.0	35.1–38.8	38.9–45.1	Above 45.1
50–59	Below 25.5	25.5–28.6	28.7–31.3	31.4–35.1	35.2–39.8	Above 39.8
60–69	Below 23.7	23.7–26.5	26.6–29.0	29.1–32.2	32.3–36.8	Above 36.8
Men						
Age: 18–29	Below 38.1	38.1–42.1	42.2–45.6	45.7–51.0	51.1–56.1	Above 56.1
30–39	Below 36.7	36.7–40.9	41.0–44.3	44.4–48.8	48.9–54.2	Above 54.2
40–49	Below 34.6	34.6–38.3	38.4–42.3	42.4–46.7	46.8–52.8	Above 52.8
50–59	Below 31.1	31.1–35.1	35.2–38.2	38.3–43.2	43.3–49.6	Above 49.6
60–69	Below 27.4	27.4–31.3	31.4–34.9	35.0–39.4	39.5–46.0	Above 46.0

SOURCE: Ratings based on norms from The Cooper Institute of Aerobic Research, Dallas, Texas; from *The Physical Fitness Specialist Manual,* Revised 2002. Used with permission.

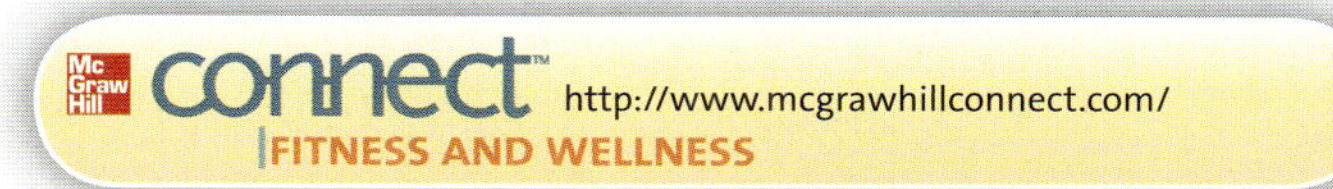

	$\dot{V}O_{2max}$	Cardiovascular Fitness Rating
1-mile walk test		
3-minute step test		
1.5-mile run-walk test		

The 12-Minute Swim Test

If you enjoy swimming and prefer to build a cardiorespiratory training program around this type of exercise, you can assess your cardiorespiratory endurance by taking the 12-minute swim test. You will receive a rating based on the distance you can swim in 12 minutes.

Note, however, that this test is appropriate only for relatively strong swimmers who are confident in the water. If you are unsure about your swimming ability, this test may not be appropriate for you. If necessary, ask your school's swim coach or a qualified swimming instructor to evaluate your ability in the water before attempting this test.

Equipment

1. A swimming pool that provides measurements in yards
2. A wall clock that is clearly visible from the pool, or someone with a watch who can time you

Preparation

You may want to practice pacing yourself before taking the test to avoid going too fast at the start and becoming prematurely fatigued. Allow yourself a day or two to recover from your practice swim before taking the test.

Instructions

1. Warm up before taking the test. Do some walking or light jogging before getting in the pool. Once in the water, swim a lap or two at an easy pace to make sure your muscles are warm and you are comfortable.
2. Try to cover the distance as fast as possible without overexerting yourself. If possible, monitor your own time, or have someone call out your time at various intervals of the test to determine whether your pace is correct.
3. Record the distance, in yards, that you were able to cover during the 12-minute period.
4. Cool down after the test by swimming a lap or two at an easy pace.
5. Use the following chart to gauge your level of cardiorespiratory fitness.

DISTANCE IN YARDS

Women	*Needs Work*	*Better*	*Fair*	*Good*	*Excellent*
Age: 13–19	Below 500	500–599	600–699	700–799	Above 800
20–29	Below 400	400–499	500–599	600–699	Above 700
30–39	Below 350	350–449	450–549	550–649	Above 650
40–49	Below 300	300–399	400–499	500–599	Above 600
50–59	Below 250	250–349	350–449	450–549	Above 550
60 and over	Below 250	250–299	300–399	400–499	Above 500
Men					
Age: 13–19	Below 400	400–499	500–599	600–699	Above 700
20–29	Below 300	300–399	400–499	500–599	Above 600
30–39	Below 250	250–349	350–449	450–549	Above 550
40–49	Below 200	200–299	300–399	400–499	Above 500
50–59	Below 150	150–249	250–349	350–449	Above 450
60 and over	Below 150	150–199	200–299	300–399	Above 400

100 yards = 91 meters

SOURCE: Cooper, K. H. 1982. *The Aerobics Program for Total Well-Being.* New York: Bantam Books.

Record your fitness rating:

	Cardiovascular Fitness Rating
12-minute swim test	

Using Your Results

How did you score? Are you surprised by your rating for cardiovascular fitness? Are you satisfied with your current rating?

If you're not satisfied, set a realistic goal for improvement: ______________________________

____

Are you satisfied with your current level of cardiovascular fitness as evidenced in your daily life—your ability to walk, run, bicycle, climb stairs, do yard work, or engage in recreational activities?

If you're not satisfied, set some realistic goals for improvement, such as completing a 5K run or 25-mile bike ride: ______________________________

____

What should you do next? Enter the results of this lab in the Preprogram Assessment column in Appendix C. If you've set goals for improvement, begin planning your cardiorespiratory endurance exercise program by completing the plan in Lab 4.2. After several weeks of your program, complete this lab again, and enter the results in the Postprogram Assessment column of Appendix C. How do the results compare? (Remember, it's best to compare $\dot{V}O_{2max}$ scores for the same test.)

SOURCES: Brooks, G. A., and T. D. Fahey. 1987. *Fundamentals of Human Performance.* New York: Macmillan. Kline, G. M., et al. 1987. Estimation of $\dot{V}O_{2max}$ from a one-mile track walk, gender, age, and body weight. *Medicine and Science in Sports and Exercise* 19(3): 253–259. McArdle, W. D., F. I. Katch, and V. L. Katch. 2010. *Exercise Physiology-. Energy, Nutrition, and Human Peformance.* Philadelphia: Lea and Febiger, pp. 243–246.

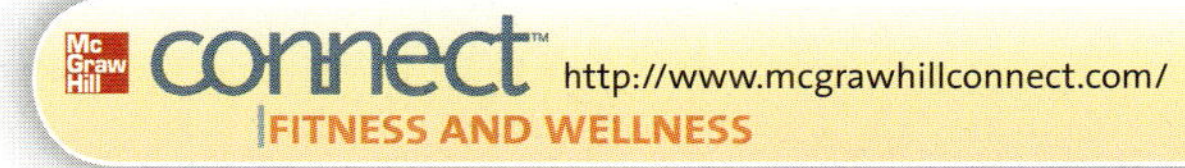

Touring the Cardiorespiratory System

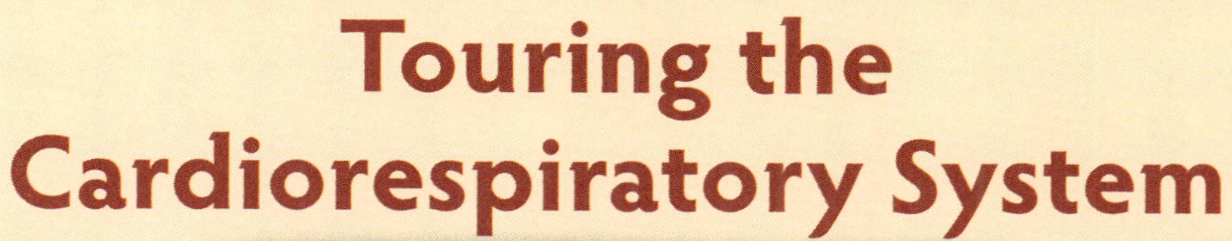

The Cardiorespiratory System

The Heart and Lungs

Atherosclerosis: The Process of Cardiovascular Disease

Diabetes: A Disorder of Metabolism

GOALS OF THE TOUR

1. **The Cardiorespiratory System.** You will be able to identify the parts of the cardiorespiratory system and the pattern of blood flow through the body.
2. **The Heart and Lungs.** You will be able to identify the chambers of the heart and describe the flow of blood through the right side of the heart to the lungs (pulmonary circulation) and through the left side of the heart to the body (systemic circulation).
3. **Atherosclerosis.** You will be able to explain the process of cardiovascular disease and compare and contrast the outcomes affecting the heart and the brain.
4. **Diabetes.** You will be able to describe how the body uses digested food for energy and growth and how this process is disrupted when a person has diabetes.

The Cardiorespiratory System

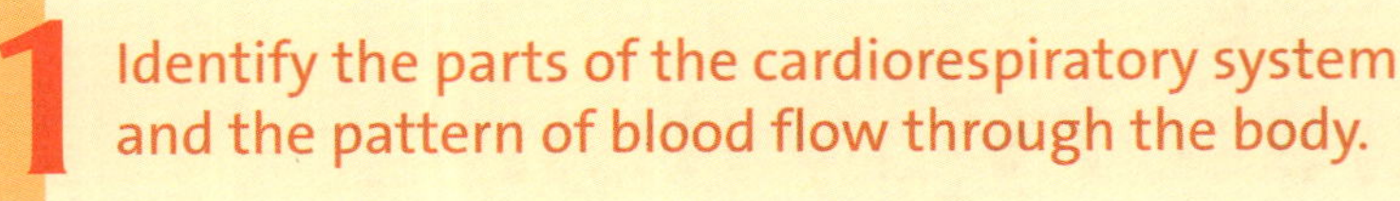

Identify the parts of the cardiorespiratory system and the pattern of blood flow through the body.

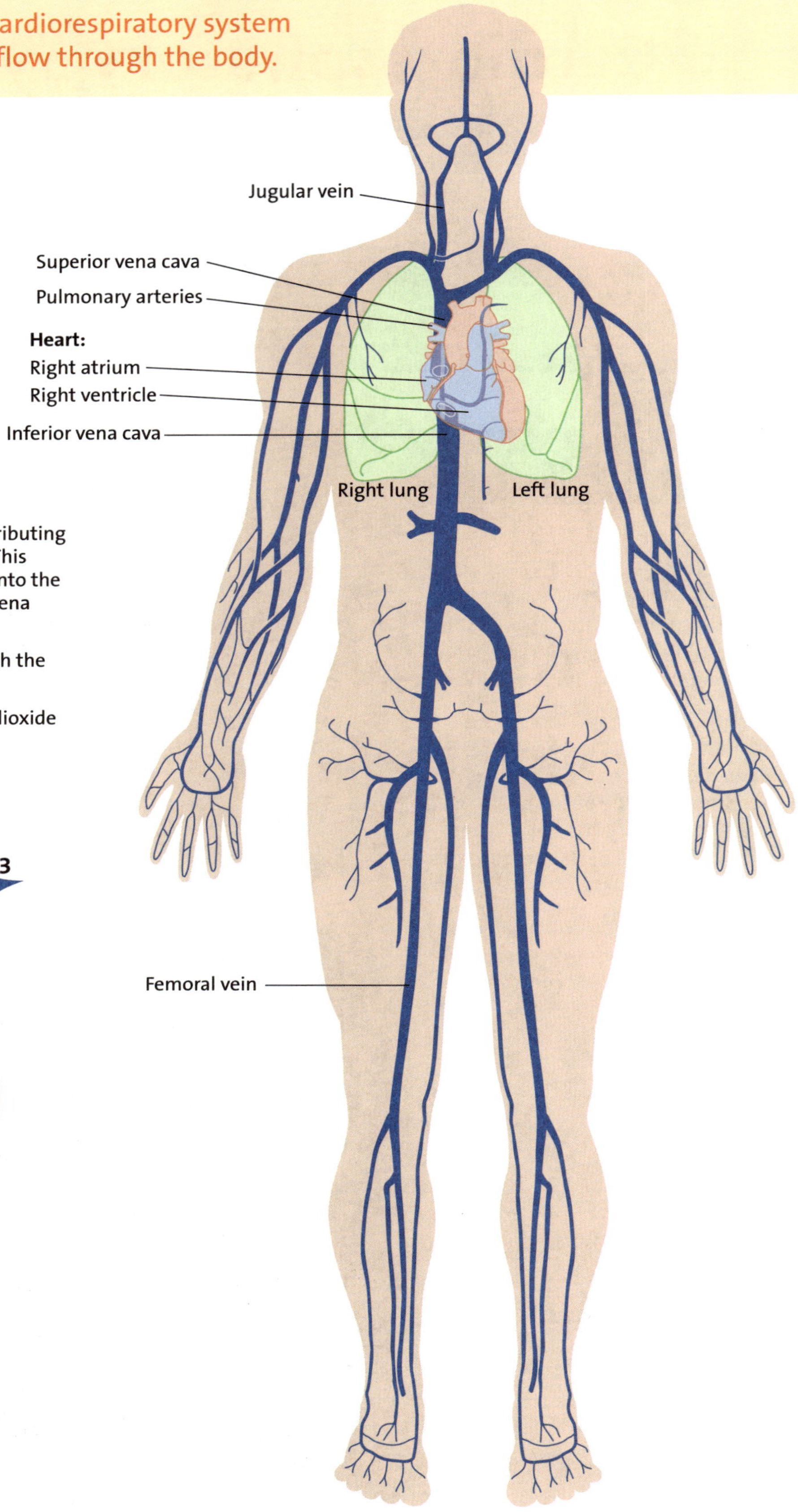

Jugular vein

Superior vena cava

Pulmonary arteries

Heart:

Right atrium

Right ventricle

Inferior vena cava

Right lung

Left lung

Femoral vein

Return of deoxygenated blood to the heart

1. Blood travels through the body, distributing oxygen and picking up carbon dioxide. This waste-laden, oxygen-poor blood flows into the right side of the heart via the superior vena cava and the inferior vena cava.

2. From there, blood is pumped through the pulmonary arteries into the lungs.

3. In the lungs, blood discards carbon dioxide and picks up oxygen.

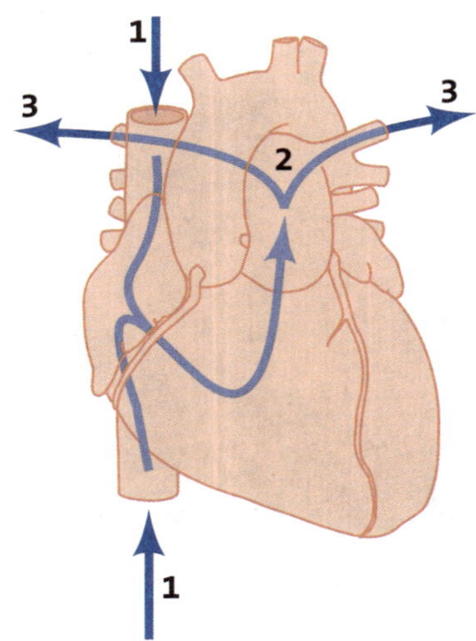

The Heart and Lungs

Identify the chambers of the heart and describe the flow of blood through the right side of the heart to the lungs (pulmonary circulation) and through the left side of the heart to the body (systemic circulation).

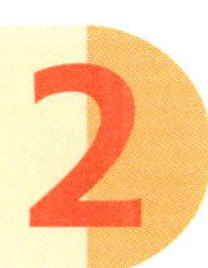

Blood is supplied to the heart muscle by the right and left coronary arteries, which branch off the aorta.

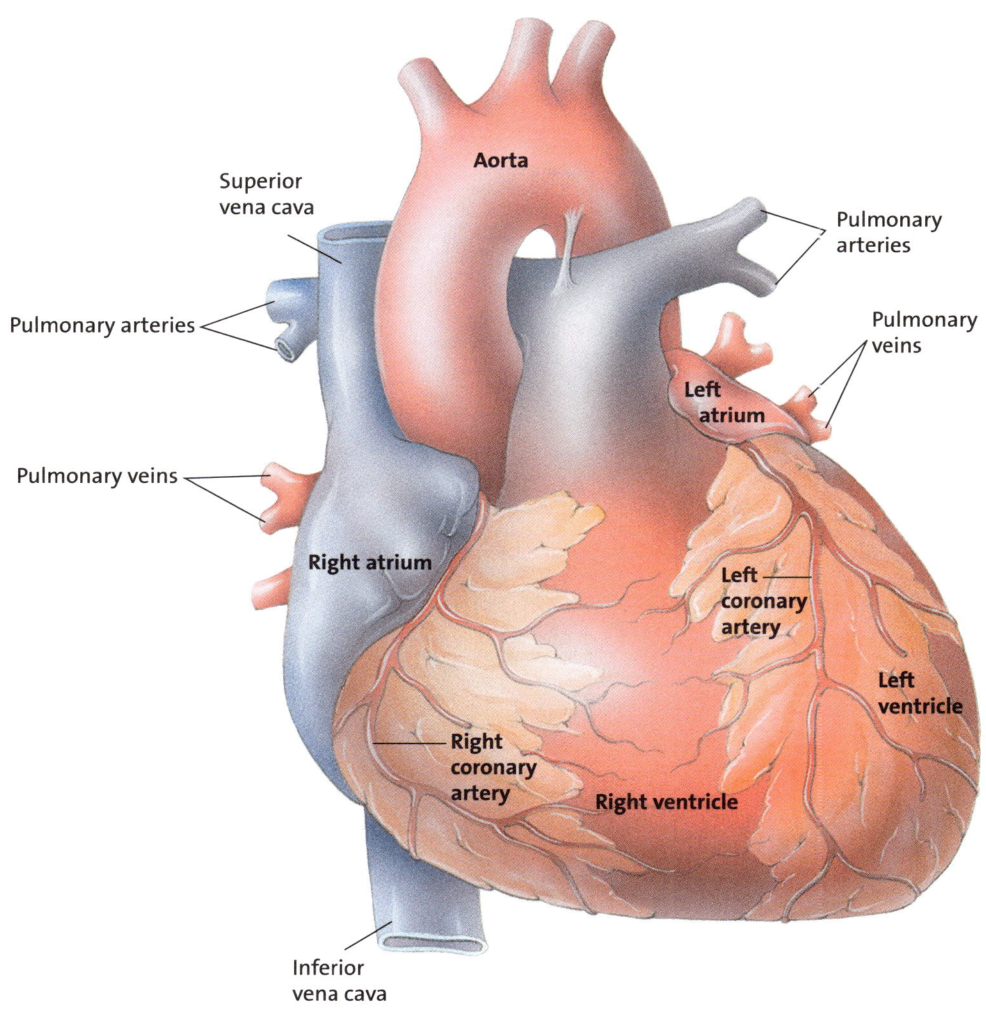

Atherosclerosis: The Process of Cardiovascular Disease

3 Explain the process of cardiovascular disease and compare and contrast the outcomes affecting the heart and the brain.

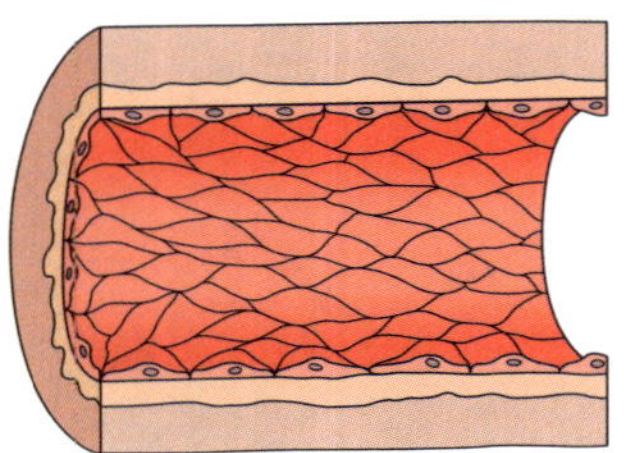

1. A healthy artery allows blood to flow through freely.

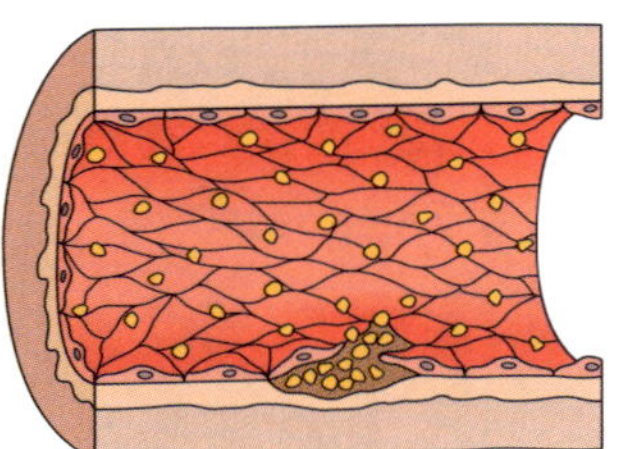

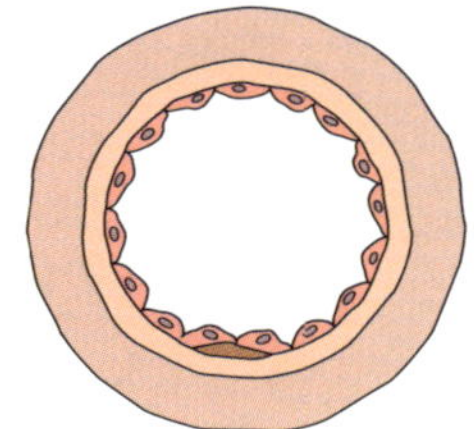

2. Plaque buildup begins when endothelial cells lining the arteries are damaged by smoking, high blood pressure, oxidized LDL cholesterol, and other causes. Excess cholesterol particles collect beneath these cells.

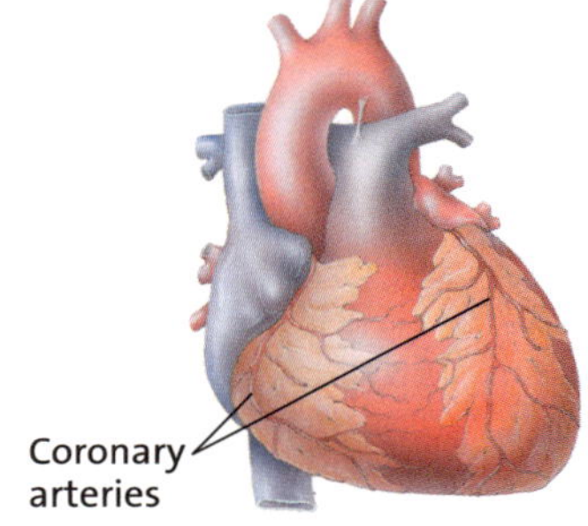

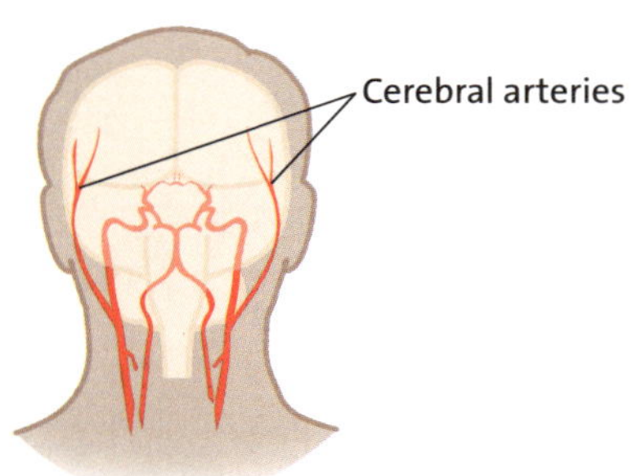

Diabetes: A Disorder of Metabolism

Describe how the body uses digested food for energy and growth and how this process is disrupted when a person has diabetes.

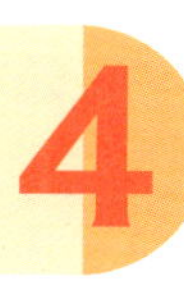

Normal metabolism

1. When a meal is consumed, food is broken down into nutrients that the body can use to produce energy and build and nourish cells. Carbohydrates are broken down into glucose, which is the body's primary source of energy.

2. When glucose enters the bloodstream, the pancreas secretes the hormone insulin, which allows glucose to enter body cells.

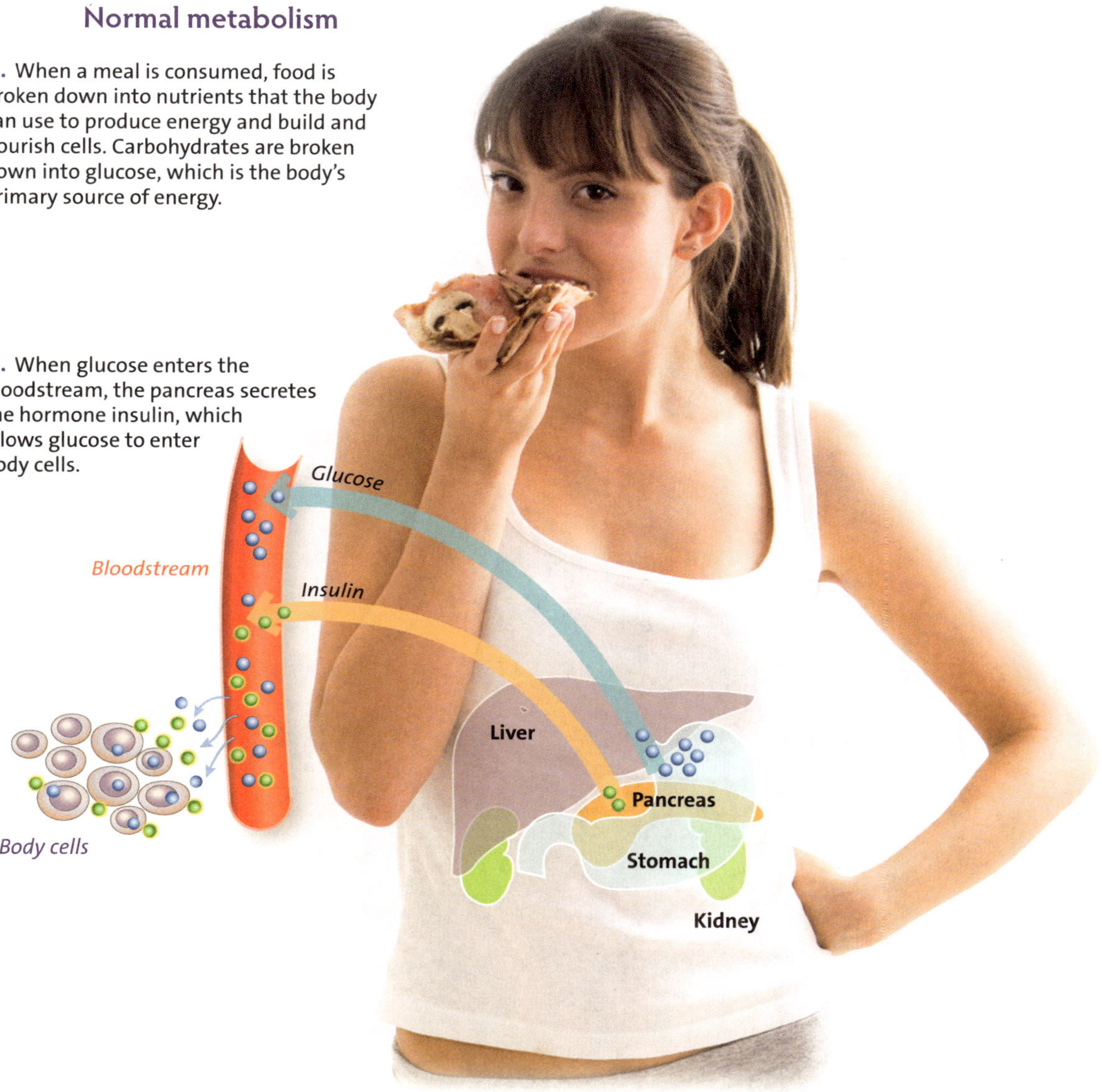

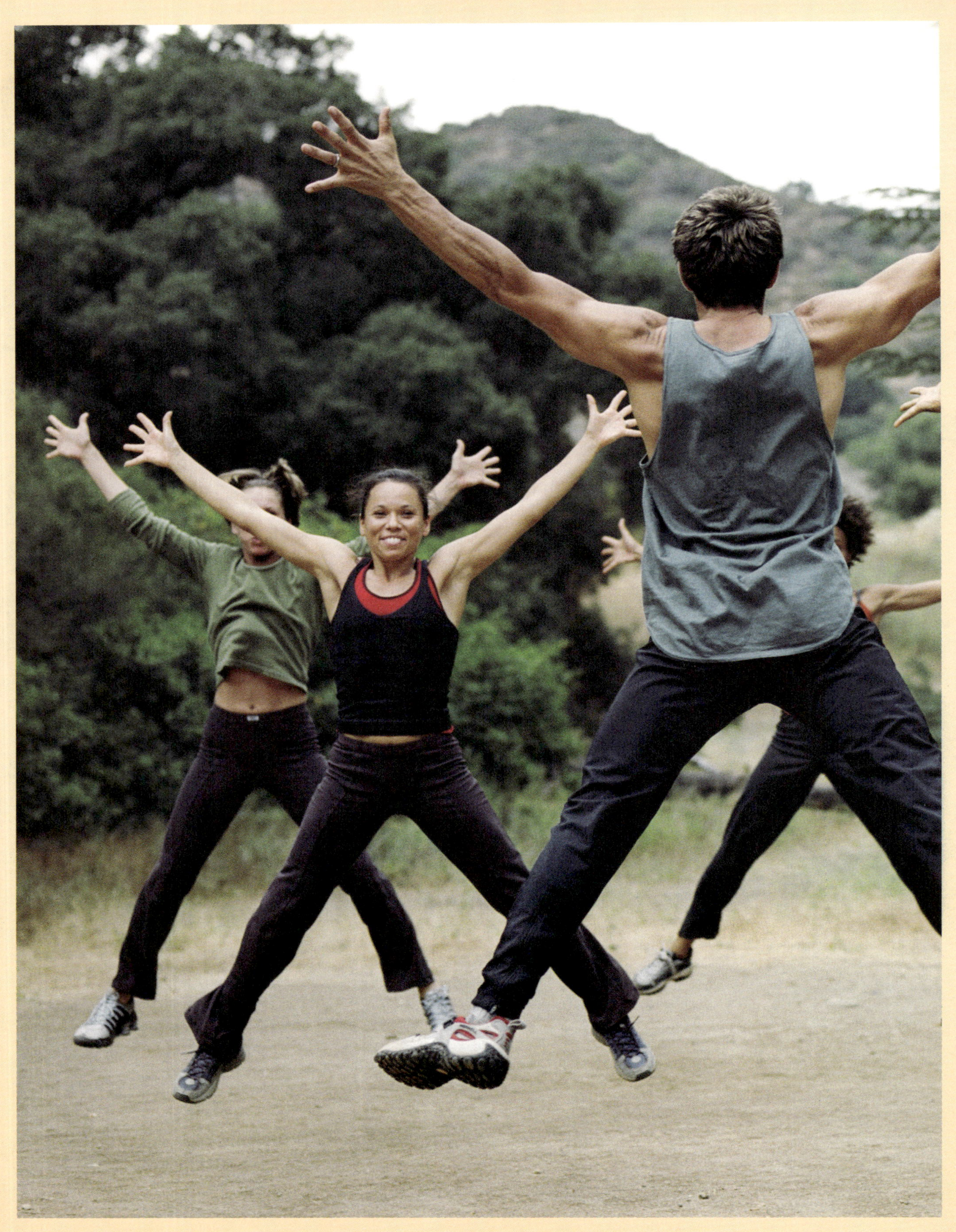

Name ______________________ Section ______________ Date ____________

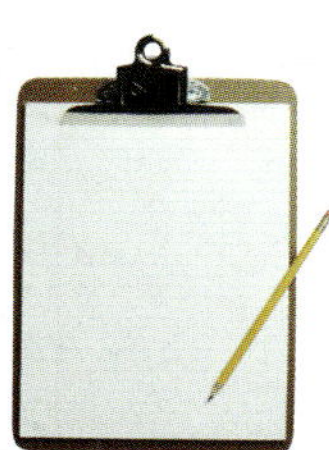

LAB 4.2 Developing an Exercise Program for Cardiorespiratory Endurance

1. *Goals.* List goals for your cardiorespiratory endurance exercise program. Your goals can be specific or general, short or long term. In the first section, include specific, measurable goals that you can use to track the progress of your fitness program. These goals might be things like raising your cardiorespiratory fitness rating from fair to good or swimming laps for 30 minutes without resting. In the second section, include long-term and more qualitative goals, such as improving self-confidence and reducing your risk for chronic disease.

   Specific Goals: Current Status ______________________ Final Goals ______________________

   ______________________ ______________________

   ______________________ ______________________

   Other goals: ____

   ____

2. *Type of Activities.* Choose one or more endurance activities for your program. These can include any activity that uses large-muscle groups, can be maintained continuously, and is rhythmic and aerobic in nature. Examples include walking, jogging, cycling, group exercise such as aerobic dance, rowing, rope skipping, stair-climbing, cross-country skiing, swimming, skating, and endurance game activities such as soccer and tennis. Choose activities that are both convenient and enjoyable. Fill in the activity names on the program plan.
3. *Frequency.* On the program plan, fill in how often you plan to participate in each activity; the ACSM recommends participating in cardiorespiratory endurance exercise 3-5 days per week.

Program Plan

Type of Activity	Frequency (check ✓)							Intensity (bpm or RPE)	Time (min)
	M	T	W	Th	F	Sa	Su		

4. *Intensity.* Determine your exercise intensity using one of the following methods, and enter it on the program plan. Begin your program at a lower intensity and slowly increase intensity as your fitness improves, so select a range of intensities for your program,

a. Target heart rate zone: Calculate target heart rate zone in beats per minute and then calculate the corresponding 10-second exercise count by dividing the total count by 6. For example, the 10-second exercise counts corresponding to a target heart rate zone of 122–180 bpm would be 20–30 beats.

   Maximum heart rate: 220 − ______________ (age (years)) = ______________ bpm

   Maximum Heart Rate Method

   65% training intensity = ______________ (maximum heart rate) bpm × 0.65 = ______________ bpm

   90% training intensity = ______________ (maximum heart rate) bpm × 0.90 = ______________ bpm

   Target heart rate zone = ____________ **to** ____________ **bpm** **10-second count =** ________ **to** ________

Heart Rate Reserve Method

Resting heart rate:________ bpm (taken after 10 minutes of complete rest)

Heart rate reserve = ______________ bpm − ______________ bpm = ____________ bpm
(maximum heart rate) (resting heart rate)

50% training intensity = (______________ bpm × 0.50) + ______________ bpm = ____________ bpm
(heart rate reserve) (resting heart rate)

85% training intensity = (______________ bpm × 0.85) + ______________ bpm = ____________ bpm
(heart rate reserve) (resting heart rate)

Target heart rate zone = ____________ to ____________ bpm

10-second count = ____________ to ______________

b. Ratings of perceived exertion (RPE): If you prefer, determine an RPE value that corresponds to your target heart rate range (see p. 126 and Figure 4.5).

5. *Time (Duration).* A total time of 20–60 minutes is recommended; your duration of exercise will vary with intensity. For developing cardiorespiratory endurance, higher-intensity activities can be performed for a shorter duration; lower intensities require a longer duration. Enter a duration (or a range of duration) on the program plan.
6. *Monitoring Your Program.* Complete a log like the one below to monitor your program and track your progress. Note the date on top, and fill in the intensity and time (duration) for each workout. If you prefer, you can also track other variables such as distance. For example, if your cardiorespiratory endurance program includes walking and swimming, you may want to track miles walked and yards swum in addition to the duration of each exercise session.

Activity/Date													
1	Intentsity												
	Time												
	Distance												
2	Intentsity												
	Time												
	Distance												
3	Intentsity												
	Time												
	Distance												
4	Intentsity												
	Time												
	Distance												

7. *Making Progress.* Follow the guidelines in the chapter and Table 4.6 to slowly increase the amount of overload in your program. Continue keeping a log, and periodically evaluate your progress.

Progress Checkup: Week ________ of program

Goals: Original Status	Current Status
______________________________	______________________________
______________________________	______________________________
______________________________	______________________________

List each activity in your program and describe how satisfied you are with the activity and with your overall progress. List any problems you've encountered or any unexpected costs or benefits of your fitness program so far.

CHAPTER 5

Cardiovascular Health

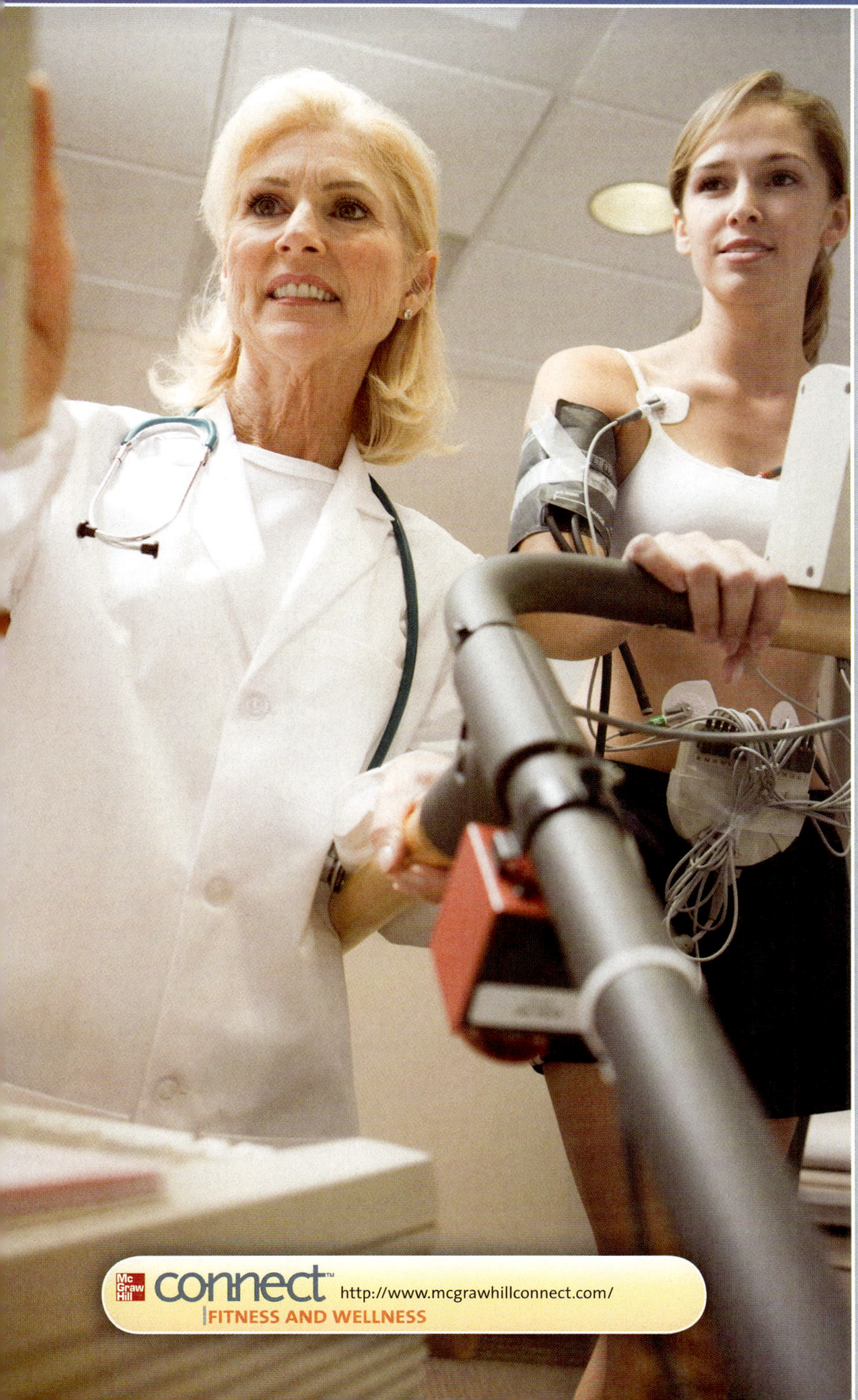

LOOKING AHEAD...

After reading this chapter, you should be able to:

- Describe the controllable and uncontrollable risk factors associated with cardiovascular disease
- Discuss the major forms of cardiovascular disease and how they develop
- List the steps you can take now to lower your personal risk of developing cardiovascular disease

TEST YOUR KNOWLEDGE

1. Women are about as likely to die of cardiovascular disease as they are to die of breast cancer. True or false?
2. On average, how much earlier does heart disease develop in people who don't exercise regularly than in people who do?
   a. 6 months
   b. 2 years
   c. 6 years
3. Which of the following foods would be a good choice for promoting heart health?
   a. whole grains
   b. salmon
   c. bananas

Answers

1. **False.** Cardiovascular disease kills far more. Among American women, nearly 1 in 3 deaths is due to cardiovascular disease and about 1 in 30 is due to breast cancer.
2. **c.** Both aerobic exercise and strength training significantly improve cardiovascular health.
3. **All three.** Whole grains (whole wheat, oatmeal, rye, barley, and brown rice), foods with omega-3 fatty acids (salmon), and foods high in potassium and low in sodium (bananas) all improve cardiovascular health.

Cardiovascular disease (CVD) affects nearly 83 million Americans and is the leading cause of death in the United States. CVD claims one life every 39 seconds—more than 2200 Americans every day. CVD is often thought to affect primarily men and older adults, but heart disease is the number-one killer of American women, and more than 18% of CVD-related deaths occur in people under age 65.

CVD is largely due to our way of life. Millions of Americans are overweight and sedentary, smoke, manage stress ineffectively, have uncontrolled high blood pressure or high cholesterol levels, and don't know the signs of CVD. Not all risk factors for CVD are controllable—some people have an inherited tendency toward high cholesterol levels, for example—but many are within your control.

This chapter explains the major forms of CVD, including hypertension, atherosclerosis, and stroke. It also considers the factors that put people at risk for CVD. Most important, it explains the steps you can take to protect your heart and promote cardiovascular health throughout your life.

RISK FACTORS FOR CARDIOVASCULAR DISEASE

Researchers have identified a variety of factors associated with an increased risk of developing CVD. They are grouped into two categories: major risk factors and contributing risk factors. Some risk factors are linked to controllable aspects of lifestyle and can therefore be changed. Others are beyond your control. (You can evaluate your personal CVD risk factors in Part I of Lab 5.1.)

Major Risk Factors That Can Be Changed

The American Heart Association (AHA) has identified six major risk factors for CVD that can be changed: tobacco use, high blood pressure, unhealthy blood cholesterol levels, physical inactivity, overweight and obesity, and diabetes. Most Americans, including young adults, have major risk factors for CVD.

Tobacco Use Nearly 1 in 5 deaths is attributable to smoking. In 2008, an estimated 71 million Americans were tobacco users, including 13.6 million college students. Smoking remains the number-one preventable cause of CVD in the United States. People who smoke a pack of cigarettes a day have twice the risk of heart attack as nonsmokers; smoking two or more packs a day triples the risk. When smokers have heart attacks, they are 2 to 3 times more likely than nonsmokers to die from them. Cigarette smoking also doubles the risk of stroke.

Smoking harms the cardiovascular system in several ways:

- It damages the lining of arteries.
- It reduces the level of *high-density lipoproteins* (*HDL*), or "good" cholesterol.
- It raises the levels of triglycerides and *low-density lipoproteins* (*LDL*), or "bad" cholesterol.
- Nicotine increases blood pressure and heart rate.
- The carbon monoxide in cigarette smoke displaces oxygen in the blood, reducing the oxygen available to the body.
- Smoking causes **platelets** to stick together in the bloodstream, leading to clotting.
- Smoking speeds the development of fatty deposits in the arteries.

You don't have to smoke to be affected. The risk of developing heart disease increases up to 30% among people exposed to environmental tobacco smoke (ETS)—also known as "secondhand smoke." Researchers estimate that about 49,000 nonsmokers die from heart disease each year as a result of exposure to ETS.

High Blood Pressure In addition to being a form of CVD in itself, high blood pressure, or **hypertension,** is a risk factor for other forms of cardiovascular disease, including heart attacks and strokes.

Blood pressure, the force exerted by the blood on the vessel walls, is created by the pumping action of the heart. High blood pressure occurs when too much force is exerted against the walls of the arteries. Short periods of high blood pressure—such as in response to excitement or exertion—are normal, but chronic high blood pressure is a health risk.

Health care professionals measure blood pressure with a stethoscope and an instrument called a *sphygmomanometer.* At home, you can track your own blood pressure by using an inexpensive blood pressure monitor (see the box "Digital Tools for Heart Health"). Blood pressure is expressed as two numbers—for example, 120 over 80—and measured in millimeters of mercury (mm Hg). The first number is systolic blood pressure; the second is diastolic blood pressure. A normal blood pressure reading for a healthy adult is below 120 systolic over 80 diastolic; CVD risk increases when blood pressure rises above this

> **Wellness Tip**
>
> Always relax a few minutes before checking your blood pressure; doing so will help your blood pressure settle to its normal level. You may get a false reading if you take your blood pressure when you're agitated or moving around.

Digital Tools for Heart Health

connect ACTIVITY DO IT ONLINE

Do you ever check your own heart rate or blood pressure? For people who have heart disease or certain risk factors, tracking these vital signs can become routine. Fortunately, there are plenty of electronic devices available that make it easy to check your heart rate and blood pressure.

Heart Rate Monitors

As described in Chapter 4, there are many kinds of commercially available heart rate monitors. Although these devices are typically meant for use while exercising, they can also give you an accurate count of your resting heart rate. Knowing your resting heart rate can be important for several reasons. For example, a consistently high resting heart rate can be a sign of trouble or indicate that you need to improve your level of cardiorespiratory fitness.

Heart rate monitors usually feature a strap that goes around the user's chest and a watch-like device worn on the arm. The strap contains one or more sensors that gauge the wearer's heartbeat and transmit the information to the wrist device. Smaller, one-piece monitors are also available; some of these devices are worn on the wrist and measure the pulse in the wrist, and even smaller monitors can be worn on a finger (your index finger, for example, has its own measurable pulse).

Simple heart rate monitors display only your current heart rate, but more full-featured models can display other types of information and recall previous readings for comparison.

Blood Pressure Monitors

A home blood pressure monitor is an electronic version of the sphygmomanometer you've seen in doctors' offices. A home monitor features an inflatable arm strap, an inflating bulb, and a monitoring device. These parts are interconnected by flexible air hoses. You place the strap around your upper arm, squeeze the bulb a few times to inflate the strap, and then wait. As the strap slowly releases air, the device checks your pulse and your blood pressure. The monitor displays your diastolic/systolic blood pressure reading on a screen, in the familiar "120/80" format, along with your pulse rate in beats per minute.

Though relatively inexpensive, home blood pressure monitors are typically accurate and widely recommended by doctors for patients with hypertension or prehypertension. If you purchase a blood pressure monitor, take it to your doctor to make sure it provides the same readings as his or her professionally calibrated equipment.

In fact, it's a good idea to talk to your doctor before monitoring your heart rate or blood pressure. Your doctor can tell if it's necessary (and it may not be if you're in overall good health); if your doctor thinks it's a good idea, he or she can give you baseline readings and advice on the proper way to monitor yourself. Your doctor will also tell you when you should be concerned about a reading, and what to do when you are concerned.

WELLNESS IN THE DIGITAL AGE

Table 5.1 Blood Pressure Classification for Healthy Adults

CATEGORY*	SYSTOLIC (mm Hg)		DIASTOLIC (mm Hg)
Normal**	below 120	and	below 80
Prehypertension	120–139	or	80–89
Hypertension⁺			
Stage 1	140–159	or	90–99
Stage 2	160 and above	or	100 and above

*When systolic and diastolic pressure fall into different categories, the higher category should be used to classify blood pressure status.

**The risk of death from heart attack and stroke begins to rise when blood pressure is above 115/75.

⁺Based on the average of two or more readings taken at different physician visits. In persons over 50, systolic blood pressure greater than 140 is a much more significant CVD risk factor than diastolic blood pressure.

SOURCE: *The Seventh Report of the Joint National Committee on Prevention, Detection, Evaluation, and Treatment of High Blood Pressure.* 2003. Bethesda, Md.: National Heart, Lung, and Blood Institute. National Institutes of Health (NIH Publication No. 03-5233).

level. High blood pressure in adults is defined as equal to or greater than 140 over 90 (Table 5.1).

High blood pressure results from an increased output of blood by the heart or from increased resistance to blood flow in the arteries. The latter condition can be caused by the constriction of smooth muscle surrounding the arteries or by **atherosclerosis,** a disease process that causes arteries to become clogged and narrowed. High blood pressure also scars and hardens arteries, making them less elastic and further increasing blood pressure. When a person has high blood pressure, the heart must work harder than normal to force blood through the

KEY TERMS

cardiovascular disease (CVD) A collective term for various diseases of the heart and blood vessels.

platelets Cell fragments in the blood that are necessary for the formation of blood clots.

hypertension Sustained abnormally high blood pressure.

atherosclerosis A form of CVD in which the inner layers of artery walls are made thick and irregular by plaque deposits; arteries become narrowed, and blood supply is reduced.

narrowed and stiffened arteries, straining both the heart and the arteries. Eventually, the strained heart weakens and tends to enlarge, which weakens it even more.

High blood pressure is often called a silent killer, because it usually has no symptoms. A person may have high blood pressure for years without realizing it. But during that time, it damages vital organs and increases the risk of heart attack, congestive heart failure, stroke, kidney failure, and blindness.

Recent research has shed new light on the importance of lowering blood pressure to improve cardiovascular health. The risk of death from heart attack or stroke begins to rise when blood pressure is above 115 over 75, well below the traditional 140 over 90 cutoff for hypertension. People with blood pressures in the prehypertension range are at increased risk of heart attack and stroke as well as at significant risk of developing full-blown hypertension.

Hypertension is common. About 33% of adults have hypertension and 30% have prehypertension (defined as systolic pressure of 120–139 and diastolic pressure of 80–89). The incidence of high blood pressure rises dramatically with increasing age, but it can occur among children and young adults. In most cases, hypertension cannot be cured, but it can be controlled. The key to avoiding complications is to have your blood pressure tested at least once every 2 years (more often if you have other CVD risk factors).

Lifestyle changes are recommended for everyone with prehypertension and hypertension. These changes include weight reduction, regular physical activity, a healthy diet, and moderation of alcohol use. The DASH diet (see Chapter 3), is recommended specifically for people with high blood pressure; it emphasizes fruits, vegetables, and whole grains—foods that are rich in potassium and fiber, both of which may reduce blood pressure. Sodium restriction is also helpful. The 2010 Dietary Guidelines for Americans recommend restricting sodium consumption to less than 1500 mg per day. This recommendation applies to all Americans, but is particularly important for people with hypertension, African Americans, and middle-aged and older adults. Adequate potassium intake is also important. For people whose blood pressure isn't controlled adequately with lifestyle changes, medication is prescribed.

Unhealthy Cholesterol Levels *Cholesterol* is a fatty, waxlike substance that circulates through the bloodstream and is an important component of cell membranes, sex hormones, vitamin D, the fluid that coats the lungs, and the protective sheaths around nerves. Adequate cholesterol is essential for the proper functioning of the body. Excess cholesterol, however, can clog arteries and increase the risk of CVD (Figure 5.1). Your liver manufactures cholesterol; you also get cholesterol from foods.

GOOD VERSUS BAD CHOLESTEROL Cholesterol is carried in the blood by protein-lipid packages called **lipoproteins. Low-density lipoproteins (LDLs)** shuttle cholesterol from the liver to the organs and tissues that require it. LDL is known as "bad" cholesterol because if there is more than the body can use, the excess is deposited in the blood vessels. LDL that accumulates and becomes trapped in artery walls may be oxidized by free radicals, speeding inflammation and damage to artery walls and increasing the likelihood that an artery will become blocked, causing a heart attack or stroke. **High-density lipoproteins (HDLs),** or "good" cholesterol, shuttle unused cholesterol back to the liver for recycling. By removing cholesterol from blood vessels, HDL helps protect against atherosclerosis.

RECOMMENDED BLOOD CHOLESTEROL LEVELS The risk for CVD increases with higher blood cholesterol levels, especially LDL. The National Cholesterol Education Program (NCEP) recommends lipoprotein testing at least once every 5 years for all adults, beginning at age 20. The recommended test measures total cholesterol, LDL cholesterol, HDL cholesterol, and triglycerides (another type of blood fat). In general, high LDL, total cholesterol, and triglyceride levels, combined with low HDL levels, are associated with a higher risk for CVD. You can reduce this risk by lowering LDL, total cholesterol, and triglycerides. Raising HDL is important because a high HDL level seems to offer protection from CVD even in cases where total cholesterol is high. This seems to be especially true for women.

As shown in Table 5.2, LDL levels below 100 mg/dl (milligrams per deciliter) and total cholesterol levels below 200 mg/dl are desirable. An estimated 33.5 million American adults (age 20 and over) have total cholesterol levels of 240 mg/dl or higher.

The CVD risk associated with elevated cholesterol levels also depends on other factors. For example, an above-optimal level of LDL would be of more concern for someone who also smokes and has high blood pressure than for someone without these additional CVD risk factors, and it is especially a concern for diabetics.

IMPROVING CHOLESTEROL LEVELS Your primary goal should be to reduce your LDL to healthy levels. Important dietary changes for reducing LDL levels include choosing unsaturated fats instead of saturated and trans fats and increasing fiber intake. Decreasing saturated and trans fats is particularly important because they promote the production and excretion of cholesterol by the liver. Exercising regularly and eating more fruits, vegetables, fish, and whole grains also help. Many experts believe that cholesterol-lowering foods may be most effective when eaten in combination rather than separately. You can raise your HDL levels by exercising regularly, losing weight if you are overweight, quitting smoking, and altering the amount and type of fat you consume.

Physical Inactivity An estimated 40–60 million Americans are so sedentary that they are at high risk

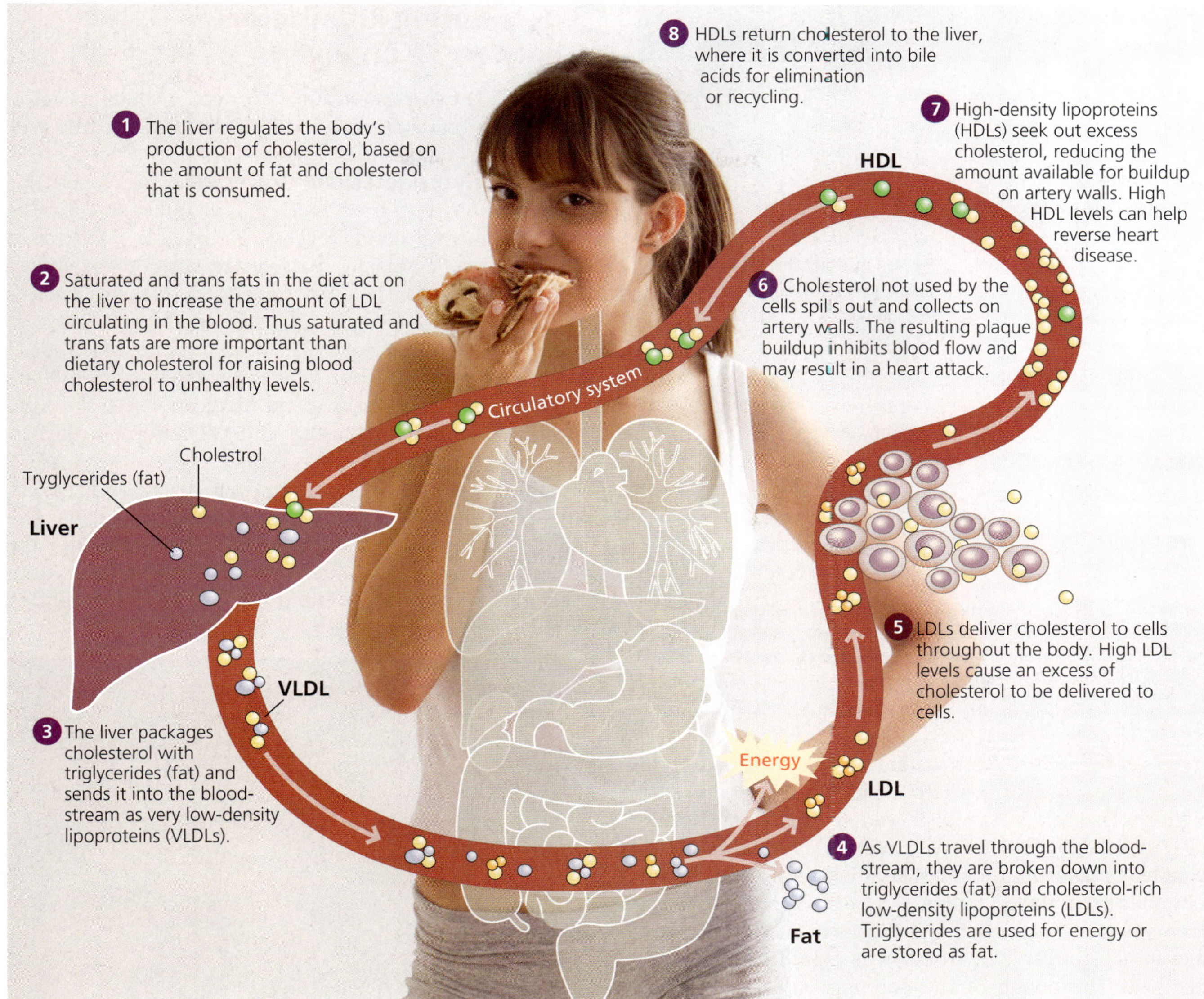

FIGURE 5.1 **Travels with cholesterol.**

for developing CVD. Exercise is thought to be the closest thing we have to a magic bullet against heart disease. It lowers CVD risk by helping to decrease blood pressure and resting heart rate, increase HDL levels, maintain desirable weight, improve the condition of the blood vessels, and prevent or control diabetes. One study found that women who accumulated at least 3 hours of brisk walking each week cut their risk of heart attack and stroke by more than half. (See Chapter 4 for more information on the benefits of cardiorespiratory exercise.)

Obesity The risk of death from CVD is 2 to 3 times higher in obese people (BMI ≥ 30) than it is in lean people (BMI 18.5–24.9), and for every 5-unit increment of BMI, a person's risk of death from coronary heart disease

Fitness Tip

Weight training should be part of any fitness program, but it can raise your blood pressure, at least temporarily. Be sure to balance weight training with aerobic exercise, which can lower blood pressure over the long term.

KEY TERMS

lipoproteins Protein-and-lipid substances in the blood that carry fats and cholesterol; classified according to size, density, and chemical composition.

low-density lipoprotein (LDL) A lipoprotein containing a moderate amount of protein and a large amount of cholesterol; "bad" cholesterol.

high-density lipoprotein (HDL) A lipoprotein containing relatively little cholesterol that helps transport cholesterol out of the arteries; "good" cholesterol.

Table 5.2 Cholesterol Guidelines

TOTAL CHOLESTEROL (mg/dl)	
Less than 200	Desirable
200–239	Borderline high
240 or more	High
LDL CHOLESTEROL (mg/dl)	
Less than 100	Optimal
100–129	Near optimal/above optimal
130–159	Borderline high
160–189	High
190 or more	Very high
HDL CHOLESTEROL (mg/dl)	
Less than 40	Low (undesirable)
60 or more	High (desirable)
TRIGLYCERIDES (mg/dl)	
Less than 150	Normal
150–199	Borderline high
200–499	High
500 or more	Very high

SOURCE: Expert Panel on Detection, Evaluation, and Treatment of High Blood Cholesterol in Adults. 2001. Executive Summary of the Third Report of the National Cholesterol Education Program (NCEP) (Adult Treatment Panel III). *Journal of the American Medical Association* 285(19).

increases by 30%. Excess weight increases the strain on the heart by contributing to high blood pressure and high cholesterol. It can also lead to diabetes, another CVD risk factor (see the next section). As discussed in Chapter 6, distribution of body fat is also significant: Fat that collects in the abdomen is more dangerous than fat that collects around the hips. Obesity in general, and abdominal obesity in particular, is significantly associated with narrowing of the coronary arteries, even in young adults in their 20s.

A sensible diet and regular exercise are the best ways to achieve and maintain a healthy body weight. For someone who is overweight, even modest weight reduction can reduce CVD risk by lowering blood pressure, improving cholesterol levels, and reducing diabetes risk.

Diabetes As described in Chapter 6, *diabetes* is a disorder in which the metabolism of glucose is disrupted, causing a buildup of glucose in the bloodstream. People with diabetes are at increased risk for CVD, partly because elevated blood glucose levels can damage the lining of arteries, making them more vulnerable to atherosclerosis. Diabetics also often have other risk factors, including hypertension, obesity, unhealthy cholesterol and triglyceride levels, and platelet and blood coagulation abnormalities. Even people whose diabetes is under control face an increased risk of CVD. Therefore, careful control of other risk factors is critical for people with diabetes. People with pre-diabetes also face a significantly increased risk of CVD.

Contributing Risk Factors That Can Be Changed

Other CVD risk factors can be changed, including triglyceride levels, psychological and social factors, and drug use.

High Triglyceride Levels *Triglycerides* are blood fats that are absorbed from food and manufactured by the body. High triglyceride levels are a reliable predictor of heart disease, especially if associated with other risk factors, such as low HDL levels, obesity, and diabetes. Factors contributing to elevated triglyceride levels include excess body fat, physical inactivity, cigarette smoking, type 2 diabetes, excess alcohol intake, very-high-carbohydrate diets, and certain diseases and medications. A full lipid profile should include testing and evaluation of triglyceride levels (see Table 5.2).

For people with borderline high triglyceride levels, increased physical activity, reduced intake of sugars, and weight reduction can help bring levels down into the healthy range. For people with high triglycerides, drug therapy may be needed. Limiting alcohol use and quitting smoking are also helpful.

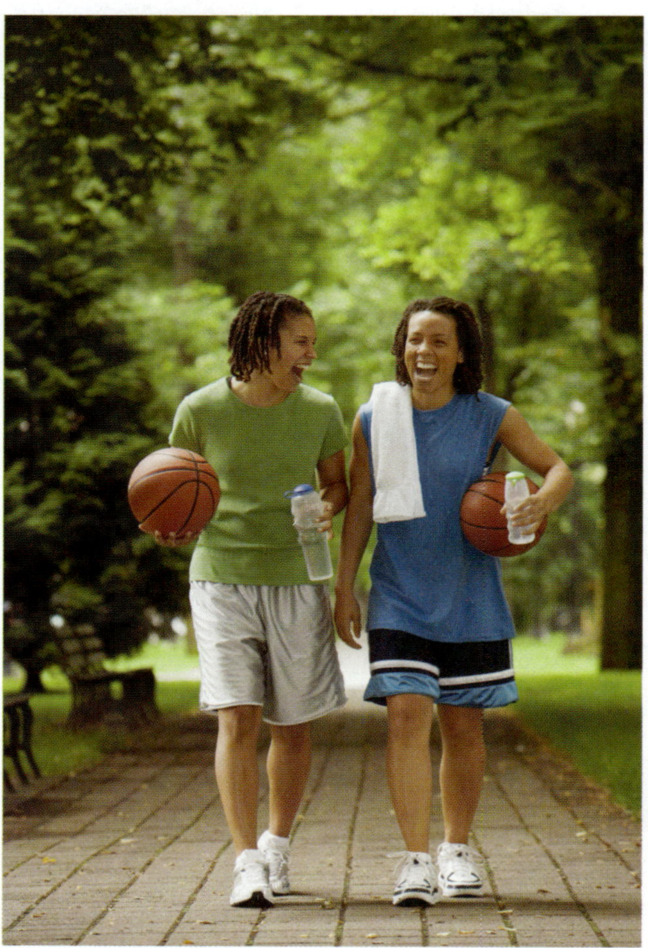

Stress and social isolation increase the risk of cardiovascular disease. A strong social support network improves both health and overall wellness.

Psychological and Social Factors Many of the psychological and social factors that influence other areas of wellness are also important risk factors for CVD. They include chronic stress, chronic hostility and anger, lack of social support, and others. The cardiovascular system is affected by both sudden, acute episodes of mental stress and the more chronic, underlying emotions of anger, anxiety, and depression.

Alcohol and Drugs Drinking too much alcohol raises blood pressure and can increase the risk of stroke and heart failure. Stimulant drugs, particularly cocaine, can also cause serious cardiac problems, including heart attack, stroke, and sudden cardiac death. Injection drug use can cause infection of the heart and stroke.

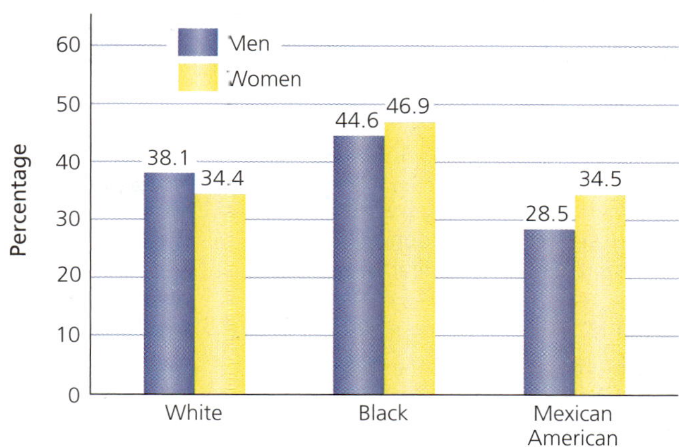

FIGURE 5.2 Percentage of adult Americans with cardiovascular disease.

SOURCE: American Heart Association. 2010. *Heart Disease and Stroke Statistics—2010 Update.* Da las, Texas: American Heart Association.

Major Risk Factors That Can't Be Changed

A number of major risk factors for CVD cannot be changed. They include heredity, aging, being male, and ethnicity.

Heredity Multiple genes contribute to the development of CVD and its risk factors. Having an unfavorable set of genes increases your risk, but risk is modifiable by lifestyle factors such as whether you smoke, exercise, or eat a healthy diet. People who inherit a tendency for CVD are not destined to develop it, but they may have to work harder than other people to prevent it.

Aging About 70% of all heart attack victims are age 65 or older, and about 75% who suffer fatal heart attacks are over 65. For people over 55, the incidence of stroke more than doubles in each successive decade. However, even people in their 30s and 40s, especially men, can have heart attacks.

Being Male Although CVD is the leading killer of both men and women in the United States, men face a greater risk of heart attack than women, especially earlier in life. Until age 55, men also have a greater risk of hypertension than women. The incidence of stroke is higher for males than females until age 65. Estrogen production, which is highest during the childbearing years, may protect premenopausal women against CVD (see the box "Gender, Ethnicity, and CVD"). By age 75, the gender gap nearly disappears.

Wellness Tip

Some medications can raise your blood pressure, especially if you take them every day. This includes a variety of over-the-counter medications, such as acetaminophen.

Ethnicity Rates of heart disease vary among ethnic groups in the United States, with African Americans having much higher rates of hypertension, heart disease, and stroke than other groups. Figure 5.2 shows how rates of CVD compare among non-Hispanic whites, blacks, and Mexican Americans in the United States. Puerto Rican Americans, Cuban Americans, and Mexican Americans are more likely to suffer from high blood pressure and angina (a warning sign of heart disease) than non-Hispanic white Americans. Asian Americans historically have had far lower rates of CVD than white Americans.

C-Reactive Protein Inflammation plays a key role in the development of CVD. When an artery is injured by smoking, cholesterol, hypertension, or other factors, the body's response is to produce inflammation. A substance called C-reactive protein (CRP) is released into the bloodstream during the inflammatory response, and high levels of CRP indicate a substantially elevated risk of heart atack and stroke. CRP may also be harmful to the coronary arteries themselves.

Lifestyle changes and certain drugs can reduce CRP levels. Statin drugs, widely prescribed to lower cholesterol, also decrease inflammation; this may be one reason that statin drugs seem to lower CVD risk even in people with normal blood lipid levels.

Possible Risk Factors Currently Being Studied

In recent years, several other possible risk factors for cardiovascular disease have been identified.

Elevated blood levels of homocysteine, an amino acid that may damage the lining of blood vessels, are associated with an increased risk of CVD. Men generally have higher homocysteine levels than women, as do individuals with diets low in folic acid, vitamin B-12, and vitamin B-6. Most

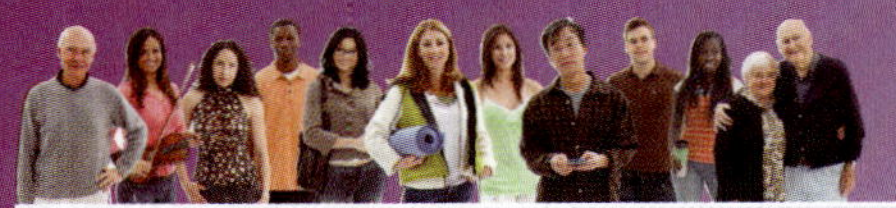

Gender, Ethnicity, and CVD

DIMENSIONS OF DIVERSITY

CVD is the leading cause of death for all Americans, but significant differences exist between men and women and between white Americans and African Americans in the incidence, diagnosis, and treatment of this deadly disease.

CVD in Women

CVD has been thought of as a "man's disease," but it actually kills more women than men. Polls indicate that women vastly underestimate their risk of dying of a heart attack and overestimate their risk of dying of breast cancer. In reality, nearly 1 in 3 women dies of CVD, while 1 in 30 dies of breast cancer. For women, CVD typically does not develop until after age 50.

The hormone estrogen, produced naturally by a woman's ovaries until menopause, improves blood lipid concentrations and reduces other CVD risk factors. For several decades, many physicians encouraged menopausal women to take hormone replacement therapy (HT) to relieve menopause symptoms and presumably to reduce their risk of CVD. However, some studies found that HT may actually *increase* a woman's risk for heart disease and other health problems, including breast cancer. Some newer studies have found that the increased risk of CVD in women who start HT may be age-dependent; women in the early stages of menopause or ages 50–59 did not appear to have excess risk. This suggests that outcomes may depend on several factors, including the timing of hormone use. The U.S. Preventive Services Task Force and the American Heart Association recommend that HT not be used to protect against CVD.

When women have heart attacks, they are more likely than men to die within a year. One reason is that because they develop heart disease at older ages, women are more likely to have other health problems that complicate treatment. Women have smaller hearts and arteries than men, possibly making diagnosis and treatment more difficult.

Women presenting with CVD are just as likely as men to report chest pain, but are also likely to report non-chest-pain symptoms, which may obscure their diagnosis. These additional symptoms include fatigue, weakness, shortness of breath, nausea, vomiting, and pain in the abdomen, neck, jaw, and back. Women are also more likely to have pain at rest, during sleep, or with mental stress. A woman who experiences these symptoms should be persistent in seeking accurate diagnosis and appropriate treatment.

Careful diagnosis of cardiac symptoms is also key in avoiding unnecessary invasive procedures in cases of stress cardiomyopathy ("broken heart syndrome"), which occurs much more commonly in women than in men. In this condition, hormones and neurotransmitters associated with a severe stress response stun the heart, producing heart-attack-like symptoms and decreased pumping function of the heart, but no damage to the heart muscle. Typically, the condition reverses quickly.

Women should be aware of their CVD risk factors and consult with a physician to assess their risk and determine the best way to prevent CVD.

CVD in African Americans

African Americans are at substantially higher risk for death from CVD than members of other ethnic groups. The rate of hypertension among African Americans is among the highest of any group in the world. Blacks tend to develop hypertension at an earlier age than whites, and their average blood pressure is much higher. They also have a higher risk of stroke, have strokes at younger ages, and have more significant stroke-related disabilities. Some experts recommend that blacks be treated with antihypertensive drugs at an earlier stage—when blood pressure reaches 130/80 rather than the typical 140/90 cutoff for hypertension.

A number of genetic and biological factors may contribute to CVD in African Americans. For example, blacks may be

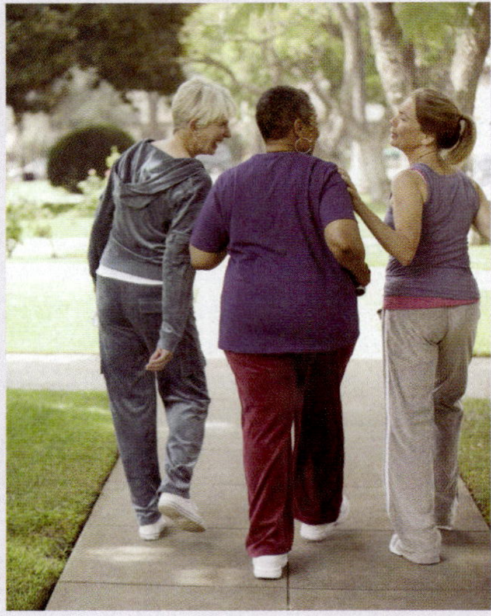

more sensitive to salt and have a physiologically different response to stress, which can lead to high blood pressure and other CVD risk factors. Low income is another factor in CVD risk and is associated with reduced access to adequate health care, insurance, and information about prevention. Discrimination may also play a role, both by increasing stress and by affecting treatment by physicians and hospitals.

Although these factors are important, some evidence favors lifestyle explanations for the higher CVD rate among African Americans. For example, black New Yorkers born in the South have a much higher CVD risk than those born in the Northeast. (Researchers speculate that some lifestyle risk factors for CVD, including smoking and a high-fat diet, may be more common in the South.) People with low incomes, who are disproportionately black, tend to smoke more, use more salt, and exercise less than those with higher incomes.

The general preventive strategies recommended for all Americans may be particularly critical for African Americans. Tailoring your lifestyle to your particular ethnic risk may also be helpful in some cases. Discuss your particular risk profile with your physician to help identify lifestyle changes most appropriate for you.

people can lower homocysteine levels easily by adopting a healthy diet rich in fruits, vegetables, and grains. Severe vitamin D deficiency has also been associated with heart dysfunction, independent of homocysteine levels.

High levels of a specific type of LDL called lipoprotein(a), or Lp(a), may be a risk factor for coronary heart disease (CHD), especially when associated with high LDL or low HDL levels. Lp(a) levels have a strong genetic component

Ask yourself

QUESTIONS FOR CRITICAL THINKING AND REFLECTION

What risk factors do you have for cardiovascular disease? Which ones are factors you have control over, and which are factors you can't change? If you have risk factors you cannot change (such as a family history of CVD), were you aware that you can make lifestyle adjustments to reduce your risk? Do you think you will make them? Why or why not?

and are difficult to treat. About 25% of the U.S. population has elevated lipoprotein(a) levels.

LDL particles differ in size and density, and people with a high proportion of small, dense LDL particles—a condition called LDL pattern B—also appear to be at greater risk for CVD. Exercise, a low-fat diet, and certain lipid-lowering drugs may help lower CVD risk in people with LDL pattern B.

Several infectious agents, including *Chlamydia pneumoniae, cytomegalovirus,* and *Helicobacter pylori,* have also been identified as possible risk factors for cardiovascular disease. Infections may damage arteries and lead to chronic inflammation.

Certain CVD risk factors are often found in a cluster referred to as *metabolic syndrome* or *insulin resistance syndrome.* It is estimated that about 34% of the adult U.S. population has metabolic syndrome. As described in Chapter 6, symptoms of metabolic syndrome include abdominal obesity, high triglycerides, low HDL cholesterol, high blood pressure, and high blood glucose levels (Table 5.3). Metabolic syndrome significantly increases the risk of CVD—more so in women than in men. Weight control, physical activity, and a diet rich in unsaturated fats and fiber are recommended for people with metabolic syndrome. Exercise is especially important because it increases insulin sensitivity even if it doesn't produce weight loss.

Table 5.3 Defining Characteristics of Metabolic Syndrome*

Abdominal obesity (waist circumference)	
Men	>40 in (>102 cm)
Women	>35 in (>88 cm)
Triglycerides	≥150 mg/dl
HDL cholesterol	
Men	<40 mg/dl or drug-treated
Women	<50 mg/dl or drug-treated
Blood pressure	≥130/ ≥ 85 mm Hg or drug-treated
Fasting glucose	≥110 mg/dl or drug-treated

*A person is diagnosed with metabolic syndrome if he or she has three or more of the risk factors listed here.

SOURCE: Grundy, S. M., et al. 2005. Diagnosis and management of the metabolic syndrome: An American Heart Association/National Heart, Lung, and Blood Institute Scientific Statement. *Circulation* 112: 2735.

MAJOR FORMS OF CARDIOVASCULAR DISEASE

Although deaths from CVD have declined drastically over the past 60 years, it remains the leading cause of death in America. According to the National Center for Health Statistics, heart disease killed nearly 600,000 Americans in 2009. The financial burden of CVD, including the costs of medical treatments and lost productivity, exceeds $286 billion annually. Although the main forms of CVD are interrelated and have elements in common, we treat them separately here for the sake of clarity. Hypertension, which is both a major risk factor and a form of CVD, was described earlier in the chapter.

Atherosclerosis

Atherosclerosis is a form of arteriosclerosis, or thickening and hardening of the arteries. In atherosclerosis, arteries become narrowed by deposits of fat, cholesterol, and other substances. The process begins when endothelial cells (the cells lining the arteries) become damaged, most likely through a combination of factors such as smoking, high blood pressure, high insulin or glucose levels, and deposits of oxidized LDL particles. The body's response to this damage results in inflammation and changes in the artery lining. Deposits, called **plaques,** accumulate on artery walls; the arteries lose their elasticity and their ability to expand and contract, restricting blood flow. Once narrowed by a plaque, an artery is vulnerable to blockage by blood clots. (See page T3-4 of the color transparency insert "Touring the Cardiorespiratory System" in Chapter 4.) The risk of life-threatening clots and heart attacks increases if the fibrous cap covering a plaque ruptures.

If the heart, brain, and/or other organs are deprived of blood and the oxygen it carries, the effects of atherosclerosis can be deadly. Coronary arteries, which supply the heart with blood, are particularly susceptible to plaque buildup, a condition called **coronary heart disease (CHD),** or *coronary artery disease (CAD).* The blockage of a coronary artery causes a heart attack. If a cerebral artery (leading to the brain) is blocked, the result is a stroke. The main risk factors for atherosclerosis are cigarette smoking, physical inactivity, high levels of blood cholesterol, high blood pressure, and diabetes.

Heart Disease and Heart Attacks

The American Heart Association estimates that 785,000 Americans have a first heart attack each year, and 470,000

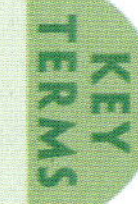

plaque A deposit of fatty (and other) substances on the inner wall of an artery.

coronary heart disease (CHD) Heart disease caused by atherosclerosis in the arteries that supply blood to the heart muscle; also called *coronary artery disease (CAD).*

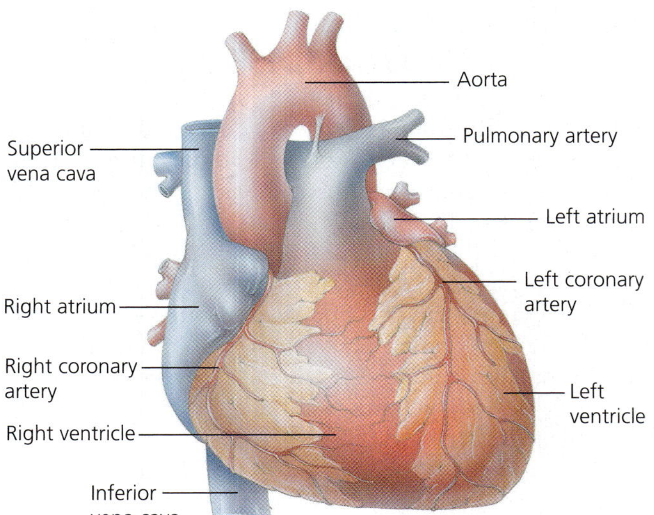

FIGURE 5.3 Blood supply to the heart.
Blood is supplied to the heart from the right and left coronary arteries, which branch off the aorta. If a coronary artery becomes blocked by plaque buildup or a blood clot, a heart attack occurs; part of the heart muscle may die due to lack of oxygen.

suffer a recurrent attack. About 195,000 people suffer a symptomless, or "silent," heart attack each year. Although a **heart attack,** or *myocardial infarction* (*MI*), may come without warning, it is usually the end result of a long-term disease process. The heart requires a steady supply of oxygen-rich blood to function properly (Figure 5.3). If one of the coronary arteries that supplies blood to the heart becomes blocked, a heart attack results. A heart attack caused by a blood clot is called a *coronary thrombosis.* During a heart attack, part of the heart muscle (myocardium) may die from lack of blood flow.

Chest pain, called **angina pectoris,** is a signal that the heart isn't getting enough oxygen to supply its needs. Although not actually a heart attack, angina—felt as an extreme tightness in the chest and heavy pressure behind the breastbone or in the shoulder, neck, arm, hand, or back—is a warning that the heart is overloaded.

If the electrical impulses that control heartbeat are disrupted, the heart may beat too quickly, too slowly, or in an irregular fashion, a condition known as **arrhythmia.** The symptoms of arrhythmia range from imperceptible to severe and even fatal. **Sudden cardiac death,** also called *cardiac arrest,* is most often caused by an arrythmia called *ventricular fibrillation,* a kind of "quivering" of the ventricle that makes it ineffective in pumping blood. If ventricular fibrillation continues for more than a few minutes, it is generally fatal. Cardiac defibrillation, in which an electrical shock is delivered to the heart, can jolt the heart into a more efficient rhythm. This shock can be administered with an automated external defibrillator (AED), a first-aid device that is available in many public places in case someone experiences a heart attack.

Heart attack symptoms may include pain or pressure in the chest; pain in the arm, neck, or jaw; difficulty breathing; excessive sweating; nausea and vomiting; and loss of consciousness. But not all heart attacks involve sharp chest pain. Women, in particular, are more likely to have different symptoms—shortness of breath, weakness, unusual fatigue, cold sweat, and dizziness.

If symptoms of heart trouble occur, it is critical to contact an emergency medical service or go immediately to the nearest hospital or clinic (see the box "What to Do in Case of a Heart Attack, Stroke, or Cardiac Arrest"). Many experts also suggest that the heart attack victim chew and swallow one adult aspirin tablet (325 mg); aspirin has an immediate anticlotting effect. If someone having a heart attack gets to the emergency department quickly enough, a clot-dissolving agent can be injected to dissolve a clot in the coronary artery, reducing the amount of damage to the heart muscle.

Physicians have a variety of diagnostic tools and treatments for heart disease. A patient may undergo a stress or exercise test, in which he or she runs on a treadmill or pedals a stationary cycle while being monitored with an electrocardiogram (ECG or EKG). Certain characteristic changes in the heart's electrical activity while it is under stress can reveal particular heart problems, such as restricted blood flow to the heart muscle. Tools that allow the physician to visualize a patient's heart and arteries include magnetic resonance imaging (MRI), electron-beam computed tomography (EBCT), echocardiograms, and others.

If tests indicate a problem or if a person has already had a heart attack, several treatments are possible. Along with a low-fat diet, regular exercise, and smoking cessation, many patients are also advised to take a low-dose aspirin tablet daily. Aspirin has an anticlotting effect, discouraging

Wellness Tip

AEDs have very simple instructions printed on them; public AEDs are so easy to use that no training is required. If you must assist a heart attack victim and an AED is nearby, use it.

KEY TERMS

heart attack Damage to, or death of, heart muscle, resulting from a failure of the coronary arteries to deliver enough blood to the heart; also known as *myocardial infarction* (*MI*).

angina pectoris A condition in which the heart muscle does not receive enough blood, causing severe pain in the chest and often in the arm and shoulder.

arrhythmia A change in the normal pattern of the heartbeat.

sudden cardiac death A nontraumatic, unexpected death from sudden cardiac arrest, most often due to arrhythmia; in most instances, victims have underlying heart disease.

stroke An impeded blood supply to some part of the brain resulting in the destruction of brain cells; also called *cerebrovascular accident* (*CVA*).

What to Do in Case of a Heart Attack, Stroke, or Cardiac Arrest

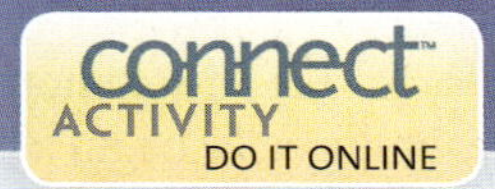

TAKE CHARGE

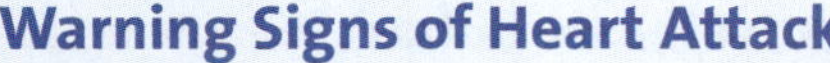

Warning Signs of Heart Attack

Some heart attacks are sudden and intense—the "movie heart attack," where no one doubts what's happening. But most heart attacks start slowly, with mild pain or discomfort. Often people affected aren't sure what's wrong and wait too long before getting help. Here are signs that can mean a heart attack is happening:

- ***Chest discomfort.*** Heart attacks often involve discomfort in the chest that lasts more than a few minutes, or that goes away and comes back. It can feel like uncomfortable pressure, squeezing, fullness, or pain.
- ***Discomfort in other areas of the upper body.*** Symptoms can include pain or discomfort in one or both arms, the back, neck, jaw, or stomach.
- ***Shortness of breath.*** May occur with or without chest discomfort.
- ***Other signs.*** These may include breaking out in a cold sweat, nausea, vomiting, or lightheadedness.

Not all of the signs occur in every heart attack. As with men, women's most common heart attack symptom is chest pain or discomfort, but women are somewhat more likely than men to experience some of the other symptoms, particularly shortness of breath, nausea/vomiting, and back or jaw pain.

If you or someone you're with has chest discomfort, especially with one or more of the other signs, don't wait longer than a few minutes (no more than 5) before calling for help.

Calling 9-1-1 is almost always the fastest way to get lifesaving treatment. Emergency medical services staff can begin treatment when they arrive—up to an hour sooner than if someone gets to the hospital by car. The staff are also trained to revive someone whose heart has stopped. Patients with chest pain who arrive by ambulance usually receive faster treatment at the hospital, too. Today, medications and treatments are available that weren't available in the past, but they must be given relatively quickly after the heart attack to be effective.

If you can't access the emergency medical services (EMS), have someone drive you to the hospital right away. If you're the one having symptoms, don't drive yourself, unless you have absolutely no other option.

Warning Signs of Stroke

- Sudden numbness or weakness of the face, arm, or leg, especially on one side of the body
- Sudden confusion, trouble speaking or understanding
- Sudden trouble seeing in one or both eyes
- Sudden trouble walking, dizziness, or loss of balance or coordination
- Sudden, severe headache with no known cause

If you or someone with you has one or more of these signs, don't delay! Immediately call 9-1-1 or the EMS number so an ambulance (ideally with advanced life support) can be sent for you. Also, check the time so you'll know when the first symptoms appeared. It's very important to take immediate action. If given within 3 hours of the start of symptoms, a clot-busting drug called tissue plasminogen activator (tPA) can reduce long-term disability from the most common type of stroke. tPA is the only FDA-approved medication for the treatment of stroke within 3 hours of symptom onset.

Signs of Cardiac Arrest

Cardiac arrest strikes immediately and without warning. Here are the signs:

- Sudden loss of responsiveness.
- No response to tapping on shoulders.
- No normal breathing.
- The victim does not take a normal breath for at least 5 seconds when you tilt the head up and check.

If these signs of cardiac arrest are present, tell someone else to call 9-1-1 and to get an AED if one is available before you begin cardiopulmonary resuscitation (CPR). Use the AED as soon as it arrives.

SOURCE: American Heart Association, 2010. *Heart Attack, Stroke, and Cardiac Arrest Warning Signs.* Reprinted with permission. www.americanheart.org. Copyright © 2010 American Heart Association.

platelets in the blood from sticking to arterial plaques and forming clots; it also reduces inflammation. Low-dose aspirin therapy appears to help prevent first heart attacks in men, second heart attacks in men and women, and strokes in women over age 65. In addition to aspirin, prescription drugs can also help reduce the strain on the heart.

Several surgical treatments are available to treat certain forms of heart disease. *Balloon angioplasty* involves threading a catheter with an inflatable balloon tip through a coronary artery until it reaches the area of blockage; the balloon is then inflated, flattening the plaque and widening the arterial opening. Many surgeons permanently implant coronary *stents*—flexible stainless steel tubes—to prop the artery open and prevent reclogging after angioplasty. In coronary bypass surgery, healthy blood vessels are grafted to coronary arteries to bypass blockages.

Stroke

A **stroke**, also called a *cerebrovascular accident* (*CVA*), occurs when the blood supply to the brain is cut off. If brain

cells are deprived of blood for more than a few minutes, they die. Once brain cells begin dying, about 2 million cells are lost every minute that blood flow is not restored. Prompt treatment of stroke can greatly decrease the risk of permanent disability. The American Heart Association estimates that 795,000 Americans suffer a stroke each year.

A stroke may be caused by a blood clot that blocks an artery (*ischemic stroke*) or by a ruptured blood vessel (*hemorrhagic stroke*). Ischemic strokes, which account for 87% of all strokes, are often caused by atherosclerosis or certain types of arrhythmia. Hemorrhagic strokes may occur if there is a weak spot in an artery wall or following a head injury. The interruption of the blood supply to any area of the brain prevents the nerve cells there from functioning, in some cases causing death. Nerve cells control sensation and most body movements; depending on the area of the brain affected, a stroke may cause paralysis, walking disability, speech impairment, memory loss, and changes in behavior.

Effective treatment requires the prompt recognition of symptoms and correct diagnosis of the type of stroke that has occurred. Treatment may involve the use of clot-dissolving and antihypertensive drugs. Even if brain tissue has been damaged or destroyed, nerve cells in the brain can make new pathways, and some functions can be taken over by other parts of the brain.

Many people have strokes without knowing it, so they do not realize they may need treatment or evaluation for the risk of a full-blown stroke in the future. These silent strokes do not cause any noticeable symptoms while they are occuring. Although they may be mild, silent strokes leave their victims at a higher risk for subsequent and more serious strokes later in life. They also contribute to loss of mental and cognitive skills. In 2008, a study of MRI scans of 2000 elderly people revealed that 11% of the subjects had brain damage from one or more strokes but did not realize they had ever had a stroke. A 2009 study suggested that silent strokes may be five times more prevalent than full-blown strokes in people under age 65.

Congestive Heart Failure

The heart's pumping mechanism can be damaged by a number of conditions, including high blood pressure, heart attack, atherosclerosis, viral infections, rheumatic fever, and birth defects. When the heart cannot maintain its regular pumping rate and force, fluids begin to back up. When extra fluid seeps through capillary walls, edema (swelling) results, usually in the legs and ankles, but sometimes in other parts of the body as well. Fluid can collect in the lungs and interfere with breathing, particularly when a person is lying down. This condition is called *pulmonary edema,* and the entire process is known as **congestive heart failure.** Treatment includes reducing the workload on the heart, modifying salt intake, and using drugs that help the body eliminate excess fluid.

KEY TERMS

congestive heart failure A condition resulting from the heart's inability to pump out all the blood that returns to it; blood backs up in the veins leading to the heart, causing an accumulation of fluid in various parts of the body.

PROTECTING YOURSELF AGAINST CARDIOVASCULAR DISEASE

You can take several important steps right now to lower your risk of developing CVD (Figure 5.4). Reducing CVD risk factors when you are young can pay off with many extra years of life and health.

Eat a Heart-Healthy Diet

For most Americans, changing to a heart-healthy diet involves cutting total fat intake, substituting unsaturated fats for saturated and trans fats, and increasing intake of whole grains and fiber. The following aspects of nutrition apply directly to heart health:

- *Decreased fat and cholesterol.* The National Cholesterol Education Program (NCEP) recommends that all Americans over age 2 adopt a diet in which fats account for no more than 30% of total daily calories, with no more than one-third of total fat calories (10% of total daily calories) coming from saturated fat. The American Heart Association and the 2010 Dietary Guidelines Advisory Committee recommend that no more than 7% of daily calories come from saturated fats. The NCEP recommends that most Americans limit dietary cholesterol intake to no more than 300 milligrams per day; for people with heart disease or high LDL levels, the suggested daily limit is 200 milligrams.
- *Fiber.* Studies have shown that a high-fiber diet is associated with a 40–50% reduction in the risk of heart attack and stroke. To get the recommended 25–38 grams of dietary fiber a day, eat whole grains, fruits, and vegetables. Good sources of fiber include oatmeal, some breakfast cereals, barley, legumes, and most fruits and vegetables.
- *Sodium and potassium.* Reducing sodium intake to recommended levels, while also increasing potassium intake, can help reduce blood pressure for many people. The American Heart Association and the 2010 Dietary Guidelines Advisory Committee recommend that sodium intake be reduced to no more than 1500 mg per day for all Americans.
- *Alcohol.* Moderate alcohol use may increase HDL cholesterol; it may also reduce stroke risk, possibly by dampening the inflammatory response or by affecting blood clotting. For most people under age 45, however, the risks of alcohol use probably outweigh any health

Do More

- Eat a diet rich in fruits, vegetables, whole grains, and low-fat or fat-free dairy products. Eat five to nine servings of fruits and vegetables each day.
- Eat several servings of high-fiber foods each day.
- Eat two or more servings of fish per week; try a few servings of nuts and soy foods each week.
- Choose unsaturated fats rather than saturated and trans fats.
- Be physically active; do both aerobic exercise and strength training on a regular basis.
- Achieve and maintain a healthy weight.
- Develop effective strategies for handling stress and anger. Nurture old friendships and family ties, and make new friends; pay attention to your spiritual side.
- Obtain recommended screening tests and follow your physician's recommendations.

Do Less

- Don't use tobacco in any form: cigarettes, spit tobacco, cigars and pipes, bidis and clove cigarettes.
- Limit consumption of fats, especially trans fats and saturated fats.
- Limit consumption of salt to no more than 2300 mg of sodium per day (1500 mg if you have or are at high risk for hypertension).
- Avoid exposure to environmental tobacco smoke.
- Avoid excessive alcohol consumption—no more than one drink per day for women and two drinks per day for men.
- Limit consumption of cholesterol, added sugars, and refined carbohydrates.
- Avoid excess stress, anger, and hostility.

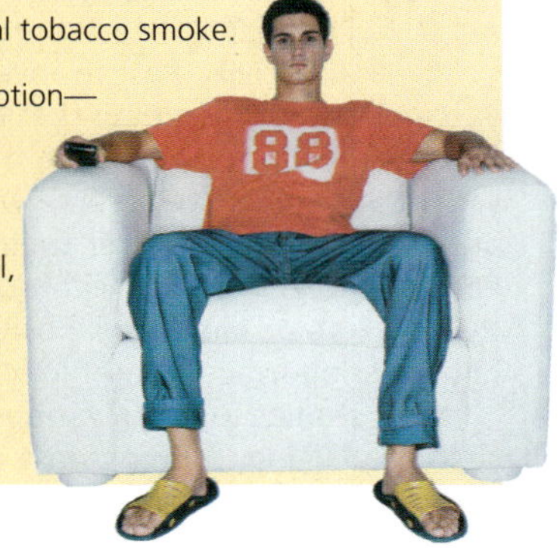

FIGURE 5.4 Strategies for reducing your risk of cardiovascular disease.

Wellness Tip

Oatmeal can actually lower your level of LDL cholesterol. Oatmeal contains soluble fiber, which prevents LDL particles from entering the bloodstream.

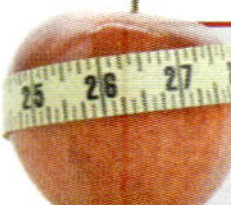

Ask Yourself

QUESTIONS FOR CRITICAL THINKING AND REFLECTION

Has anyone you know ever had a heart attack? If so, was the onset gradual or sudden? Were appropriate steps taken to help the person (for example, call 9-1-1, give CPR, or use an AED)? Do you feel comfortable dealing with a cardiac emergency? If not, what can you do to improve your readiness?

benefit. Excessive alcohol consumption increases the risk of a variety of serious health problems, including hypertension, stroke, some cancers, liver disease, alcohol dependence, and injuries.

Exercise Regularly

You can significantly reduce your risk of CVD with a moderate amount of physical activity (see the box "How Does Exercise Affect CVD Risk?"). A formal exercise program can provide even greater benefits. The information in Chapters 2, 4, 6, 8 and 9 can help you create and implement a complete exercise program that meets your needs for fitness and prevention of chronic disease.

Avoid Tobacco

The number-one risk factor for CVD that you can control is smoking. If you smoke, quit. If you don't, don't start. If you live or work with people who smoke, encourage them to quit—for their sake and yours. If you find yourself breathing in smoke, take steps to prevent or stop this exposure.

Know and Manage Your Blood Pressure

If you have no CVD risk factors, have your blood pressure measured at least once every 2 years; yearly tests are recommended if you have other risk factors. If your blood pressure is high, follow your physician's advice on lowering it.

Ask Yourself

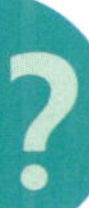

QUESTIONS FOR CRITICAL THINKING AND REFLECTION

Do you know what your blood pressure and cholesterol levels are? If not, is there a reason you don't know? Is there something preventing you from getting this information about yourself? How can you motivate yourself to have these easy but important health checks?

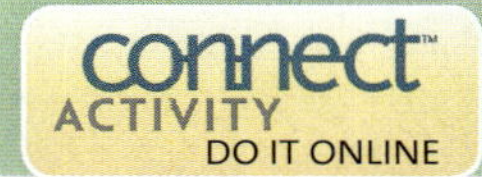

THE EVIDENCE FOR EXERCISE

How Does Exercise Affect CVD Risk?

Regular exercise directly and indirectly benefits your cardiovascular health and can actually help you avoid having a heart attack or stroke. The evidence comes from dozens of large-scale, population-based studies conducted over the past several decades. There is so much evidence about the cardiovascular health benefits of exercise, in fact, that physicians regard physical activity as a magic bullet against heart disease.

Physical activity has an inverse relationship with cardiovascular disease, meaning that the more exercise you get, the less likely you are to develop or die from CVD. Compared to sedentary individuals, people who engage in regular, moderate physical activity lower their risk of CVD by 20% or more. People who get regular, vigorous exercise reduce their risk of CVD by 30% or more. This positive benefit applies regardless of gender, age, race, or ethnicity.

Most studies focus on various aerobic endurance exercises, such as walking, running on a treadmill, or biking. As noted in Chapter 1, the type of exercise performed is less important than the amount of energy expended during the activity. The greater the energy expenditure, the greater the health benefits. In three different studies conducted between 1999 and 2002, for example, researchers focused on women of various ages who walked for exercise. All three studies showed that the women's relative risk of CVD dropped as they expended more and more energy by walking.

Exercise affects heart health via many mechanisms, all of which are being studied. For example, exercise helps people lose weight and improve body composition. Weight loss can improve heart health by reducing the amount of stress on the heart. Changing body composition to a more positive ratio of fat to fat-free mass boosts resting metabolic rate. Exercise directly strengthens the heart muscle itself, and it improves the balance of fats in the blood by boosting HDL and reducing LDL and triglyceride levels.

Exercise can also prevent metabolic syndrome and reverse many of its negative effects on the body. For example, exercise improves the health and function of the endothelial cells—the inner lining of the arteries. These cells secrete nitric oxide, which regulates blood flow, improves nerve function, strengthens the immune system, enhances reproductive health, and suppresses inflammation. Exercise training also improves the function of cell sodium-potassium pumps, which regulate fluid and electrolyte balance and cellular communication throughout the body.

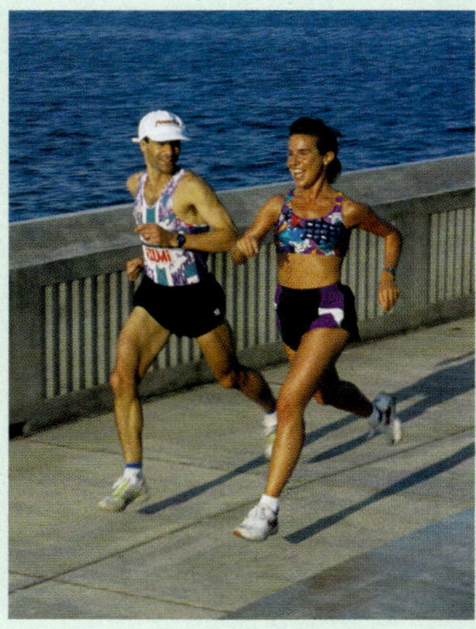

One of the clearest positive effects of exercise is on hypertension. Many studies, involving thousands of people, have shown that physical activity reduces both systolic and diastolic blood pressure. These studies showed that people who engaged in regular aerobic exercise lowered their resting blood pressure by 2–4%, on average. Lowered blood pressure itself reduces the risk of other kinds of cardiovascular disease.

Fewer studies have been conducted on exercise and risk of stroke. Even with limited evidence, however, there appears to be a similar inverse relationship between physical activity and stroke. According to a handful of studies, the most physically active people reduced their risk of both ischemic and hemorrhagic strokes by up to 30%. Although this benefit appears to apply equally to men and women, there is not sufficient evidence that it applies equally across races or ethnicities.

Of course, exercise isn't possible for everyone and may actually be dangerous for some people. People with CVD or serious risk factors for heart disease should work with their physician to determine whether or how to exercise.

SOURCES: Cornelissen, V. A., and R. H. Fagard. 2005. Effect of resistance training on resting blood pressure: A meta-analysis of randomized controlled trials. *Journal of Hypertension* 23(2): 251–259; Physical Activity Guidelines Advisory Committee. 2008. *Physical Activity Guidelines Advisory Committee Report, 2008*. Washington, D.C.: U.S. Department of Health and Human Services; Schnohr, P., et al. 2006. Long-term physical activity in leisure time and mortality from coronary heart disease, stroke, respiratory diseases, and cancer. The Copenhagen City Heart Study. *European Journal of Cardiovascular Prevention and Rehabilitation* 13(2): 173–179; Williams, M. A., et al. 2007. Resistance exercise in individuals with and without cardiovascular disease: 2007 update: A scientific statement from the American Heart Association Council on Clinical Cardiology and Council on Nutrition, Physical Activity, and Metabolism. *Circulation* 116(5): 572–584.

Know and Manage Your Cholesterol Levels

All people age 20 and over should have their cholesterol checked at least once every 5 years. The NCEP recommends a fasting lipoprotein profile that measures total cholesterol, HDL, LDL, and triglyceride levels. Once you know your baseline numbers, you and your physician can develop an LDL goal and lifestyle plan.

Develop Ways to Handle Stress and Anger

To reduce the psychological and social risk factors for CVD, develop effective strategies for handling the stress in your life. Shore up your social support network, and try some of the techniques described in this chapter for managing stress and anger.

Getting to Know Your Pulse Rate

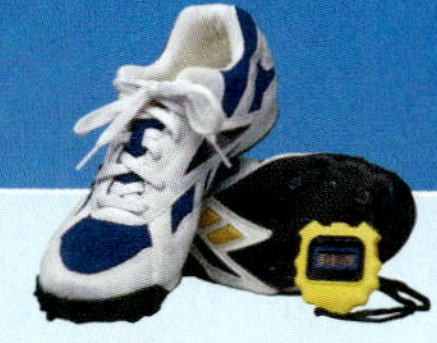

PERSONAL CHALLENGE

Do you know what your resting pulse rate is? It's easy to find out, and it can be useful information for you and your doctor. Chapter 4 provides instructions for checking your own pulse. Practice a few times, and then check your resting pulse rate each day for 7 consecutive days. Write the results here:

Day	Time	Pulse
1.	____________	____________
2.	____________	____________
3.	____________	____________
4.	____________	____________
5.	____________	____________
6.	____________	____________
7.	____________	____________

Be sure to rest for at least 10 minutes before checking your resting pulse rate, and don't check your pulse right after eating (some foods can increase your heart rate temporarily). For most people, a resting pulse rate between 60 and 100 beats per minute is considered normal. Very fit people may have a slower resting pulse rate.

TIPS FOR TODAY AND THE FUTURE

Because cardiovascular disease is a long-term process that can begin when you're young, it's important to develop heart-healthy habits early in life.

RIGHT NOW YOU CAN

- Make an appointment to have your blood pressure and cholesterol levels checked.
- List the key stressors in your life, and decide what to do about the ones that bother you most.
- Plan to replace one high-fat item in your diet with one that is high in fiber. For example, replace a doughnut with a bowl of whole-grain cereal.

IN THE FUTURE YOU CAN

- Track your eating habits for one week, then compare them to the DASH eating plan. Make adjustments to bring your diet closer to the DASH recommendations.
- Sign up for a class in CPR. A CPR certification equips you with valuable lifesaving skills you can use to help someone who is choking, having a heart attack, or experiencing cardiac arrest.

SUMMARY

- The major controllable risk factors for CVD are smoking, hypertension, unhealthy cholesterol levels, inactivity, overweight and obesity, and diabetes.
- Contributing factors for CVD that can be changed include high triglyceride levels, inadequate stress management, a hostile personality, depression, anxiety, lack of social support, poverty, and alcohol and drug use.
- Major risk factors for CVD that can't be changed are heredity, aging, being male, and ethnicity.
- Hypertension weakens the heart and scars and hardens arteries, causing resistance to blood flow. It is defined as blood pressure equal to or higher than 140 over 90.
- Atherosclerosis is a progressive hardening and narrowing of arteries that can lead to restricted blood flow and even complete blockage.
- Heart attacks, strokes, and congestive heart failure are the results of a long-term disease process; hypertension and atherosclerosis are usually involved.
- Reducing heart disease risk involves eating a heart-healthy diet, exercising regularly, avoiding tobacco, managing blood pressure and cholesterol levels, and handling stress and anger.

FOR FURTHER EXPLORATION

BOOKS

Heller, M. 2007. *The DASH Diet Action Plan, Based on the National Institutes of Health Research: Dietary Approaches to Stop Hypertension.* Northbrook, Ill.: Amidon Press. *Provides background information and guidelines for adopting the DASH diet; also includes meal plans to suit differing caloric needs and recipes.*

COMMON QUESTIONS ANSWERED

Q I know what foods to avoid to prevent CVD, but are there any foods I should eat to protect myself from CVD?

A The most important dietary change for CVD prevention is a negative one: cutting back on foods high in saturated and trans fat. However, certain foods can be helpful. The positive effects of unsaturated fats, soluble fiber, and alcohol on heart health were discussed earlier in the chapter. Other potentially beneficial foods include those rich in the following:

- ***Omega-3 fatty acids.*** Found in fish, shellfish, and some nuts and seeds, omega-3 fatty acids reduce clotting and inflammation and may lower the risk of fatal arrhythmia.
- ***Folic acid, vitamin B-6, and vitamin B-12.*** These vitamins may affect CVD risk by lowering homocysteine levels; see Table 3.4 for a list of food sources.
- ***Plant stanols and sterols.*** Plant stanols and sterols, found in some types of trans fat–free margarines and other products, reduce the absorption of cholesterol in the body and help lower LDL levels.
- ***Soy protein.*** Replacing some animal protein with soy protein can lower LDL cholesterol. Soy-based foods include tofu, tempeh, and soy-based beverages.
- ***Calcium.*** Diets rich in calcium may help prevent hypertension and possibly stroke by reducing insulin resistance and platelet aggregation. Low-fat and fat-free dairy products are rich in calcium; refer to Chapter 3 for other sources.

Q The advice I hear from the media about protecting myself from CVD seems to be changing all the time. What am I supposed to believe?

A Health-related research is now described in popular newspapers and magazines rather than just medical journals, meaning that more and more people have access to the information. Researchers do not deliberately set out to mislead or confuse people. However, news reports may oversimplify the results of research studies, leaving out some of the qualifications and questions the researchers present with their findings. In addition, news reports may not differentiate between a preliminary finding and a result that has been verified by a large number of long-term studies. And researchers themselves must strike a balance between reporting promising preliminary findings to the public, thereby allowing people to act on them, and waiting 10–20 years until long-term studies confirm (or disprove) a particular theory.

Although you cannot become an expert on all subjects, there are some strategies you can use to assess the health advice that appears in the media; see the box "Evaluating Health News."

Q What's a heart murmur, and is it dangerous?

A A heart murmur is an extra or altered heart sound heard during a routine medical exam. The source is often a problem with one of the heart valves that separate the chambers of the heart. Congenital defects and

Lipsky, M. S., et al. 2008. *American Medical Association Guide to Preventing and Treating Heart Disease.* New York: Wiley. *A team of doctors provides advice to consumers on heart health.*

Manger, W. M., and N. M. Kaplan. 2011. *101 Questions and Answers about Hypertension.* Alameda, Calif.: Hunter House. *A team of doctors answers questions about preventing, treating, and living with high blood pressure.*

Mostyn, B. 2007. *Pocket Guide to Low Sodium Foods*, 2nd ed. Olympia, Wash.: InData Publishing. *Lists thousands of low-sodium products that can be purchased in supermarkets, as well as low-sodium choices available in many restaurants.*

ORGANIZATIONS AND WEB SITES

American Heart Association. Provides information on hundreds of topics relating to the prevention and control of CVD.

http://www.heart.org (general information)

The Human Heart: An On-Line Exploration. An online museum exhibit containing information on the structure and function of the heart, how to monitor your heart's health, and how to maintain a healthy heart.

http://www.fi.edu/learn/heart/index.html

MedlinePlus: Blood, Heart and Circulation Topics. Provides links to reliable sources of information on cardiovascular health.

http://www.nlm.nih.gov/medlineplus/bloodheartandcirculation.html

National Cholesterol Education Program (NCEP): Cholesterol Counts for Everyone. Provides information on cholesterol for people with heart disease and people who want to avoid it.

http://rover.nhlbi.nih.gov/chd

National Heart, Lung, and Blood Institute. Provides information on a variety of topics relating to cardiovascular health and disease, including cholesterol, smoking, obesity, hypertension, and the DASH diet.

http://www.nhlbi.nih.gov

National Stroke Association. Provides information and referrals for stroke victims and their families; the Web site has a stroke risk assessment.

http://www.stroke.org

See also the listings for Chapters 7 and 10.

SELECTED BIBLIOGRAPHY

Albert, C. M., et al. 2008. Effect of folic acid and B vitamins on risk of cardiovascular events and total mortality among women at high risk for cardiovascular disease: A randomized trial. *Journal of the American Medical Association* 299(17): 2027–2036.

American Cancer Society. 2011. *Cancer Facts and Figures, 2011.* Atlanta, Ga.: American Cancer Society.

American Heart Association. 2011. *Heart Disease and Stroke Statistics—2011 Update.* Dallas, Texas: American Heart Association.

certain infections can cause abnormalities in the valves. The most common heart valve disorder is mitral valve prolapse (MVP), which occurs in about 4% of the population. MVP is characterized by a "billowing" of the mitral valve, which separates the left ventricle and left atrium, during ventricular contraction. In some cases, blood leaks from the ventricle into the atrium. Most people with MVP have no symptoms; they have the same ability to exercise and live as long as people without MVP.

MVP can be confirmed with echocardiography. Treatment is usually unnecessary, although surgery may be needed in the rare cases where leakage through the faulty valve is severe. Experts disagree over whether patients with MVP should take antibiotics prior to dental procedures, a precautionary step used to prevent bacteria, which may be dislodged into the bloodstream during some types of dental and surgical procedures, from infecting the defective valve. Most often, only those patients with significant blood leakage are advised to take antibiotics.

Although MVP usually requires no treatment, more severe heart valve disorders can impair blood flow through the heart. Treatment depends on the location and severity of the problem. More serious defects may be treated with surgery to repair or replace a valve.

Q How does stress contribute to cardiovascular disease?

A With stress, the brain tells the adrenal glands to secrete cortisol and other hormones and neurotransmitters, which in turn activate the sympathetic nervous system—causing the fight-or-flight response. This response increases heart rate and blood pressure so that more blood is distributed to the heart and other muscles in anticipation of physical activity. Blood glucose concentrations and cholesterol also increase to provide a source of energy, and the platelets become activated so that they will be more likely to clot in case of injury. Such a response can be adaptive if you're being chased by a hungry lion but may be more detrimental than useful if you're sitting at a desk taking an exam or feeling frustrated by a task given to you by your boss.

If you are healthy, you can tolerate the cardiovascular responses that take place during stress, but if you already have CVD, stress can lead to adverse outcomes such as abnormal heart rhythms, heart attacks, and sudden cardiac death. It has long been known that an increase in heart rhythm problems and deaths is associated with acute mental stress. For example, the rate of potentially life-threatening arrhythmias in patients who already had underlying heart disease doubled during the month after the September 11 terrorist attacks; this increase was not limited to people in proximity to Manhattan.

Because avoiding all stress is impossible, having healthy mechanisms to cope with it is your best defense. Instead of adopting unhealthy habits such as smoking, drinking, or overeating to deal with stress, try healthier coping techniques such as exercising, getting enough sleep, and talking to family and friends.

COMMON QUESTIONS ANSWERED

For more Common Questions Answered about heart health, visit the Online Learning Center at www.mhhe.com/fahey.

Bibbins-Doming, K., et al. 2010. Projected effect of dietary salt reductions on future cardiovascular disease. *New England Journal of Medicine* 362(7): 590–599.

Berger, J. S., et al. 2006. Aspirin for the primary prevention of cardiovascular events in women and men: A sex-specific meta-analysis of randomized controlled trials. *Journal of the American Medical Association* 295(3): 306–313.

Bonaa, K. H., et al. 2006. Homocysteine lowering and cardiovascular events after acute myocardial infarction. *New England Journal of Medicine* 354(15): 1578–1588.

Centers for Disease Control and Prevention. 2008. Awareness of stroke warning symptoms—13 states and the District of Columbia, 2005. *Morbidity and Mortality Weekly Report* 57(18): 481–485.

Centers for Disease Control and Prevention. 2009. Application of lower sodium intake recommendations to adults—United States, 1999–2006. *Morbidity and Mortality Weekly Report* 58(11): 281–283.

de Torbal, A., et al. 2006. Incidence of recognized and unrecognized myocardial infarction in men and women aged 55 and older: The Rotterdam Study. *European Heart Journal* 27(6): 729–736.

Elliott, P., et al. 2006. Association between protein intake and blood pressure: The INTERMAP study. *Archives of Internal Medicine* 166(1): 79–87.

Giovannucci, E., et al. 2008. 25-hydroxyvitamin D and risk of myocardial infarction in men: A prospective study. *Archives of Internal Medicine* 168(11): 1174–1180.

Gommans, J., et al. 2009. Preventing strokes: The assessment and management of people with transient ischemic attack. *New Zealand Medical Journal* 122(1293): 50–60.

Gurfinkel, E. P., et al. 2007. Invasive vs. non-invasive treatment in acute coronary syndromes and prior bypass surgery. *International Journal of Cardiology* 119(1): 65–72.

Harvard Medical School. 2008. The status of statins. *Harvard Women's Health Watch* 15(6): 1–3.

Jenkins, D. J., et al. 2006. Assessment of the longer-term effects of a dietary portfolio of cholesterol-lowering foods in hypercholesterolemia. *American Journal of Clinical Nutrition* 83(3): 582–591.

Kidambi, S., et al. 2009. Hypertension, insulin resistance, and aldosterone: Sex-specific relationships. *Journal of Clinical Hypertension* 11(3): 130–137.

Marshall, D. A., et al. 2009. Achievement of heart health characteristics through participation in an intensive lifestyle change program (Coronary Artery Disease Reversal Study). *Journal of Cardiopulmonary Rehabilitation and Prevention* 29(2): 84–94.

Mirmiran, P., et al. 2009. Fruit and vegetable consumption and risk factors for cardiovascular disease. *Metabolism* 58(4): 460–468.

Muller, D., et al. 2006. How sudden is sudden cardiac death? Circulation 114(11): 1146–1150.

National Center for Health Statistics. 2011. Deaths: Preliminary data for 2009. *National Vital Statistics Reports* 59(4).

Nita, C., et al. 2008. Hypertensive waist: First step of the screening for metabolic syndrome. *Metabolic Syndriome and Related Disorders* 7(2): 105–110.

Ostrom, M. P., et al. 2008. Mortality incidence and the severity of coronary atherosclerosis assessed by computed tomography angiography. *Journal of the American College of Cardiology* 52(16): 1335–1343.

Pickering, T. G., et al. 2008. Call to action on use and reimbursement for home blood pressure monitoring: A joint scientific statement from the

CRITICAL CONSUMER

Evaluating Health News

Americans face an avalanche of health information from newspapers, magazines, books, and television programs. It's not always easy to decide what to believe. The following questions can help you evaluate health news:

- ***Is the report based on research or on an anecdote?*** Information or recommendations based on one or more carefully designed research studies have more validity than one person's experiences.
- ***What is the source of the information?*** A study in a respected publication has been reviewed by editors and other researchers in the field—people who are in a position to evaluate the merits of the study and its results. Information put forth by government agencies and national research organizations is also usually considered reliable.
- ***How big was the study?*** A study that involves many subjects is more likely to yield reliable results than a study involving only a few people. Another indication that a finding is meaningful is if several different studies yield the same results.
- ***Who were the people involved in the study?*** Research findings are more likely to apply to you if you share important characteristics with the subjects of the study. For example, the results of a study on men over age 50 who smoke may not be particularly meaningful for a 30-year-old nonsmoking woman. Even less applicable are studies done in test tubes or on animals.
- ***What kind of study was it?*** Epidemiological studies involve observation or interviews in order to trace the relationships among lifestyle, physical characteristics, and diseases. Although epidemiological studies can suggest links, they cannot establish cause-and-effect relationships. Clinical or interventional studies involve testing the effects of different treatments on groups of people who have similar lifestyles and characteristics. They are more likely to provide conclusive evidence of a cause-and-effect relationship. The best interventional studies share the following characteristics:
    - ***Controlled.*** A group of people who receive the treatment is compared with a matched group who do not receive the treatment.
    - ***Randomized.*** The treatment and control groups are selected randomly.
    - ***Double-blind.*** Researchers and participants are unaware of who is receiving the treatment.
    - ***Multicenter.*** The experiment is performed at more than one institution.
- ***What do the statistics really say?*** First, are the results described as statistically significant? If a study is large and well designed, its results can be deemed statistically significant, meaning there is less than a 5% chance that the findings resulted from chance. Second, are the results stated in terms of relative or absolute risk? Many findings are reported in terms of *relative risk*, how a particular treatment or condition affects a person's disease risk. Consider the following examples of relative risk:
    - According to some estimates, taking estrogen without progesterone can increase a postmenopausal woman's risk of dying from endometrial cancer by 233%.
    - Giving antiviral medication to HIV-infected pregnant women reduces prenatal transmission of HIV by 90%.

The first of these two findings seems far more dramatic than the second—until one also considers *absolute risk*, the actual risk of the illness in the population being considered. The absolute risk of endometrial cancer is 0.3%; a 233% increase based on the effects of estrogen raises it to 1%, a change of 0.7%. Without treatment, about 25% of infants born to HIV-infected women will be infected with HIV; with treatment, the absolute risk drops to about 2%, a change of 23%. Because the absolute risk of an HIV-infected mother's passing the virus to her infant is so much greater than a woman's risk of developing endometrial cancer (25% compared with 0.3%), a smaller change in relative risk translates into a much greater change in absolute risk.

- ***Is new health advice being offered?*** If the media report new guidelines for health behavior or medical treatment, examine the source. Government agencies and national research foundations usually consider a great deal of evidence before offering health advice. Above all, use common sense, and check with your physician before making a major change in your health habits based on news reports.

American Heart Association, American Society of Hypertension, and Preventive Cardiovascular Nurses Association. *Hypertension* 52(1): 10–29.

Raggi, P., et al. 2008. Coronary artery calcium to predict all-cause mortality in elderly men and women. *Journal of the American College of Cardiology* 52(1): 17–23.

Refsum, H., et al. 2006. The Hordaland Homocysteine Study: A community-based study of homocysteine, its determinants, and associations with disease. *Journal of Nutrition* 136(6 Suppl.): 1731S–1740S.

Rho, R. W., and R. L. Page. 2007. The automated external defibrillator. *Journal of Cardiovascular Electrophysiology* 18: 1–4.

Ridker, P. M., et al. 2008. Rosuvastatin to prevent vascular events in men and women with elevated C-reactive protein. *New England Journal of Medicine* 359(21): 2195–2207.

Sesso, H. D., et al. 2008. Vitamins E and C in the prevention of cardiovascular disease in men: Physician's Health Study II randomized controlled trial. *Journal of the American Medical Association* 300(18): 2123–2133.

Sui, X., et al. 2007. Cardiorespiratory fitness and the risk of nonfatal cardiovascular disease in women and men with hypertension. *American Journal of Hypertension* 20(6): 608–615.

Tufts University. 2006. Pendulum swings on estrogen and women's heart health risk. *Health & Nutrition Newsletter* 24(3): 1–2.

University of California, Berkeley. 2008. Heart tests: Low- to high-tech. University of California, Berkeley, *Wellness Letter*, August, 5.

Wang, X., et al. 2007. Efficacy of folic acid supplementation in stroke prevention: A meta-analysis. *Lancet* 369(9576): 1876–1882.

Name ______________________ Section ____________ Date __________

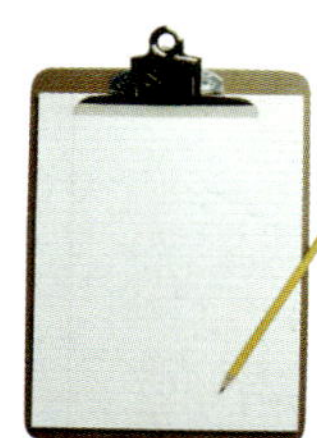

LAB 5.1 Cardiovascular Health

Part I CVD Risk Assessment

Your chances of suffering a heart attack or stroke before age 55 depend on a variety of factors, many of which are under your control. To help identify your risk factors, circle the response for each risk category that best describes you.

1. Sex and Age
   - 0 Female age 55 or younger; male age 45 or younger
   - 2 Female over age 55; male over age 45
2. Heredity/Family History
   - 0 Neither parent suffered a heart attack or stroke before age 60.
   - 3 One parent suffered a heart attack or stroke before age 60.
   - 7 Both parents suffered a heart attack or stroke before age 60.
3. Smoking
   - 0 Never smoked
   - 3 Quit more than 2 years ago and lifetime smoking is less than 5 pack-years*
   - 6 Quit less than 2 years ago and/or lifetime smoking is greater than 5 pack-years*
   - 8 Smoke less than 1/2 pack per day
   - 13 Smoke more than 1/2 pack per day
   - 15 Smoke more than 1 pack per day
4. Environmental Tobacco Smoke
   - 0 Do not live or work with smokers
   - 2 Exposed to ETS at work
   - 3 Live with smoker
   - 4 Both live and work with smokers
5. Blood Pressure
   (If available, use the average of the last three readings.)
   - 0 120/80 or below
   - 1 121/81–130/85
   - 3 Don't know blood pressure
   - 5 131/86–150/90
   - 9 151/91–170/100
   - 13 Above 170/100
6. Total Cholesterol
   - 0 Lower than 19 0
   - 1 190–210
   - 2 Don't know
   - 3 211–240
   - 4 241–270
   - 5 271–300
   - 6 Over 300
7. HDL Cholesterol
   - 0 Over 60 mg/dl
   - 1 55–60
   - 2 Don't know HDL
   - 3 45–54
   - 5 35–44
   - 7 25–34
   - 12 Lower than 25
8. Exercise
   - 0 Exercise three times a week
   - 1 Exercise once or twice a week
   - 2 Occasional exercise less than once a week
   - 7 Rarely exercise
9. Diabetes
   - 0 No personal or family history
   - 2 One parent with diabetes
   - 6 Two parents with diabetes
   - 9 Type 2 diabetes
   - 13 Type 1 diabetes
10. Body Mass Index (kg/m2)
    - 0 <23.0
    - 1 23.0–24.9
    - 2 25.0–28.9
    - 3 29.0–34.9
    - 5 35.0–39.9
    - 7 ≥40
11. Stress
    - 0 Relaxed most of the time
    - 1 Occasionally stressed and angry
    - 2 Frequently stressed and angry
    - 3 Usually stressed and angry

Scoring

Total your risk factor points. Refer to the list below to get an approximate rating of your risk of suffering an early heart attack or stroke.

Score	*Estimated Risk*
Less than 20	Low risk
20–29	Moderate risk
30–45	High risk
Over 45	Extremely high risk

*Pack-years can be calculated by multiplying the number of packs you smoked per day by the number of years you smoked. For example, if you smoked a pack and a half a day for 5 years, you would have smoked the equivalent of 1.5 × 5 = 7.5 pack-years.

Part II Hostility Assessment

Are you too hostile? To help answer that question, Duke University researcher Redford Williams, M.D., has devised a short self-test. It's not a scientific evaluation, but it does offer a rough measure of hostility. Are the following statements true or false for you?

1. I often get annoyed at checkout cashiers or the people in front of me when I'm waiting in line.
2. I usually keep an eye on the people I work or live with to make sure they do what they should.
3. I often wonder how homeless people can have so little respect for themselves.
4. I believe that most people will take advantage of you if you let them.
5. The habits of friends or family members often annoy me.
6. When I'm stuck in traffic, I often start breathing faster and my heart pounds.
7. When I'm annoyed with people, I really want to let them know it.
8. If someone does me wrong, I want to get even.
9. I'd like to have the last word in any argument.
10. At least once a week, I have the urge to yell at or even hit someone.

According to Williams, five or more "true" statements suggest that you're excessively hostile and should consider taking steps to mellow out.

Using Your Results

How did you score? (1) What is your CVD risk assessment score? Are you surprised by your score?

Are you satisfied with your CVD risk rating? If not, set a specific goal:

(2) What is your hostility assessment score? Are you surprised by the result?

Are you satisfied with your hostility rating? If not, set a specific goal:

What should you do next? Enter the results of this lab in the Preprogram Assessment column in Appendix C. (1) If you've set a goal for the overall CVD risk assessment score, identify a risk area that you can change, such as smoking, exercise, or stress. Then list three steps or strategies for changing the risk area you've chosen.
Risk area:
Strategies for change:

(2) If you've set a goal for the hostility assessment score, begin by keeping a log of your hostile responses. Review the anger management strategies in Chapter 10, and select several that you will try to use to manage your angry responses. Strategies for anger management:

Next, begin to put your strategies into action. After several weeks of a program to reduce CVD risk or hostility, do this lab again and enter the results in the Postprogram Assessment column of Appendix C. How do the results compare?

SOURCES: Hostility quiz from *Life Skills* by Virginia Williams and Redford Williams. New York: Times Books. Reprinted by permission of the authors.

Body Composition

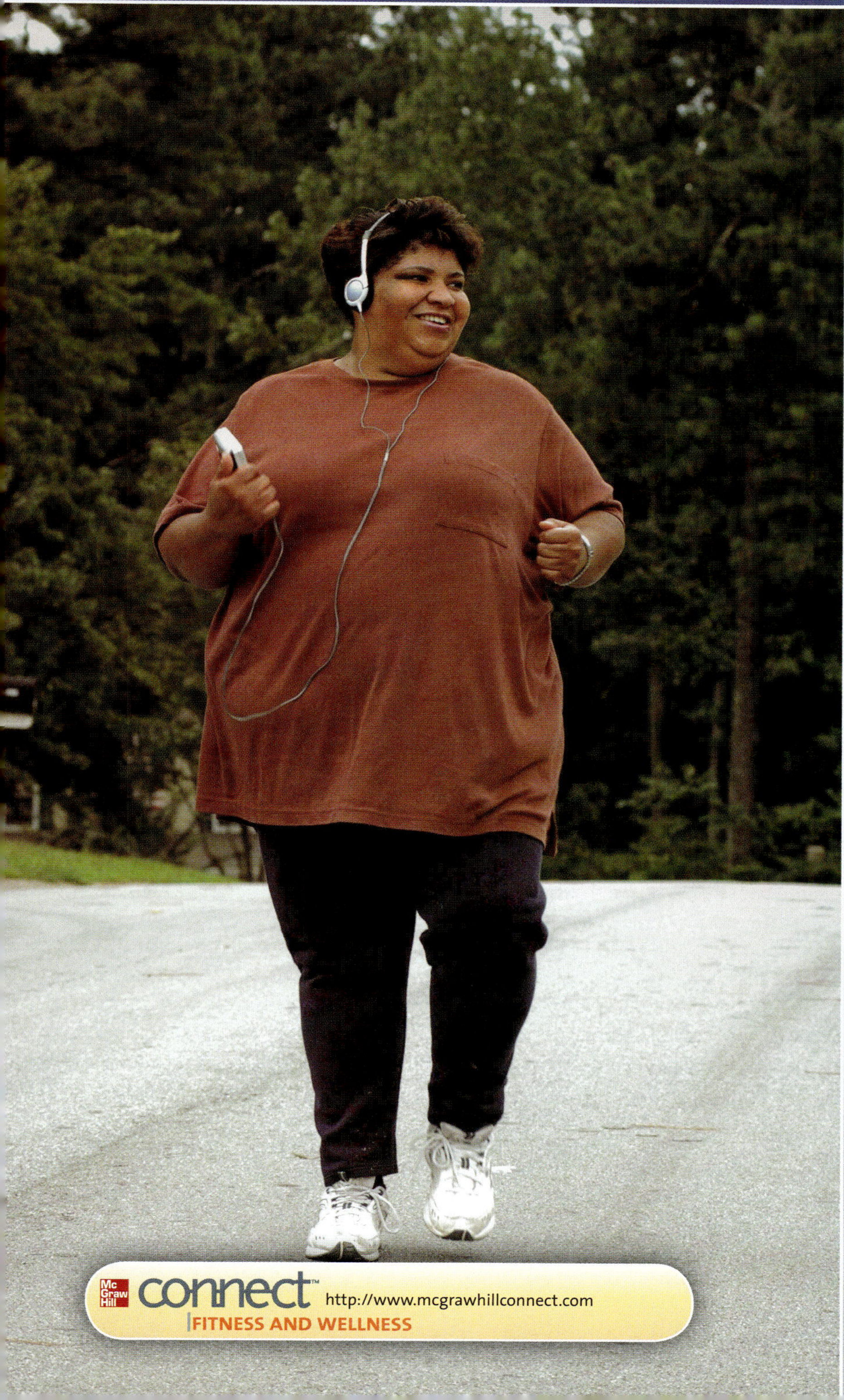

LOOKING AHEAD...

After reading this chapter, you should be able to:

- Define fat-free mass and body fat, and describe their functions in the body
- Explain how body composition affects overall health and wellness
- Describe how body mass index, body composition, and body fat distribution are measured and assessed
- Explain how to determine recommended body weight and body fat distribution

TEST YOUR KNOWLEDGE

1. Exercise helps reduce the risks associated with overweight and obesity even if it doesn't result in improvements in body composition. True or false?
2. Which of the following is the most significant risk factor for the most common type of diabetes (type 2 diabetes)?
   a. smoking
   b. low-fiber diet
   c. overweight or obesity
   d. inactivity
3. In women, excessive exercise and low energy (calorie) intake can cause which of the following?
   a. unhealthy reduction in body fat levels
   b. amenorrhea (absent menstruation)
   c. bone density loss and osteoporosis
   d. muscle wasting and fatigue

Answers

1. **True.** Regular physical activity provides protection against the health risks of overweight and obesity. It lowers the risk of death for people who are overweight or obese as well as for those at a normal weight.
2. **c.** All four are risk factors for diabetes, but overweight/obesity is the most significant. It's estimated that 90% of cases of type 2 diabetes could be prevented if people adopted healthy lifestyle behaviors.
3. **All four.** Very low levels of body fat, and the behaviors used to achieve them, have serious health consequences for both men and women.

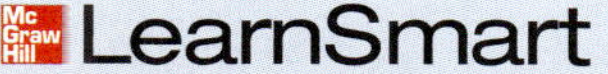

Body composition, the body's relative amounts of fat and fat-free mass, is an important component of fitness for health and wellness. People with an optimal body composition tend to be healthier, to move more efficiently, and to feel better about themselves. They also have a lower risk of many chronic diseases.

Many people, however, don't succeed in their efforts to obtain a fit and healthy body because they set unrealistic goals and emphasize short-term weight loss rather than permanent lifestyle changes that lead to fat loss and a healthy body composition. Successful management of body composition requires the long-term, consistent coordination of many aspects of a wellness program. Even in the absence of changes in body composition, an active lifestyle improves wellness and decreases the risk of disease and premature death (see the box "Why Is Physical Activity Important Even if Body Composition Doesn't Change?").

This chapter focuses on defining and measuring body composition. The aspects of lifestyle that affect body composition are discussed in detail in other chapters: physical activity and exercise in Chapters 2, 4, 8, and 9, nutrition in Chapter 3, weight management in Chapter 7, and stress management in Chapter 10.

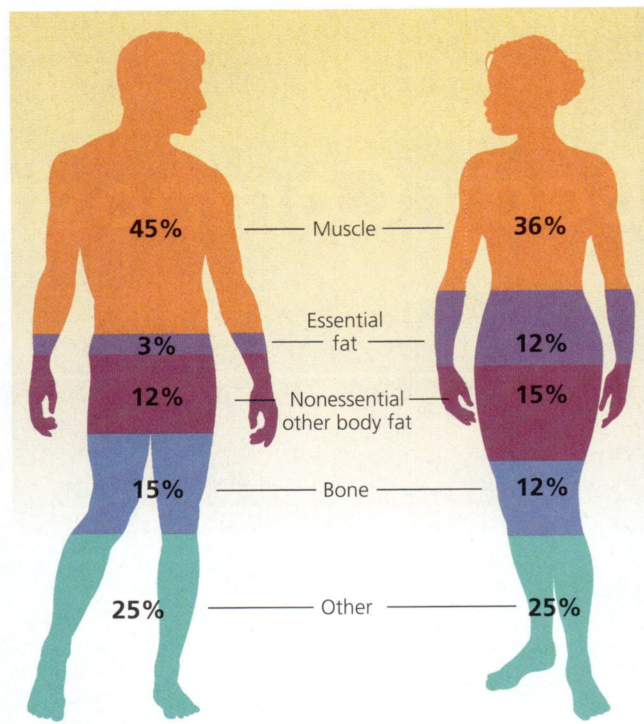

FIGURE 6.1 Body composition of a typical man and woman, 20–24 years old.

SOURCE: Adapted from Brooks, G. A., et al. 2005. *Exercise Physiology: Human Bioenergetics and Its Applications*, 4th ed. New York: McGraw-Hill.

WHAT IS BODY COMPOSITION, AND WHY IS IT IMPORTANT?

The human body can be divided into fat-free mass and body fat. As defined in Chaper 2, fat-free mass is composed of all the body's nonfat tissues: bone, water, muscle, connective tissue, organ tissues, and teeth.

A certain amount of body fat is necessary for the body to function. Fat is incorporated into the nerves, brain, heart, lungs, liver, mammary glands, and other body organs and tissues. It is the main source of stored energy in the body; it also cushions body organs and helps regulate body temperature. This **essential fat** makes up about 3–5% of total body weight in men and about 8–12% in women (Figure 6.1). The percentage is higher in women due to fat deposits in the breasts, uterus, and other sex-specific sites.

Most of the fat in the body is stored in fat cells, or **adipose tissue,** located under the skin (**subcutaneous fat**) and around major organs (**visceral** or **intra-abdominal fat**). People have a genetically determined number of fat cells, but these cells can become larger or smaller depending on how much fat is being stored. The amount of stored fat depends on several factors, including age, sex, metabolism, diet, and activity level. The primary source of excess body fat is excess calories consumed in the diet—that is, calories consumed in excess of calories expended in metabolism, physical activity, and exercise. A pound of body fat is equal to 3500 calories, so an intake of just 100 calories a day in excess of calories expended will result in a 10-pound weight gain over the course of a year. Excess stored body fat is associated with increased risk of chronic diseases like diabetes and cardiovascular disease, as described later in this chapter.

Overweight and Obesity Defined

Some of the most commonly used methods of assessing and classifying body composition are described later in this chapter. Some methods are based on body fat and others on total body weight. Methods based on total body weight are less accurate than those based on body fat, but they are commonly used because body weight is easier to measure than body fat.

In the past, many people relied on height/weight tables (which were based on insurance company mortality statistics) to determine whether they were at a healthy weight. Such tables, however, can be highly inaccurate for some people. Because muscle tissue is denser and heavier than fat, a fit person can easily weigh more than the recommended weight on a height/weight table. For the same reason, an unfit person may weigh less than the table's recommended weight.

When looking at body composition, the most important consideration is the proportion of the body's total weight that is fat—the **percent body fat.** For example, two women may both be 5 feet, 5 inches tall and weigh 130 pounds. But one woman may have only 15%

Why Is Physical Activity Important Even if Body Composition Doesn't Change?

connect ACTIVITY DO IT ONLINE

THE EVIDENCE FOR EXERCISE

Physical activity is important for health even if it produces no changes in body composition—that is, even if a person remains overweight or obese. Physical activity confers benefits no matter how much you weigh; conversely, physical inactivity operates as a risk factor for health problems independently of body composition.

Regular physical activity and exercise block many of the destructive effects of obesity. For example, physical activity improves blood pressure, blood glucose levels, cholesterol levels, and body fat distribution. It also lowers the risk of cardiovascular disease, diabetes, and premature death. Although physical activity and exercise produce these improvements quickly in some people and slowly in others, due to genetic differences, the improvements do occur. Physical activity is particularly important for the many people who have metabolic syndrome or pre-diabetes, both of which are characterized by insulin resistance. Exercise encourages the body's cells to take up and use insulin efficiently for converting nutrients into usable energy. Being physically inactive for just one day decreases the capacity of the cells to take up and use blood sugar.

Although being physically active and not being sedentary may sound identical, experts describe them as different dimensions of the same health issue. Data suggest that it is important not only to be physically active but also to avoid prolonged sitting. In one study, people who watched TV or used a computer 4 or more hours a day had twice the risk of having metabolic syndrome as those who spent less than 1 hour a day in these activities; other studies reported similar results. Thus, in addition to increasing physical activity, avoiding or reducing sedentary behavior is an important—and challenging—health goal.

Although physical activity is important even if it doesn't change body composition, at a certain level, physical activity and exercise do improve body composition (meaning less fat and more lean muscle mass). Evidence supports a *dose-response* relation between exercise and fat loss: The more you exercise, the more fat you will lose. This includes both total body fat and abdominal fat. Additionally, the more body fat a person has, the greater is the loss of abdominal fat with exercise. Studies show that, even without calorie reduction, walking 150 minutes per week at a pace of 4 miles per hour, or jogging 75 minutes a week at 6 miles per hour, produces a decrease in total fat and abdominal fat that is associated with improved metabolic health.

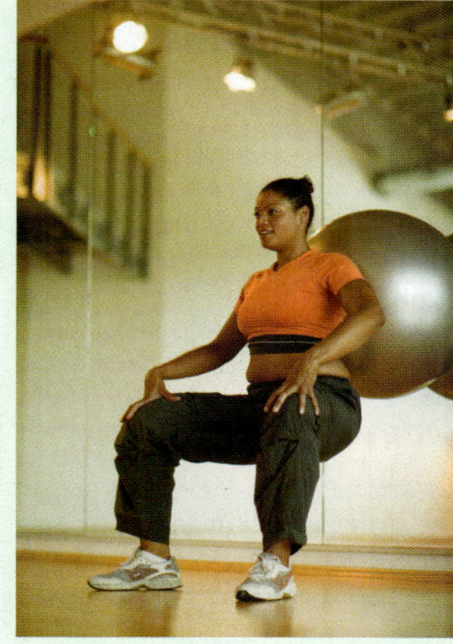

Studies also show, however, that combining exercise with an appropriate reduction in calories is an even better way to reduce levels of body fat and increase lean muscle mass. The results of combining exercise and calorie reduction may not show up as expected on the scale, because the weight of body fat lost is partially offset by the weight of muscle mass gained. Still, your body composition, physical fitness, and overall health have improved.

The question is sometimes asked, Which is more important in combating the adverse health effects of obesity—physical activity or physical fitness? Many studies suggest that both are important; the more active and fit you are, the lower your risk of having health problems and dying prematurely. Of the two, however, physical activity appears to be more important for health than physical fitness.

SOURCES: Baer, H. J., et al. 2011. Risk factors for mortality in the nurses' health study: A competing risks analysis. *American Journal of Epidemiology* 173(3): 319–329; Farrell, S. W. 2010. Cardiorespiratory fitness, adiposity, and all-cause mortality in women. *Medicine and Science in Sports and Exercise* 42(11): 2006–2012; Physical Activity Guidelines Advisory Committee. 2008. *Physical Activity Guidelines Advisory Committee Report, 2008*. Washington, D.C.: U.S. Department of Health and Human Services; Stephens, B. R., et al. 2011. Effects of 1 day of inactivity on insulin action in healthy men and women: interaction with energy intake. *Metabolism Clinical and Experimental*. 60: 941–949.

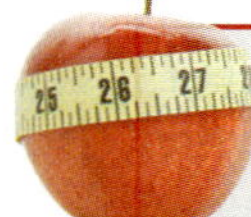

Wellness Tip

Sleep problems increase the risk of obesity, especially in children and young adults. Sleep loss increases production of the hormone ghrelin, which boosts appetite and slows metabolic rate. Fatigue can also make it hard to live a healthy lifestyle and maintain a healthy weight.

KEY TERMS

essential fat Fat incorporated in various tissues of the body; critical for normal body functioning.

adipose tissue Tissue in which fat is stored; fat cells.

subcutaneous fat Fat located under the skin.

visceral fat Fat located around major organs; also called *intra-abdominal fat*.

percent body fat The percentage of total body weight that is composed of fat.

of her body weight as fat, whereas the other woman could have 34% body fat. Although neither woman is overweight by most standards, the second woman is overfat. Too much body fat (not just total weight) has a negative effect on health and well-being. Just as the amount of body fat is important, so is its location on your body. Visceral fat is more harmful to health than subcutaneous fat.

Overweight is usually defined as total body weight above the recommended range for good health as determined by large-scale population surveys. **Obesity** is defined as a more serious degree of overweight that carries multiple major health risks. The cutoff point for obesity may be set in terms of percent body fat or in terms of some measure of total body weight.

Prevalence of Overweight and Obesity Among Americans

By any measure, Americans are getting fatter. Since 1960, the average American man's weight has increased from 166 to 191 pounds, and the average American woman's weight has increased from 140 to 164 pounds. The prevalence of obesity has increased from about 13% in 1960 to about 34% today, and about 67% of adult Americans are now overweight (Figures 6.2 and 6.3). In June 2010, the National Center for Health Statistics reported that for the first time ever, more Americans are obese than overweight. According to these statistics, about 33% of adult men and 35% of adult women are obese. Experts predict that, by 2015, 75% of adults will be overweight and 41% will be obese.

Possible explanations for this increase include more time spent in sedentary work and leisure activities, fewer short trips on foot and more by automobile, fewer daily gym classes for students, more meals eaten outside the home, greater consumption of fast food, increased portion sizes, and increased consumption of soft drinks and convenience foods. According to the USDA, average calorie intake among Americans increased by more than 500 calories per day between 1970 and 2010. Further, the CDC says that nearly 40% of adult Americans are physically inactive and get no exercise at all.

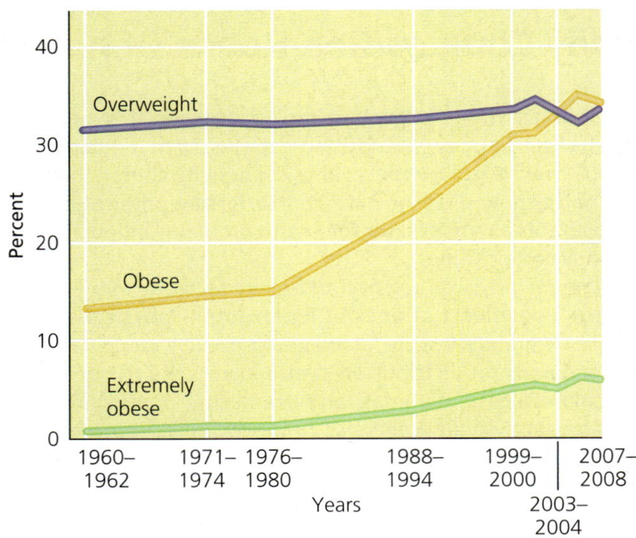

FIGURE 6.2 Trends in overweight, obesity, and extreme obesity in adults aged 20–74 in the United States, 1960–2008.
SOURCE: National Center for Health Statistics. 2010. *2007-2008 National Health and Nutrition Examination Survey (NHANES)*. Hyattsville, Md.: National Center for Health Statistics.

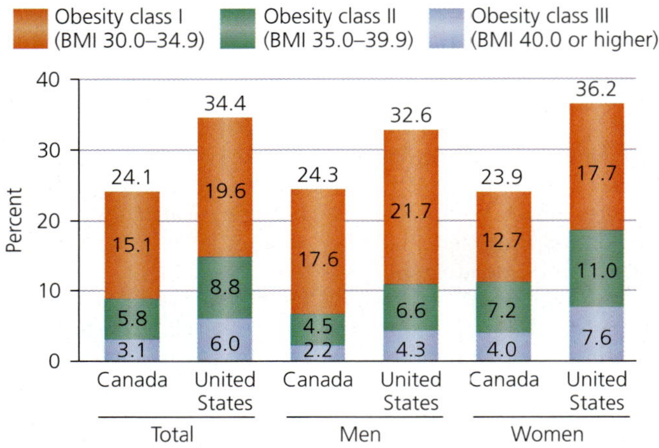

FIGURE 6.3 Prevalence of obesity in people aged 20–79, by sex, in the U.S. and Canada, 2007–2009.
SOURCE: National Center for Health Statistics. March 2011.

Excess Body Fat and Wellness

As rates of overweight and obesity increase, so do the problems associated with them. Obesity doubles mortality rates and can reduce life expectancy by 10–20 years. In fact, if the current trends in overweight and obesity (and their related health problems) continue, scientists believe the average American's life expectancy will soon decline by 5 years.

Metabolic Syndrome, Diabetes, and Premature Death

Many overweight and obese people—especially those who are sedentary and eat a poor diet—suffer from a group of symptoms called **metabolic syndrome** (or *insulin resistance syndrome*). Symptoms include a resistance to the effects of insulin, high blood pressure, high blood glucose levels, abnormal blood fat levels (high triglycerides and low HDLs, or "good" cholesterol), **chronic inflammation**, and fat deposits in the abdominal region. Metabolic syndrome increases the risk of heart disease, more so in men than in women. According to the American Heart Association, about 34% of adult Americans have metabolic syndrome.

Even mild to moderate overweight is associated with a substantial increase in the risk of type 2 diabetes. Obese people are more than three times as likely as nonobese people to develop type 2 diabetes, and the incidence of this disease among Americans has increased dramatically as the

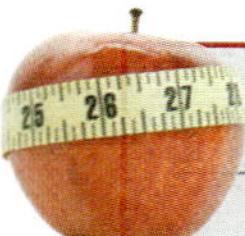

Wellness Tip

As obesity rates have increased, so have rates of infertility. Obese men and women are both at greater risk of infertility because obesity interferes with normal hormone levels and functions.

rate of obesity has climbed (see the box "Diabetes" and the depiction of diabetes on page T3-5 of the color transparency insert "Touring the Cardiorespiratory System" in Chapter 4).

Obesity is also associated with increased risk of death from many types of cancer. Other health problems associated with obesity include hypertension, impaired immune function, gallbladder and kidney diseases, skin problems, sleep and breathing disorders, erectile dysfunction, pregnancy complications, back pain, arthritis, and other bone and joint disorders.

Body Fat Distribution and Health The distribution of body fat (the locations of fat on the body) is also an important indicator of health. Men and postmenopausal women tend to store fat in the upper regions of their bodies, particularly in the abdominal area (the "apple shape"). Premenopausal women usually store fat in the hips, buttocks, and thighs (the "pear shape"). Excess fat in the abdominal area increases risk of high blood pressure, diabetes, early-onset heart disease, stroke, certain cancers, and mortality. The reason for this increase in risk is not entirely clear, but it appears that abdominal fat is more easily mobilized and sent into the bloodstream, increasing disease-related blood fat levels.

The risks from body fat distribution are usually assessed by measuring waist circumference. A total waist measurement of more than 40 inches (102 cm) for men and more than 35 inches (88 cm) for women is associated with a significantly increased risk of disease. In the United States, waist circumference increased by about 1 inch in men and women between 1999 and 2008. Waist circumference tends to be higher in taller people, so waist-to-height ratio is a more accurate measure than waist circumference alone. Your waist measurement should be less than half your height. Using this index, a person who is 5 feet 8 inches (68 inches) tall should have a waist circumference of less than 34 inches. A person who is 6 feet 4 inches (76 inches) tall should have a waist circumference of less than 38 inches.

Performance of Physical Activities Too much body fat makes physical activity difficult because moving the body through everyday activities means working harder and using more energy. In general, overfat people are less fit than others and don't have the muscular strength, endurance, and flexibility that make normal activity easy. Because exercise is more difficult, they do less of it, depriving themselves of an effective way to improve body composition.

Ask Yourself

QUESTIONS FOR CRITICAL THINKING AND REFLECTION

How do you view your own body composition? Where do you think you've gotten your ideas about how your body should look and perform? In light of what you've learned in this chapter, do the ideals and images promoted in our culture seem reasonable? Do they seem healthy?

Emotional Wellness and Self-Image Obesity can affect psychological as well as physical wellness. Being perceived as fat can be a source of judgment, ostracism, and sometimes discrimination by others; it can contribute to psychological problems such as depression, anxiety, and low self-esteem.

The popular image of the "ideal" body has changed greatly in the past 50 years, evolving from slightly plump to unhealthily thin. The ideal body—as presented by the media—is an unrealistic goal for most Americans. This is because one's ability to change body composition depends on heredity as well as diet and exercise. Body image, problems with body image, and unhealthy ways of dealing with a negative body image are all discussed in Chapter 7.

Problems Associated with Very Low Levels of Body Fat

Though not as prevalent a problem as overweight or obesity, having too little body fat is also dangerous. Essential fat is necessary for the functioning of the body, and health experts generally view too little body fat—less than 8–12% for women and 3–5% for men—as a threat to health. Extreme leanness is linked with reproductive, respiratory, circulatory, and immune system disorders and with premature death. Extremely lean people may experience muscle wasting and fatigue. They are also more likely to have eating disorders, which are described in more detail

KEY TERMS

overweight Body weight above the recommended range for good health; sometimes defined as a body mass index between 25 and 29.9.

obesity Severely overweight, characterized by an excessive accumulation of body fat; may also be defined in terms of some measure of total body weight or a body mass index of 30 or more.

metabolic syndrome A cluster of symptoms present in many overweight and obese people that greatly increases their risk of heart disease, diabetes, and other chronic illnesses; symptoms include insulin resistance, abnormal blood fats, abdominal fat deposition, type 2 diabetes, high blood pressure, and chronic inflammation.

chronic inflammation A response of blood vessels to harmful substances, such as germs, damaged cells, or irritants that can lead to heart disease, cancer, allergies, and muscle degeneration.

connect ACTIVITY DO IT ONLINE

Diabetes

Diabetes mellitus is a disease that causes a disruption of normal metabolism. The pancreas normally secretes the hormone insulin, which stimulates cells to take up glucose (blood sugar) to produce energy. Diabetes disrupts this process, causing a buildup of glucose in the bloodstream. Diabetes is associated with kidney failure, nerve damage, circulation problems, retinal damage and blindness, and increased rates of heart attack, stroke, and hypertension. The incidence of diabetes among Americans has increased dramatically as the rate of obesity has climbed. Diabetes is currently the seventh leading cause of death in the United States.

Types of Diabetes

About 25.8 million Americans (8.3% of the population) have one of two major forms of diabetes. About 5–10% of people with diabetes have the more serious form, known as *type 1 diabetes.* In this type of diabetes, the pancreas produces little or no insulin, so daily doses of insulin are required, and people with type 1 diabetes may require other medications to control their blood sugar levels and other complications of the disease. (Without insulin, a person with type 1 diabetes can lapse into a coma.) Type 1 diabetes usually strikes before age 30.

The remaining 90–95% of Americans with diabetes have *type 2 diabetes.* This condition can develop slowly, and about 25% of affected individuals are unaware of their condition. In type 2 diabetes, the pancreas doesn't produce enough insulin, cells are resistant to insulin, or both. This condition is usually diagnosed in people over age 40, although there has been a tenfold increase in type 2 diabetes in children in the past two decades. About one-third of people with type 2 diabetes must take insulin; others may take medications that increase insulin production or stimulate cells to take up glucose.

A third type of diabetes occurs in 2–10% of women during pregnancy. *Gestational diabetes* usually disappears after pregnancy, but 5–10% of women with gestational diabetes go on to have type 2 diabetes immediately after pregnancy. Women who had gestational diabetes during pregnancy have up to a 60% chance of developing diabetes in the next 10–20 years.

The term *pre-diabetes* describes blood glucose levels that are higher than normal but not high enough for a diagnosis of full-blown diabetes. According to 2010 estimates from the American Diabetes Association, about 79 million Americans have pre-diabetes; experts warn that most people with the condition will develop type 2 diabetes unless they adopt preventive lifestyle measures.

The major factors involved in the development of diabetes are age, obesity, physical inactivity, a family history of diabetes, and lifestyle. Excess body fat reduces cell sensitivity to insulin, and insulin resistance is usually a precursor of type 2 diabetes. Ethnicity also plays a role. According to the CDC, the rate of diagnosed diabetes cases is highest among Native Americans and Alaska Natives, followed by blacks, Hispanics, Asian Americans, and white Americans. Across all races, about 27% of Americans age 60 and older have diabetes, either diagnosed or undiagnosed.

Treatment

There is no cure for diabetes, but it can be managed successfully by keeping blood sugar levels within safe limits through diet, exercise, and, if necessary, medication. Blood sugar levels can be monitored using a home test, and close control of glucose levels can significantly reduce the rate of serious complications.

Nearly 90% of people with type 2 diabetes are overweight when diagnosed, including 55% who are obese. An important step in treatment is to lose weight. Even a small amount of exercise and weight loss can be beneficial. Regular exercise and a healthy diet are often sufficient to control type 2 diabetes.

Prevention

It is estimated that 90% of cases of type 2 diabetes could be prevented if people adopted healthy lifestyle behaviors, including regular physical activity, a moderate diet, and modest weight loss. For people with pre-diabetes, lifestyle measures are more effective than medication for delaying or preventing the development of diabetes. Studies of people with pre-diabetes show that a 5–7% weight loss can lower diabetes onset by nearly 60%. Exercise (endurance and/or strength training) makes cells more sensitive to insulin and helps stabilize blood glucose levels; it also helps keep body fat at healthy levels.

A moderate diet to control body fat is perhaps the most important dietary recommendation for the prevention of diabetes. However, the composition of the diet may also be important. Studies have linked diets low in fiber and high in sugar, refined carbohydrates, saturated fat, red meat, and high-fat dairy products to increased risk of diabetes; diets rich in whole grains, fruits, vegetables, legumes, fish, and poultry may be protective. Specific foods linked to higher diabetes risk include soft drinks, white bread, white rice, french fries, processed meats, and sugary desserts.

Warning Signs and Testing

Be alert for the warning signs of diabetes:

- Frequent urination
- Extreme hunger or thirst
- Unexplained weight loss
- Extreme fatigue
- Blurred vision
- Frequent infections
- Cuts and bruises that are slow to heal
- Tingling or numbness in the hands or feet
- Generalized itching with no rash

The best way to avoid complications is to recognize these symptoms and get early diagnosis and treatment. Type 2 diabetes is often asymptomatic in the early stages, however, and major health organizations now recommend routine screening for people over age 45 and anyone younger who is at high risk, including anyone who is obese.

Screening involves a blood test to check glucose levels after either a period of fasting or the administration of a set dose of glucose. A fasting glucose level of 126 mg/dl or higher indicates diabetes; a level of 100–125 mg/dl indicates pre-diabetes. If you are concerned about your risk for diabetes, talk with your physician about being tested.

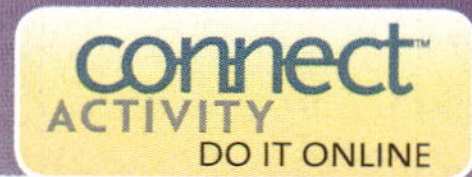

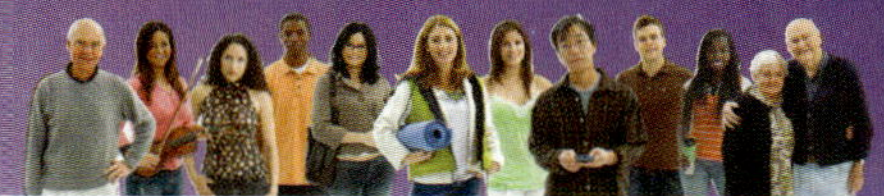

The Female Athlete Triad

DIMENSIONS OF DIVERSITY

Excess exercise and disordered eating

Absent or infrequent menstruation

Decreased bone density

While obesity is at epidemic levels in the United States, many girls and women strive for unrealistic thinness in response to pressure from peers and a society obsessed with appearance. This quest for thinness has led to an increasingly common, underreported condition called the **female athlete triad.**

The triad consists of three interrelated disorders: abnormal eating patterns (and excessive exercising), followed by lack of menstrual periods (amenorrhea), followed by decreased bone density (premature osteoporosis). Left untreated, the triad can lead to decreased physical performance, increased incidence of bone fractures, disturbances of heart rhythm and metabolism, and even death.

Abnormal eating is the event from which the other two components of the triad flow. Abnormal eating ranges from moderately restricting food intake, to binge eating and purging (bulimia), to severely restricting food intake (anorexia nervosa). Whether serious or relatively mild, eating disorders prevent women from getting enough calories to meet their bodies' needs.

Disordered eating, combined with intense exercise and emotional stress, can suppress the hormones that control the menstrual cycle. If the menstrual cycle stops for three consecutive months, the condition is called amenorrhea. Prolonged amenorrhea can lead to osteoporosis. Bone density may erode to the point that a woman in her twenties has the bone density of a woman in her sixties. Women with osteoporosis have fragile, easily fractured bones. Some researchers have found that even a few missed menstrual periods can decrease bone density.

All physically active women and girls have the potential to develop one or more components of the female athlete triad. For example, it is estimated that 5–20% of women who exercise regularly and vigorously may develop amenorrhea. But the triad is most prevalent among athletes who participate in certain sports: those in which appearance is highly important, those that emphasize a prepubertal body shape, those that require contour-revealing clothing for competition, those that require endurance, and those that use weight categories for participation. Such sports include gymnastics, figure skating, swimming, distance running, cycling, cross-country skiing, track, volleyball, rowing, horse racing, and cheerleading.

The female athlete triad can be life-threatening. Typical signs of the eating disorders that trigger the condition are extreme weight loss, dry skin, loss of hair, brittle fingernails, cold hands and feet, low blood pressure and heart rate, swelling around the ankles and hands, and weakening of the bones. Female athletes who have repeated stress fractures may be suffering from the condition.

Early intervention is the key to stopping this series of interrelated conditions. Unfortunately, once the condition has progressed, long-term consequences, especially bone loss, are unavoidable. Teenagers may need only to learn about good eating habits; college-age women with a long-standing problem may require psychological counseling.

SOURCES: Ackerman, K. E., et al. 2011. Bone health and the female athlete triad in adolescent athletes. *Physician Sportsmedicine* 39(1): 131–141; Nattiv, A., et al. 2007. American College of Sports Medicine position stand: The female athlete triad. *Medicine and Science in Sports and Exercise* 39(10): 1867–1882; Witkop, C. T., et al. 2010. Understanding the spectrum of the female athlete triad. *Obstetrics and Gynecology* 116(6): 1444–1448.

in Chapter 7. For women, an extremely low percentage of body fat is associated with **amenorrhea** and loss of bone mass (see the box "The Female Athlete Triad").

ASSESSING BODY MASS INDEX, BODY COMPOSITION, AND BODY FAT DISTRIBUTION

Although a scale can tell your total weight, it can't reveal whether a fluctuation in weight is due to a change in muscle, body water, or fat. Most important, a scale can't differentiate between overweight and overfat.

There are a number of simple, inexpensive ways to estimate healthy body weight and healthy body composition. These assessments can provide you with information about the health risks associated with your current body weight and body composition. They can also help you establish

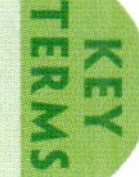
KEY TERMS

amenorrhea Absent or infrequent menstruation, sometimes related to low levels of body fat and excessive quantity or intensity of exercise.

female athlete triad A condition consisting of three interrelated disorders: abnormal eating patterns (and excessive exercising) followed by lack of menstrual periods (amenorrhea) and decreased bone density (premature osteoporosis).

reasonable goals and set a starting point for current and future decisions about weight loss and weight gain.

Calculating Body Mass Index

Body mass index (BMI) is a measure of body weight that is useful for classifying the health risks of body weight if you don't have access to more sophisticated methods. Though more accurate than height-weight tables, body mass index is also based on the concept that weight should be proportional to height. BMI is a fairly accurate measure of the health risks of body weight for average (nonathletic) people, and it is easy to calculate and rate. Researchers frequently use BMI in conjunction with waist circumference in studies that examine the health risks associated with body weight (Table 6.1).

Because BMI doesn't distinguish between fat weight and fat-free weight, however, it is inaccurate for some groups. For example, athletes who weight train have more muscle mass—and thus weigh more—than average people and may be classified as overweight by the BMI scale. Because their "excess" weight is in the form of muscle, however, it is healthy. Further, BMI is not particularly useful for tracking changes in body composition—gains in muscle mass and losses of fat. Women are likely to have more body fat for a given BMI than men. BMI measurements have also over- and underestimated the prevalence of obesity in several ethnic groups. If you are an athlete, a serious weight trainer, or a person of short stature, do not use BMI as your primary means of assessing whether your current weight is healthy. Instead, try one of the methods described in the next section for estimating percent body fat.

BMI is calculated by dividing your body weight (expressed in kilograms) by the square of your height (expressed in meters). The following example is for a person who is 5 feet, 3 inches tall (63 inches) and weighs 130 pounds:

1. Divide body weight in pounds by 2.2 to convert weight to kilograms:
   $130 \div 2.2 = 59.1$
2. Multiply height in inches by 0.0254 to convert height to meters:
   $63 \times 0.0254 = 1.6$
3. Multiply the result of step 2 by itself to get the square of the height measurement:
   $1.6 \times 1.6 = 2.56$
4. Divide the result of step 1 by the result of step 3 to determine BMI:
   $59.1 \div 2.56 = 23$

An alternative equation, based on pounds and inches, is

$$BMI = [weight/(height \times height)] \times 703$$

Space for your own calculations can be found in Lab 6.1, and a complete BMI chart appears in Lab 6.2.

Under separate standards from the National Institutes of Health (NIH) and the World Health Organization (WHO), a BMI between 18.5 and 24.9 is considered healthy. A person with a BMI of 25 or above is classified as overweight, and someone with a BMI of 30 or above is classified as obese (Table 6.1). A person with a BMI below 18.5 is classified as underweight, although low BMI values may be healthy in some cases if they are not the result of smoking, an eating disorder, or an underlying disease. A BMI of 17.5 or less is sometimes used as a diagnostic criterion for the eating disorder anorexia nervosa (Chapter 7).

In classifying the health risks associated with overweight and obesity, the NIH and WHO guidelines consider body fat distribution and other disease risk factors in addition to BMI. As described earlier, excess fat in the abdomen is of greater concern than excess fat in other areas. Methods of assessing body fat distribution are discussed later in the chapter; the NIH and WHO guidelines use measurement of waist circumference (see Table 6.1). At a given level of overweight, people with a large waist circumference and/or additional disease risk factors are at greater risk for health problems. For example, a man with a BMI of 27, a waist circumference of more than 40 inches, and high blood pressure is at greater risk for health problems than another man who

Table 6.1 Classifications from the World Health Organization

Body Mass Index (BMI) Classifications

WEIGHT STATUS CLASSIFICATION	BODY MASS INDEX
Underweight	<18.5
Severe thinness	<16.0
Moderate thinness	16.0–16.9
Mild thinness	17.0–18.4
Normal	18.5–24.9
Overweight	25.0–29.9
Obese, Class I	30.0–34.9
Obese, Class II	35.0–39.9
Obese, Class III	≥40.0

Waist Circumference Classifications

CLASSIFICATION	WAIST CIRCUMFERENCE IN INCHES (CENTIMETERS)	
	WOMEN	MEN
Normal	<32 in. (80 cm)	<37 in. (94 cm)
Increased	≥32 in. (80 cm)	≥37 in. (94 cm)
Substantially increased	≥35 in. (88 cm)	≥40 in. (102 cm)

SOURCE: Wormser, D., et al. 2011. Separate and combined associations of body-mass index and abdominal adiposity with cardiovascular disease: Collaborative analysis of 58 prospective studies. *Lancet.* 377(9771): 1085–1095; table adapted from World Health Organization. 2000. *Obesity: Preventing and Managing the Global Epidemic. Report of a WHO Consultation.* Geneva: World Health Organization Technical Report Series 894: i–xii, 1.

has a BMI of 27 but has a smaller waist circumference and no other risk factors.

Thus, optimal BMI for good health depends on many factors; if your BMI is 25 or above, consult a physician for help in determining a healthy BMI for you. While BMI and waist circumference are important measures of health, they must be considered with other factors such as high blood pressure, diabetes, blood fats, and insulin resistance.

Estimating Percent Body Fat

Assessing body composition involves estimating percent body fat. The only method for directly measuring the percentage of body weight that is fat is an autopsy—the dissection and chemical analysis of the body. However, there are indirect techniques that can provide an estimate of percent body fat. One of the most accurate is underwater weighing. Other techniques include skinfold measurements, the Bod Pod, bioelectrical impedance analysis, and dual-energy X-ray absorptiometry.

All of these methods have a margin of error, so it is important not to focus too much on precise values. For example, underwater weighing has a margin of error of about ±3%, meaning that if a person's percent body fat is actually 17%, the test result may be between 14% and 20%. The results of different methods may also vary, so if you plan to track changes in body composition over time, be sure to perform the assessment using the same method each time. See Table 6.2 for body composition ratings based on percent body fat. As with BMI, the percent body fat ratings indicate cutoff points for health risks associated with underweight and obesity.

Underwater Weighing In hydrostatic (underwater) weighing, an individual is submerged and weighed under water. The percentages of fat and fat-free weight are calculated from body density. Muscle has a higher density and fat a lower density than water (1.1 grams per cubic centimeter for fat-free mass, 0.91 gram per cubic centimeter for fat, and 1 gram per cubic centimeter for water). Therefore, people with more body fat tend to float and weigh less under water, and lean people tend to sink and weigh more under water. Most university exercise physiology departments or sports medicine laboratories have an underwater weighing facility. For an accurate assessment of your body composition, find a place that does underwater weighing or has a BodPod (described in the next section).

Table 6.2 Percentage of Body Fat as the Criterion for Obesity

CATEGORY	PERCENT BODY FAT MALES	PERCENT BODY FAT FEMALES
Normal	12–20%	20–30%
Borderline	21–25%	31–33%
Obese	> 25%	> 33%

SOURCE: Bray, G. A. 2003. *Contemporary Diagnosis and Management of Obesity and the Metabolic Syndrome,* 3rd ed. Newton, Pa.: Handbooks in Health Care.

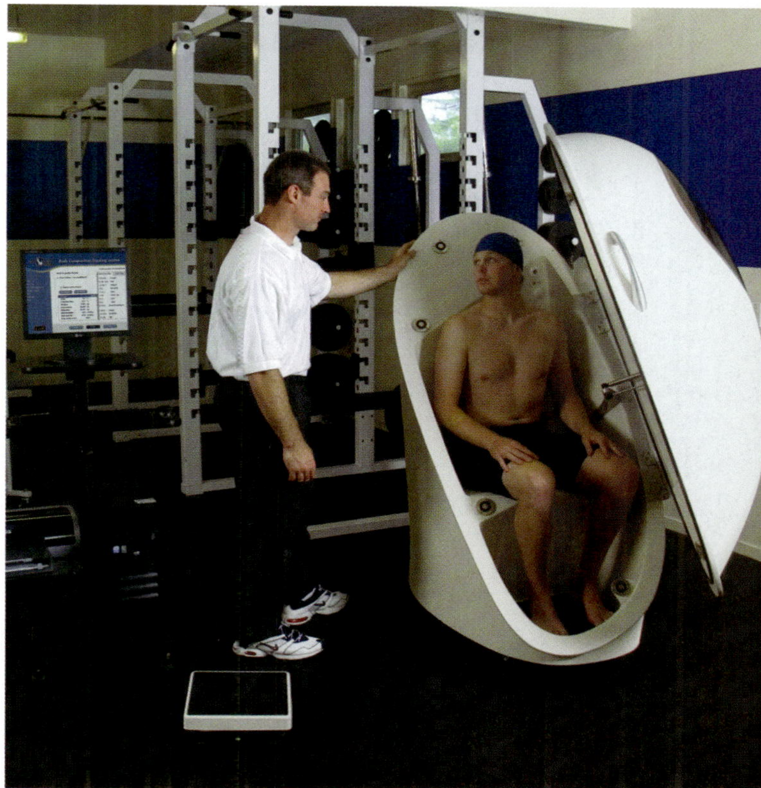

The Bod Pod.

The Bod Pod The Bod Pod, a small chamber containing computerized sensors, measures body composition by air displacement. The technique's technical name is *plethysmography.* It determines the percentage of fat by calculating body density from how much air is displaced by the person sitting inside the chamber. The Bod Pod has an error rate of about ± 2–4% in determining percent body fat.

Skinfold Measurements Skinfold measurement is a simple, inexpensive, and practical way to assess body composition. Skinfold measurements can be used to assess body composition because equations can link the thickness of skinfolds at various sites to percent body fat calculations from more precise laboratory techniques.

Skinfold assessment typically involves measuring the thickness of skinfolds at several different sites on the body.

body mass index (BMI) A measure of relative body weight correlating highly with more direct measures of body fat, calculated by dividing total body weight (in kilograms) by the square of body height (in meters).

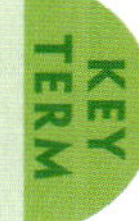

WELLNESS IN THE DIGITAL AGE

Using BIA at Home

Scientists can use several techniques to accurately measure body composition. As described in the chapter, these techniques include underwater weighing, air displacement, and Dual-energy X-ray absorptiometry (DEXA). These methods, however, are costly and require technical expertise.

You can estimate your body fat and fat-free weight simply and accurately, at home, without the help of a technician. All you need is a digital home scale with a built-in bioelectrical impedance analyzer (BIA). BIA works by measuring the resistance in the body to a small electric current. Electricity flows more slowly through fat tissue than through muscle, so the more fat you have, the more slowly such a current will flow through your body. Conversely, a current will pass through your body more quickly if you have more fat-free (muscle) weight.

To use a BIA scale, just stand on the scale with bare feet. As it checks your weight, the scale sends a low-voltage electrical current through your body and analyzes the speed at which the current travels. Checking your weight and body composition takes no longer than checking your weight alone. Most BIA scales can remember your last weight and body composition measurement, making it easy to compare the measurements from day to day or week to week. Some scales can remember measurements for multiple people, as well.

A study of 22 weight-trained men showed that BIA compared favorably to underwater weighing for measuring body composition. Measurements of fat and lean mass are most valuable for measuring changes in body composition during diet and exercise programs.

Popular BIA scales are manufactured by Taylor, Whynter, Omron, RemedyT, and Tanita. These scales are available in most department stores and online, and cost between $50 and $200 depending on features.

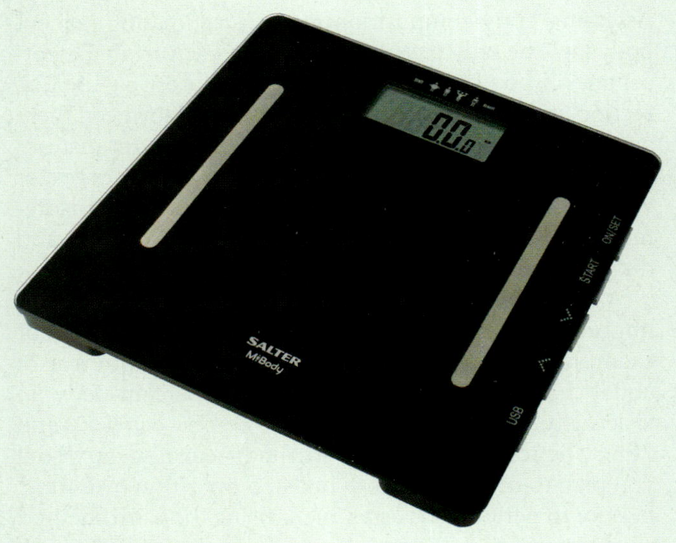

You can sum the skinfold values as an indirect measure of body fatness. For example, if you plan to create a fitness (and dietary change) program to improve body composition, you can compare the sum of skinfold values over time as an indicator of your program's progress and of improvements in body composition. You can also plug your skinfold values into equations like those in Lab 6.1 that predict percent body fat. When using these equations, however, remember that they have a fairly substantial margin of error (±4% if performed by a skilled technician), so don't focus too much on specific values. The sum represents only a relative measure of body fatness.

Skinfolds are measured with a device called a **caliper,** which is a pair of spring-loaded, calibrated jaws. High-quality calipers are made of metal and have parallel jaw surfaces and constant spring tension. Inexpensive plastic calipers are also available; to ensure accuracy, plastic calipers should be spring-loaded and have metal jaws. Refer to Lab 6.1 for instructions on how to take skinfold measurements.

Taking accurate measurements with calipers requires patience, experience, and considerable practice. It's best to take several measurements at each site (or have several different people take each measurement) to help ensure accuracy. Be sure to take the measurements in the exact

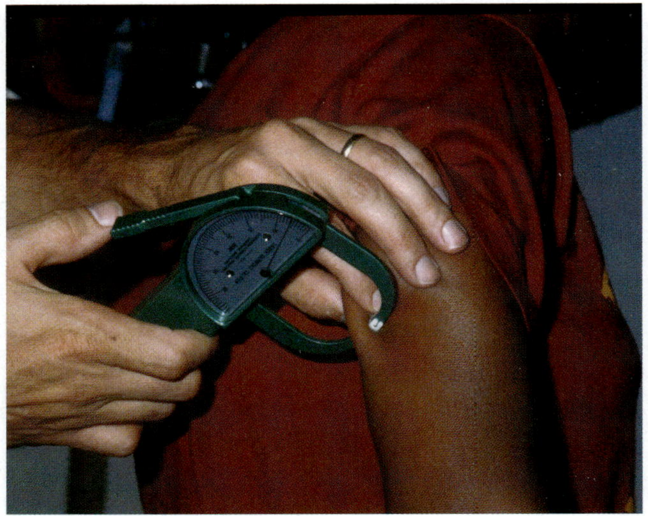

Taking skinfold measurements with calipers.

caliper A pressure-sensitive measuring instrument with two jaws that can be adjusted to determine thickness.

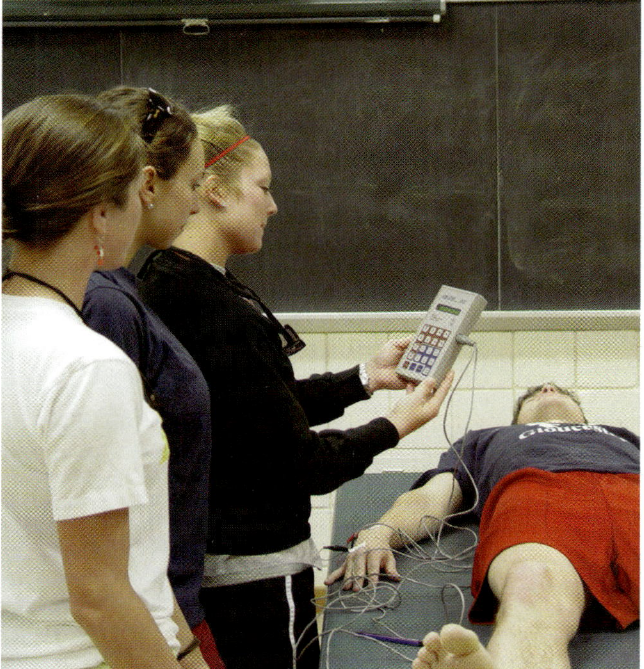

Using bioelectrical impedance analysis to estimate percent body fat.

location called for in the procedure. Because the amount of water in your body changes during the day, skinfold measurements taken in the morning and evening often differ. If you repeat the measurements in the future to track changes in your body composition, measure skinfolds at approximately the same time of day.

Bioelectrical Impedance Analysis (BIA) The BIA technique works by sending a small electrical current through the body and measuring the body's resistance to it. Fat-free tissues, where most body water is located, are good conductors of electrical current, whereas fat is not (see the box "Using BIA at Home"). Thus, the amount of resistance to electrical current is related to the amount of fat-free tissue in the body (the lower the resistance, the greater the fat-free mass) and can be used to estimate percent body fat.

Bioelectrical impedance analysis has an error rate of about ± 4–5%. To reduce error, follow the manufacturer's instructions carefully and avoid overhydration or underhydration (more or less body water than normal). Because measurement varies with the type of BIA analyzer, use the same instrument to compare measurements over time.

Advanced Techniques: DEXA and TOBEC Dual-energy X-ray absorptiometry (DEXA) works by measuring the tissue absorption of high- and low-energy X-ray beams. The procedure has an error rate of about ± 2%. Total body electrical conductivity (TOBEC) estimates lean body mass by passing a body through a magnetic field. Some fitness centers and sports medicine research facilities offer these body composition assessment techniques.

Ask Yourself

QUESTIONS FOR CRITICAL THINKING AND REFLECTION

Calculate your BMI using the formula given in the chapter, and compare it with the BMIs of several of your classmates. Do the results surprise you? How well do you think BMI reflects body composition? Why do you think it is such a commonly used measure?

Assessing Body Fat Distribution

Researchers have studied many different methods for measuring body fat distribution. Two of the simplest to perform are waist circumference measurement and waist-to-hip ratio calculation. In the first method, you measure your waist circumference; in the second, you divide your waist circumference by your hip circumference. Waist circumference has been found to be a better indicator of abdominal fat than waist-to-hip ratio. More research is needed to determine the precise degree of risk associated with specific values for these two assessments of body fat distribution. However, as noted earlier, a total waist measurement of more than 40 inches (102 cm) for men and 35 inches (88 cm) for women and a waist-to-hip ratio above 0.94 for young men and 0.82 for young women are associated with a significantly increased risk of heart disease and diabetes. Lab 6.1 shows you how to measure your body fat distribution.

SETTING BODY COMPOSITION GOALS

If assessment tests indicate that fat loss would be beneficial for your health, your first step is to establish a goal. You can use the ratings in Table 6.1 or Table 6.2 to choose a target value for BMI or percent body fat (depending on which assessment you completed).

Make sure your goal is realistic and will ensure good health. Heredity limits your capacity to change your body composition, and few people can expect to develop the body of a fashion model or competitive bodybuilder. However, you can improve your body composition through a

Fitness Tip

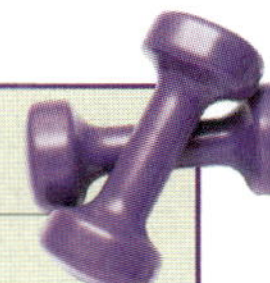

For most people, walking and running are better activities for weight loss than swimming. But this might not be true for older women. Recent research revealed that older women who swam lost more weight and controlled their blood sugar better than similar-aged women who walked.

PERSONAL CHALLENGE

Tracking Your Weight

Some studies have found that recording body weight every day helps keep you accountable to your weight-loss program and helps you make faster progress. An easy way to track your weight daily is to write it down in a table like the following:

1. ________	11. ________	21. ________
2. ________	12. ________	22. ________
3. ________	13. ________	23. ________
4. ________	14. ________	24. ________
5. ________	15. ________	25. ________
6. ________	16. ________	26. ________
7. ________	17. ________	27. ________
8. ________	18. ________	28. ________
9. ________	19. ________	29. ________
10. ________	20. ________	30. ________

To make things more interesting, track your weight like this for a few weeks, and then convert the information into a line chart. A chart can help you visualize the data and make it easier for you to gauge your progress. You can easily track daily weights and convert them into charts in a spreadsheet program.

program of regular exercise and a healthy diet. If your body composition is in or close to the recommended range, you may want to set a lifestyle goal rather than a specific percent body fat or BMI goal. For example, you might set a goal of increasing your daily physical activity from 20 to 60 minutes or beginning a program of weight training, and then let any improvements in body composition occur as a secondary result of your primary target (physical activity). Remember, a lifestyle that includes regular exercise may be more important for health than trying to reach any ideal weight.

If you are significantly overfat or if you have known risk factors for disease (such as high blood pressure or high cholesterol), consult your physician to determine a body composition goal for your individual risk profile. For people who are obese, small losses of body weight (5–15%) over a 6–12 month period can result in significant health improvements.

Once you've established a body composition goal, you can then set a target range for body weight. Although body weight is not an accurate method of assessing body composition, it's a useful method for tracking progress in a program to change body composition. If you're losing a small or moderate amount of weight and exercising, you're probably losing fat while building muscle mass. Lab 6.2 will help you determine a range for recommended body weight.

Using percent body fat or BMI will generate a fairly accurate target body weight for most people. However, it's best not to stick rigidly to a recommended body weight calculated from any formula; individual genetic, cultural, and lifestyle factors are also important. Decide whether the body weight that the formulas generate for you is realistic, meets all your goals, is healthy, *and* is reasonable for you to maintain.

MAKING CHANGES IN BODY COMPOSITION

Chapter 7 includes specific strategies for losing or gaining weight and improving body composition. In general, lifestyle should be your focus—regular physical activity, endurance exercise, strength training, and a moderate energy intake. Making significant cuts in food intake in order to lose weight and body fat is a difficult strategy to maintain; focusing on increased physical activity is a better approach for many people. In studies of people who have lost weight and maintained the loss, physical activity was the key to long-term success.

You can track your progress toward your target body composition by checking your body weight regularly. Also, focus on how much energy you have and how your clothes fit.

To get a more accurate idea of your progress, you should directly reassess your body composition occasionally during your program: Body composition changes as weight changes. Losing a lot of weight usually includes losing some muscle mass no matter how hard a person exercises, partly because carrying less weight requires the muscular system to bear a smaller burden. Conversely, a large gain in weight without exercise still causes some gain in muscle mass because muscles are working harder to carry the extra weight.

TIPS FOR TODAY AND THE FUTURE

A wellness lifestyle can lead naturally to a body composition that is healthy and appropriate for you.

RIGHT NOW YOU CAN

- Find out what types of body composition assessment techniques are available at facilities on your campus or in your community.
- Do 30 minutes of physical activity—walk, jog, bike, swim, or climb stairs.
- Drink a glass of water instead of a soda, and include a high-fiber food such as whole-grain bread or cereal, popcorn, apples, berries, or beans in your next snack or meal.

IN THE FUTURE YOU CAN

- Think about your image of the ideal body type for your sex. Consider where your idea comes from, whether you use this image to judge your own body, and whether it is a realistic goal for you.
- Be aware of media messages (especially visual images) that make you feel embarrassed or insecure about your body. Remind yourself that these messages are usually designed to sell a product; they should not form the basis of your body image.

SUMMARY

- The human body is composed of fat-free mass (which includes bone, muscle, organ tissues, and connective tissues) and body fat.
- Having too much body fat has negative health consequences, especially in terms of cardiovascular disease and diabetes. Distribution of fat is also a significant factor in health.
- A fit and healthy-looking body, with the right body composition for a particular person, develops from habits of proper nutrition and exercise.
- Measuring body weight is not an accurate way to assess body composition because it does not differentiate between muscle weight and fat weight.
- Body mass index (calculated from weight and height measurements) and waist circumference can help classify the health risks associated with overweight. BMI is sometimes inaccurate, however, particularly in muscular people.
- Techniques for estimating percent body fat include underwater weighing, skinfold measurements, the Bod Pod, bioelectrical impedance analysis, DEXA, and TOBEC.
- Body fat distribution can be assessed through waist measurement or the waist-to-hip ratio.
- Recommended body composition and weight can be determined by choosing a target BMI or target body fat percentage. Keep heredity in mind when setting a goal, and focus on positive changes in lifestyle.

FOR FURTHER EXPLORATION

BOOKS

Acevedo, E., and M. Starks. 2011. *Exercise Testing and Prescription Lab Manual,* 2nd ed. Champaign, Ill.: Human Kinetics. *A book on physical fitness measurement techniques for students in kinesiology and physical education.*

American College of Sports Medicine. 2009. *ACSM's Health Related Physical Fitness Assessment Manual.* Philadelphia: Lippincott Williams and Wilkins. *A book written for professionals on assessing physical fitness in healthy adults.*

Bagchi, D., and H. G. Preuss. 2007. *Obesity: Epidemiology, Pathophysiology, and Prevention.* London: CRC Press. *A comprehensive guide for health professionals on the incidence, health risks, and prevention of obesity.*

Heyward, V. H. 2006. *Advanced Fitness Assessment and Exercise Prescription,* 5th ed. Champaign, Ill.: Human Kinetics. *Detailed coverage of assessing body composition, fitness, flexibility, and other aspects of fitness.*

Korbonit, M. 2008. *Obesity and Metabolism.* Basel, Switzerland: S Karger Pub. *Describes the physiology of weight control and metabolism.*

Lean, M., et al. 2007. *ABC of Obesity.* Boston: Blackwell Publishing Limited. *Examines the impact of obesity on the average person's life and discusses some of the most current options for preventing and treating obesity.*

ORGANIZATIONS AND WEB SITES

American Diabetes Association. Provides information, a free newsletter, and referrals to local support groups; the Web site includes an online diabetes risk assessment.

http://www.diabetes.org

American Heart Association: Body Composition Tests. Offers detailed information about body composition, testing and analysis, and the impact of body composition on heart health.

http://www.heart.org/HEARTORG/GettingHealthy/NutritionCenter/Body-Composition-Tests_UCM_305883_Article.jsp

Methods of Body Composition Analysis Tutorials. Provides information about body composition assessment techniques, including underwater weighing, BIA, and DEXA.

http://nutrition.uvm.edu/bodycomp

National Heart, Lung, and Blood Institute: Obesity Education Initiative. Provides information on the latest federal obesity standards and a BMI calculator.

http://www.nhlbi.nih.gov/about/oei/index.htm

National Institute of Diabetes and Digestive and Kidney Diseases Weight-Control Information Network. Provides information about adult obesity: how it is defined and assessed, the risk factors associated with it, and its causes.

http://win.niddk.nih.gov

National Health and Nutrition Examination Survey (NHANES). Ongoing survey and assessment of health status and practices in the United States.

http://www.cdc.gov/nchs/nhanes/new_nhanes.htm

Robert Wood Johnson Foundation. Promotes the health and health care of Americans through research and distribution of information on healthy lifestyles.

http://www.rwjf.org

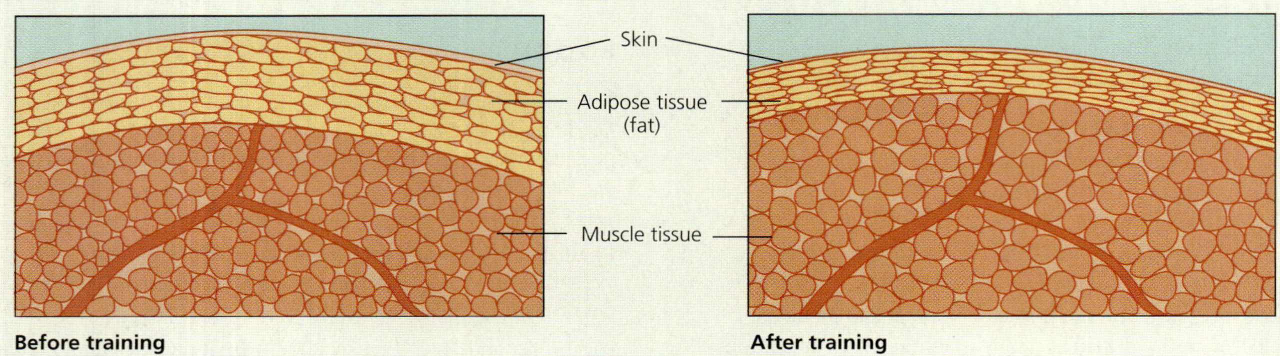

EFFECTS OF EXERCISE ON BODY COMPOSITION. Endurance exercise and strength training both reduce body fat and increase muscle mass.

Q Is spot reducing effective?

A *Spot reducing* refers to attempts to lose body fat in specific parts of the body by doing exercises for those parts. Danish researchers have shown that fat use increases in adipose tissue surrounding active muscle, but it is not known if short-term fat use helps reduce fat in specific sites. Most studies show that spot-reducing exercises contribute to fat loss only to the extent that they burn calories. The best way to reduce fat in any specific area is to create an overall negative energy balance: Take in less energy (food) than you use through exercise and metabolism.

Q How does exercise affect body composition?

A Cardiorespiratory endurance exercise burns calories, thereby helping create a negative energy balance. Weight training does not use many calories and therefore is of little use in creating a negative energy balance. However, weight training increases muscle mass, which maintains a higher metabolic rate (the body's rate of energy use) and helps improve body composition. To minimize body fat and increase muscle mass, thereby improving body composition, combine cardiorespiratory endurance exercise and weight training (see figure).

Q Are people who have a desirable body composition physically fit?

A Having a healthy body composition is not necessarily associated with overall fitness. For example, many bodybuilders have very little body fat but have poor cardiorespiratory capacity and flexibility. Some athletes, such as NFL linemen, weigh 300 pounds or more; they have to lose the weight when they retire if they don't want to jeopardize their health.To be fit, you must rate high on all the components of fitness.

Q What is liposuction, and will it help me lose body fat?

A Suction lipectomy, popularly known as *liposuction*, has become the most popular type of elective surgery in the world. The procedure involves removing limited amounts of fat from specific areas. Typically, no more than 2.5 kilograms (5.5 pounds) of adipose tissue are removed at a time. The procedure is usually successful if the amount of excess fat is limited and skin elasticity is good. The procedure is most effective if integrated into a program of dietary restriction and exercise. Side effects include infection, dimpling, and wavy skin contours. Liposuction has a death rate of 1 in 5000 patients, primarily from pulmonary thromboembolism (a blood clot in the lungs) or fat embolism (circulatory blockage caused by a dislodged piece of fat). Other serious complications include shock, bleeding, and impaired blood flow to vital organs.

Q What is cellulite, and how do I get rid of it?

A *Cellulite* is the name commonly given to ripply, wavy fat deposits that collect just under the skin. The "cottage cheese" appearance stems from the breakdown of tissues supporting the fat. These rippling fat deposits are really the same as fat deposited anywhere else in the body. The only way to control them is to create a negative energy balance—that is, burn more calories than you take in. There are no creams or lotions that will rub away surface (subcutaneous) fat deposits, and spot reducing is also ineffective. The solution is sensible eating habits and exercise.

For more Common Questions Answered about body composition, visit the Online Learning Center at www.mhhe.com/fahey.

USDA Food and Nutrition Information Center: Weight and Obesity. Provides links to recent reports and studies on the issue of obesity among Americans.

http://fnic.nal.usda.gov/nal_display/index.php?info_center=4&tax_level=1&tax_subject=271

See also the listings for Chapters 2, 3, and 7.

SELECTED BIBLIOGRAPHY

Ackerman, K. E., et al. 2011. Bone health and the female athlete triad in adolescent athletes. *Physician Sportsmedicine* 39(1): 131–141.

Alexander, S. C., et al. 2011. Do the five As work when physicians counsel about weight loss? *Family Medicine* 43(3): 179–184.

Allen, T. W., et al. 2010. Body size, body composition, and cardiovascular disease risk factors in NFL players. *Physician Sportsmedicine* 38(1): 21–27.

American College of Sports Medicine. 2009. *ACSM's Resource Manual for Guidelines for Exercise Testing and Prescription*, 6th ed. Philadelphia: Lippincott Williams and Wilkins.

American Heart Association. 2011. *Heart Disease and Stroke Statistics—2011 Update.* Dallas, Tx.: American Heart Association.

Baer, H. J., et al. 2011. Risk factors for mortality in the Nurses' Health Study: A competing risks analysis. *American Journal of Epidemiology* 173(3): 319–329.

Beeson, W. L., et al. 2010. Comparison of body composition by bioelectrical impedance analysis and dual-energy X-ray absorptiometry in Hispanic diabetics. *International Journal of Body Composition Research* 8(2): 45–50.

Blair, S. N. 2009. Physical inactivity: The biggest public health problem of the 21st century. *British Journal of Sports Medicine* 43(1): 1–2.

Borrud, L. G., et al. 2010. Body composition data for individuals 8 years of age and older: U.S. population, 1999–2004. *Vital Health Statistics* 11(250): 1–87.

Bouchla, A., et al. 2011. The addition of strength training to aerobic interval training: Effects on muscle strength and body composition in CHF patients. *Journal of Cardiopulmonary Rehabilitation and Prevention* 31(1): 47–51.

Caldwell, K., et al. 2010. Developing mindfulness in college students through movement-based courses: Effects on self-regulatory self-efficacy, mood, stress, and sleep quality. *Journal of American College of Health* 58(5): 433–442.

Centers for Disease Control and Prevention. 2011. *National diabetes fact sheet: National estimates and general information on diabetes and prediabetes in the United States, 2011.* Atlanta: Centers for Disease Control and Prevention.

Farrell, S. W., et al. 2010. Cardiorespiratory fitness, adiposity, and all-cause mortality in women. *Medicine and Science in Sports and Exercise* 42(11): 2006–2012.

Flegal, K. M., et al. 2007. Cause-specific excess deaths associated with underweight, overweight, and obesity. *Journal of the American Medical Association* 298 (17): 2028–2037.

Ford, E. S., et al. 2011. Trends in obesity and abdominal obesity among adults in the United States from 1999–2008. *International Journal of Obesity* 35: 736–743.

Gallagher, K. M., et al. 2011. When 'fit' leads to fit, and when 'fit' leads to fat: How message framing and intrinsic vs. extrinsic exercise outcomes interact in promoting physical activity. *Psychological Health* 1–16.

Hainer, V., et al. 2009. Fat or fit: What is more important? *Diabetes Care* 32 (Suppl 2): S392–S397.

Harvey, S. B., et al. 2010. Physical activity and common mental disorders. *British Journal of Psychiatry*. 197: 357–364.

Hjgaard, B., et al. 2008. Waist circumference and body mass index as predictors of health care costs. *PLoS ONE* 3(7): e2619.

Hurvitz, M., et al. 2009. The young female athlete. *Pediatrics Endocrinology Reviews* 7(2): 123–129.

Lee, D. C., et al. 2009. Does physical activity ameliorate the health hazards of obesity? *British Journal of Sports Medicine* 43(1): 49–51.

Malina, R. M. 2007. Body composition in athletes: Assessment and estimated fatness. *Clinics in Sports Medicine* 26(1): 37–68.

Mattsson, S., and B. J. Thomas. 2006. Development of methods for body composition studies. *Physics in Medicine and Biology* 51(13): R203–R228.

Moon, J. R. 2008. Percent body fat estimations in college men using field and laboratory methods: A three-compartment model approach. *Dynamic Medicine* 7:7.

Murphy, M. H., et. al. 2009. Accumulated versus continuous exercise for health benefit: A review of empirical studies. *Sports Medicine* 39(1): 29–43.

Ode, J. J., et al. 2007. Body mass index as a predictor of percent fat in college athletes and nonathletes. *Medicine and Science in Sports and Exercise* 39(3): 403–409.

Pauli, S. A., et al. 2010. Athletic amenorrhea: Energy deficit or psychogenic challenge? *Annals of the New York Academy of Sciences* 1205: 33–38.

Puterman, E., et al. 2010. The power of exercise: Buffering the effect of chronic stress on telomere length. *PLoS One* 5(5): e10837.

Romero-Corral, A., et al. 2008. Accuracy of body mass index in diagnosing obesity in the adult general population. *International Journal of Obesity* 32(6): 959–966.

Stephens, B. R., et al. 2011 Effects of 1 day of inactivity on insulin action in healthy men and women: Interaction with energy intake. *Metabolism Clinical and Experimental* 60: 941–949.

Varady, K., et al. 2007. Validation of hand-held bioelectrical impedance analysis with magnetic resonance imaging for the assessment of body composition in overweight women. *American Journal of Human Biology* 19(3): 429–433.

Wada, R., et al. 2010. Body composition and wages. *Economics and Human Biology* 8(2): 242–254.

Wang, X., et al. 2008. Weight regain is related to decreases in physical activity during weight loss. *Medicine and Science in Sports and Exercise* 40(10): 1781–1788.

Wormser, D., et al. 2011. Separate and combined associations of body-mass index and abdominal adiposity with cardiovascular disease: Collaborative analysis of 58 prospective studies. *Lancet* 377(9771): 1085–1095.

Zanovec, M., et al. 2009. Self-reported physical activity improves prediction of body fatness in young adults. *Medicine and Science in Sports and Exercise* 41(2): 328–335.

Name ______________________ Section ______________ Date ____________

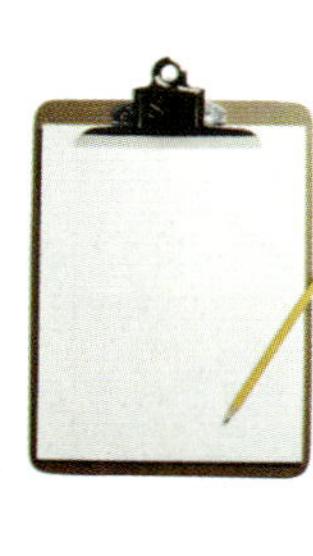

LAB 6.1 Assessing Body Mass Index and Body Composition

Body Mass Index

Equipment

1. Weight scale
2. Tape measure or other means of measuring height

Instructions

Measure your height and weight, and record the results. Be sure to record the unit of measurement.

Height: ____________ Weight: ____________

Calculating BMI (see also the shortcut chart of BMI values in Lab 6.2)

1. Convert your body weight to kilograms by dividing your weight in pounds by 2.2.

   Body weight ____________ lb ÷ 2.2 lb/kg = body weight ____________ kg
2. Convert your height measurement to meters by multiplying your height in inches by 0.0254.

   Height ____________ in. × 0.0254 m/in. = height ____________ m
3. Square your height measurement.

   Height ____________ m × height ____________ m = height ____________ m^2
4. BMI equals body weight in kilograms divided by height in meters squared (kg/m^2).

   Body weight ____________ (from step 1) kg ÷ height ____________ (from step 3) m^2 = BMI ____________ kg/m^2

Rating Your BMI

Refer to the table for a rating of your BMI. Record the results below and on the final page of this lab.

Classification	BMI (kg/m^2)
Underweight	<18.5
Normal	18.5–24.9
Overweight	25.0–29.9
Obesity (I)	30.0–34.9
Obesity (II)	35.0–39.9
Extreme obesity (III)	≥ 40.0

BMI ____________ kg/m^2

Classification ____________

Skinfold Measurements

Equipment

1. Skinfold calipers
2. Partner to take measurements
3. Marking pen (optional)

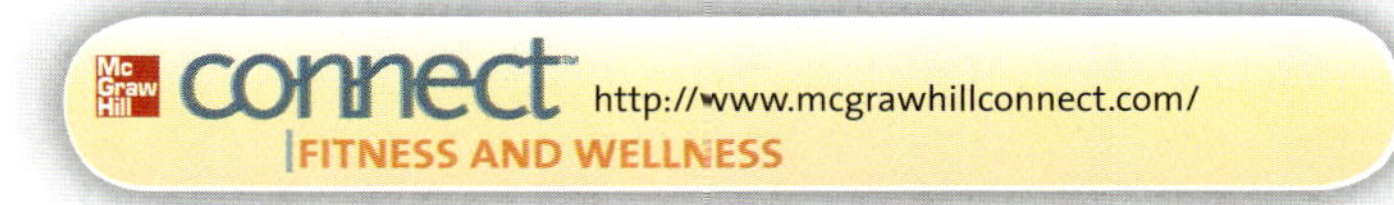

LABORATORY ACTIVITIES

Instructions

1. *Select and locate the correct sites for measurement.* All measurements should be taken on the right side of the body with the subject standing. Skinfolds are normally measured on the natural fold line of the skin, either vertically or at a slight angle. The skinfold measurement sites for males are chest, abdomen, and thigh; for females, triceps, suprailium, and thigh. If the person taking skinfold measurements is inexperienced, it may be helpful to mark the correct sites with a marking pen.

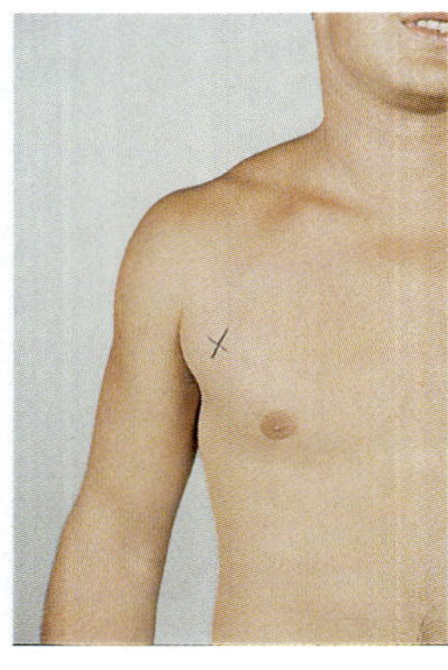

(a) Chest

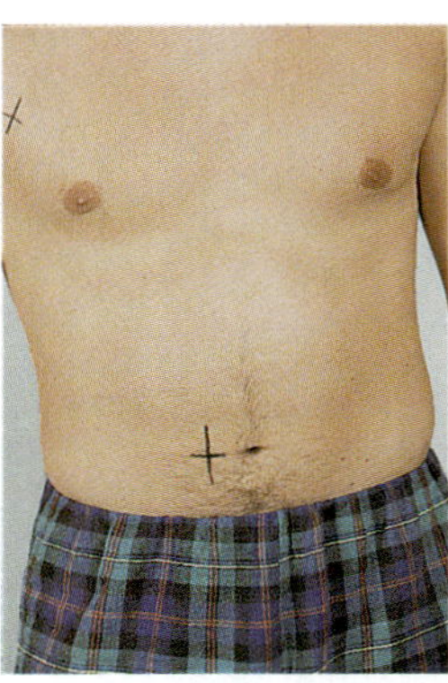

(b) Abdomen

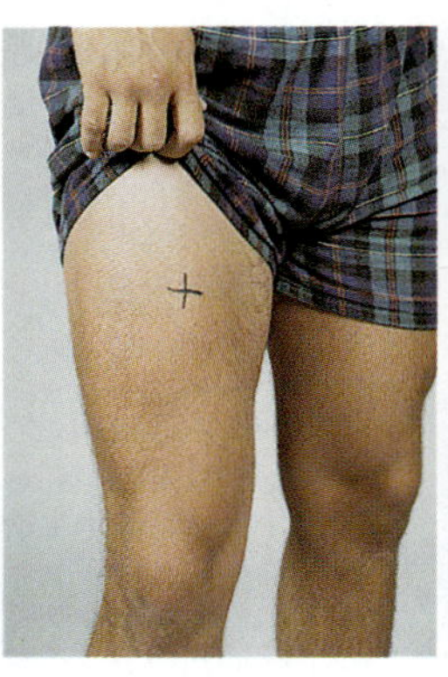

(c) Thigh

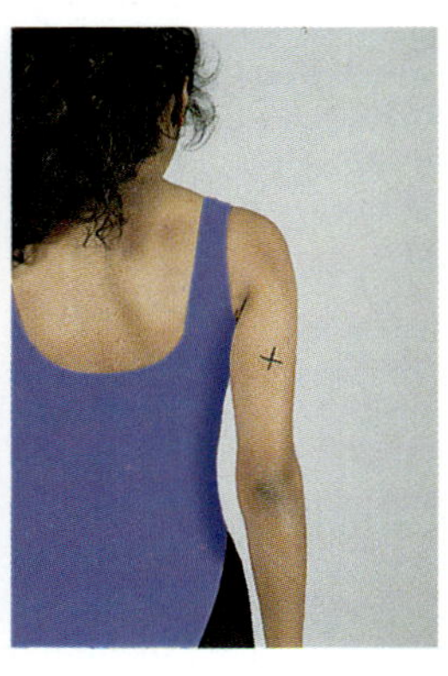

(d) Triceps

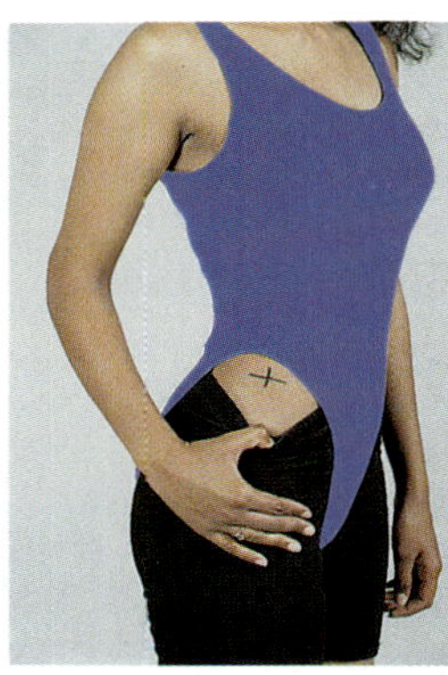

(e) Suprailium

   (a) Chest. Pinch a diagonal fold halfway between the nipple and the shoulder crease. *(b) Abdomen.* Pinch a vertical fold about 1 inch to the right of the umbilicus (navel). *(c) Thigh.* Pinch a vertical fold midway between the top of the hipbone and the kneecap. *(d) Triceps.* Pinch a vertical skinfold on the back of the right arm midway between the shoulder and elbow. The arm should be straight and should hang naturally. *(e) Suprailium.* Pinch a fold at the top front of the right hipbone. The skinfold here is taken slightly diagonally according to the natural fold tendency of the skin.

2. *Measure the appropriate skinfolds.* Pinch a fold of skin between your thumb and forefinger. Pull the fold up so that no muscular tissue is included; don't pinch the skinfold too hard. Hold the calipers perpendicular to the fold and measure the skinfold about 0.25 inch away from your fingers. Allow the tips of the calipers to close on the skinfold and let the reading settle before marking it down. Take readings to the nearest half-millimeter. Continue to repeat the measurements until two consecutive measurements match, releasing and repinching the skinfold between each measurement. Make a note of the final measurement for each site.

   Time of day of measurements: ___________

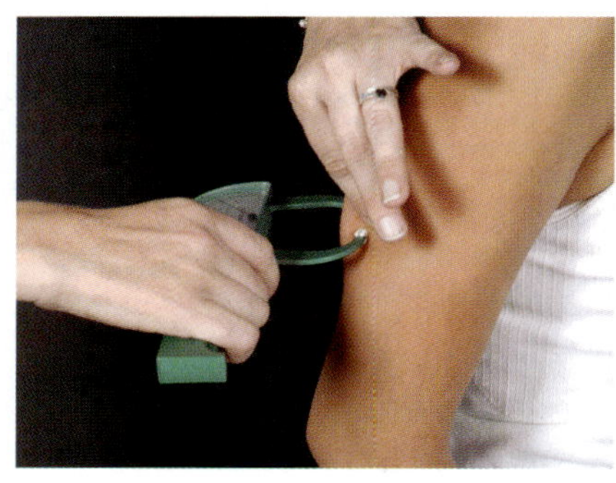

Men		*Women*	
Chest: ______________	mm	Triceps: ______________	mm
Abdomen: ___________	mm	Suprailium: ___________	mm
Thigh: ______________	mm	Thigh: _______________	mm

Determining Percent Body Fat

Add the measurements of your three skinfolds. Use this sum as a point of comparison for future assessments and/or to find the percent body fat that corresponds to your total in the appropriate table. For example, a 20-year-old female with measurements of 17 mm, 21 mm, and 22 mm would have a skinfold sum of 60 mm; according to the following table her percent body fat is 23.5.

Sum of three skinfolds: ______________ mm   Percent body fat: ______________ %

Prediction of Fat Percentage in Females from the Sum of Three Skinfolds

Sum of Skinfolds (mm)	Age (Years)								
	20	*25*	*30*	*35*	*40*	*45*	*50*	*55*	*60 and over*
20	9.3	9.6	9.9	10.2	10.5	10.8	11.1	11.4	11.7
25	11.2	11.5	11.8	12.1	12.4	12.7	13.0	13.3	13.6
30	13.1	13.4	13.7	14.0	14.3	14.6	14.9	15.2	15.5
35	14.9	15.2	15.5	15.8	16.1	16.4	16.7	17.0	17.3
40	16.7	17.0	17.3	17.6	17.9	18.2	18.5	18.8	19.1
45	18.4	18.8	19.1	19.4	19.7	20.0	20.3	20.6	20.9
50	20.2	20.5	20.8	21.1	21.4	21.7	22.0	22.4	22.7
55	21.9	22.2	22.5	22.8	23.1	23.4	23.7	24.1	24.4
60	23.5	23.8	24.1	24.4	24.8	25.1	25.4	25.7	26.0
65	25.1	25.4	25.7	26.1	26.4	26.7	27.0	27.3	27.7
70	26.7	27.0	27.3	27.6	27.9	28.3	28.6	28.9	29.2
75	28.2	28.5	28.8	29.1	29.5	29.8	30.1	30.4	30.8
80	29.7	30.0	30.3	30.6	31.0	31.3	31.6	31.9	32.3
85	31.1	31.4	31.7	32.1	32.4	32.7	33.0	33.4	33.7
90	32.5	32.8	33.1	33.5	33.8	34.1	34.4	34.8	35.1
95	33.8	34.1	34.5	34.8	35.1	35.5	35.8	36.1	36.5
100	35.1	35.4	35.8	36.1	36.4	36.8	37.1	37.4	37.8
105	36.3	36.7	37.0	37.3	37.7	38.0	38.3	38.7	39.0
110	37.5	37.9	38.2	38.5	38.9	39.2	39.5	39.9	40.2
115	38.7	39.0	39.3	39.7	40.0	40.4	40.7	41.0	41.4
120	39.8	40.1	40.4	40.8	41.1	41.5	41.8	42.1	42.5
125	40.8	41.2	41.5	41.8	42.2	42.5	42.9	43.2	43.5
130	41.8	42.1	42.5	42.8	43.2	43.5	43.9	44.2	44.5
135	42.7	43.1	43.4	43.8	44.1	44.5	44.8	45.1	45.5

SOURCES: Table generated from equations in Jackson, A. S., and M. L. Pollock. 1978. Generalized equations for predicting body density in men, *British Journal of Nutrition* 40: 497–504; Jackson, A. S., M. L. Pollock, and A. Ward. 1980. Gerneralized equations for predicting body density in women, *Medicine and Science in Sports and Exercise* 12: 175–182; Seri, W. E. 1956. Gross composition of the body. In J. H. Lawrence and C. A. Tobias. (eds.), *Advances in Biological and Medical Physics,* IV. New York: Academic Press.

Prediction of Fat Percentage in Males from the Sum of Three Skinfolds

Sum of Skinfolds (mm)	Age (Years)								
	20	*25*	*30*	*35*	*40*	*45*	*50*	*55*	*60 and over*
10	1.6	2.1	2.7	3.2	3.7	4.3	4.8	5.3	5.9
15	3.2	3.8	4.3	4.8	5.4	5.9	6.4	7.0	7.5
20	4.8	5.4	5.9	6.4	7.0	7.5	8.1	8.6	9.2
25	6.4	6.9	7.5	8.0	8.6	9.1	9.7	10.2	10.8
30	8.0	8.5	9.1	9.6	10.2	10.7	11.3	11.8	12.4
35	9.5	10.0	10.6	11.2	11.7	12.3	12.8	13.4	13.9
40	11.0	11.6	12.1	12.7	13.2	13.8	14.4	14.9	15.5
45	12.5	13.1	13.6	14.2	14.7	15.3	15.9	16.4	17.0
50	14.0	14.5	15.1	15.6	16.2	16.8	17.3	17.9	18.5
55	15.4	16.0	16.5	17.1	17.7	18.2	18.8	19.4	19.9
60	16.8	17.4	17.9	18.5	19.1	19.7	20.2	20.8	21.4
65	18.2	18.8	19.3	19.9	20.5	21.1	21.6	22.2	22.8
70	19.5	20.1	20.7	21.3	21.9	22.4	23.0	23.6	24.2
75	20.9	21.5	22.0	22.6	23.2	23.8	24.4	24.9	25.5
80	22.2	22.8	23.3	23.9	24.5	25.1	25.7	26.3	26.9
85	23.4	24.0	24.6	25.2	25.8	26.4	27.0	27.6	28.2
90	24.7	25.3	25.9	26.5	27.0	27.6	28.2	28.8	29.4
95	25.9	26.5	27.1	27.7	28.3	28.9	29.5	30.1	30.7
100	27.1	27.7	28.3	28.9	29.5	30.1	30.7	31.3	31.9
105	28.2	28.8	29.4	30.0	30.6	31.2	31.8	32.4	33.0
110	29.3	29.9	30.5	31.1	31.7	32.4	33.0	33.6	34.2
115	30.4	31.0	31.6	32.2	32.8	33.5	34.1	34.7	35.3
120	31.5	32.1	32.7	33.3	33.9	34.5	35.1	35.7	36.4
125	32.5	33.1	33.7	34.3	34.9	35.6	36.2	36.8	37.4

SOURCES: Table generated from equations in Jackson, A. S., and M. L. Pollock, 1978. Generalized equations for predicting body density in men, *British Journal of Nutrition* 40: 497–504; Jackson, A. S., M. L. Pollock, and A. Ward. 1980. Generalized equations for predicting body density in women, *Medicine and Science in Sports and Exercise* 12: 175–182; Seri, W. E. 1956. Gross composition of the body. In J. H. Lawrence and C. A. Tobias. (eds.), *Advances in Biological and Medical Physics,* IV. New York: Academic Press.

Rating Your Body Composition

Refer to the chart to rate your percent body fat. Record it below and in the chart at the end of this lab.

Rating: ________________

Percent Body Fat Classification

	Percent Body Fat (%)		
	20–39 Years	*40–59 Years*	*60–79 Years*
Women			
Essential*	8–12	8–12	8–12
Low/athletic**	13–20	13–22	13–23
Recommended	21–32	23–33	24–35
Overfat†	33–38	34–39	36–41
Obese†	≥39	≥40	≥42

	Percent Body Fat (%)		
	20–39 Years	*40–59 Years*	*60–79 Years*
Men			
Essential*	3–5	3–5	3–5
Low/athletic**	6–7	6–10	6–12
Recommended	8–19	11–21	13–24
Overfat†	20–24	22–27	25–29
Obese†	≥25	≥28	≥30

NOTE: The cutoffs for recommended, overfat, and obese ranges in this table are based on a study that linked body mass index classifications from the National Institutes of Health with predicted percent body fat (measured using dual-energy X-ray absorptiometry).

*Essential body fat is necessary for the basic functioning of the body.
**Percent body fat in the low/athletic range may be appropriate for some people as long as it is not the result of illness or disordered eating habits.
†Health risks increase as percent body fat exceeds the recommended range.

SOURCES: Gallagher, D., et al. 2009. Healthy percentage body fat ranges: An approach for developing guidelines based on body mass index. *American Journal of Clinical Nutrition* 72: 694–701. American College of Sports Medicine. 2009. *ACSM's Resource Manual for Guidelines for Exercise Testing and Prescription*, 6th ed. Philadelphia: Lippincott Williams and Wilkins.

Other Methods of Assessing Percent Body Fat

If you use a different method, record the name of the method and the result below and in the chart at the end of this lab. Find your body composition rating on the chart above.

Method used: ________________ Percent body fat: ________________ % Rating (from chart above): ________________

Waist Circumference and Waist-to-Hip Ratio

Equipment

1. Tape measure
2. Partner to take measurements

Preparation

Wear clothes that will not add significantly to your measurements.

Instructions

Stand with your feet together and your arms at your sides. Raise your arms only high enough to allow for taking the measurements. Your partner should make sure the tape is horizontal around the entire circumference and pulled snugly against your skin. The tape shouldn't be pulled so tight that it causes indentations in your skin. Record measurements to the nearest millimeter or one-sixteenth of an inch.

Waist. Measure at the smallest waist circumference. If you don't have a natural waist, measure at the level of your navel.

Waist measurement: ____________

Hip. Measure at the largest hip circumference. Hip measurement: ____________

Waist-to-Hip Ratio: You can use any unit of measurement (for example, inches or centimeters) as long as you're consistent. Waist-to-hip ratio equals waist measurement divided by hip measurement.

Waist-to-hip ratio: ____________ (waist measurement) ÷ ____________ (hip measurement) = ____________

Determining Your Risk

The table below indicates values for waist circumference and waist-to-hip ratio above which the risk of health problems increases significantly. If your measurement or ratio is above either cutoff point, put a check on the appropriate line below and in the chart at the end of this lab.

Waist circumference: _____________ (✓ high risk) Waist-to-hip ratio: _____________ (✓ high risk)

Body Fat Distribution

Cutoff Points for High Risk

	Waist Circumference	*Waist-to-Hip Ratio*
Men	More than 40 in. (102 cm)	More than 0.94
Women	More than 35 in. (88 cm)	More than 0.82

SOURCE: National Heart, Lung, and Blood Institute. 1998. *Clinical Guidelines on the Identification, Evaluation, and Treatment of Overweight and Obesity in Adults: The Evidence Report. Bethesda*, Md.: National Institutes of Health. Heyward, V. H., and D. R. Wagner. 2004. *Applied Body Composition Assessment*, 2nd ed. Champaign, Ill.: Human Kinetics.

Rating Your Body Composition

Assessment	*Value*	*Classification*
BMI	_____________ kg/m^2	_____________
Skinfold measurements or alternative method of determining percent body fat Specify method: _____________	_____________ % body fat	_____________
Waist circumference Waist-to-hip ratio	_____________ in. or cm _____________ (ratio)	_____________ (✓ high risk) _____________ (✓ high risk)

Using Your Results

How did you score? Are you surprised by your ratings for body composition and body fat distribution? Are your current ratings in the range for good health? Are you satisfied with your current body composition? Why or why not?

If you're not satisfied, set a realistic goal for improvement:

What should you do next? Enter the results of this lab in the Preprogram Assessment column in Appendix C. If you've determined that you need to improve your body composition, set a specific goal by completing Lab 6.2, and then plan your program using the labs in Chapters 3 and 7. After several weeks or months of an exercise and/or dietary change program, complete this lab again and enter the results in the Postprogram Assessment column of Appendix C. How do the results compare?

Name ______________________ Section ______________ Date ____________

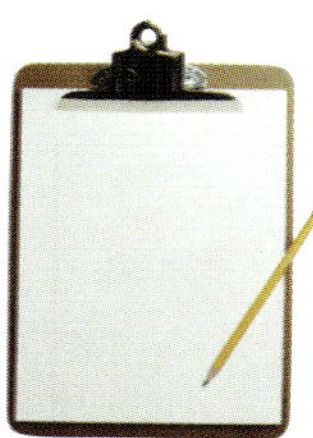

LAB 6.2 Setting Goals for Target Body Weight

This lab is designed to help you set body weight goals based on a target BMI or percent body fat. If the results of Lab 6.1 indicate that a change in body composition would be beneficial for your health, you may want to complete this lab to help you set goals.

Remember, though, that a wellness lifestyle—including a balanced diet and regular exercise—is more important for your health than achieving any specific body weight, BMI, or percent body fat. You may want to set goals for improving your diet and increasing physical activity and let your body composition change as a result. If so, use the labs in Chapters 3, 4, and 8 as your guides.

Equipment

Calculator (or pencil and paper for calculations)

Preparation

Determine percent body fat and/or calculate BMI as described in Lab 6.1. Keep track of height and weight as measured for these calculations.

Height: ______________ Weight: ______________

Instructions: Target Body Weight from Target BMI

Use the chart below to find the target body weight that corresponds to your target BMI. Find your height in the left column, and then move across the appropriate row until you find the weight that corresponds to your target BMI. Remember, BMI is only an indirect measurement of body composition. It is possible to improve body composition without any significant change in weight. For example, a weight training program may result in increased muscle mass and decreased fat mass without any change in overall weight. For this reason, you may want to set alternative or additional goals, such as improving the fit of your clothes or decreasing your waist measurement.

	<18.5 Underweight		18.5–24.9 Normal						25–29.9 Overweight					30–34.9 Obesity (Class I)					35–39.9 Obesity (Class II)					≥40 Extreme Obesity
BMI	17	18	19	20	21	22	23	24	25	26	27	28	29	30	31	32	33	34	35	36	37	38	39	40
Height	Body Weight (pounds)																							
4' 10"	81	86	91	96	101	105	110	115	120	124	129	134	139	144	148	153	158	163	168	172	177	182	187	192
4' 11"	84	89	94	99	104	109	114	119	124	129	134	139	144	149	154	159	163	168	173	178	183	188	193	198
5'	87	92	97	102	108	113	118	123	128	133	138	143	149	154	159	164	169	174	179	184	190	195	200	205
5' 1"	90	95	101	106	111	117	122	127	132	138	143	148	154	159	164	169	175	180	185	191	196	201	207	212
5' 2"	93	98	104	109	115	120	126	131	137	142	148	153	159	164	170	175	181	186	191	197	202	208	213	219
5' 3"	96	102	107	113	119	124	130	136	141	147	153	158	164	169	175	181	186	192	198	203	209	215	220	226
5' 4"	99	105	111	117	122	128	134	140	146	152	157	163	169	175	181	187	192	198	204	210	216	222	227	233
5' 5"	102	108	114	120	126	132	138	144	150	156	162	168	174	180	186	192	198	204	210	216	222	229	235	241
5' 6"	105	112	118	124	130	136	143	149	155	161	167	174	180	186	192	198	205	211	217	223	229	236	242	248
5' 7"	109	115	121	128	134	141	147	153	160	166	173	179	185	192	198	204	211	217	224	230	236	243	249	256
5' 8"	112	118	125	132	138	145	151	158	165	171	178	184	191	197	204	211	217	224	230	237	244	250	257	263
5' 9"	115	122	129	136	142	149	156	163	169	176	183	190	197	203	210	217	224	230	237	244	251	258	264	271
5' 10"	119	126	133	139	146	153	160	167	174	181	188	195	202	209	216	223	230	237	244	251	258	265	272	279
5' 11"	122	129	136	143	151	158	165	172	179	187	194	201	208	215	222	230	237	244	251	258	265	273	280	287
6'	125	133	140	148	155	162	170	177	184	192	199	207	214	221	229	236	243	251	258	266	273	280	288	295
6' 1"	129	137	144	152	159	167	174	182	190	197	205	212	220	228	235	243	250	258	265	273	281	288	296	303
6' 2"	132	140	148	156	164	171	179	187	195	203	210	218	226	234	242	249	257	265	273	281	288	296	304	312
6' 3"	136	144	152	160	168	176	184	192	200	208	216	224	232	240	248	256	264	272	280	288	296	304	312	320
6' 4"	140	148	156	164	173	181	189	197	206	214	222	230	238	247	255	263	271	280	288	296	304	312	321	329

SOURCE: Ratings from the National Heart, Lung, and Blood Institute. 1998. *Clinical Guidelines on the Identification, Evaluation, and Treatment of Overweight and Obesity in Adults.* Bethesda, Md.: National Institutes of Health.

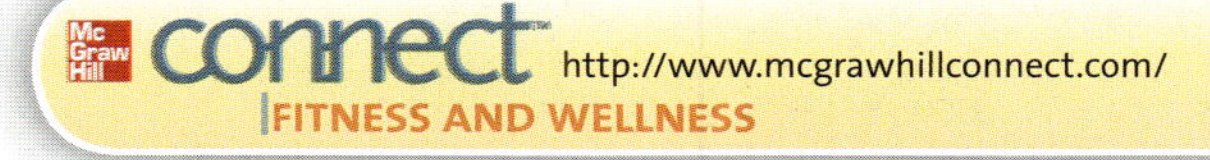

Current BMI: _____________ Target BMI: _____________ Target body weight (from chart): _____________

Alternative/additional goals: ____

____

Note: You can calculate target body weight from target BMI more precisely by using the following formula: (1) convert your height measurement to meters, (2) square your height measurement, (3) multiply this number by your target BMI to get your target weight in kilograms, and (4) convert your target weight from kilograms to pounds:

1. Height _____________ in. × 0.0254 m/in. = height _____________ m
2. Height _____________ m × height _____________ m = _____________ m^2
3. Target BMI _____________ × height _____________ m^2 = target weight _____________ kg
4. Target weight _____________ kg × 2.2 lb/kg = target weight _____________ lb

Instructions: Target Body Weight from Target Body Fat Percentages

Use the formula below to determine the target body weight that corresponds to your target percent body fat.

Current percent body fat: _____________ Target percent body fat: _____________

Formula	*Example: 180-lb male, current percent body fat of 24%, goal of 21%*
1. To determine the fat weight in your body, multiply your current weight by percent body fat (determined through skinfold measurements and expressed as a decimal).	180 lb × 0.24 = 43.2 lb
2. Subtract the fat weight from your current weight to get your current fat-free weight.	180 lb − 43.2 lb = 136.8 lb
3. Subtract your target percent body fat from 1 to get target percent fat-free weight.	1 − 0.21 = 0.79
4. To get your target body weight, divide your fat-free weight by your target percent fat-free weight.	136.8 lb ÷ 0.79 = 173 lb

Note: Weight can be expressed in either pounds or kilograms, as long as the unit of measurement is used consistently.

1. Current body weight _____________ × percent body fat _____________ = fat weight _____________
2. Current body weight _____________ − fat weight _____________ = fat-free weight _____________
3. 1 − target percent body fat _____________ = target percent fat-free weight _____________
4. Fat-free weight _____________ ÷ target percent fat-free weight _____________ = target body weight_____________

Setting a Goal

Based on these calculations and other factors (including heredity, individual preference, and current health status), select a target weight or range of weights for yourself.

Target body weight: _____________

CHAPTER 7

Weight Management

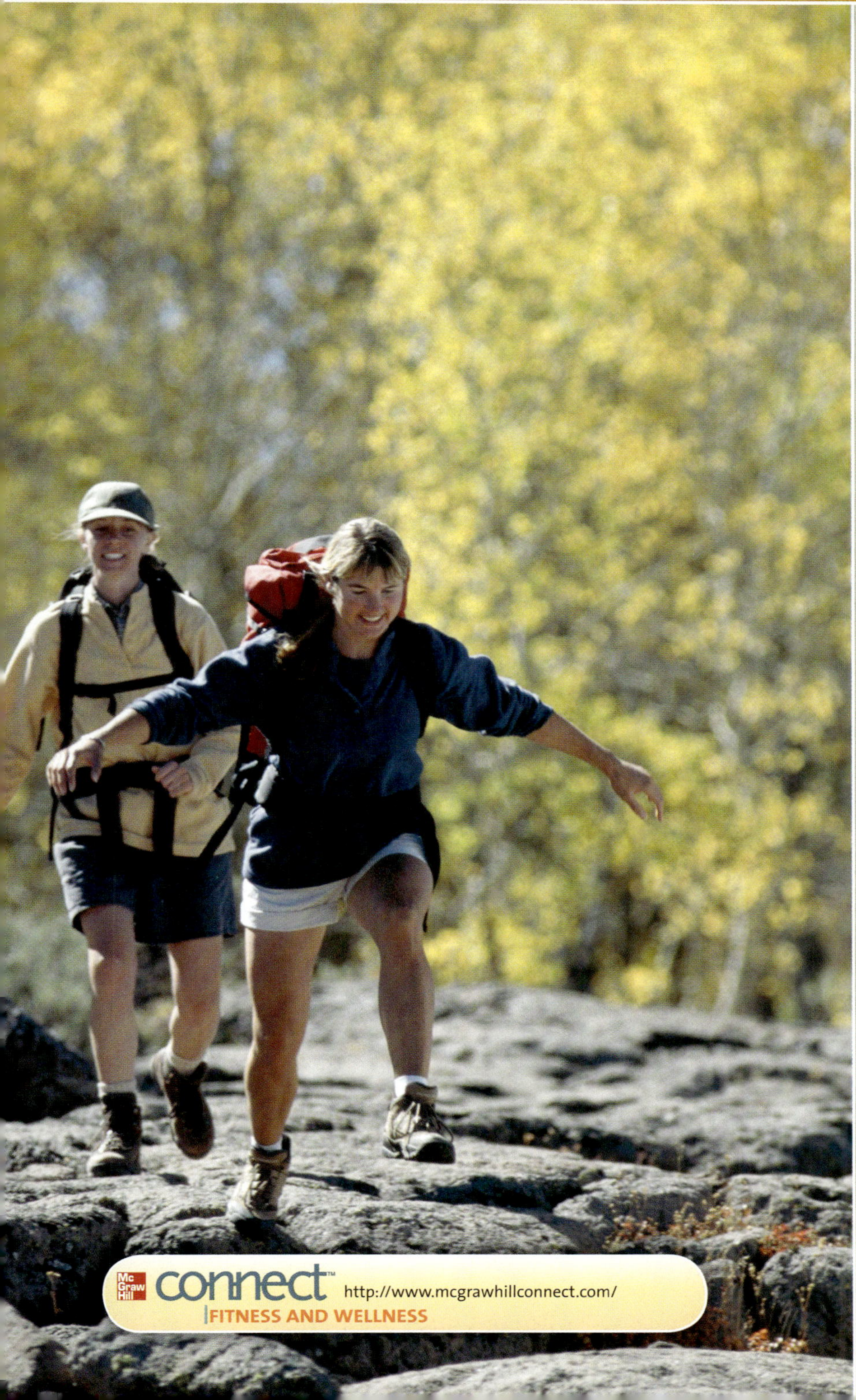

LOOKING AHEAD...

After reading this chapter, you should be able to:

- Explain the health risks associated with overweight and obesity
- Explain the factors that may contribute to a weight problem, including genetic, physiological, lifestyle, and psychosocial factors
- Describe lifestyle factors that contribute to weight gain and loss, including the role of diet, exercise, and emotional factors
- Identify and describe the symptoms of eating disorders and the health risks associated with them
- Design a personal plan for successfully managing body weight

TEST YOUR KNOWLEDGE

1. About what percentage of American adults are overweight?
   a. 15%
   b. 35%
   c. 65%
2. The consumption of low-calorie sweeteners has helped Americans control their weight. True or false?
3. Approximately how many female high school and college students have either anorexia or bulimia?
   a. 0%
   b. 1%
   c. 2%

Answers

1. **c.** About 68% of American adults are overweight, including 32.2% of adult men and 35.5% of adult women who are obese.
2. **False.** Since the introduction of low-calorie sweeteners, both total calorie and sugar intake have increased, as has the proportion of Americans who are overweight.
3. **c.** About 2–4% of female students suffer from bulimia or anorexia, and many more occasionally engage in behaviors associated with these eating disorders.

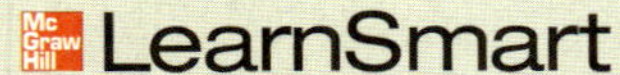

Achieving and maintaining a healthy body weight is a serious public health challenge in the United States and a source of distress for many Americans. Under standards developed by the National Institutes of Health, about 68% of American adults are overweight, including more than 33.8% who are obese (Table 7.1 and Figure 7.1). In 2007–2008, 32.2% of adult men and 35.5% of adult women were obese. The problems of overweight and obesity affect Americans of all ages. According to the National Center for Health Statistics, 24% of Americans age 18–29 are obese. The American Medical Association says that one-third of American children are at risk of becoming overweight. And while millions struggle to lose weight, others fall into dangerous eating patterns such as binge eating or self-starvation.

Table 7.1 Vital Statistics: Weight of Americans Age 20 and Older: 2007–2008

GROUP	PERCENT OVERWEIGHT*	PERCENT OBESE
Both sexes	68.0	33.8
All races, male	72.3	32.2
All races, female	64.1	35.5
White, male	72.6	31.9
White, female	61.2	33.0
African American, male	68.5	37.3
African American, female	78.2	49.6
Latino, male	79.3	34.3
Latino, female	76.1	43.0

*Includes obesity

SOURCE: Flegal, K. M., et al. 2010. Prevalence and Trends in Obesity Among US Adults, 1999–2008. *Journal of the American Medical Association* 303(3): 235–241.

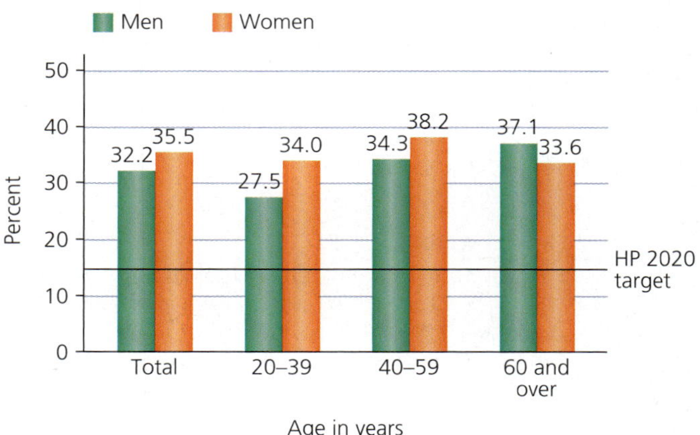

FIGURE 7.1 Obesity pevalence, by age and sex of American adults, 2007–2008.

Healthy People 2020 sets a target obesity prevalence of not greater than 15% for all adults.

SOURCE: Flegal, K. M., et al. 2010. Prevalence and Trends in Obesity Among US Adults, 1999–2008. *Journal of the American Medical Association* 303(3): 235–241.

Controlling body weight is a matter of controlling body fat. As explained in Chapter 6, the most important consideration for health is not total weight but body composition—the proportion of fat to fat-free mass. Many people who are "overweight" are also "overfat," and the health risks they face are due to the latter condition. Although this chapter uses the common terms ***weight management*** and ***weight loss,*** the goal for wellness is to adopt healthy behaviors and achieve an appropriate body composition, not to conform to rigid standards of total body weight.

Although not completely understood, managing body weight is not a mysterious process. The "secret" is balancing calories consumed with calories expended in daily activities—in other words, eating a moderate diet and getting regular physical activity.

This chapter explores the factors that contribute to the development of overweight and obesity as well as to eating disorders. It also takes a closer look at weight management through lifestyle and suggests specific strategies for reaching and maintaining a healthy weight.

HEALTH IMPLICATIONS OF OVERWEIGHT AND OBESITY

As rates of overweight and obesity have risen in the United States, so has the prevalence of the health conditions associated with overweight—including a more than 33% rise in the rate of type 2 diabetes in just the past decade. It is estimated that inactivity and overweight account for more than 100,000 premature deaths annually in the United States, second only to tobacco-related deaths. More than $75 billion per year is spent treating obesity-related health problems.

Obesity is one of six major controllable risk factors for heart disease; it also increases the risk for other forms of cardiovascular disease (CVD), hypertension, certain forms of cancer, diabetes, gallbladder disease, respiratory problems, joint diseases, skin problems, impaired immune function, and sleep disorders. Obesity doubles mortality rates and can reduce life expectancy by 10–20 years. In fact, if current trends in overweight and obesity (and their related health problems) continue, some experts predict that the average American's life expectancy will soon decline by 5 years.

Gaining weight over the years also has been found to be dangerous. A recent study showed that women who gained more than 22 pounds since they were 18 years old had a sevenfold increase in the risk of heart disease. Many studies have confirmed that obesity and—to a lesser extent—overweight shorten lives.

At the same time, even modest weight loss can have a significant positive impact on health. A weight loss of just 5–10% in obese individuals can reduce the risk of weight-related health conditions and increase life expectancy.

Beating the "Freshman 15"

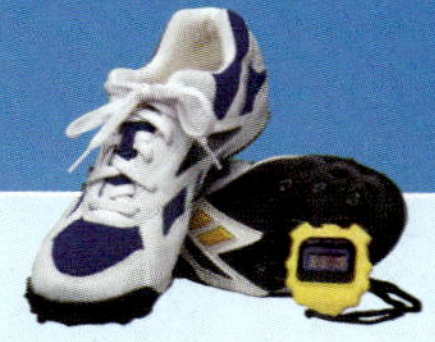

PERSONAL CHALLENGE

How much weight have you put on since you started going to college? It isn't unusual for first-year college students to gain some weight (often called the "Freshman 15"), and many students continue gaining weight throughout their college years.

If you've gained weight since starting college, write down the number of pounds you've gained: __________ pounds

Next, think of five reasons why you have gained this weight, and list them below:

1: ______________________________

2: ______________________________

3: ______________________________

4: ______________________________

5: ______________________________

Now, think of five things you can start doing right now either to stop gaining weight or start losing weight:

1: ______________________________

2: ______________________________

3: ______________________________

4: ______________________________

5: ______________________________

Keep these lists in mind as you work through this chapter, its labs, and the Behavior Change Workbook at the end of the text. The lists may become the starting point for creating a personal weight-management plan, should you decide you need one.

FACTORS CONTRIBUTING TO EXCESS BODY FAT

Several factors determine body weight and composition. These factors can be grouped into genetic, physiological, lifestyle, and psychosocial factors.

Genetic Factors

Estimates of the genetic contribution to obesity vary widely, from about 25–40% of an individual's body fat. More than 600 genes have been linked to obesity, but their actions are still under study. Genes influence body size and shape, body fat distribution, and metabolic rate. Genetic factors also affect the ease with which weight is gained as a result of overeating and where on the body extra weight is added.

If both parents are obese, their children have an 80% risk of being obese; children with one obese parent face a 40% risk of becoming obese. In studies that compared adoptees and their biological parents, the weights of the adoptees were found to be more like those of the biological parents than the adoptive parents, indicating a strong genetic link.

Hereditary influences, however, must be balanced against the contribution of environmental factors. Not all children of obese parents become obese, and normal-weight parents can have overweight children. Environmental factors like diet and exercise are probably responsible for such differences. Thus, the *tendency* to develop obesity may be inherited, but the expression of this tendency is affected by environmental influences.

Physiological Factors

Metabolism is a key physiological factor in the regulation of body fat and body weight. Hormones also play a role. A few other physiological factors have been proposed as causes for weight gain, such as carbohydrate craving due to low levels of the neurotransmitter serotonin, but research on this and other theories has so far been inconclusive.

Metabolism and Energy Balance Metabolism is the sum of all the vital processes by which food energy and nutrients are made available to and used by the body. The largest component of metabolism, **resting metabolic rate (RMR)**, is the energy required to maintain vital body functions, including respiration, heart rate, body temperature,

resting metabolic rate (RMR) The energy required (in calories) to maintain vital body functions, including respiration, heart rate, body temperature, and blood pressure, while the body is at rest.

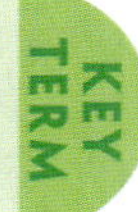

ENERGY IN
Food calories
ENERGY OUT
Physical activity 20–30%
Food digestion ±10%
Resting metabolism 65–70%

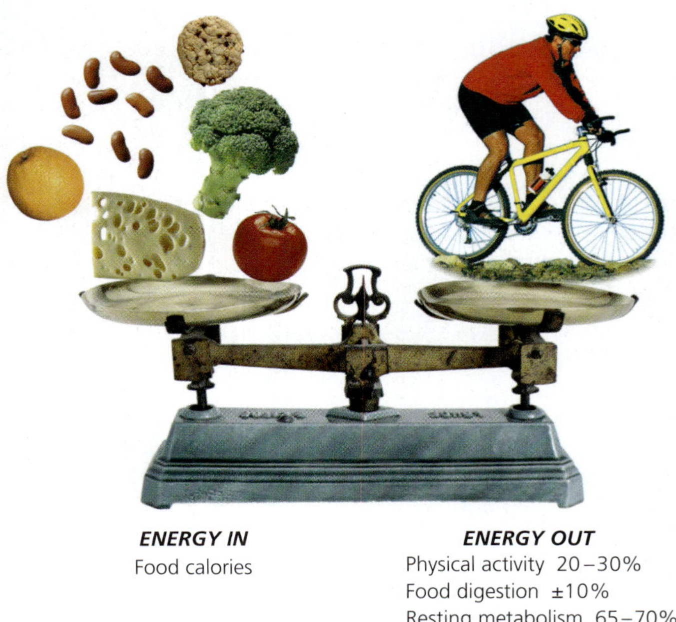

FIGURE 7.2 The energy-balance equation

and blood pressure, while the body is at rest. As shown in Figure 7.2, RMR accounts for about 65–70% of daily energy expenditure. The energy required to digest food accounts for an additional ±10% of daily energy expenditure. The remaining 20–30% is expended during physical activity.

Both heredity and behavior affect metabolic rate. Men, who have a higher proportion of muscle mass than women, have a higher RMR (muscle tissue is more metabolically active than fat). Also, some individuals inherit a higher or lower RMR than others. A higher RMR means that a person burns more calories while at rest and can therefore take in more calories without gaining weight.

Weight loss or gain also affects metabolic rate. When a person loses weight, both RMR and the energy required to perform physical tasks decrease. The reverse occurs when weight is gained. One reason exercise is so important during a weight-loss program is that exercise, especially resistance training, helps maintain muscle mass and metabolic rate.

Exercise has a positive effect on metabolism. When people exercise, they slightly increase their RMR—the number of calories their bodies burn at rest. In fact, a 2011 study of college-age men showed that following 45 minutes of vigorous exercise, the participants' resting metabolic rate remained elevated for 14 hours—during which the men burned an additional 200 calories while at rest or performing normal, everyday activities. People who regularly exercise also increase their muscle mass, which is associated with a higher metabolic rate. The exercise itself also burns calories, raising total energy expenditure. The higher the energy expenditure, the more the person can eat without gaining weight.

The energy-balance equation is the key to weight management. If you burn the same amount of energy as you take in (a *neutral* energy balance), your weight remains constant. If you consume more calories than you expend (a *positive* energy balance), your weight increases. If you burn more calories than you consume (a *negative* energy balance), your weight decreases.

To create a negative energy balance and lose weight and body fat, you can increase the amount of energy you burn by increasing your level of physical activity and/or decrease the amount of energy you take in by consuming fewer calories.

Hormones Hormones clearly play a role in the accumulation of body fat, especially for women. Hormonal changes at puberty, during pregnancy, and at menopause contribute to the amount and location of fat accumulation. For example, during puberty, hormones cause the development of secondary sex characteristics, including larger breasts, wider hips, and a fat layer under the skin. This addition of body fat at puberty is normal and healthy.

One hormone thought to be linked to obesity is *leptin*. Secreted by the body's fat cells, leptin is carried to the brain, where it appears to let the brain know how big or small the body's fat stores are. With this information, the brain can regulate appetite and metabolic rate accordingly. Researchers hope to use leptin and other hormones to develop treatments for obesity based on appetite control. As most of us will admit, however, hunger is often *not* the primary reason we overeat. Cases of obesity based solely or primarily on hormone abnormalities do exist, but they are rare.

Lifestyle Factors

Genetic and physiological factors may increase the risk for excess body fat, but they are not sufficient to explain the increasingly high rate of obesity in the United States. The gene pool has not changed dramatically in the past 40 years, but the rate of obesity among Americans has more than doubled. Clearly, other factors are at work—particularly lifestyle factors such as increased energy intake and decreased physical activity.

Eating Americans have access to plenty of calorie-dense foods, and many have eating habits that contribute to weight gain. Most overweight adults will admit to eating more than they should of high-fat, high-sugar, high-calorie foods. Americans eat out more frequently now than in the past, and we rely more heavily on fast food and packaged convenience foods. Restaurant and convenience food portion sizes tend to be large, and the foods themselves are likely to be high in fat, sugar, and calories and low in nutrients.

Studies have consistently found that people underestimate portion sizes by as much as 25%. When participants in one study were asked to report their food intake over the previous 24 hours, the majority underestimated their actual intake by about 600 calories. Many Americans are unaware of how many calories they actually consume each day.

Americans' average calorie intake has increased by 18% since 1983. Many of those extra calories come from carbohydrates, such as refined sugars. The popularity of sugar-free soft drinks does not appear to be helping people lose weight. The result has been a substantial increase in the number of overweight and obese Americans.

Physical Activity Activity levels among Americans are declining, beginning in childhood and continuing throughout life. Many schools have cut back on physical education classes and even recess. Most adults drive to work, sit all day, and then relax in front of the TV (or continue working) at night. One study found that 60% of the incidence of overweight can be linked to excessive television viewing. On average, Americans exercise 15 minutes per day and watch 170 minutes of TV and movies.

Psychosocial Factors Many people have learned to use food as a means of coping with stress and negative emotions. Eating can provide a powerful distraction from difficult feelings—loneliness, anger, boredom, anxiety, shame, sadness, inadequacy. It can be used to combat low moods, low energy levels, and low self-esteem. When eating becomes the primary means of regulating emotions, **binge eating** or other unhealthy eating patterns can develop.

Obesity is strongly associated with socioeconomic status. The prevalence of obesity goes down as income level goes up. More women than men are obese at lower income levels, but men are somewhat more obese at higher levels. These differences may reflect the greater sensitivity and concern for a slim physical appearance among upper-income women, as well as greater access to information about nutrition and to low-fat and low-calorie foods. It may also reflect the greater acceptance of obesity among certain ethnic groups, as well as different cultural values related to food choices.

In some families and cultures, food is used as a symbol of love and caring. It is an integral part of social gatherings and celebrations. In such cases, it may be difficult to change established eating patterns because they are linked to cultural and family values.

> **Ask Yourself**
>
> **QUESTIONS FOR CRITICAL THINKING AND REFLECTION**
>
> Is anyone in your family overweight? If so, can you identify factors that may contribute to this weight problem, such as heredity, eating patterns, or psychosocial factors? Has the person tried to address the problem? How is the issue handled in your family? How do family members help the situation or make it worse?

> **Wellness Tip**
>
> Looking for an easy way to cut calories? Cut down on soda or beer. A 12-ounce can of regular soda or beer contains about 150 calories. Reduce your consumption by just one can a day, and you can lose about 15 pounds in a year!

ADOPTING A HEALTHY LIFESTYLE FOR SUCCESSFUL WEIGHT MANAGEMENT

When all the research is assessed, it becomes clear that most weight problems are lifestyle problems. Even though more and more young people are developing weight problems, most arrive at early adulthood with the advantage of having a normal body weight—neither too fat nor too thin. In fact, many young adults get away with very poor eating and exercise habits and don't develop a weight problem. But as the rapid growth of adolescence slows and family and career obligations increase, maintaining a healthy weight becomes a greater challenge. Slow weight gain is a major cause of overweight and obesity, so weight management is important for everyone, not just for people who are currently overweight. A good time to develop a lifestyle for successful weight management is during early adulthood, when healthy behavior patterns have a better chance of taking hold.

Permanent weight loss is not something you start and stop. You need to adopt healthy behaviors that you can maintain throughout your life, including eating habits, physical activity and exercise, an ability to think positively and manage your emotions effectively, and the coping strategies you use to deal with the stresses and challenges in your life.

Diet and Eating Habits

In contrast to dieting, which involves some form of food restriction, the term *diet* refers to your daily food choices. Everyone has a diet, but not everyone is dieting. It's important to develop a diet that you enjoy and that enables you to maintain a healthy body composition.

Use MyPlate or DASH as the basis for planning a healthy diet (Chapter 4), and choose the healthiest

> **binge eating** A pattern of eating in which normal food consumption is interrupted by episodes of high consumption.

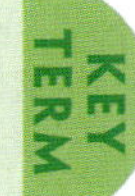

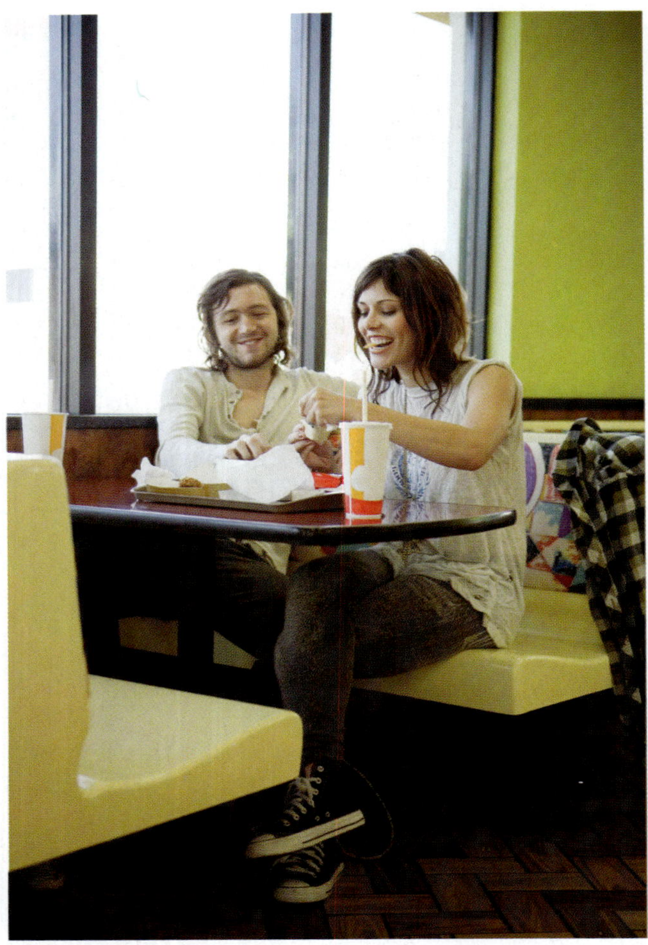

When fast food is the only available option, it can be difficult to make healthy lifestyle changes.

options within each food group. For weight management, you may need to pay special attention to total calories, portion sizes, energy density, fat and carbohydrate intake, and eating habits.

Total Calories The USDA suggests approximate daily energy intakes based on gender, age, and activity level. However, the precise number of calories needed to maintain weight will vary from one person to another based on heredity, fitness status, level of physical activity, and other factors. It may be more important to focus on individual energy balance than on a general recommendation for daily calorie intake. To calculate your approximate daily caloric needs, complete Lab 7.1.

The best approach for weight loss is combining an increase in physical activity with moderate calorie restriction. Don't go on a crash diet. You need to eat and drink enough to meet your need for essential nutrients. To maintain weight loss, you will probably have to maintain some degree of the calorie restriction you used to lose the weight. Therefore, it is important that you adopt a level of food intake that you can live with over the long term. For most people, maintaining weight loss is more difficult than losing the weight in the first place. To identify weight-loss goals and ways to meet them, complete Lab 7.2.

Portion Sizes Overconsumption of total calories is closely tied to portion sizes. Many Americans are unaware that the portion sizes of packaged foods and of foods served at restaurants have increased in size, and most of us significantly underestimate the amount of food we eat. Studies have found that the larger the meal, the greater the underestimation of calories. Limiting portion sizes is critical for weight management. For many people, concentrating on portion sizes is easier than counting calories. See Chapter 4 for more information and hints on choosing appropriate portion sizes.

Energy (Calorie) Density Experts also recommend that you pay attention to *energy density*—the number of calories per ounce or gram of weight in a food. Studies suggest that it isn't consumption of a certain amount of fat or calories in food that reduces hunger and leads to feelings of fullness and satisfaction. Rather, it is consumption of a certain weight of food. Foods that are low in energy density have more volume and bulk; that is, they are relatively heavy but have few calories (Table 7.2). For example, for the same 100 calories, you could eat 20 baby carrots or four pretzel twists. You are more likely to feel full after eating the serving of carrots because it weighs ten times as much as the serving of pretzels (10 ounces versus 1 ounce).

Fresh fruits and vegetables, with their high water and fiber content, are low in energy density, as are wholegrain foods. Fresh fruits contain fewer calories and more fiber than fruit juices or drinks. Meat, ice cream, potato chips, croissants, crackers, and cakes and cookies are examples of foods high in energy density. Strategies

Table 7.2 Examples of Foods Low in Energy Density

FOOD	AMOUNT	CALORIES
Carrot, raw	1 medium	25
Popcorn, air popped	2 cups	62
Apple	1 medium	72
Vegetable soup	1 cup	72
Plain instant oatmeal	½ cup	80
Fresh blueberries	1 cup	80
Corn on the cob (plain)	1 ear	80
Cantaloupe	½ melon	95
Light (fat-free) yogurt with fruit	6 oz.	100
Unsweetened apple sauce	1 cup	100
Pear	1 medium	100
Corn flakes	1 cup	101
Sweet potato, baked	1 medium	120

Evaluating Fat and Sugar Substitutes

CRITICAL CONSUMER

Foods made with fat and sugar substitutes are often promoted for weight loss. But what are fat and sugar substitutes? And can they really contribute to weight management?

Fat Substitutes

A variety of substances are used to replace fats in processed foods and other products. Some contribute calories, protein, fiber, and/or other nutrients; others do not. Fat replacers can be classified into three general categories:

- *Carbohydrate-based fat replacers* include starch, fibers, gums, cellulose, polydextrose, and fruit purees. They are found in dairy and meat products, baked goods, salad dressing, and many other prepared foods. Newer types such as Oatrim, Z-trim, and Nu-trim are made from types of dietary fiber that may actually lower cholesterol levels. Carbohydrate-based fat replacers contribute up to 4 calories per gram.
- *Protein-based fat replacers* are typically made from milk, egg whites, soy, or whey; trade names include Simplesse, Dairy-lo, and Supro. They are used in cheese, sour cream, mayonnaise, margarine spreads, frozen desserts, salad dressings, and baked goods. These substances contribute 1–4 calories per gram.
- *Fat-based fat replacers* include glycerides, olestra, and other types of fatty acids. Some of these compounds are not absorbed well by the body and so provide fewer calories per gram (5 calories compared with the standard 9 for fats); others are impossible for the body to digest and so contribute no calories at all. Olestra, marketed under the trade name Olean and used in fried snack foods, is an example of the latter type of compound. Concerns have been raised about the safety of olestra because it reduces the absorption of fat-soluble nutrients and certain antioxidants and because it causes gastrointestinal distress in some people.

Nonnutritive Sweeteners and Sugar Alcohols

Sugar substitutes are often referred to as nonnutritive sweeteners because they provide no calories or essential nutrients. The Food and Drug Administration (FDA) has approved five types of nonnutritive sweeteners for use in the United States: acesulfame-K (Sunett, Sweet One), aspartame (NutraSweet, Equal, NatraTaste), saccharin (Sweet 'N Low), sucralose (Splenda), and neotame. They are used in beverages, desserts, baked goods, yogurt, chewing gum, and products such as toothpaste, mouthwash, and cough syrup. Another sweetener, stevia, is an extract of a South American shrub. The FDA has not objected to the use of stevia or sweeteners made from a highly processed component of stevia, called rebaudioside-A. Several such products are available.

Sugar alcohols are made by altering the chemical form of sugars extracted from fruits and other plant sources; they include erythritol, isomalt, lactitol, maltitol, mannitol, sorbitol, and zylitol. Sugar alcohols provide 0.2–2.5 calories per gram, compared to 4 calories per gram in standard sugar. They have typically been used to sweeten sugar-free candies but are now being added to many sweet foods (candy, cookies, and so on) promoted as low-carbohydrate products, often combined with other sweeteners. Sugar alcohols are digested in a way that can create gas, cramps, and diarrhea if they are consumed in large amounts—more than about 10 grams in one meal.

Fat and Sugar Substitutes in Weight Management

Whether fat and sugar substitutes help you achieve and maintain a healthy weight depends on your eating and activity habits. The increase in the availability of fat-free and sugar-free foods in the United States has *not* been associated with a drop in calorie consumption. When evaluating foods containing fat and sugar substitutes, consider these issues:

- ***Is the food lower in calories or just lower in fat?*** Reduced-fat foods often contain extra sugar to improve the taste and texture lost when fat is removed, so such foods may be as high or even higher in total calories than their fattier counterparts.
- ***Are you choosing foods with fat and/or sugar substitutes instead of foods you typically eat or in addition to foods you typically eat?*** If you consume low-fat, no-sugar-added ice cream instead of regular ice cream, you may save calories. But if you add such ice cream to your daily diet simply because it is lower in fat and sugar, your overall calorie consumption—and your weight—may increase.

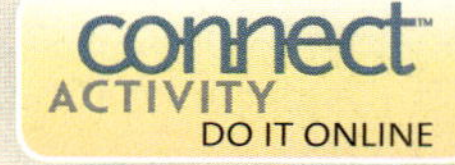

- ***Is an even healthier choice available?*** Many of the foods containing fat and sugar substitutes are low-nutrient snack foods. Fruits, vegetables, and whole grains are healthier snack choices.

for lowering the energy density of your diet include the following:

- Eat fruit with breakfast and for dessert.
- Add extra vegetables to sandwiches, casseroles, stir-fry dishes, pizza, pasta dishes, and fajitas.
- Start meals with a bowl of broth-based soup; include a green salad or fruit salad.
- Snack on fresh fruits and vegetables rather than crackers, chips, or other energy-dense snack foods.
- Limit serving sizes of energy-dense foods such as butter, mayonnaise, cheese, chocolate, fatty meats, croissants, and snack foods that are fried, are high in added sugars (including reduced-fat products), or contain trans fat.
- Avoid processed foods, which can be high in fat and sodium. Even processed foods labeled "fat-free" or "reduced fat" may be high in calories. Such products may contain sugar and fat substitutes (see the box "Evaluating Fat and Sugar Substitutes").

Eating Habits Equally important to weight management is eating small, frequent meals—four to five meals per day, including breakfast and snacks—on a regular schedule.

Nutrition Facts
Serving Size 1 cup (59g)
Servings per Container about 10

Amount per Serving	Cereal	Cereal with 1/2 cup Fat Free Milk
Calories	190	230
Calories from Fat	10	10
	% Daily Value**	
Total Fat 1g*	2%	2%
Saturated Fat 0g	0%	0%
Trans Fat 0g		
Polyunsaturated Fat 0.5g		
Monounsaturated Fat 0g		
Cholesterol 0mg	0%	0%
Sodium 775mg	13%	32%
Potassium 330mg	9%	15%
Total Carbohydrate 32g	15%	11%
Dietary Fiber 8g	32%	32%
Soluble Fiber 1g		
Sugars 4g		
Other Carbohydrate 19g		
Protein 4g		

Vitamin A	15%	20%
Vitamin C	2%	2%
Calcium	2%	15%
Iron	60%	60%
Vitamin D	10%	25%
Thiamin	25%	30%
Riboflavin	25%	35%
Niacin	25%	25%
Vitamin B6	25%	25%
Folic Acid	50%	50%
Vitamin B12	25%	35%
Phosphorus	20%	30%
Magnesium	25%	30%
Zinc	15%	20%
Copper	15%	15%

*Amount in Cereal. One half cup fat free milk contributes an additional 40 calories, 65mg sodium, 200mg potassium, 6g total carbohydrate (6g sugars), and 4g protein.
*Percent Daily Values are based on a 2,000 calorie diet. Your daily values may be higher or lower depending on your calorie needs:

	Calories	2,000	2,500
Total Fat	Less than	65g	80g
Sat Fat	Less than	20g	25g
Cholesterol	Less than	300mg	300mg
Sodium	Less than	2,400mg	2,400mg
Potassium		3,500mg	3,500mg
Total Carbohydrate		300g	375g
Dietary Fiber		25g	30g

INGREDIENTS: WHOLE WHEAT FLOUR, RAISINS, CORN SYRUP, SALT, MALTED BARLEY FLOUR.
VITAMINS AND MINERALS: REDUCED IRON, NIACINAMIDE, ZINC OXIDE (SOURCE OF ZINC), VITAMIN B_6, VITAMIN A PALMITATE, RIBOFLAVIN (VITAMIN B_2), THIAMIN MONONITRATE (VITAMIN B_1), FOLIC ACID, VITAMIN B_{12}, VITAMIN D.
MAY CONTAIN TRACES OF SOY.

FIGURE 7.3 High-fiber, low-calorie breakfast cereal. Many breakfast cereals are excellent sources of fiber, complex carbohydrates, and essential nutrients and are low in fat and cholesterol.

Skipping meals leads to excessive hunger, feelings of deprivation, and increased vulnerability to binge eating or snacking. Establish a regular pattern of eating, and set some rules governing food choices. Rules governing breakfast might be these, for example: Choose a low-sugar, high-fiber cereal (Figure 7.3) with nonfat milk and fruit most of the time; have a hard-boiled egg no more than three times a week; save pancakes and waffles for special occasions. For effective weight management, it is better to consume the majority of calories during the day rather than in the evening.

Decreeing some foods off-limits generally sets up a rule to be broken. A more sensible rule is "everything in moderation." No foods need to be entirely off-limits, though some should be eaten judiciously.

PHYSICAL ACTIVITY AND EXERCISE

Regular physical activity is another important lifestyle factor in weight management. Physical activity and exercise burn calories and keep the metabolism geared to using food for energy instead of storing it as fat. Making significant cuts in food intake in order to lose weight is a difficult strategy to maintain; increasing your physical activity is a much better approach. Regular physical activity also protects against weight gain and is essential for maintaining weight loss.

Physical Activity All physical activity will help you manage your weight. The first step in becoming more active is to incorporate more physical activity into your daily life. If you are currently sedentary, start by accumulating short bouts of moderate-intensity physical activity—walking, gardening, doing housework, and so on—for a total of 150 minutes or more per week. Even a small increase in activity level can help maintain your current weight or help you lose a moderate amount of weight. In fact, research suggests that fidgeting—stretching, squirming, standing up, and so on—may help prevent weight gain in some people. Short bouts of activity spread throughout the day can produce many of the same health benefits as continuous physical activity.

If you are overweight and want to lose weight, or if you are trying to maintain a lower weight following weight loss, a greater amount of physical activity can help. Researchers have found that people who lose weight and don't regain it typically burn about 2800 calories per week in physical activity—the equivalent of about 1 hour of brisk walking per day.

Exercise Once you become more active every day, begin a formal exercise program that includes cardiorespiratory endurance exercise, resistance training, and stretching exercises (see the box "What Is the Best Way to Exercise for Weight Loss?"). Moderate-intensity endurance exercise, if performed frequently for a relatively long duration, can burn a significant number of calories. Endurance training also increases the rate at which your body uses calories after your exercise session is over—burning an additional 5–180 extra calories, depending on the intensity of exercise. Resistance training builds muscle mass, and more muscle translates into a higher metabolic rate. Resistance training can also help you maintain your muscle mass during a period of weight loss, helping you avoid the significant drop in RMR associated with weight loss.

Regular physical activity, maintained throughout life, makes weight management easier. The sooner you establish good habits, the better. The key to success is making exercise an integral part of a lifestyle you can enjoy now and will enjoy in the future.

Fitness Tip

When you watch TV, turn commercial breaks into exercise breaks. When commercials come on, get off the couch and move: Do jumping jacks, push-ups, curl-ups, run in place, or just walk around. During a 2-hour program, you can accumulate about 30 minutes of physical activity this way!

What Is the Best Way to Exercise for Weight Loss?

THE EVIDENCE FOR EXERCISE

If weight loss is your primary goal, the guidelines for planning a fitness program can vary depending on your weight, body composition, and current level of fitness. For example, there is some dispute among fitness experts about the best target heart rate (THR) zone to use when exercising for weight loss. Some experts recommend exercising at a moderate THR (55–69% of maximum heart rate) because the body burns fat at a slightly more efficient rate at this level of exertion. Others recommend exercising vigorously (70–90% of maximum heart rate) because exercise at this intensity burns more calories overall. According to some estimates, for example, a 30-minute workout at 80–85% of maximum heart rate burns about 30% more calories overall than a 30-minute workout at 60–65% maximum heart rate—but the lower-intensity workout burns roughly 20% more fat calories than the higher-intensity workout.

Regardless, if you are obese or your fitness level is very low, start with a lower-intensity workout (55% of maximum heart rate), and stick with it until your cardiorespiratory fitness level improves enough to support short bouts of higher-intensity exercise. This way, you will burn more fat, reduce the risk of injury and strain on your heart, and improve your chances of staying with your program. Even if your primary goal is to lose weight, you are also improving your cardiorespiratory fitness. Any amount of exercise, even at low to moderate intensity, will help you achieve both goals. But patience is required, especially if you need to lose a great deal of weight.

For weight loss to occur, exercise at lower intensities has to be offset by longer and/or more frequent exercise sessions. Experts recommend 60–90 minutes of daily exercise for anyone who needs to lose weight or maintain weight loss. If you cannot fit such a large block of activity into your daily schedule, break your workouts into short segments—as little as 10–15 minutes each. This approach is probably best for someone who has been sedentary, because it allows the body to become accustomed to exercise at a gradual pace while preventing injury and avoiding strain on the heart.

Many research studies have shown that walking is an ideal form of exercise for losing weight and avoiding weight gain. A landmark 15-year study by the University of North Carolina at Charlotte showed that, over time, people who walked only 30 minutes per day gained 18 pounds less than people who did not walk. Those who regularly walked farther were better able to lose or maintain weight. Other studies found that people who walked 30 minutes five times per week lost an average of 5 pounds in 6–12 months, without dieting, watching what they ate, or exercising intensely. You can lose even more weight if you eat sensibly and walk farther and faster.

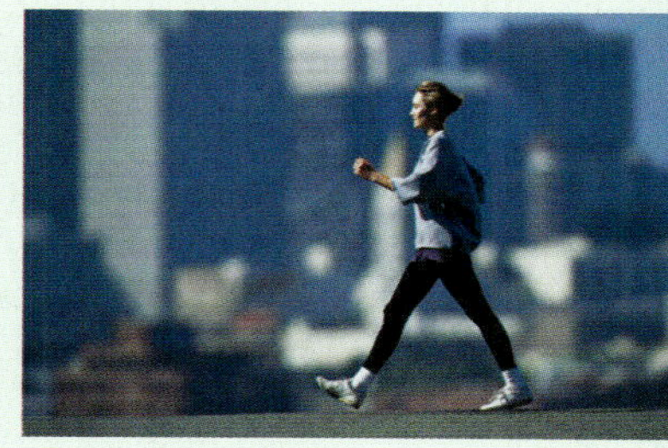

A 165-pound adult who walks at a speed of 3 miles per hour for 60 minutes a day, 5 days a week, can lose about one-half pound of body weight per week. Regular walking is the simplest and most effective health habit for controlling body weight and promoting health. Even if you're sedentary, a few months of walking can increase your fitness level to the point where more vigorous types of exercise—and even greater health benefits—are possible.

SOURCES: Gordon-Larsen, P., et al. 2009. Fifteen-year longitudinal trends in walking patterns and their impact on weight change. *American Journal of Clinical Nutrition* 89(1): 19–26. Levine, J. A., et al. 2008. The role of free-living daily walking in human weight gain and obesity. *Diabetes* 57(3): 548–554. Nelson, M. E., and S. C. Folta. 2009. Further evidence for the benefits of walking. *American Journal of Clinical Nutrition* 89(1): 15–16. Physical Activity Guidelines Advisory Committee. 2008. *Physical Activity Guidelines Advisory Committee Report, 2008*. Washington, D.C.: U.S. Department of Health and Human Services.

THOUGHTS AND EMOTIONS

The way you think about yourself and your world influences, and is influenced by, how you feel and how you act. In fact, research on people who have a weight problem indicates that low self-esteem and the negative emotions that accompany it are significant problems. People with low self-esteem mentally compare the actual self to an internally held picture of the "ideal self," an image based on perfectionist goals and beliefs about how they and others should be. The more these two pictures differ, the larger the impact on self-esteem and the more likely the presence of negative emotions.

Besides the internal picture we carry of ourselves, all of us carry on an internal dialogue about events happening to us and around us. This *self-talk* can be either self-deprecating or positively motivating, depending on our beliefs and attitudes. Having realistic beliefs and goals and engaging in positive self-talk and problem solving support a healthy lifestyle. (Chapter 10 and Activity 11 in the Behavior Change Workbook at the end of the text include strategies for developing realistic self-talk.)

Coping Strategies

Appropriate coping strategies help you deal with the stresses of life; they are also an important lifestyle factor

Ask Yourself

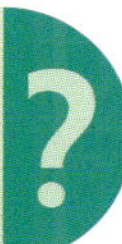

QUESTIONS FOR CRITICAL THINKING AND REFLECTION

Have you ever used food as an escape when you were stressed out or distraught? Were you aware of what you were doing at the time? How can you avoid using food as a coping mechanism in the future?

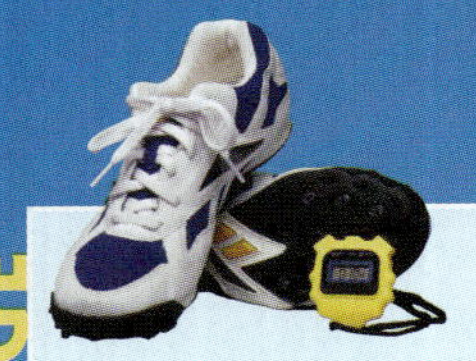

PERSONAL CHALLENGE

If you're trying to lose weight or maintain your current weight, it's a good idea to write down everything you eat, including how many calories it contains. Researchers have found that writing down the food choices you make every day increases your commitment and helps you stick to your diet, especially during high-risk times such as holidays, parties, and family gatherings.

Writing every day also serves as a reminder to you that losing weight is important. In a multicenter study conducted over 6 months in 2008, dieters who kept a daily food journal lost twice as much weight as those who didn't track what they ate.

Besides tracking what you eat, keep track of your formal exercise program and other daily physical activities so you can begin increasing either their intensity or duration. People who succeed in their health program expend lots of energy in physical activity—according to one study, an average of 2700 calories a week. Tracking your physical activities and daily exercise routines provides all the same benefits as tracking your eating habits. Your log will help you see your progress, track fitness improvements and weight loss, and maintain a positive perspective on your efforts. All this will help you take your program seriously over the long term.

in weight management. Many people use eating as a way to cope; others may use drugs, alcohol, smoking, or gambling. Those who overeat might use food to alleviate loneliness or to serve as a pickup for fatigue, as an antidote to boredom, or as a distraction from problems. Some people even overeat to punish themselves for real or imagined transgressions.

Those who recognize that they are misusing food in such ways can analyze their eating habits with fresh eyes. They can consciously attempt to find new coping strategies and begin to use food appropriately—to fuel life's activities, to foster growth, and to bring pleasure, but *not* to manage stress. For a summary of the components of weight management through healthy lifestyle choices, see the box "Lifestyle Strategies for Successful Weight Management."

APPROACHES TO OVERCOMING A WEIGHT PROBLEM

Each year, Americans spend more than $40 billion on various weight-loss plans and products. If you are overweight, you may already be creating a plan to lose weight and keep it off. You have many options.

Doing It Yourself

If you need to lose weight, focus on adopting the healthy lifestyle described throughout this book. The "right" weight for you will evolve naturally, and you won't have to diet. Combine modest cuts in energy intake with exercise, and avoid very-low-calorie diets. (In general, a low-calorie diet should provide 1200–1500 calories per day.) By achieving a negative energy balance of 250–1000 calories per day, you'll produce the recommended weight loss of ½–2 pounds per week.

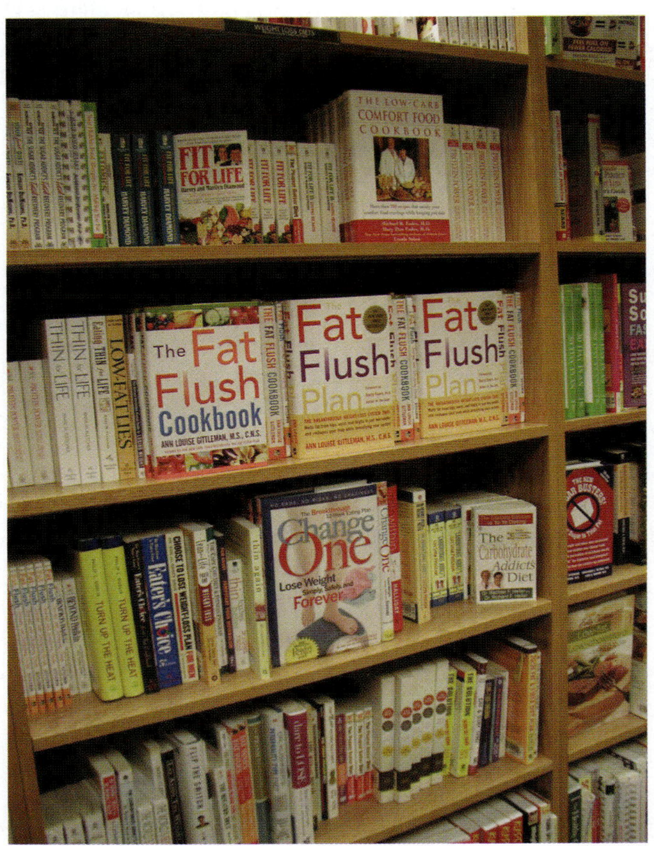

There are many plans and supplements promoted for weight loss, but few have any research supporting their effectiveness for long-term weight management.

Most low-calorie diets cause a rapid loss of body water at first. When this phase passes, weight loss declines. As

Lifestyle Strategies for Successful Weight Management

TAKE CHARGE

Food Choices

• Focus on making good choices from each food group.

• Favor foods with a *low energy (calorie) density* and a *high nutrient density*.

• Check labels for serving sizes, calories, and nutrients.

• Watch for hidden calories. Reduced-fat foods often have as many calories as their full-fat versions.

• Drink fewer calories in the form of soda, fruit drinks, sports drinks, alcohol, and specialty coffees and teas.

Planning and Serving

• Keep a log of what you eat, as described earlier in the text.

• Eat four to five meals/snacks daily, *including breakfast*, to distribute calories throughout your day.

• Fix more meals yourself and eat out less often.

• Keep low-calorie snacks on hand to combat the "munchies." Fresh fruits and vegetables are good choices.

• When shopping, make a list and stick to it. Don't shop when you're hungry. Avoid aisles that contain problem foods.

• Consume the majority of your daily calories during the day, not in the evening.

• Pay attention to portion sizes. Use measuring cups and spoons and a food scale to become familiar with portion sizes.

• Serve meals on small plates and in small bowls to help you eat smaller portions without feeling deprived.

• Eat only in specifically designated spots. Remove food from other areas of your home.

• When you eat, just eat. Don't do anything else.

• Avoid late-night eating, a behavior specifically associated with weight gain among college students.

• Eat slowly. It takes time for your brain to get the message that your stomach is full. Take small bites and chew food thoroughly. Pay attention to every bite, and enjoy your food.

Special Occasions

• When you eat out, choose a restaurant where you can make healthy food choices. Ask the server not to put bread and butter on the table before the meal, and request that sauces and salad dressings be served on the side. If portion sizes are large, take half your food home for a meal later in the week. Don't choose supersized meals.

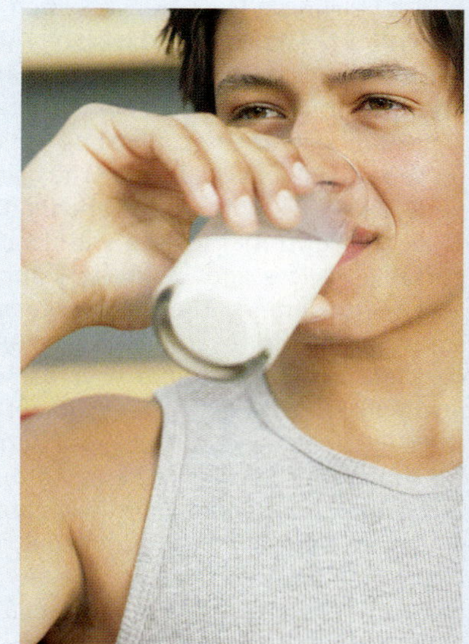

• If you cook a large meal for friends, send leftovers home with your guests.

• If you're eating at a friend's home, eat a little and leave the rest. Don't eat to be polite.

Physical Activity and Stress Management

• Increase your level of daily physical activity, as slowly as necessary based on your current fitness level.

• Begin an exercise program that includes cardiorespiratory endurance exercise, strength training, and stretching.

• Develop techniques for handling stress. See Chapter 10 for more on stress management.

• Develop strategies for coping with nonhunger cues to eat, such as boredom, sleepiness, or anxiety. Try calling a friend, taking a shower, or reading a magazine.

• Tell family members and friends that you're changing your eating and exercise habits. Ask them to be supportive.

Visit the Small Steps site for more tips (www.smallstep.gov).

a result, dieters are often misled into believing that their efforts are not working. They give up, not realizing that smaller losses later in the diet are actually more significant than the initial big losses, because later loss is mostly fat loss, whereas initial loss is primarily fluid. For someone who is overweight, reasonable weight loss is 8–10% of body weight over 6 months.

For many Americans, maintaining weight loss is a bigger challenge than losing weight. Most weight lost during a period of dieting is regained. When planning a weight-management program, you need to include strategies that you can maintain over the long term, both for food choices and for physical activity. Weight management is a lifelong project. A registered dietitian or nutritionist can recommend an appropriate plan for you when you want to lose weight on your own. For more tips on losing weight on your own, refer to the section later in the chapter on creating an individual weight-management plan.

Diet Books

Many people who try to lose weight by themselves fall prey to one or more of the dozens of diet books on the market. Although some books contain useful advice and

WELLNESS IN THE DIGITAL AGE

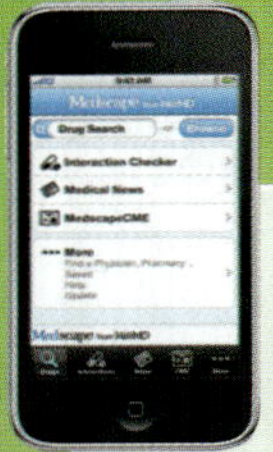

High-Tech Weight Management

Technology is making inroads into the area of weight management at an ever-quickening pace. Once the domain of clinical weight-loss programs, digital tools are now available for consumers who want to lose weight or keep it off.

At the clinical level, new research shows that overweight patients who are equipped with high-tech monitoring devices (which monitor their energy intake and output) lose at least as much weight as patients who participate only in in-person weight-management counseling sessions. When person-to-person counseling is added to the use of digital monitors, patients lose even more weight and manage to keep it off longer.

At the consumer level, a wide and ever-growing range of portable devices and weight-loss applications are also available to consumers. There are dozens of "apps" that run on smart phones, for example, which can help you keep a nutrition journal and calculate your daily intake of calories and nutrients. Such apps often pair with other programs that can help you track your physical activity level and calculate the number of calories you burn throughout the day. Some of these apps can upload your daily data to a Web site that lets you track energy intake and output over the course of time. Many such programs can also help with goal-setting, provide dietary or exercise advice, or let you join communities of users who are also trying to manage their weight.

Internet-based weight-loss programs have proliferated over the last decade. Most such Web sites offer a cross between self-help and group support through chat rooms, bulletin boards, and e-newsletters. Many sites offer online self-assessment for diet and physical activity habits as well as a meal plan; some provide access to a staff professional for individualized help. Many are free, but some charge a weekly or monthly fee.

Research suggests that this type of program provides an alternative to in-person diet counseling and can lead to weight loss for some people. Studies found that people who logged on more frequently tended to lose more weight; weekly online contact in terms of behavior therapy proved most successful for weight loss. The criteria used to evaluate commercial programs can also be applied to Internet-based programs. If you're interested in joining an online weight-loss program, make sure the service offers member-to-member support and access to staff professionals.

An example of a particularly successful online weight-management program is the National Weight Control

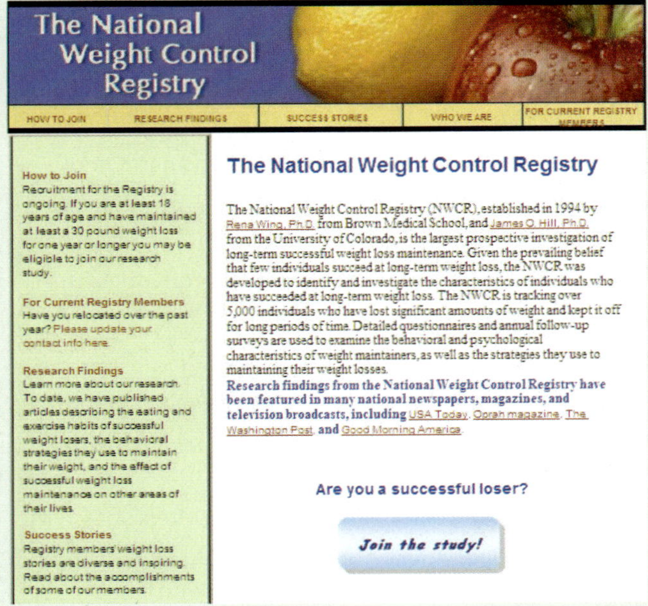

Registry. This site is part of an ongoing study of people who have lost significant amounts of weight and kept it off. The average participant in the registry has lost 71 pounds and kept the weight off for more than 5 years. Nearly all participants use a combination of diet and exercise to manage their weight. Most follow moderate-calorie diets that are relatively low in fat and fried foods; users monitor their body weight and their food intake frequently. Participants engage in an average of 60 minutes of moderate physical activity daily. The National Weight Control Registry study illustrates that to lose weight and keep it off, you must decrease daily calorie intake and/or increase daily physical activity—and continue to do so over your lifetime. And this fact is an important lesson: Even with the help of digital devices and programs, weight management is still primarily a matter of personal effort, perseverance, and a commitment to lifestyle changes that last for life.

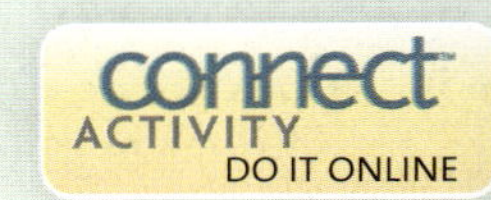

SOURCE: The National Weight Control Registry, www.nwcr.ws. Screen reprinted by permission.

motivational tips, most make empty promises. Accept books that advocate a balanced approach to diet plus exercise and sound nutritional advice, but reject any book that:

- Advocates an unbalanced way of eating, such as a high-carbohydrate-only diet or a low-carbohydrate, high-protein diet, or that promotes a single food, such as cabbage or grapefruit.
- Claims to be based on a "scientific breakthrough" or to have the "secret to success."
- Uses gimmicks, such as matching eating to blood type, hyping insulin resistance as the cause of obesity, or combining foods in special ways to achieve weight loss.
- Promises quick weight loss or limits the selection of foods.

Many diets cause weight loss if maintained. The real difficulty is finding a safe and healthy pattern of food choices and physical activity that results in long-term maintenance of a healthy body weight and reduced risk of chronic disease (see the box "High-Tech Weight Management").

Dietary Supplements and Diet Aids

The number of dietary supplements and other weight-loss aids on the market has also increased in recent years. Promoted in advertisements, magazines, direct mail campaigns, infomercials, and on Web sites, these products typically promise a quick and easy path to weight loss. Most of these products are marketed as dietary supplements and so are subject to fewer regulations than over the counter (OTC) medications. A 2002 report from the Federal Trade Commission stated that more than half of advertisements for weight-loss products made representations that are likely to be false.

In late 2008, the FDA identified more than 25 weight-loss pill products that consumers should not purchase or use and ordered the products recalled from stores. Such recalls are becoming more common. Studies revealed that some of the recalled supplements contained prescription medications, including sibutramine (a weight-loss medication sold under the brand name Meridia) and phenytoin, an antiseizure medication. In its consumer alert, the FDA noted that a number of the recalled supplements contained pharmaceuticals in amounts far exceeding FDA-recommended levels. Some of the supplements contained substances that are not approved for sale in the United States, including rimonabant (a prescription weight-loss drug sold in Europe) and phenolphthalein, which is thought to be a carcinogen. The use of these drugs could lead to complications such as heart attack, stroke, suicide, and even cancer. The prescription medications were not listed on any of the supplements' labels, meaning consumers could be taking lethal doses of prescription drugs without knowing it.

The following sections describe some commonly marketed OTC products for weight loss.

Formula Drinks and Food Bars Canned diet drinks, powders used to make shakes, and diet food bars and snacks are designed to achieve weight loss by substituting for some or all of a person's daily food intake. However, most people find it difficult to use these products for long periods, and muscle loss and other serious health problems may result if they are used as the sole source of nutrition for an extended period. Use of such products sometimes results in rapid short-term weight loss, but the weight is typically regained because users don't learn to change their eating and lifestyle behaviors.

Wellness Tip

If you're tempted to start taking an OTC weight-loss supplement, do your homework first. Ask for your doctor's opinion, and check the FDA's supplement Web page at http://www.fda.gov/Food/DietarySupplements/default.htm.

Herbal Supplements As described in Chapter 3, herbs are marketed as dietary supplements, so there is little information about effectiveness, proper dosage, drug interactions, and side effects. In addition, labels may not accurately reflect the ingredients and dosages present, and safe manufacturing practices are not guaranteed. For example, the substitution of a toxic herb for another compound during the manufacture of a Chinese herbal weight-loss preparation caused more than 100 cases of kidney damage and cancer among users in Europe.

The FDA has banned the sale of ephedra (*ma huang*), stating that it presented a significant and unreasonable risk to human health. Ephedrine, the active ingredient in ephedra, is structurally similar to amphetamine and was widely used in weight-loss supplements. It may suppress appetite, but adverse effects have included elevated blood pressure, panic attacks, seizures, insomnia, and increased risk of heart attack or stroke, particularly when combined with another stimulant, such as caffeine. The FDA banned the synthetic stimulant phenylpropanolamine for similar reasons. Other herbal stimulants still on the market are described in Table 7.3.

Other Supplements Fiber is another common ingredient in OTC diet aids, promoted for appetite control. However, dietary fiber acts as a bulking agent in the large intestine, not the stomach, so it doesn't have a pronounced effect on appetite. In addition, many diet aids contain only 3 or fewer grams of fiber, which does not contribute much toward the recommended daily intake of 25–38 grams.

Other popular dietary supplements include conjugated linoleic acid, carnitine, chromium, pyruvate, calcium, B vitamins, chitosan, and a number of products labeled "fat absorbers," "fat blockers," or "starch blockers." Research has not found these products to be effective, and many have potentially adverse side effects.

Weight-Loss Programs

Weight-loss programs come in a variety of types, including noncommercial support organizations, commercial programs, Web sites, and clinical programs.

A study lasting from 2008 to 2011 revealed an interesting phenomenon regarding weight-loss interventions among college students: Groups of students who shared certain characteristics did better at losing and managing weight than groups of dissimilar students. The study grouped students according to common eating habits or common psychosocial characteristics, both of which contribute to weight gain. These "clusters" of similar students were able to lose more weight and keep more weight off than were "nonclustered" groups of students who did not share common dietary or psychosocial characteristics. The findings of this study may help shape group-oriented weight-loss programs in the future, whether such programs are commercial, noncommercial, or clinical.

Table 7.3 Ingredients Commonly Found in Weight-Loss Products

COMMON NAME	USE/CLAIM	EVIDENCE/EFFICACY	SAFETY ISSUES
Bitter orange extract (*Citrus aurantium*)	CNS stimulant	Limited evidence	Highly concentrated extracts may increase blood pressure; should not be used by people with cardiac problems
Caffeine	CNS stimulant; increases fat metabolism	Amplifies effects of ephedra	Generally considered safe; caution advised in caffeine-sensitive individuals
Garcinia cambogia	May interfere with fat metabolism or suppress appetite	Inconclusive evidence	Short-term use (<12 weeks) generally considered safe when used as directed
Green tea extract	Diuretic; increases metabolism	Limited evidence	Generally considered safe
Guarana	CNS stimulant; diuretic	Few clinical trials	Same as for caffeine; overdose can cause painful urination, abdominal spasms, and vomiting
Senna, cascara, aloe, buckthorn berries	Stimulant, laxative	Not effective for weight loss	Chronic use decreases muscle tone in large intestine, causes electrolyte imbalances, and leads to dependence on laxatives
Tea, kola, dandelion, bucho, uva-ursi, damiana, juniper	Diuretic	Not effective for weight loss	Chronic use can cause possible electrolyte imbalance in some people
Yerba mate	Stimulant, laxative, diuretic	Limited evidence	Long-term use as a beverage may increase the risk of oral cancer

SOURCE: Adapted from Leslie, K. K. 2003. Herbal weight-loss products: Effective and appropriate? *Today's Dietician* 5(8).

Noncommercial Weight-Loss Programs Noncommercial programs such as TOPS (Take Off Pounds Sensibly) and Overeaters Anonymous (OA) mainly provide group support. They do not advocate any particular diet, but they do recommend seeking professional advice for creating an individualized diet and exercise plan. Like Alcoholics Anonymous, OA is a 12-step program with a spiritual orientation that promotes abstinence from compulsive overeating. These types of programs are generally free. Your physician or a registered dietitian can also provide information and support for weight loss.

Commercial Weight-Loss Programs Commercial weight-loss programs typically provide group support, nutrition education, physical activity recommendations, and behavior modification advice. Some also make packaged foods available to assist in following dietary advice.

A responsible and safe weight-loss program should have the following features:

- The recommended diet should be safe and balanced, include all the food groups, and meet the Dietary Reference Intakes (DRIs) for all nutrients. Physical activity and exercise should be strongly encouraged.
- The program should promote slow, steady weight loss averaging ½–2 pounds per week. (There may be rapid weight loss initially due to fluid loss.)
- If a participant plans to lose more than 20 pounds, has any health problems, or is taking medication on a regular basis, the program should offer physician evaluation and monitoring. The program's staff should include qualified counselors and health professionals.
- The program should include plans for weight maintenance after the weight-loss phase is over.
- The program should provide information on all fees and costs, including those of supplements and prepackaged foods, as well as data on risks and expected outcomes of participating in the program.

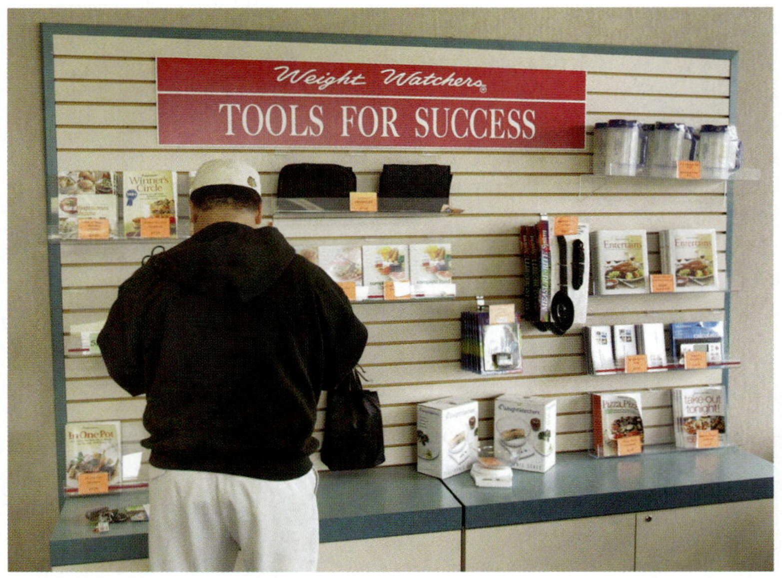

A variety of commercial weight-loss programs are available. These programs yield mixed results, but most provide nutritional counseling and support for people who are serious about losing weight.

You should also consider whether a program fits your lifestyle and whether you are truly ready to make a commitment to it. A strong commitment and a plan for maintenance are especially important because only 10–15% of program participants maintain their weight loss; the rest gain back all or more than they had lost. One study of participants found that regular exercise was the best predictor of maintaining weight loss, and frequent television viewing was the best predictor of weight gain.

Clinical Weight-Loss Programs Medically supervised clinical programs are usually located in a hospital or other medical setting. Designed to help those who are severely obese, these programs typically involve a closely monitored very-low-calorie diet. The cost of a clinical program is usually high, but insurance often covers part of the fee.

Prescription Drugs

For a medicine to cause weight loss, it must reduce energy consumption, increase energy expenditure, and/or interfere with energy absorption. The medications most often prescribed for weight loss are appetite suppressants that reduce feelings of hunger or increase feelings of fullness. Appetite suppressants usually work by increasing levels of catecholamine or serotonin, two brain chemicals that affect mood and appetite.

All prescription weight-loss drugs have potential side effects. Those that affect catecholamine levels, including phentermine (Ionamin, Obenix, Fastin, and Adipex-P), diethylpropion (Tenuate), and mazindol (Sanorex), may cause sleeplessness, nervousness, and euphoria.

Most appetite suppressants are approved by the FDA only for short-term use. One drug—orlistat (Xenical)—is approved for longer-term use. Orlistat lowers calorie consumption by blocking fat absorption in the intestines; it prevents about 30% of the fat in food from being digested. Similar to the fat substitute olestra, orlistat also reduces the absorption of fat-soluble vitamins and antioxidants.

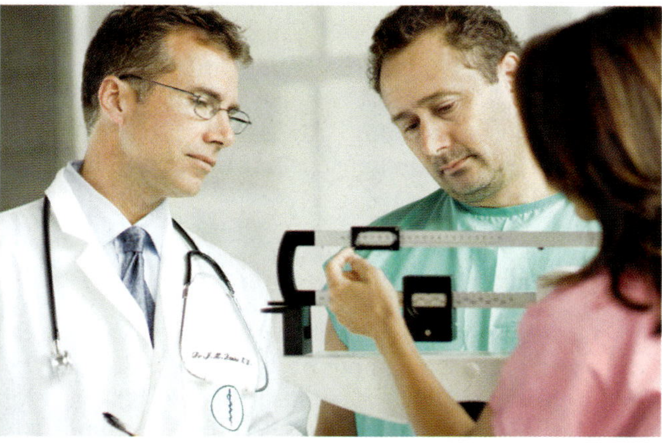

Very obese people may get the most benefit from a clinical weight-loss program, where diet and activity are monitored closely by health professionals.

Therefore, taking a vitamin supplement is highly recommended if taking orlistat. Side effects include diarrhea, cramping, and other gastrointestinal problems if users do not follow a low-fat diet. In 2007, the FDA approved Alli, a lower-dose version of orlistat that is sold over the counter.

All of these medications work best in conjunction with behavior modification. Appetite suppressants produce modest weight loss—about 5–22 pounds above the loss expected with nondrug obesity treatments. Individuals respond differently, however, and some experience more weight loss than others. Weight loss tends to level off or reverse after 4–6 months on a medication, and many people regain the weight they've lost when they stop taking the drug.

Prescription weight-loss drugs are not for people who just want to lose a few pounds. The latest federal guidelines advise people to try lifestyle modification for at least 6 months before trying drug therapy. Prescription drugs are recommended only in certain cases: for people who have been unable to lose weight with nondrug options and who have a body mass index (BMI) over 30 (or over 27 if two or more additional risk factors such as diabetes and high blood pressure are present). For severely obese people who have been unable to lose weight by other methods, prescription drugs may provide a good option.

Surgery

It is estimated that 5.7% of adult Americans have a BMI grreater than 40, qualifying them as severely or "morbidly" obese. The number of severely obese people has nearly doubled in the last two decades. Severe obesity is a serious medical condition that is often complicated by other health problems such as diabetes, sleep disorders, heart disease, and arthritis. Surgical intervention—known as *bariatric surgery*—may be necessary as a treatment of last resort. Bariatric surgery may be recommended for patients with a BMI greater than 40, or greater than 35 with obesity-related illnesses.

Due to the increasing prevalence of severe obesity, surgical treatment of obesity is growing worldwide. Obesity-related health conditions, as well as risk of premature death, generally improve after surgical weight loss. Surgery, however, is not without risks. A 2006 study found that patients with poor cardiorespiratory fitness prior to surgery experienced more postoperative complications, including stroke, kidney failure, and even death, than patients with higher fitness levels.

Bariatric surgery modifies the gastrointestinal tract by changing the size of the stomach by partitioning the stomach with staples or a band, or by modifying the way the stomach drains (gastric bypass). In either type of surgical intervention, the goal is to promote weight loss by reducing the amount of food the patient can eat. The two most common surgeries are the Roux-en-Y gastric bypass and the vertical banded gastroplasty (VGB/Lap-Band). Potential complications from surgery include nutritional deficiencies, fat intolerance, nausea,

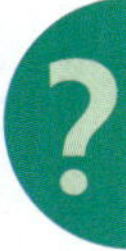

Ask Yourself

QUESTIONS FOR CRITICAL THINKING AND REFLECTION

Why do you think people continue to buy into fad diets and weight-loss gimmicks, even though they are constantly reminded that the key to weight management is lifestyle change? Have you ever tried a fad diet or dietary supplement? If so, what were your reasons for trying it? What were the results?

vomiting, and reflux. As many as 10–20% of patients may require follow-up surgery to address complications. According to a 2009 study by the Agency for Healthcare Research and Quality, however, the rate of complications in bariatric surgery patients fell more than 20% from 2002–2006. This drop in complications has reduced the number of rehospitalizations for bariatric surgery patients, and has also helped bring down the overall cost of these procedures.

Weight loss from surgery generally ranges between 40% and 70% of total body weight over the course of a year. The key to success is to have adequate follow-up and to stay motivated so that life behaviors and eating patterns are changed permanently.

The surgical technique of liposuction involves the removal of small amounts of fat from specific locations. Liposuction is not a method for treating obesity.

Psychological Help

When concerns about body weight and shape have developed into an eating disorder, professional help is recommended. Therapists who help people with these disorders should have experience in weight management, body image issues, eating disorders, addictions, and abuse issues.

BODY IMAGE

The collective picture of the body as seen through the mind's eye, **body image** consists of perceptions, images, thoughts, attitudes, and emotions. A negative body image is characterized by dissatisfaction with the body in general or some part of the body in particular.

More and more people are becoming unhappy with their bodies and obsessed with their weight. In recent surveys, more than half of Americans have stated that they are dissatisfied with their weight; only about 10% report being completely satisfied with their bodies. Dissatisfaction with body weight and shape is associated with dangerous eating patterns, such as binge eating or self-starvation, and with eating disorders.

Fitness Tip

It may not be possible to be "too fit," but it is possible to exercise too much. This is a common problem among people who are obsessed with their weight or body image. Track your exercise habits for a week; if they seem excessive and you can't seem to cut back, talk to a professional counselor or your doctor to find out if you have a body image problem.

Severe Body Image Problems

Poor body image can cause significant psychological distress. A person can become preoccupied by a perceived defect in appearance, thereby damaging self-esteem and interfering with relationships. Adolescents and adults who have a negative body image are more likely to diet restrictively, eat compulsively, or develop some other form of disordered eating.

When dissatisfaction becomes extreme, the condition is called *body dysmorphic disorder (BDD)*. BDD affects about 2% of Americans, males and females in equal numbers. BDD usually begins before age 18 but can begin in adulthood. Sufferers are overly concerned with physical appearance, often focusing on slight flaws that are not obvious to others. Individuals with BDD may spend hours every day thinking about their flaws and looking at themselves in mirrors; they may desire and seek repeated cosmetic surgeries. BDD is related to obsessive-compulsive disorder and can lead to depression, social phobia, and suicide if left untreated. Medication and therapy can help people with BDD.

In some cases, body image may bear little resemblance to fact. A person with the eating disorder anorexia nervosa typically has a severely distorted body image, believing herself to be fat even when she has become emaciated (see the next section for more on anorexia). Distorted body image is also a hallmark of *muscle dysmorphia,* a disorder experienced by some bodybuilders and other active people who see themselves as small and out of shape despite being very muscular. People with muscle dysmorphia may let obsessive weight training interfere with their work and relationships. They may also use potentially dangerous muscle-building drugs.

To assess your body image, complete the body image self-test in Lab 7.3.

Acceptance and Change

There are limits to the changes that can be made to body weight and body shape, both of which are influenced by heredity. Knowing when the limits to healthy change have been reached—and learning to accept those limits—is crucial for overall wellness. Women in particular tend to measure self-worth in terms of their appearance. When they don't measure up to an unrealistic cultural ideal,

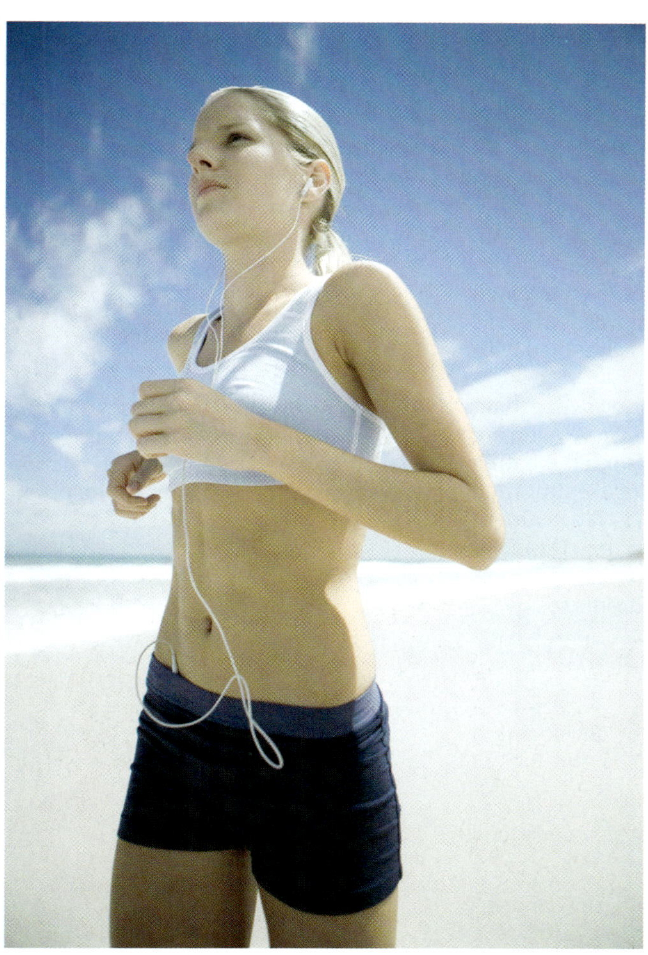

Exercise is a healthy practice, but people with eating disorders sometimes exercise compulsively, building their lives around their workouts. Compulsive exercise can lead to injuries, low body fat, and other health problems.

they see themselves as defective, and their self-esteem falls. The result can be negative body image, disordered eating, or even a full-blown eating disorder (see the box "Gender, Ethnicity, and Body Image").

Weight management needs to take place in a positive and realistic atmosphere. For an obese person, losing as few as 10 pounds can reduce blood pressure and improve mood. The hazards of excessive dieting and overconcern about body weight need to be countered by a change in attitude. A reasonable weight must take into account a person's weight history, social circumstances, metabolic profile, and psychological well-being.

EATING DISORDERS

Problems with body weight and weight control are not limited to excessive body fat. A growing number of people, especially adolescent girls and young women, experience **eating disorders,** characterized by severe disturbances in body image, eating patterns, and eating-related behavior. The major eating disorders are anorexia nervosa, bulimia nervosa, and binge-eating disorder. Eating disorders affect about 10 million American females and 1 million males. Many more people have abnormal eating habits and attitudes about food that, although not meeting the criteria for a major eating disorder, do disrupt their lives. To assess your eating habits, complete Lab 7.3.

Although many different explanations for the development of eating disorders have been proposed, they share one central feature: a dissatisfaction with body image and body weight. Such dissatisfaction is created by distorted thinking, including perfectionist beliefs, unreasonable demands for self-control, and excessive self-criticism. Dissatisfaction with body weight leads to dysfunctional attitudes about eating, such as fear of fat, preoccupation with food, and problematic eating behaviors. Eating disorders are classified as mental disorders.

Anorexia Nervosa

A person with **anorexia nervosa** does not eat enough food to maintain a reasonable body weight. Anorexia affects 1% of Americans, or about 3 million people, 95% of them female. Although it can occur later, anorexia typically develops between ages 12 and 18.

People with anorexia have an intense fear of gaining weight or becoming fat. Their body image is distorted so that, even when emaciated, they think they are fat. People with anorexia may engage in compulsive behaviors or rituals that help them keep from eating. They also commonly use vigorous and prolonged physical activity to reduce body weight. Although they may express a great interest in food, their diet becomes more and more extreme.

People with anorexia are typically introverted, emotionally reserved, and socially insecure. Their entire sense of self-esteem may be tied up in their evaluation of their body shape and weight.

Anorexia nervosa has been linked to a variety of medical complications, including disorders of the cardiovascular, gastrointestinal, and endocrine systems. Because of extreme weight loss, females with anorexia often stop menstruating. When body fat is virtually gone and muscles are severely wasted, the body turns to its organs in a desperate search for protein. Death can occur from heart failure caused by electrolyte imbalances. About one in ten

body image The mental representation a person holds about her or his body at any given moment in time, consisting of perceptions, images, thoughts, attitudes, and emotions about the body.

eating disorder A serious disturbance in eating patterns or eating-related behavior, characterized by a negative body image and concerns about body weight or body fat.

anorexia nervosa An eating disorder characterized by a refusal to maintain body weight at a minimally healthy level and an intense fear of gaining weight or becoming fat; self-starvation.

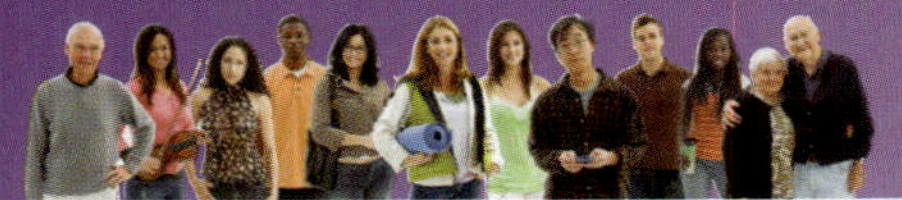

DIMENSIONS OF DIVERSITY

Gender, Ethnicity, and Body Image

Body Image and Gender

Women are much more likely than men to be dissatisfied with their bodies, often wanting to be thinner than they are. In one study, only 30% of eighth-grade girls reported being content with their bodies, while 70% of their male classmates expressed satisfaction with their looks. Girls and women are much more likely than boys and men to diet, develop eating disorders, and be obese.

The image of the ideal woman presented in the media is often unrealistic and even unhealthy. In a review of BMI data for Miss America pageant winners since 1922, researchers noted a significant decline in BMI over time, with an increasing number of recent winners having BMIs in the "underweight" category. The average fashion model is 4–7 inches taller and almost 50 pounds lighter than the average American woman. Most fashion models are thinner than 98% of American women.

Our culture may be promoting an unattainable masculine ideal as well. Researchers have found that media consumption is positively associated with a desire for thinness and muscularity. Researchers studying male action figures note that they have become increasingly muscular. Such media messages can be demoralizing; although not as commonly as girls and women, boys and men also suffer from body image problems.

Body Image and Ethnicity

Although some groups espouse thinness as an ideal body type, others do not. In many traditional African societies, for example, full-figured women's bodies are seen as symbols of health, prosperity, and fertility. African American teenage girls have a more positive body image than white girls; in one survey, two-thirds of them defined beauty as "the right attitude," whereas white girls were more preoccupied with weight and body shape.

Nevertheless, recent evidence indicates that African American women are as likely to engage in disordered eating behavior—especially binge eating and vomiting—as their Latina, Native American, and white counterparts. This finding underscores the complex nature of eating disorders and body image.

Avoiding Body-Image Problems

To minimize your risk of developing a body-image problem, keep the following strategies in mind:

- Focus on healthy habits and good physical health.
- Put concerns about physical appearance in perspective. Your worth as a human being does not depend on how you look.
- Practice body acceptance. You can influence your body size and type through lifestyle to some degree, but the fact is that some people are genetically designed to be bigger or heavier than others.
- Find things to appreciate in yourself besides an idealized body image. People who can learn to value other aspects of themselves are more accepting of the physical changes that occur naturally with age.
- View eating as a morally neutral activity—eating dessert isn't "bad" and doesn't make you a bad person.
- See the beauty and fitness industries for what they are. Realize that their goal is to prompt dissatisfaction with yourself so that you will buy their products.

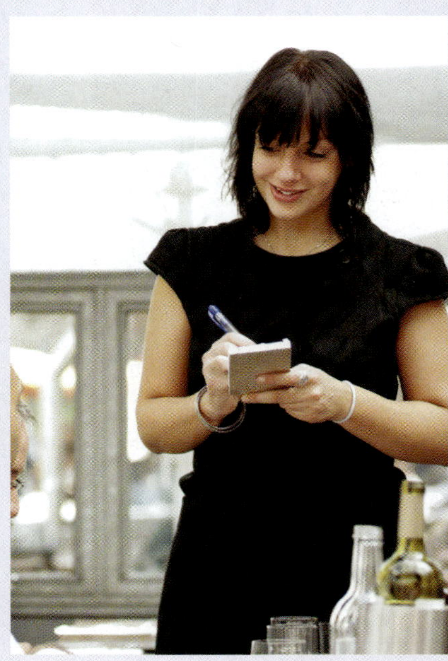

women with anorexia dies of starvation, cardiac arrest, or other medical complications—one of the highest death rates for any psychiatric disorder. Depression is also a serious risk, and about half the fatalities relating to anorexia are suicides.

Bulimia Nervosa

A person with **bulimia nervosa** engages in recurrent episodes of binge eating followed by **purging.** Although bulimia usually begins in adolescence or young adulthood, it has recently begun to emerge at increasingly younger (11–12 years) and older (40–60 years) ages. Research suggests that about 5% of college-age women have bulimia.

During a binge, a bulimic person may rapidly consume thousands of calories. This is followed by an attempt to get rid of the food by purging, usually by vomiting or using laxatives or diuretics. During a binge, bulimics feel as though they have lost control and cannot stop or limit how much they eat. Some binge and purge only occasionally; others do so many times every day. Binges may be triggered by a major life change or other stressful event. Binge eating and purging may become a way of dealing with difficult feelings such as anger and disappointment.

The binge-purge cycle of bulimia places a tremendous strain on the body and can have serious health effects, including tooth decay, esophageal damage and chronic hoarseness, menstrual irregularities, depression, liver

Ask yourself

QUESTIONS FOR CRITICAL THINKING AND REFLECTION

Do you know someone you suspect may be suffering from an eating disorder? Does the advice in this chapter seem helpful to you? Do you think you could follow it? Why or why not? Have you ever experienced disordered eating patterns yourself? If so, can you identify your reasons for it?

and kidney damage, and cardiac arrhythmia. Bulimia is often difficult to recognize because bulimics conceal their eating habits and usually maintain a normal weight, although they may experience fluctuations of 10–15 pounds.

Binge-Eating Disorder

Binge-eating disorder affects about 2% of American adults. It is characterized by uncontrollable eating without any compensatory purging behaviors. Common eating patterns are eating more rapidly than normal, eating until uncomfortably full, eating when not hungry, and preferring to eat alone. Uncontrolled eating is usually followed by weight gain and feelings of guilt, shame, and depression. Many people with binge-eating disorder mistakenly see rigid dieting as the only solution to their problem, but this usually causes feelings of deprivation and a return to overeating.

Compulsive overeaters rarely eat because of hunger. Instead, they use food to cope with stress, conflict, and other difficult emotions or to provide solace or entertainment. Binge eaters are almost always obese, so they face all the health risks associated with obesity. In addition, binge eaters may have higher-than-average rates of depression and anxiety.

Borderline Disordered Eating

People with *borderline disordered eating* have some symptoms of eating disorders—for example, excessive dieting or occasional bingeing or purging—but do not meet the full diagnostic criteria for anorexia, bulimia, or binge-eating disorder. Some experts estimate, however, that as many as one-quarter of people with borderline disordered eating will eventually develop a full eating disorder.

Meaningful statistics about borderline disordered eating are hard to come by, in part because it is difficult to define exactly when eating habits cross the line between normal and disordered. However, many experts feel that the majority of Americans, particularly women, have at least some unhealthy attitudes and behaviors in relation to food and self-image. Concerns about weight and dieting are so common as to be considered culturally normal for many Americans.

Ideally, our relationship to food should be a happy one. The biological urge to satisfy hunger is one of our most basic drives, and eating is associated with many pleasurable sensations. For some of us, food triggers pleasant memories of good times, family, holidays, and fun. But for too many people, food is a source of anguish rather than pleasure. Eating results in feelings of guilt and self-loathing rather than satisfaction, causing tremendous disruption in the lives of affected individuals.

How do you know if you have disordered eating habits? When thoughts about weight and food dominate your life, you have a problem. If you're convinced that your worth as a person hinges on how you look and how much you weigh, it's time to get help. Self-induced vomiting or laxative use after meals, even if only once in a while, is reason for concern. Do you feel compelled to overexercise to compensate for what you've eaten? Do you routinely restrict your food intake and sometimes eat nothing in an effort to feel more in control? These are all danger signs and could mean that you are developing a serious problem. Lab 7.3 can help you determine whether you are at risk for an eating disorder.

Treating Eating Disorders

The treatment of eating disorders must address both problematic eating behaviors and the misuse of food to manage stress and emotions. Treatment for anorexia nervosa first involves averting a medical crisis by restoring adequate body weight; then the psychological aspects of the disorder can be addressed. The treatment of bulimia nervosa or binge-eating disorder involves first stabilizing the eating patterns, then identifying and changing the patterns of thinking that lead to disordered eating. Treatment usually involves a combination of psychotherapy, medication, and medical management. Friends and family members often want to know what they can do to help; for suggestions, see the box "If Someone You Know Has an Eating Disorder."

People with milder patterns of disordered eating may benefit from getting a nutrition checkup with a registered dietitian. A professional can help determine appropriate body weight and calorie intake and offer advice on how to budget calories into a balanced, healthy diet.

KEY TERMS

bulimia nervosa An eating disorder characterized by recurrent episodes of binge eating and then purging to prevent weight gain.

purging The use of vomiting, laxatives, excessive exercise, restrictive dieting, enemas, diuretics, or diet pills to compensate for food that has been eaten and that the person fears will produce weight gain.

binge-eating disorder An eating disorder characterized by binge eating and a lack of control over eating behavior in general.

TAKE CHARGE

If Someone You Know Has an Eating Disorder . . .

Secrecy and denial are two hallmarks of eating disorders, so it can be hard to know if someone has anorexia or bulimia. Signs that someone may have anorexia include sudden weight loss, excessive dieting or exercise, guilt or preoccupation with food or eating, frequent weighing, fear of becoming fat despite being thin, and baggy or layered clothes to conceal weight loss. Signs that someone may have bulimia include excessive eating without weight gain, secretiveness about food (stealing, hiding, or hoarding food), self-induced vomiting (bathroom visits during or after a meal), swollen glands or puffy face, erosion of tooth enamel, and use of laxatives, diuretics, or diet pills to control weight.

If you decide to approach a friend with your concerns, here are some tips to follow:

- Find out about treatment resources in your community (see the For Further Exploration section for suggestions). You may want to consult a professional at your school clinic or counseling center about the best way to approach the situation.
- Arrange to speak with your friend in a private place, and allow enough time to talk.
- Express your concerns, with specific observations of your friend's behavior. Expect him or her to deny or minimize the problem and possibly to become angry with you. Stay calm and nonjudgmental, and continue to express your concern.
- Avoid giving simplistic advice about eating habits. Listen if your friend wants to talk, and offer your support and understanding. Give your friend the information you found about where he or she can get help, and offer to go along.
- If the situation is an emergency—if your friend has fainted, for example, or attempted suicide—call 911 for help immediately.
- If you are upset about the situation, consider talking to someone yourself. The professionals at the clinic or counseling center are there to help you. Remember, you are not to blame for another person's eating disorder.

TIPS FOR TODAY AND THE FUTURE

Many approaches work, but the simplest formula for weight management is moderate food intake coupled with regular exercise.

RIGHT NOW YOU CAN

- Assess your weight-management needs. Do you need to gain weight, lose weight, or stay at your current weight?
- List five things you can do to add more physical activity (not exercise) to your daily routine.
- Identify the foods you regularly eat that may be sabotaging your ability to manage your weight.

IN THE FUTURE YOU CAN

- Make an honest assessment of your body image. Is it accurate and fair, or is it unduly negative and unhealthy? If your body image presents a problem, consider getting professional advice on how to view yourself realistically.
- Keep track of your energy needs to determine whether your energy-balance equation is correct. Use this information as part of your long-term weight-management efforts.

SUMMARY

- Excess body weight increases the risk of numerous diseases, particularly cardiovascular disease, cancer, and diabetes.
- Although genetic factors help determine a person's weight, the influence of heredity can be overcome to an extent.
- Physiological factors involved in the regulation of body weight and body fat include metabolic rate and hormones.
- Energy-balance components that an individual can control are calories taken in and calories expended in physical activity.
- Nutritional guidelines for weight management and wellness include controlling consumption of total calories, unhealthy fats and carbohydrates, and protein; monitoring portion sizes and calorie density; increasing consumption of whole grains, fruits, and vegetables; and developing an eating schedule based on rules.
- Activity guidelines for weight control emphasize engaging in moderate-intensity physical activity for 60–90 minutes or more per day; regular, prolonged endurance exercise and weight training can burn a significant number of calories while maintaining muscle mass.
- The sense of well-being that results from a well-balanced diet can reinforce commitment to weight control; improve self-esteem; and lead to realistic, as opposed to negative, self-talk. Successful weight management results in not using food as a way to cope with stress.
- In cases of extreme obesity, weight loss requires medical supervision; in less extreme cases, people can set up individual programs, perhaps getting guidance from reliable books or by joining a formal weight-loss program.
- Dissatisfaction with body image and body weight can lead to physical problems and serious eating disorders, including anorexia nervosa, bulimia nervosa, and binge-eating disorder.

COMMON QUESTIONS ANSWERED

Q How can I safely gain weight?

A Just as for losing weight, a program for weight gain should be gradual and should include both exercise and dietary changes. The foundation of a successful and healthy program for weight gain is a combination of strength training and a high-carbohydrate, high-calorie diet. Strength training will help you add weight as muscle rather than fat.

Energy balance is also important in a program for gaining weight. You need to consume more calories than your body requires in order to gain weight, but you need to choose those extra calories wisely. Fatty, high-calorie foods may seem like an obvious choice, but consuming additional calories as fat can jeopardize your health and your weight-management program. A diet high in fat carries health risks, and your body is more likely to convert dietary fat into fat tissue than into muscle mass. A better strategy is to consume additional calories as complex carbohydrates from whole grains, fruits, and vegetables.

A diet for weight gain should contain about 60–65% of total daily calories from carbohydrates. You probably do not need to be concerned with protein. Although protein requirements increase when you exercise, the protein consumption of most Americans is already well above the DRI.

In order to gain primarily muscle weight instead of fat, a gradual program of weight gain is your best bet. Try these strategies for consuming extra calories:

- Don't skip any meals.
- Add two or three snacks to your daily eating routine.
- Try a sports drink or supplement that has at least 60% of calories from carbohydrates, as well as significant amounts of protein, vitamins, and minerals. (But don't use supplements to replace meals, because they don't contain all of the components of food.)

Q How can I achieve a "perfect" body?

A The current cultural ideal of an ultratoned, ultrafit body is impossible for most people to achieve. A reasonable goal for body weight and body shape must take into account your heredity, weight history, social circumstances, metabolic rate, and psychological well-being. Don't set goals based on movie stars or fashion models. Modern photographic techniques can make people look much different on film or in magazines than they do in person. Many of these people are also genetically endowed with body shapes that are impossible for most of us to emulate. The best approach is to work with what you've got. Adopting a wellness lifestyle that includes regular exercise and a healthy diet will naturally result in the best possible body shape for you. Obsessively trying to achieve unreasonable goals can lead to problems such as eating disorders, overtraining, and injuries.

For more Common Questions Answered about weight management, visit the Online Learning Center at www.mhhe.com /fahey.

FOR FURTHER EXPLORATION

BOOKS

American Heart Association. 2011. *American Heart Association No-Fad Diet, 2nd Edition: A Personal Plan for Healthy Weight Loss.* New York: Clarkson Potter. *Provides guidelines for successful weight management.*

Dillon, E. 2009. *Issues That Concern You: Obesity.* New York: Greenhaven Press. *A collection of perspectives on the causes of obesity, its management, and its impact on individuals and society* .

Gaesser, G. A., and K. Katrina. 2006. *It's the Calories, Not the Carbs.* Victoria, B.C.: Trafford. *Provides a detailed look at the facts behind successful weight loss by shunning fad diets and practicing sound energy balance* .

Hochstrasser, A., and S. R. Fox. 2010. *The Patient's Guide to Weight Loss Surgery, Revised ed.* New York: Hatherleigh. *An easy-to-read guide to the benefits and risks of weight-loss surgery.*

Mayo Clinic. 2009. *Mayo Clinic's Essential Diabetes Book.* Rochester, Minn.: Mayo Clinic. *A user-friendly guide to diabetes.*

Smolin, L. A., and M. B. Grosvenor. 2010. *Nutrition and Eating Disorders.* New York: Chelsea House Publications. *An easy-to-understand guide to eating disorders.*

ORGANIZATIONS AND WEB SITES

Calorie Control Council. Includes a variety of interactive calculators, including an Exercise Calculator that estimates the calories burned from various forms of physical activity.

http://www.caloriecontrol.org

Frontline: Fat. Information from a PBS Frontline special that looked at how society, genetics, and biology have influenced our relationship with food and at current problems with obesity and eating disorders.

http://www.pbs.org/wgbh/pages/frontline/shows/fat

MedlinePlus: Obesity and Weight Loss. Provides reliable information from government agencies and key professional associations.

http://www.nlm.nih.gov/medlineplus/obesity.html

http://www.nlm.nih.gov/medlineplus/weightcontrol.html

National Heart, Lung, and Blood Institute (NHLBI): Aim for a Healthy Weight. Provides information and tips on diet and physical activity, as well as a BMI calculator.

http://www.nhlbi.nih.gov/health/public/heart/obesity/lose_wt

SmallStep.gov. Provides resources for increasing activity and improving diet through small changes in daily habits.

http://www.smallstep.gov

Weight-control Information Network (WIN). A service of the National Institute of Diabetes and Digestive and Kidney Diseases, serves as an online clearinghouse of weight-management information.

http://win.niddk.nih.gov/

WHO: Obesity and Overweight. Provides information on WHO's global strategy on diet and physical activity.

http://www.who.int/dietphysicalactivity/en

There are also many resources for people concerned about body image and eating disorders:

Something Fishy Website on Eating Disorders

http://www.something-fishy.org

MedlinePlus:Eating Disorders

http://www.nlm.nih.gov/medlineplus/eatingdisorders.html

National Association of Anorexia Nervosa and Associated Eating Disorders

http://www.anad.org

National Eating Disorders Association

http://www.nationaleatingdisorders.org

Women's Body Image and Health

http://www.womenshealth.gov/bodyimage

See also the listings in Chapters 1, 3, and 6.

SELECTED BIBLIOGRAPHY

Anton, S. D., et al. 2010. Effects of stevia, aspartame, and sucrose on food intake, satiety, and postprandial glucose and insulin levels. *Appetite* 55(1): 37–43.

Balkon, N., et al. 2001. Overweight and obesity: Pharmacotherapeutic considerations. *Journal of the American Academy of Nurse Practitioners* 23(2): 61–66.

Basen-Engquist, K., and M. Chang. 2011. Obesity risk and cancer: Recent review and evidence. *Current Oncology Reports* 13(1): 71–76.

Beverages total 22% of US calories—but who's counting? 2007. *Tufts Health & Nutrition Letter,* March.

Chandon, P., and B. Wansink. 2007. The biasing health halos of fast-food restaurant health claims: Lower calorie estimates and higher side-dish consumption intentions. *Journal of Consumer Research* 34(3): 301–304.

Dahlman, I., and P. Arner. 2007. Obesity and polymorphisms in genes regulating human adipose tissue. *International Journal of Obesity* 31(11): 1629–1641.

Dhingra, R., et al. 2007. Soft drink consumption and risk of developing cardiometabolic risk factors and the metabolic syndrome in middle-aged adults in the community. *Circulation* 116(5): 480–488.

Donnelly, J. E., et al. 2009. American College of Sports Medicine Position Stand: Appropriate physical activity intervention strategies for weight loss and prevention of weight regain for adults. *Medicine and Science in Sports and Medicine* 41(2): 459–471.

Drewnowski, A., and F. Bellisle. 2007. Liquid calories, sugar and body weight. *American Journal of Clinical Nutrition* 85(3): 651–661.

Greene, G. W., et al. 2011. Identifying clusters of college students at elevated health risk based on eating and exercise behaviors and psychosocial determinants of body weight. *Journal of the American Dietetic Association* 111(3): 394–400.

Hamilton, M., et al. 2007. Role of low energy expenditure and sitting in obesity, metabolic syndrome, type 2 diabetes, and cardiovascular disease. *Diabetes* 56(11): 2655–2667.

Hollis, J. F., et al. 2008. Weight loss during the intensive intervention phase of the Weight-Loss Maintenance Trial. *American Journal of Preventive Medicine* 35(2): 18–126.

Hudson, J. I., et al. 2007. The prevalence and correlates of eating disorders in the National Comorbidity Survey Replication. *Biological Psychiatry* 61(3): 348–358.

Huizinga, M. M., et al. 2009. Literacy, numeracy, and portion-size estimation skills. *American Journal of Preventive Medicine* 36(4): 324–328.

Hutchinson, D. M., and R. M. Rapee. 2007. Do friends share similar body image and eating problems? The role of social networks and peer influences in early adolescence. *Behavior Research and Therapy* 45(7): 1557–1577.

Idelevich, E., et al. 2009. Current pharmacotherapeutic concepts for the treatment of obesity in adults. *Therapeutic Advances in Cardiovascular Disease* 3(1): 75–90.

Janiszewski, P. M., and R. Ross. 2007. Physical activity in the treatment of obesity: Beyond body weight reduction. *Applied Physiology, Nutrition and Metabolism* 32(3): 512–522.

Kirk, E. P., et al. 2009. Minimal resistance training improves daily energy expenditure and fat oxidation. *Medicine and Science in Sports and Exercise,* April (published online).

Knab, A. M., et al. 2011. A 45-minute vigorous exercise bout increases metabolic rate for 14 hours. *Medicine and Science in Sports and Exercise,* February (published online).

Kulie, T., et al. 2011. Obesity and women's health: An evidence-based review. *Journal of the American Board of Family Medicine* 24(1): 75–85.

Kumanyika, S. K., et al. 2008. Population-based prevention of obesity: The need for comprehensive promotion of healthful eating, physical activity, and energy balance: A scientific statement from the American Heart Association Council on Epidemiology and Prevention, Interdisciplinary Committee for Prevention (formerly the Expert Panel on Population and Prevention Science). *Circulation* 118(4): 428–464.

Leone, J. E., and J. V. Fetro. 2007. Perceptions and attitudes toward androgenic-anabolic steroid use among two age categories: A qualitative study. *Journal of Strength and Conditioning Research* 21(2): 532–537.

Moore, S. C., et al. 2008. Past body mass index and risk of mortality among women. *International Journal of Obesity* 32(5): 730–739.

Narayan, K. M., et al. 2007. Effect of BMI on lifetime risk for diabetes in the U.S. *Diabetes Care* 30(6): 1562–1566.

Ogden, C. L., et al. 2007. Obesity among adults in the United States: No statistically significant change since 2003–2004. *National Center for Health Statistics Data Brief* 1: 1–8.

Ogden, C. L., et al. 2007. The epidemiology of obesity. *Gastroenterology* 132(6): 2087–2102.

Pellegrini, C. A., et al. 2011. The comparison of a technology-based system and an in-person behavioral weight loss intervention. *Obesity,* February (published online).

Pereira, M. A., et al. 2005. Fast-food habits, weight gain, and insulin resistance (the CARDIA study): 15-year prospective analysis. *Lancet* 365(9453): 36–42.

Ritchie, S. A., and J. M. Connell. 2007. The link between abdominal obesity, metabolic syndrome and cardiovascular disease. *Nutrition, Metabolism, and Cardiovascular Diseases* 17(4): 319–326.

Schroder, K. E. 2011. Computer-assisted dieting: Effects of a randomized nutrition intervention. *American Journal of Health Behavior* 35(2): 175–188.

U.S. Department of Health and Human Services. 2011. *Dietary Guidelines for Americans, 2010* (http://health.gov/dietaryguidelines/2010.asp; retrieved February 26, 2011).

Whitlock, G. et al. 2009. Body-mass index and cause-specific mortality in 900,000 adults: Collaborative analysis of 57 prospective studies. *Lancet* 373(9669): 1083–1096).

Name ______________________ Section ______________ Date ____________

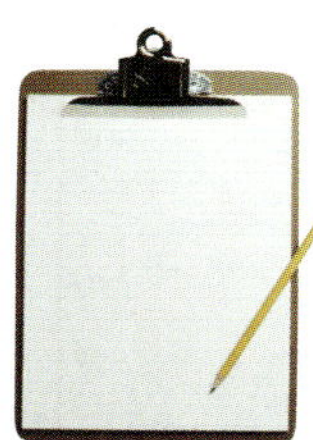

LAB 7.1 Calculating Daily Energy Needs

Part I Estimating Current Energy Intake from a Food Record

If your weight is stable, your current daily energy intake is the number of calories you need to consume to maintain your weight at your current activity level. If you completed Lab 3.2, you should have a record of your current energy intake; if you didn't complete the lab, keep a careful and complete record of everything you eat for one day, and then total the calories in all the foods and beverages you consumed. Record your total energy intake below:

Current energy intake (from food record): ______________ calories per day

Part II Estimating Daily Energy Requirements Using Food and Nutrition Board Formulas

Many people underestimate the size of their food portions, and so energy goals based on estimates of current calorie intake from food records can be inaccurate. You can also estimate your daily energy needs using the formulas listed below. To use the appropriate formula for your sex, you'll need to plug in the following:

- Age (in years)
- Height (in inches)
- Weight (in pounds)
- Physical activity coefficient (PA) from the table below.

To help estimate your physical activity level, consider the following guidelines: Someone who typically engages in 30 minutes of moderate-intensity activity, equivalent to walking 2 miles in 30 minutes, in addition to the activities involved in maintaining a sedentary lifestyle, is considered "low active"; someone who typically engages in the equivalent of 90 minutes of moderate-intensity activity is rated as "active." You might find it helpful to refer back to Lab 2.2 to estimate your physical activity level.

	Physical Activity Coefficient (PA)	
Physical Activity Level	*Men*	*Women*
Sedentary	1.00	1.00
Low active	1.12	1.14
Active	1.27	1.27
Very active	1.54	1.45

Estimated Daily Energy Requirement for Weight Maintenance in Men

$$864 - (9.72 \times \text{age}) + (\text{PA} \times [(6.39 \times \text{weight}) + (12.78 \times \text{height})])$$

1. 9.72 × __________ age (years) = __________
2. 864 − __________ result from step 1 = __________ [*result may be a negative number*]
3. 6.39 × __________ weight (pounds) = __________
4. 12.78 × __________ height (inches) = __________
5. __________ result from step 3 + __________ result from step 4 = __________
6. __________ PA (from table) × __________ result from step 5 = __________
7. __________ result from step 2 + __________ result from step 6 = __________ calories per day

Estimated Daily Energy Requirement for Weight Maintenance in Women

$$387 - (7.31 \times \text{age}) + (\text{PA} \times [(4.91 \times \text{weight}) + (16.78 \times \text{height})])$$

1. 7.31 × __________ age (years) = __________
2. 387 − __________ result from step 1 = __________ [*result may be a negative number*]
3. 4.91 × __________ weight (pounds) = __________
4. 16.78 × __________ height (inches) = __________

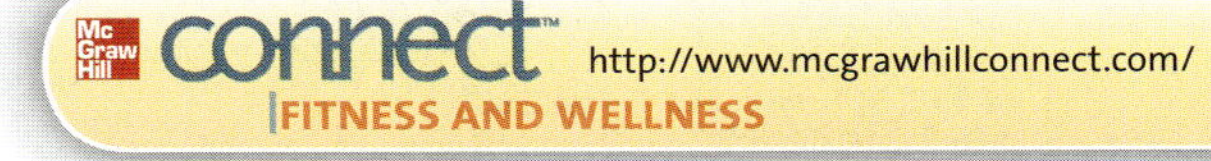

5. __________ result from step 3 + __________ result from step 4 = __________
6. __________ PA (from table) × __________ result from step 5 = __________
7. __________ result from step 2 + __________ result from step 6 = __________ calories per day

Daily energy needs for weight maintenance (from formula): _______ calories/day

Part III Determining an Individual Daily Energy Goal for Weight Maintenance

If you calculated values for daily energy needs based on both methods, examine the two values. Some difference is likely—people tend to underestimate their food intake and overestimate their level of physical activity—but if the two values are very far off, check your food record and your physical activity estimate for accuracy, and make any necessary adjustments. For an individualized estimate of daily calorie needs, average the two values:

Daily energy needs = (food record result __________ calories/day + formula result __________ calories/day) ÷ 2 __________ calories/day

Using Your Results

How did you score? Are you surprised by the value you calculated for your approximate daily energy needs? If so, is the value higher or lower than you expected?

What should you do next? Enter the results of this lab in the Preprogram Assessment column in Appendix C. (If your goal is weight gain, see p. 211 for basic guidelines.) One of the best ways to tip your energy balance toward weight loss is to increase your daily physical activity. If you include increases in activity as part of your program, then you can use the results of this lab to chart changes in your daily energy expenditure (and needs). Look for ways to increase the amount of time you spend in physical activity, thus increasing your physical activity coefficient. After several weeks of your program, complete this lab again, and enter the results in the Postprogram Assessment column of Appendix C. How do the results compare? Did your program for increasing physical activity show up as an increase in your daily energy expenditure and need?

Name ______________________ Section ______________ Date ____________

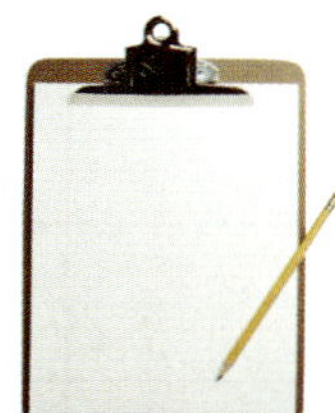

LAB 7.2 Identifying Weight-Loss Goals

Negative Calorie Balance

Complete the following calculations to determine your weekly and daily negative calorie balance goals and the number of weeks to achieve your target weight.

Current weight ________ lb − target weight (from Lab 6.2) ________ lb

= total weight to lose ________ lb

Total weight to lose ________ lb ÷ weight to lose each week ________ lb

= time to achieve target weight ________ weeks

Weight to lose each week ________ lb × 3500 cal/lb = weekly negative calorie balance ________ cal/week

Weekly negative calorie balance ________ cal/week ÷ 7 days/week

= daily negative calorie balance ________ cal/day

To keep your weight-loss program on schedule, you must achieve the daily negative calorie balance by either decreasing your calorie consumption (eating less) or increasing your calorie expenditure (being more active). Combining the two strategies may be most successful.

Changes in Activity Level

Adding a few minutes of exercise every day is a good way of expending calories. Use the calorie costs for different activities listed in the following table.

Activity	Cal/lb/min	×	Body weight	×	min	=	Total calories
Aerobic dance	.046		______		____		______
Basketball (half ct.)	.045		______		____		______
Bicycling (casual)	.049		______		____		______
Bicycling (13 mph)	.071		______		____		______
Elliptical exercise	.049		______		____		______
Football (touch)	.049		______		____		______
Hiking	.051		______		____		______
Housework	.029		______		____		______
Jogging	.060		______		____		______
Rope skipping	.071		______		____		______
Rowing	.032		______		____		______
Skating	.049		______		____		______
Soccer	.052		______		____		______
Swimming	.032		______		____		______
Walking (normal pace)	.029		______		____		______
Walking (briskly)	.048		______		____		______

Activity	Duration	Calories Used
______________	______________	______________
______________	______________	______________
______________	______________	______________

Total calories expended: ______________

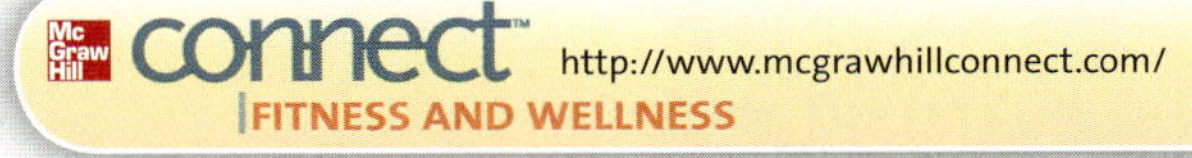

Changes in Diet

Look closely at your diet from one day, as recorded in Lab 3.2. Identify ways to cut calorie consumption by eliminating certain items or substituting lower-calorie choices. Be realistic in your cuts and substitutions; you need to develop a plan you can live with.

Food Item	Substitute Food Item	Calorie Savings
__________	__________	__________
__________	__________	__________
__________	__________	__________
	Total calories cut:	__________

Total calories expended _______ **+ total calories cut** _______ **= total negative calorie balance** _______

Common Problem Eating Behaviors

For each of the groups of statements that appear below, check those that are true for you. If you check several statements for a given pattern or problem, it will probably be a significant factor in your weight-management program. One possible strategy for dealing with each type of problem is given. For those eating problems you identify as important, add your own ideas to the strategies listed.

1. _____ I often skip meals.
   _____ I often eat a number of snacks in place of a meal.
   _____ I don't have a regular schedule of meal and snack times.
   _____ I make up for missed meals and snacks by eating more at the next meal.

Problem: Irregular eating habits
Possible solutions:

- Write out a plan for each day's meals in advance. Carry it with you and stick to it.
- ______________________________
- ______________________________

2. _____ I eat more than one sweet dessert or snack each day.
   _____ I usually snack on foods high in calories and fat (chips, cookies, ice cream).
   _____ I drink regular (not sugar-free) soft drinks.
   _____ I choose types of meat that are high in fat.
   _____ I consume more than one alcoholic beverage a day.

Problem: Poor food choices

Possible solutions:

- Keep a supply of raw fruits and vegetables handy for snacks.
- ______________________________
- ______________________________

3. _____ I always eat everything on my plate.
   _____ I often go back for seconds and thirds.
   _____ I take larger helpings than most people.
   _____ I eat up leftovers instead of putting them away.

Problem: Portion sizes too large

Possible solutions:

- Measure all portions with a scale or measuring cup.
- ______________________________
- ______________________________

Name ______________________________ Section ______________ Date __________

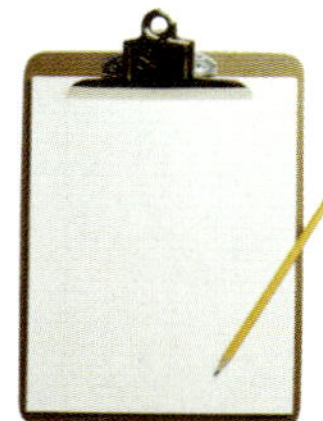

LAB 7.3 Checking for Body Image Problems and Eating Disorders

Assessing Your Body Image

	Never	Sometimes	Often	Always
1. I dislike seeing myself in mirrors.	0	1	2	3
2. When I shop for clothing, I am more aware of my weight problem, and consequently I find shopping for clothes somewhat unpleasant.	0	1	2	3
3. I'm ashamed to be seen in public.	0	1	2	3
4. I prefer to avoid engaging in sports or public exercise because of my appearance.	0	1	2	3
5. I feel somewhat embarrassed about my body in the presence of someone of the other sex.	0	1	2	3
6. I think my body is ugly.	0	1	2	3
7. I feel that other people must think my body is unattractive.	0	1	2	3
8. I feel that my family or friends may be embarrassed to be seen with me.	0	1	2	3
9. I find myself comparing myself with other people to see if they are heavier than I am.	0	1	2	3
10. I find it difficult to enjoy activities because I am self-conscious about my physical appearance.	0	1	2	3
11. Feeling guilty about my weight problem occupies most of my thinking.	0	1	2	3
12. My thoughts about my body and physical appearance are negative and self-critical.	0	1	2	3
Now add up the number of points you have circled in each column: _____	0	+ _______	+ _______	+ _______

Score Interpretation

The lowest possible score is 0, and this indicates a positive body image. The highest possible score is 36, and this indicates an unhealthy body image. A score higher than 14 suggests a need to develop a healthier body image.

SOURCE: Nash, J. D. 1997. *The New Maximize Your Body Potential.* Palo Alto, Calif.: Bull Publishing. Reprinted with permission from Bull Publishing. All rights reserved.

Eating Disorder Checklist

	Always	Very Often	Often	Sometimes	Rarely	Never
1. I like eating with other people.	0	0	0	1	2	3
2. I like my clothes to fit tightly.	0	0	0	1	2	3
3. I enjoy eating meat.	0	0	0	1	2	3
4. I have regular menstrual periods.	0	0	0	1	2	3
5. I enjoy eating at restaurants.	0	0	0	1	2	3
6. I enjoy trying new rich foods.	0	0	0	1	2	3
7. I prepare foods for others, but do not eat what I cook.	3	2	1	0	0	0
8. I become anxious prior to eating.	3	2	1	0	0	0
9. I am terrified about being overweight.	3	2	1	0	0	0
10. I avoid eating when I am hungry.	3	2	1	0	0	0
11. I find myself preoccupied with food.	3	2	1	0	0	0

	Always	Very Often	Often	Sometimes	Rarely	Never
12. I have gone on eating binges where I feel that I may not be able to stop.	3	2	1	0	0	0
13. I cut my food into small pieces.	3	2	1	0	0	0
14. I am aware of the calorie content of foods that I eat.	3	2	1	0	0	0
15. I particularly avoid foods with a high carbohydrate content (bread, potatoes, rice, etc.).	3	2	1	0	0	0
16. I feel bloated after meals.	3	2	1	0	0	0
17. I feel others would prefer me to eat more.	3	2	1	0	0	0
18. I vomit after I have eaten.	3	2	1	0	0	0
19. I feel extremely guilty after eating.	3	2	1	0	0	0
20. I am preoccupied with a desire to be thinner.	3	2	1	0	0	0
21. I exercise strenuously to burn off calories.	3	2	1	0	0	0
22. I weigh myself several times a day.	3	2	1	0	0	0
23. I wake up early in the morning.	3	2	1	0	0	0
24. I eat the same foods day after day.	3	2	1	0	0	0
25. I think about burning up calories when I exercise.	3	2	1	0	0	0
26. Other people think I am too thin.	3	2	1	0	0	0
27. I am preoccupied with the thought of having fat on my body.	3	2	1	0	0	0
28. I take longer than others to eat my meals.	3	2	1	0	0	0
29. I take laxatives.	3	2	1	0	0	0
30. I avoid foods with sugar in them.	3	2	1	0	0	0
31. I eat diet foods.	3	2	1	0	0	0
32. I feel that food controls my life.	3	2	1	0	0	0
33. I display self-control around foods.	3	2	1	0	0	0
34. I feel that others pressure me to eat.	3	2	1	0	0	0
35. I give too much time and thought to food.	3	2	1	0	0	0
36. I suffer from constipation.	3	2	1	0	0	0
37. I feel uncomfortable after eating sweets.	3	2	1	0	0	0
38. I engage in dieting behavior	3	2	1	0	0	0
39. I like my stomach to be empty.	3	2	1	0	0	0
40. I have the impulse to vomit after meals.	3	2	1	0	0	0
Now add up the number of points in each column for statements 1 through 40: ______	______ +	______ +	______ +	______ +	______ +	______

Score Interpretation

The possible range is 0–120. A score higher than 50 suggests an eating disorder. A score between 30 and 50 suggests a borderline eating disorder. A score less than 30 is within the normal range. Among those with normal eating habits, the average score is 15.4.

SOURCE: Garner, D. M., Olmstead, M., Polivy, J., Development and Validation of a Multidimensional Eating Disorder Inventory for Anorexia Nervosa and Bulimia. *International Journal of Eating Disorders* 2: 15–33, 1983.

Using Your Results

How did you score? Are you surprised by your scores? Do the results of either assessment indicate that you may have a problem with body image or disordered eating?

What should you do next? If your results are borderline, consider trying some of the self-help strategies suggested in the chapter. If body image or disordered eating is a significant problem for you, get professional advice; a physician, therapist, and/or registered dietitian can help. Make an appointment today.

CHAPTER 8

Muscular Strength and Endurance

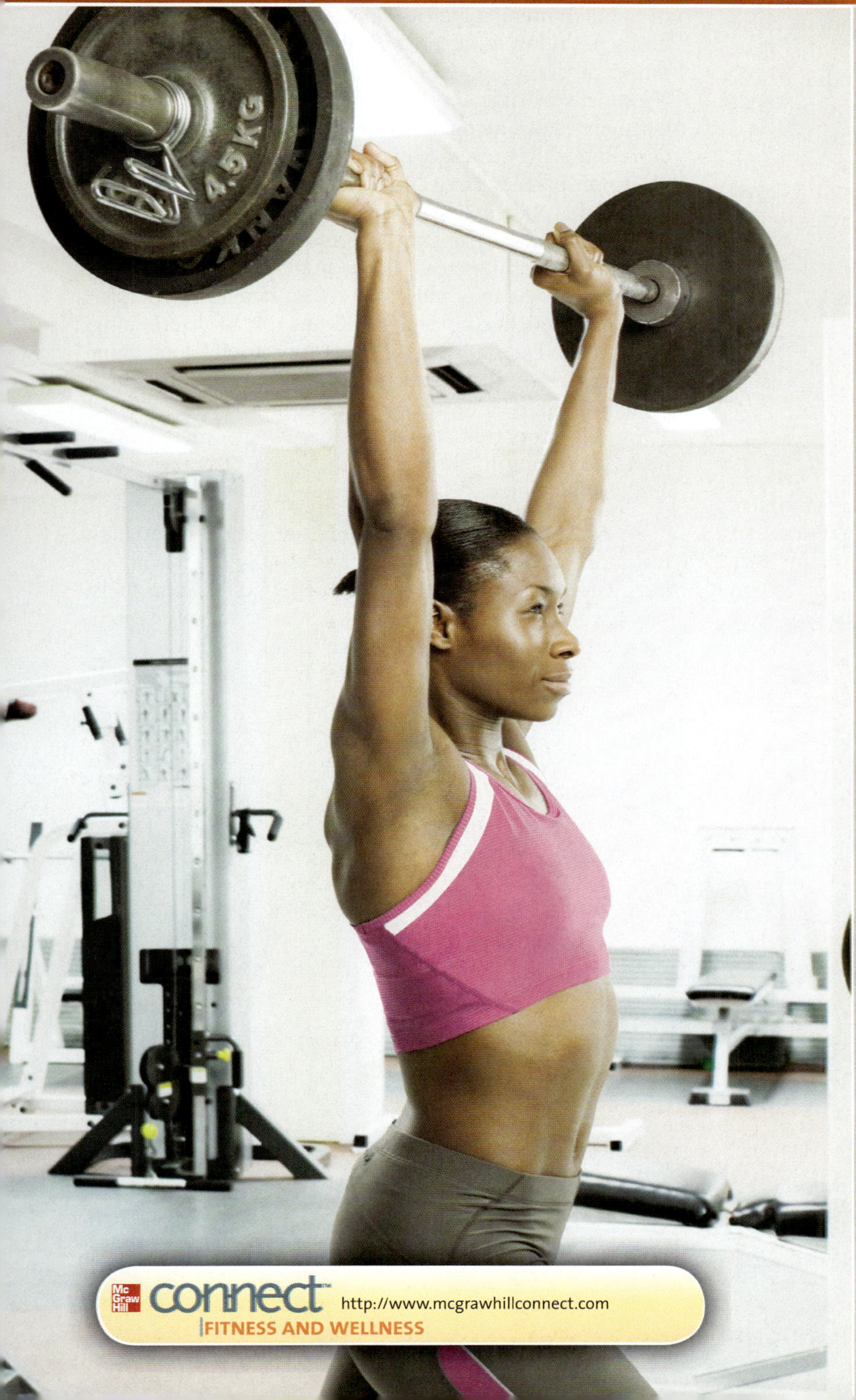

LOOKING AHEAD...

After reading this chapter, you should be able to:

- Describe the basic physiology of muscles and explain how strength training affects muscles
- Define muscular strength and endurance, and describe how they relate to wellness
- Assess muscular strength and endurance
- Apply the FITT principle to create a safe and successful strength training program
- Describe the effects of supplements and drugs that are marketed to active people and athletes
- Explain how to safely perform common strength training exercises using free weights and weight machines

TEST YOUR KNOWLEDGE

1. For women, weight training typically results in which of the following?
   a. bulky muscles
   b. significant increases in body weight
   c. improved body image
2. To maximize strength gains, it is a good idea to hold your breath as you lift a weight. True or false?
3. Regular strength training is associated with which of the following benefits?
   a. denser bones
   b. reduced risk of heart disease
   c. improved body composition
   d. fewer injuries
   e. improved metabolic health
   f. Increased longevity

Answers

1. **c.** Because the vast majority of women have low levels of testosterone, they do not develop large muscles or gain significant amounts of weight in response to a moderate-intensity weight training program. Men have higher levels of testosterone, so they can build large muscles more easily.
2. **False.** Holding one's breath while lifting weights can significantly elevate blood pressure; it also reduces blood flow to the heart and may cause faintness. You should breathe smoothly and normally while weight training. Some experts recommend that you exhale during the most difficult part of each exercise.
3. **All six.** Regular strength training has many benefits for both men and women.

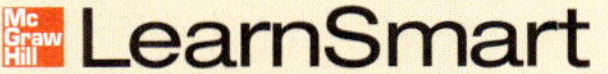

Muscles make up more than 40% of your body mass. You depend on them for movement, and, because of their mass, they are the site of a large portion of the energy reactions (metabolism) that take place in your body. Strong, well-developed muscles help you perform daily activities with greater ease, protect you from injury, and enhance your well-being in other ways.

As described in Chapter 2, muscular strength is the amount of force a muscle can produce with a single maximum effort; muscular endurance is the ability to hold or repeat a muscular contraction for a long time. This chapter explains the benefits of strength training (also called *resistance training* or *weight training*) and describes methods of assessing muscular strength and endurance. It then explains the basics of strength training and provides guidelines for setting up your own training program. The musculoskeletal system is depicted on pages T4-2 and T4-3 of the color transparency insert "Touring the Musculoskeletal System" in this chapter. You can refer to this illustration as you set up your program.

BASIC MUSCLE PHYSIOLOGY AND THE EFFECTS OF STRENGTH TRAINING

Muscles move the body and enable it to exert force because they move the skeleton. When a muscle contracts (shortens), it moves a bone by pulling on the tendon that attaches the muscle to the bone, as shown in Figure 8.1. When a muscle relaxes (lengthens), the tension placed on the tendon is released and the bone moves back to—or closer to—its starting position.

Muscle Fibers

Muscles consist of individual muscle cells, or **muscle fibers,** connected in bundles (see Figure 8.1). A single muscle is made up of many bundles of muscle fibers and is covered by layers of connective tissue that hold the fibers together. Muscle fibers, in turn, are made up of smaller protein structures called **myofibrils.** Myofibrils are made up of a series of contractile units called *sarcomeres,* which are composed largely of actin and myosin molecules. Muscle cells contract when the myosin molecules glide across the actin molecules in a ratchetlike movement.

Strength training increases the size and number of myofibrils, resulting in larger individual muscle fibers. Larger muscle fibers mean a larger and stronger muscle. The development of large muscle fibers is called **hypertrophy;** inactivity causes **atrophy,** the reversal of this process. For a depiction of the process of hypertrophy, see page T4-4 of the color transparency insert "Touring the Musculoskeletal System" in this chapter. In some species, muscles can increase in size through a separate process called **hyperplasia,** which involves an increase in the number of muscle fibers rather than the size of muscle fibers. In humans, hyperplasia is not thought to play a significant role in determining muscle size. Each muscle cell has many **nuclei** containing genes that direct the production of enzymes and structural proteins required for muscle contraction.

Muscle fibers are classified as slow-twitch or fast-twitch fibers according to their strength, speed of contraction, and energy source.

- **Slow-twitch muscle fibers** are relatively fatigue-resistant, but they don't contract as rapidly or strongly as fast-twitch fibers. The principal energy system that fuels slow-twitch fibers is aerobic (oxidative). Slow-twitch muscle fibers are typically reddish in color.

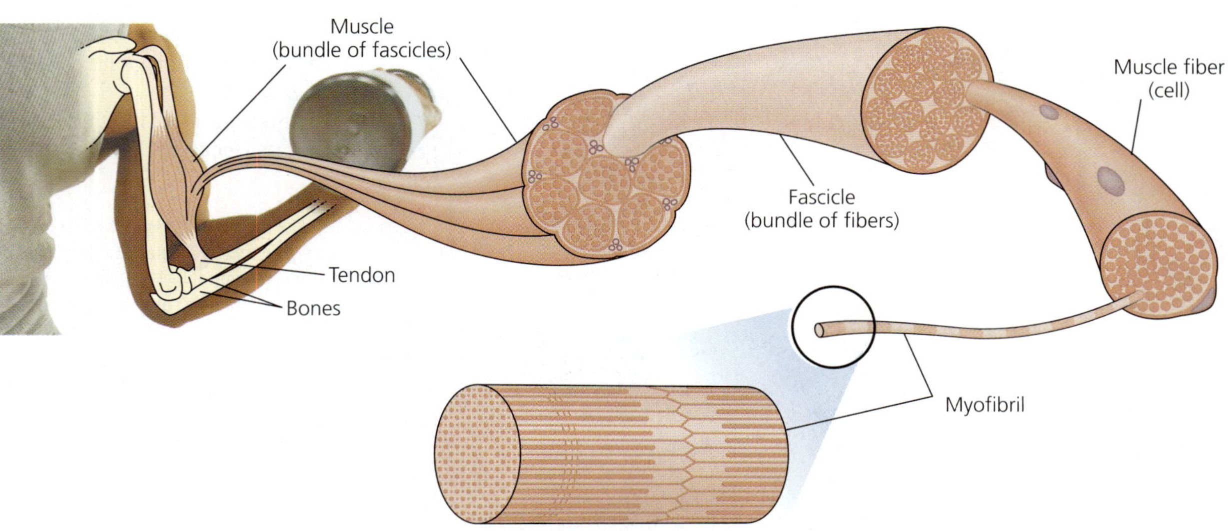

FIGURE 8.1 Components of skeletal muscle tissue.

Table 8.1 Physiological Changes and Benefits from Strength Training

CHANGE	BENEFITS
Increased muscle mass* and strength	Increased muscular strength Improved body composition Higher rate of metabolism Improved capacity to regulate fuel use with aging Toned, healthy-looking muscles Increased longevity Improved quality of life
Increased utilization of motor units during muscle contractions	Increased muscular strength and power
Improved coordination of motor units	Increased muscular strength and power
Increased strength of tendons, ligaments, and bones	Lower risk of injury to these tissues
Increased storage of fuel in muscles	Increased resistance to muscle fatigue
Increased size of fast-twitch muscle fibers (from a high-resistance program)	Increased muscular strength and power
Increased size of slow-twitch muscle fibers (from a high-repetition program)	Increased muscular endurance
Increased blood supply to muscles (from a high-repetition program) and improved blood vessel health	Increased delivery of oxygen and nutrients Faster elimination of wastes
Biochemical improvements (for example, increased sensitivity to insulin)	Enhanced metabolic health
Improved blood fat levels	Reduced risk of heart disease
Increased muscle endurance	Enhanced ability to exercise for long periods and maintain good body posture

*Due to genetic and hormonal differences, men will build more muscle mass than women, but both genders make about the same percent gains in strength through a good program.

- **Fast-twitch muscle fibers** contract more rapidly and forcefully than slow-twitch fibers but fatigue more quickly. Although oxygen is important in the energy system that fuels fast-twitch fibers, they rely more on anaerobic (nonoxidative) metabolism than do slow-twitch fibers. (See Chapter 4 for a discussion of energy systems.) Fast-twitch muscle fibers are typically whitish in color.

Most muscles contain both slow-twitch and fast-twitch fibers. The proportion of the types of fibers varies significantly among different muscles and different individuals, and that proportion is largely fixed at birth, although fibers can contract faster or slower following a period of training or a period of inactivity. The type of fiber that acts during a particular activity depends on the type of work required. Endurance activities like jogging tend to use slow-twitch fibers, whereas strength and **power** activities like sprinting use fast-twitch fibers. Strength training can increase the size and strength of both fast-twitch and slow-twitch fibers, although fast-twitch fibers are preferentially increased.

Motor Units

To exert force, a muscle recruits one or more motor units to contract. A **motor unit** is made up of a nerve connected to a number of muscle fibers. The number of muscle fibers in a motor unit varies from two to hundreds. Small motor units contain slow-twitch fibers, whereas large motor units contain fast-twitch fibers. When a motor unit calls on its fibers to contract, all fibers contract to their full capacity. The number of motor units recruited depends on the amount of strength required: When you pick up a small weight, you use fewer and smaller motor units than when picking up a large weight.

Strength training improves the body's ability to recruit motor units—a phenomenon called **muscle learning**—which increases strength even before muscle size increases. The physiological changes and benefits that result from strength training are summarized in Table 8.1.

KEY TERMS

muscle fiber A single muscle cell, usually classified according to strength, speed of contraction, and energy source.

myofibrils Protein structures that make up muscle fibers.

hypertrophy An increase in the size of muscle fibers, usually stimulated by muscular overload, as occurs during strength training.

atrophy A decrease in the size of muscle fibers.

hyperplasia An increase in the number of muscle fibers.

nucleus A cell structure containing DNA and genes that direct the production of proteins; plural, *nuclei*.

slow-twitch muscle fibers Red muscle fibers that are fatigue resistant but have a slow contraction speed and a lower capacity for tension; usually recruited for endurance activities.

fast-twitch muscle fibers White muscle fibers that contract rapidly and forcefully but fatigue quickly; usually recruited for actions requiring strength and power.

power The ability to exert force rapidly.

motor unit A motor nerve (one that initiates movement) connected to one or more muscle fibers.

muscle learning The improvement in the body's ability to recruit motor units, brought about through strength training.

Does Muscular Strength Reduce the Risk of Premature Death?

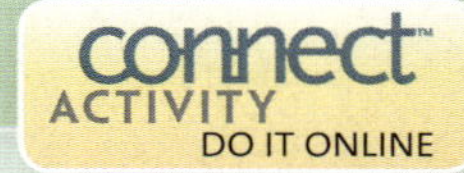

Strength training can make you stronger, but can it also help you live longer? According to a growing body of evidence, the answer is yes—especially for men.

A number of studies have associated greater muscular strength with lower rates of death from all causes, including cancer and cardiovascular disease. According to the results of a study that followed nearly 9000 men over 18 years, the stronger a man is, the lower his risk of premature death from a variety of causes. This study gauged participants' strength through exercises such as bench and leg presses; other studies have measured strength using a handgrip test, with similar outcomes. The resulting data showed significant differences in death rates among the participants, with the strongest men having the lowest death rates. This effect was particularly important for older and overweight men.

When participants in the study died, researchers analyzed causes of death and correlated the numbers of dead and surviving participants with data about their muscular fitness, the amount of time they spent exercising, and other factors (such as metabolic data, cardiovascular health, smoking status, and age). The findings revealed that, compared to men with the lowest levels of muscular strength, stronger men were

- 1.5 times less likely to die from all causes
- 1.6 times less likely to die from cardiovascular disease
- 1.25 times less likely to die from cancer

These correlations held across all age groups (ranging from age 20 to 82) and body mass indexes. They were particularly striking in older men (age 60 and older), who were more than four times more likely to die from cancer than similar-age men with greater muscular strength.

Similarly, an earlier study of more than 3000 men demonstrated an inverse relationship between muscular strength and metabolic syndrome, a cluster of symptoms that includes high blood pressure, high blood glucose levels, high triglyceride levels, low HDL cholesterol levels, and abdominal obesity. Metabolic syndrome increases risk for diabetes, heart disease, and other illnesses. The results were true regardless of participants' age, weight, or waist circumference. The findings led researchers to suggest that weight training may be a valuable way for men to avoid metabolic syndrome. Protection against metabolic syndrome is also provided by cardiorespiratory fitness, according to a 2004 study of 8570 men, in which scientists measured each participant's level of muscular strength and cardiorespiratory fitness.

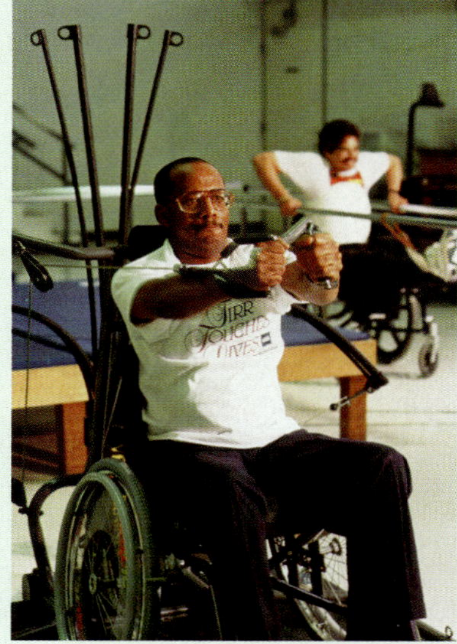

You don't have to be a power lifter or bodybuilder to enjoy the benefits of strength training. In the first study, for example, participants were advised on basic fitness techniques and healthy lifestyle behaviors. Although participants were encouraged to incorporate weight training into their fitness routine, each man chose the type and amount of weight training he felt most comfortable doing. Many researchers believe that the basic minimum recommendation of doing weight training on 2 nonconsecutive days per week may be enough to lower the average male's risk of premature death, provided he is not obese and does not already have risk factors such as diabetes, hypertension, or preexisting cancer. At the same time, as noted in Chapter 4, strength training can have negative effects on the cardiovascular system in some men, at least temporarily, if not followed by aerobic exercise. To date, only small-scale studies have been performed on women, so more research is needed to see if the same conclusions apply to women.

SOURCES: Physical Activity Guidelines Advisory Committee. 2008. *Physical Activity Guidelines Advisory Committee Report, 2008*. Washington, D.C.: U.S. Department of Health and Human Services; Ruiz, J. R., et al. 2008. Association between muscular strength and mortality in men: Prospective cohort study. *BMJ* 337: a439; Ruiz, J. R., et al. 2009. Muscular strength and adiposity as predictors of adulthood cancer mortality in men. *Cancer Epidemiology, Biomarkers, and Prevention* 18: 1468; Rantanen, T., et al. 2011. Midlife muscle strength and human longevity up to age 100 years: A 44-year prospective study among a decedent cohort. *Age* published online: DOI 10.1007/s11357-011-9256-y.

BENEFITS OF MUSCULAR STRENGTH AND ENDURANCE

Enhanced muscular strength and endurance can lead to improvements in the areas of performance, injury prevention, body composition, self-image, lifetime muscle and bone health, and metabolic health. Most important, greater muscular strength and endurance reduce the risk of premature death. Stronger people—particularly men—have a lower death rate due to all causes, including cardiovascular disease and cancer (see the box "Does Muscular Strength Reduce the Risk of Premature Death?"). The link between strength and death rate is independent of age, physical activity, smoking, alcohol intake, body composition, and family history of cardiovascular disease.

Improved Performance of Physical Activities

A person with a moderate to high level of muscular strength and endurance can perform everyday tasks—such as climbing stairs and carrying groceries—with ease. Increased strength can enhance your enjoyment of recreational sports by making it possible to achieve high levels of performance and to handle advanced techniques. Strength training also results in modest improvements in maximal oxygen consumption. People with poor muscle strength tire more easily and are less effective in both everyday and recreational activities.

Injury Prevention

Increased muscular strength and endurance help protect you from injury in two key ways:

- By enabling you to maintain good posture
- By encouraging proper body mechanics during everyday activities such as walking and lifting

Good muscle strength and, particularly, endurance in the abdomen, hips, lower back, and legs, maintain the spine in proper alignment and help prevent low-back pain, which afflicts more than 85% of Americans at some time in their lives. (Prevention of low-back pain is discussed in Chapter 9.)

Training for muscular strength and endurance also makes the **tendons, ligaments,** and **cartilage** cells stronger and less susceptible to injury. Resistance exercise prevents injuries best when the training program is gradual and progressive and builds all the major muscle groups.

Improved Body Composition

As Chapter 2 explained, healthy body composition means that the body has a high proportion of fat-free mass (composed primarily of muscle) and a relatively small proportion of fat. Strength training improves body composition by increasing muscle mass, thereby tipping the body composition ratio toward fat-free mass and away from fat.

Building muscle mass through strength training also helps with losing fat because metabolic rate is related to muscle mass: The greater your muscle mass, the higher your metabolic rate. A high metabolic rate means that a nutritionally sound diet coupled with regular exercise will not lead to an increase in body fat. Strength training can boost resting metabolic rate by up to 15%, depending on how hard you train. Resistance exercise also increases muscle temperature, which in turn slightly increases the rate at which you burn calories over the hours following a weight training session.

Enhanced Self-Image and Quality of Life

Strength training leads to an enhanced self-image in both men and women by providing stronger, firmer-looking muscles and a toned, healthy-looking body. Women tend to lose inches, increase strength, and develop greater muscle definition. Men tend to build larger, stronger muscles. The larger muscles in men combine with high levels of the hormone **testosterone** for a strong tissue-building effect; see the box "Gender Differences in Muscular Strength."

Because strength training involves measurable objectives (pounds lifted, repetitions accomplished), a person can easily recognize improved performance, leading to greater self-confidence and self-esteem. Strength training also improves quality of life by increasing energy, preventing injuries, and making daily activities easier and more enjoyable.

Improved Muscle and Bone Health with Aging

Research has shown that good muscular strength helps people live healthier lives. A lifelong program of regular strength training prevents muscle and nerve degeneration that can compromise the quality of life and increase the risk of hip fractures and other potentially life-threatening injuries.

In the general population, people begin to lose muscle mass after age 30, a condition called *sarcopenia*. At first they may notice that they cannot play sports as well as they could in high school. After more years of inactivity and strength loss, people may have trouble performing even the simple movements of daily life, such as walking up a flight of stairs or doing yard work. By age 75, about 25% of men and 75% of women cannot lift more than 10 pounds overhead. Although aging contributes to decreased strength, inactivity causes most of the loss. Poor strength makes it much more likely that a person will be injured during everyday activities.

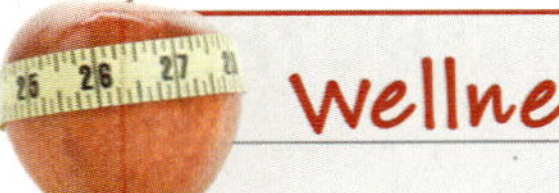

Wellness Tip

Circuit training involves a series of exercises with minimal rest in between. Circuits can include almost any kind of exercises. Circuit training is an excellent way to develop strength and endurance at the same time.

KEY TERMS

tendon A tough band of fibrous tissue that connects a muscle to a bone or other body part and transmits the force exerted by the muscle.

ligament A tough band of tissue that connects the ends of bones to other bones or supports organs in place.

cartilage Tough, resilient tissue that acts as a cushion between the bones in a joint.

testosterone The principal male hormone, responsible for the development of secondary sex characteristics and important in increasing muscle size.

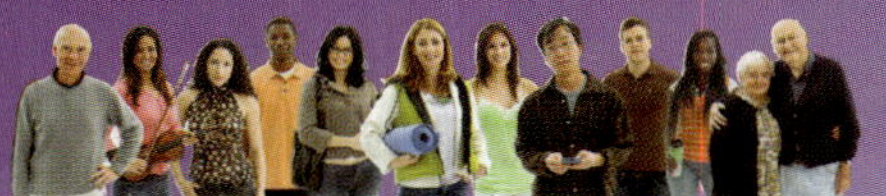

Gender Differences in Muscular Strength

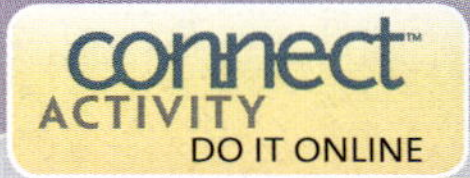

DIMENSIONS OF DIVERSITY

Men are generally stronger than women because they typically have larger bodies and a larger proportion of their total body mass is made up of muscle. But when strength is expressed per unit of cross-sectional area of muscle tissue, men are only 1–2% stronger than women in the upper body and about equal to women in the lower body. Men have a larger proportion of muscle tissue in the upper body, so they can more easily build upper-body strength than women can. Individual muscle fibers are larger in men, but the metabolism of cells within those fibers is the same in both sexes.

Two factors that help explain these disparities are testosterone levels and the speed of nervous control of muscle. Testosterone promotes the growth of muscle tissue in both males and females. Testosterone levels are 5–10 times higher in men than in women, so men tend to have larger muscles. Also, because the male nervous system can activate muscles faster, men tend to have more power.

Women are often concerned that they will develop large muscles from strength training. Because of hormonal differences, most women do not develop big muscles unless they train intensely over many years or take anabolic steroids. Women do gain muscle and improve body composition through strength training, but they don't develop bulky muscles or gain significant amounts of weight. A study of average women who weight trained 2–3 days per week for 8 weeks found that they gained about 1.75 pounds of muscle and lost about 3.5 pounds of fat. Losing muscle over time is a much greater health concern for women than small gains in muscle weight, especially because any gains in muscle weight are typically more than offset by loss of fat weight. Both men and women lose muscle mass and power as they age, but because men start out with more muscle and don't lose power as quickly, older women tend to have greater impairment of muscle function than older men. This may partially account for the higher incidence of life-threatening falls in older women.

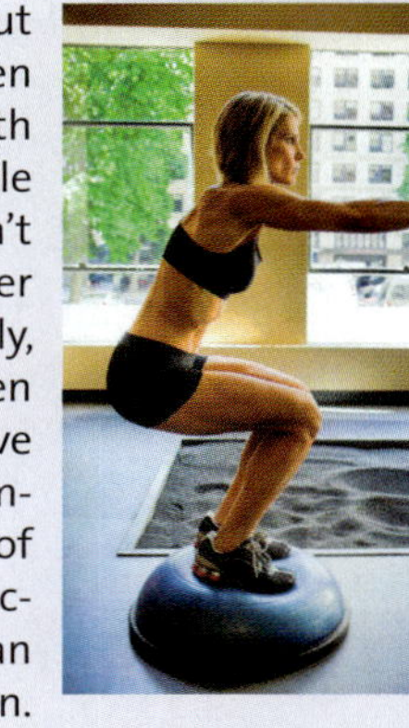

The bottom line is that both men and women can increase strength through strength training. Women may not be able to lift as much weight as men, but pound for pound of muscle, they have nearly the same capacity to gain strength as men.

As a person ages, motor nerves can become disconnected from the portion of muscle they control. By age 70, 15% of the motor nerves in most people are no longer connected to muscle tissue. Aging and inactivity also cause muscles to become slower and therefore less able to perform quick, powerful movements. Strength training helps maintain motor nerve connections and the quickness of muscles.

Osteoporosis (bone loss) is common in people over age 55, particularly postmenopausal women. Osteoporosis leads to fractures that can be life-threatening. Hormonal changes from aging account for much of the bone loss that occurs, but lack of bone mass due to inactivity and a poor diet are contributing factors. Strength training can lessen bone loss even if it is taken up later in life, and if practiced regularly, strength training may even build bone mass in postmenopausal women and older men. Increased muscle strength can also help prevent falls, which are a major cause of injury in people with osteoporosis.

Ask Yourself

QUESTIONS FOR CRITICAL THINKING AND REFLECTION

What benefits of strength training are most important to you? Are you more interested in improved physical performance? Better body composition and appearance? Long-term health benefits? How can you define your goals so they are most meaningful and motivating for you?

Metabolic and Heart Health

Strength training helps prevent and manage both cardiovascular disease (CVD) and diabetes by:

- Improving glucose metabolism
- Increasing maximal oxygen consumption
- Reducing blood pressure
- Increasing HDL cholesterol and reducing LDL cholesterol (in some people)
- Improving blood vessel health

Stronger muscles reduce the demand on the heart during ordinary daily activities such as lifting and carrying objects. The benefits of resistance exercise to the heart are so great that the American Heart Association recommends that healthy adults and many low-risk cardiac patients do strength training 2–3 days per week. Resistance training may not be appropriate for people with some types of heart disease.

ASSESSING MUSCULAR STRENGTH AND ENDURANCE

Muscular strength is usually assessed by measuring the maximum amount of weight a person can lift one time. This single maximum effort is called a **repetition maximum (RM).** You can assess the strength of your major muscle groups by taking the one–repetition maximum (1 RM) test

How Strong Are You?

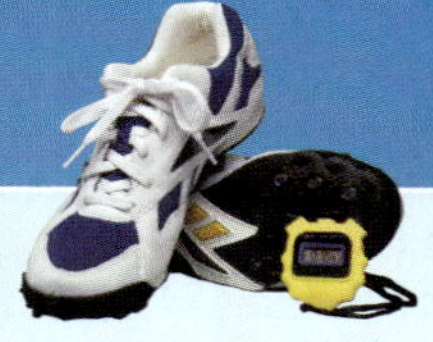

PERSONAL CHALLENGE

Tests of strength have challenged humans since the dawn of history. Strength is highly specific; one type of strength does not necessarily predict another. Strength tests help you determine your current fitness level and help you set achievable goals. You could test your capacity doing almost any exercise. Test your maximum performance on as many of the following tests as you can.

TEST	MAXIMUM REPETITIONS OR TIME	GOAL
Push-ups (Modified Or Regular)	______	______
Pull-ups or bent-arm bar hang	______	______
One-arm kettlebell snatches	______	______
Two-arm kettlebell swings	______	______
Bench press for reps (at a specific weight; e.g., 135 pounds, 225 pounds)	______	______

Write down your performance for each exercise in the second column of the list. (Note that you should wait at least a few minutes between tests.) If you aren't happy with the results, set a reasonable goal for each exercise in the third column. If you aren't sure what a reasonable goal would be, talk to your instructor or a certified personal trainer. Use these goals as a starting point for a broad-ranging strength training program.

for the bench press and by taking functional leg strength tests. You can measure 1 RM directly or estimate it by doing multiple repetitions with a submaximal (lighter) weight. It is best to train for several weeks before attempting a direct 1 RM test; once you have a baseline value, you can retest after 6–12 weeks to check your progress. See Lab 8.1 for guidelines on taking these tests. For more accurate results, avoid strenuous weight training for 48 hours beforehand.

Muscular endurance is usually assessed by counting the maximum number of **repetitions** of an exercise a person can do (such as in push-ups or kettlebell snatches) or the maximum amount of time a person can hold a muscular contraction (such as in the flexed-arm hang). You can test the muscular endurance of major muscle groups in your body by taking the curl-up test, the push-up test, and the squat endurance test. See Lab 8.2 for complete instructions on taking these assessment tests.

Ask yourself

QUESTIONS FOR CRITICAL THINKING AND REFLECTION

Considering your lifestyle and the physical activities you most commonly do, which is more important to you—muscular strength or muscular endurance? Why is this the case? Do you think your priority may change some day?

CREATING A SUCCESSFUL STRENGTH TRAINING PROGRAM

When the muscles are stressed by a greater load than they are used to, they adapt and improve their function. The type of adaptation that occurs depends on the type of stress applied.

Static Versus Dynamic Strength Training Exercises

Strength training exercises are generally classified as static or dynamic. Each involves a different way of using and strengthening muscles.

Static Exercise Also called **isometric** exercise, **static exercise** involves a muscle contraction without a change in the length of the muscle or the angle in the joint on which the muscle acts. In isometrics, the muscle contracts, but there is no movement. To perform an isometric exercise, a

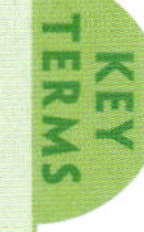

repetition maximum (RM) The maximum amount of resistance that can be moved a specified number of times.

repetitions The number of times an exercise is performed during one set.

static (isometric) exercise Exercise involving a muscle contraction without a change in the muscle's length.

person can use an immovable object like a wall to provide resistance, or simply tighten a muscle while remaining still (for example, tightening the abdominal muscles while sitting at a desk). The spine extension and the side bridge, shown on pp. 241–242, are both isometric exercises.

Static exercises are not used as widely as dynamic exercises because they don't develop strength throughout a joint's entire range of motion. During almost all movements, however, some muscles contract statically to support the skeleton so that other muscles can contract dynamically. For example, when you throw, hit a ball, or ski, the core muscles in the abdomen and back stabilize the spine. This stability allows more powerful contractions in the lower- and upper-body muscles. The core muscles contract statically during dynamic exercises, such as squats, lunges, and overhead presses.

Static exercises are useful in strengthening muscles after an injury or surgery, when movement of the affected joint could delay healing. Isometrics are also used to overcome weak points in an individual's range of motion. Statically strengthening a muscle at its weakest point will allow more weight to be lifted with that muscle during dynamic exercise. Certain types of calisthenics and Pilates exercises (described in more detail later in the chapter) also involve static contractions. For maximum strength gains, hold the isometric contraction maximally for 6 seconds; do 2–10 repetitions.

Dynamic Exercise Also called **isotonic** exercise, **dynamic exercise** involves a muscle contraction with a change in the length of the muscle. Dynamic exercises are the most popular type of exercises for increasing muscle strength and seem to be most valuable for developing strength that can be transferred to other forms of physical activity. They can be performed with weight machines, free weights, or a person's own body weight (as in curl-ups or push-ups).

There are two kinds of dynamic muscle contractions:

- A **concentric muscle contraction** occurs when the muscle applies enough force to overcome resistance and shortens as it contracts.
- An **eccentric muscle contraction** (also called a *pliometric contraction*) occurs when the resistance is greater than the force applied by the muscle and the muscle lengthens as it contracts.

For example, in an arm curl, the biceps muscle works concentrically as the weight is raised toward the shoulder and eccentrically as the weight is lowered.

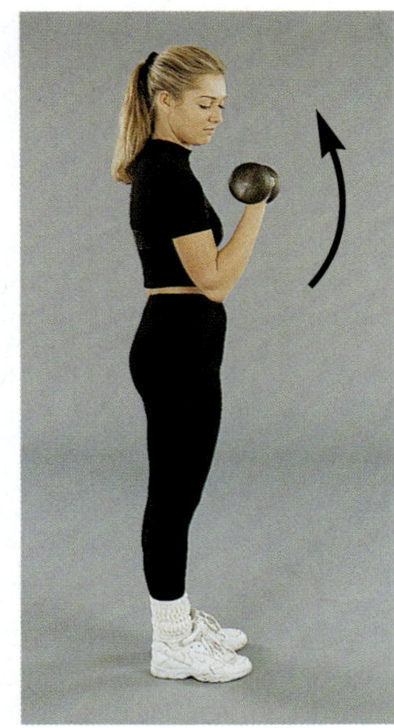
A concentric contraction.

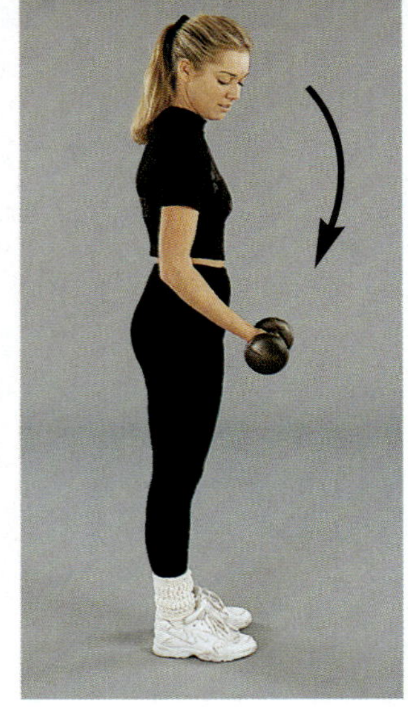
An eccentric contraction.

CONSTANT AND VARIABLE RESISTANCE Two of the most common dynamic exercise techniques are constant resistance exercise and variable resistance exercise.

- **Constant resistance exercise** uses a constant load (weight) throughout a joint's full range of motion. Training with free weights is a form of constant resistance exercise. A problem with this technique is that, because of differences in leverage, there are points in a joint's range of motion where the muscle controlling the movement is stronger and points where it is weaker. The amount of weight a person can lift is limited by the weakest point in the range.
- In **variable resistance exercise,** the load is changed to provide maximum load throughout the entire range of motion. This form of exercise uses machines that place more stress on muscles at the end of the range of motion, where a person has better leverage and can exert more force. Use elastic bands and chains with free weights to add variable resistance to the exercises.

Constant and variable resistance exercises are both extremely effective for building strength and endurance.

Pneumatic strength training machines use air pressure for resistance and are popular in many gyms and health clubs. They build strength in beginners but are less effective for more advanced strength trainers. The machines provide resistance only during the concentric (muscle shortening) phase of the exercise and not during the eccentric (muscle lengthening) phase. Such machines do not preload the muscles with resistance; they provide resistance only after the movement has been started.

OTHER DYNAMIC EXERCISE TECHNIQUES Athletes use four other kinds of isotonic techniques, primarily for training and rehabilitation.

- **Eccentric (pliometric) loading** involves placing a load on a muscle as it lengthens. The muscle contracts eccentrically in order to control the weight. Eccentric loading is practiced during most types of resistance training. For example, you are performing an eccentric movement as you lower the weight to your chest during a bench press in preparation for the active movement. You can also perform exercises designed specifically to overload muscle eccentrically, a technique called *negatives*.

- **Plyometrics** is the sudden eccentric loading and stretching of muscles followed by a forceful concentric contraction. An example would be the action of the lower-body muscles when jumping from a bench to the ground and then jumping back onto the bench. This type of exercise is used to develop explosive strength; it also helps build and maintain bone density.
- **Speed loading** involves moving a weight as rapidly as possible in an attempt to approach the speeds used in movements like throwing a softball or sprinting. In the bench press, for example, speed loading might involve doing five repetitions as fast as possible using a weight that is half the maximum load you can lift. You can gauge your progress by timing how fast you can perform the repetitions.

Training with **kettlebells** is a type of speed loading. Kettlebell training is highly ballistic, meaning that many exercises involve fast, pendulum-type motions, extreme decelerations, and high-speed eccentric muscle contractions. Kettlebell swings require dynamic concentric muscle contractions during the upward phase of the exercise followed by high-speed eccentric contractions to control the movement when returning to the starting position. Kettlebell training is very popular around the world, but more research is needed to better understand its effects on strength, power, and fitness.

- **Isokinetic** exercise involves exerting force at a constant speed against an equal force exerted by a special strength training machine. The isokinetic machine provides variable resistance at different points in the joint's range of motion, matching the effort applied by the individual while keeping the speed of the movement constant. Isokinetic exercises are excellent for building strength and endurance.

Comparing Static and Dynamic Exercise Static exercises require no equipment, so they can be done virtually anywhere. They build strength rapidly and are useful for rehabilitating injured joints. On the other hand, they have to be performed at several different angles for each joint to improve strength throughout its entire range of motion. Dynamic exercises can be performed without equipment (calisthenics) or with equipment (weight training). They are excellent for building strength and endurance, and they tend to build strength through a joint's full range of motion. Most people develop muscular strength and endurance using dynamic exercises. Ultimately, the type of exercise a person chooses depends on individual goals, preferences, and access to equipment.

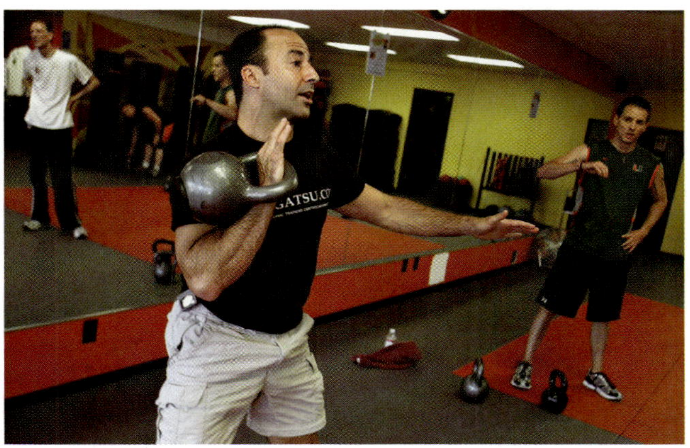

Kettlebells are growing in popularity. They provide a fast, effective workout when used properly.

Fitness Tip

As you create a personalized weight training program, focus on specificity and eliminate training methods that do not help you achieve your goal. Follow a well-designed training program that builds strength gradually and progressively. Don't adopt the program of the week just because it's popular.

Weight Machines Versus Free Weights

Muscles get stronger when made to work against resistance. Resistance can be provided by free weights, your own body weight, or exercise machines. Many people prefer weight machines because they are safe, convenient,

KEY TERMS

dynamic (isotonic) exercise Exercise involving a muscle contraction with a change in the muscle's length.

concentric muscle contraction A dynamic contraction in which the muscle gets shorter as it contracts.

eccentric muscle contraction A dynamic contraction in which the muscle lengthens as it contracts; also called a *pliometric contraction*.

constant resistance exercise A type of dynamic exercise that uses a constant load throughout a joint's full range of motion.

variable resistance exercise A type of dynamic exercise that uses a changing load, providing a maximum load at the strongest point in the affected joint's range of motion.

eccentric (pliometric) loading Loading the muscle while it is lengthening; sometimes called *negatives*.

plyometrics Rapid stretching of a muscle group that is undergoing eccentric stress (the muscle is exerting force while it lengthens), followed by a rapid concentric contraction.

speed loading Moving a load as rapidly as possible.

kettlebell A large iron weight with a connected handle; used for ballistic weight training exercises such as swings and one-arm snatches.

isokinetic The application of force at a constant speed against an equal force.

and easy to use. You just set the resistance, sit down at the machine, and start working. Machines make it easy to isolate and work specific muscles. You don't need a **spotter**—someone who stands by to assist when free weights are used—and you don't have to worry about dropping a weight on yourself. Many machines provide support for the back.

Free weights require more care, balance, and coordination to use, but they strengthen your body in ways that are more adaptable to real life. They are also more popular with athletes for developing functional strength for sports, especially sports that require a great deal of strength. Free weights are widely available, inexpensive, and convenient for home use.

Other Training Methods and Types of Equipment

You don't need a fitness center or expensive equipment to strength train. If you prefer to train at home or like low-cost alternatives, consider the following options.

Resistance Bands Resistance or exercise bands are elastic strips or tubes of rubber material that are inexpensive, lightweight, and portable. They are available in a variety of styles and levels of resistance. Some are sold with instructional guides or DVDs, and classes may be offered at fitness centers. Many free weight exercises can be adapted for resistance bands. For example, you can do biceps curls by standing on the center of the band and holding one end of the band in each hand; the band provides resistance when you stretch it to perform the curl.

Exercise (Stability) Balls The exercise or stability ball is an extra-large inflatable ball. It was originally developed for use in physical therapy but has become a popular piece of exercise equipment for use in the home or gym. It can be used to work the entire body, but it is particularly effective for working the core stabilizing muscles in the abdomen, chest, and back—muscles that are important for preventing back problems. The ball's instability forces the exerciser to use the stability muscles to balance the body, even when just sitting on the ball. Moves such as crunches are more effective when performed with an exercise ball.

When choosing a ball, make sure that your thighs are parallel to the ground when you sit on it; if you are a beginner or have back problems, choose a larger ball so that your thighs are at an angle, with hips higher than knees. Beginners should use caution until they feel comfortable with the movements and take care to avoid poor form due to fatigue.

Pilates Pilates (*pil LAH teez*) was developed by German gymnast and boxer Joseph Pilates early in the twentieth century. It often involves the use of specially designed

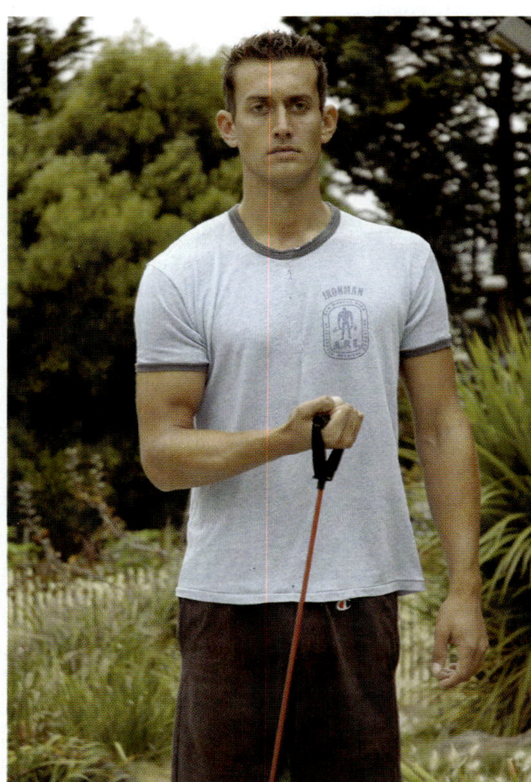

Resistance bands are a popular and inexpensive alternative to training with weights or machines.

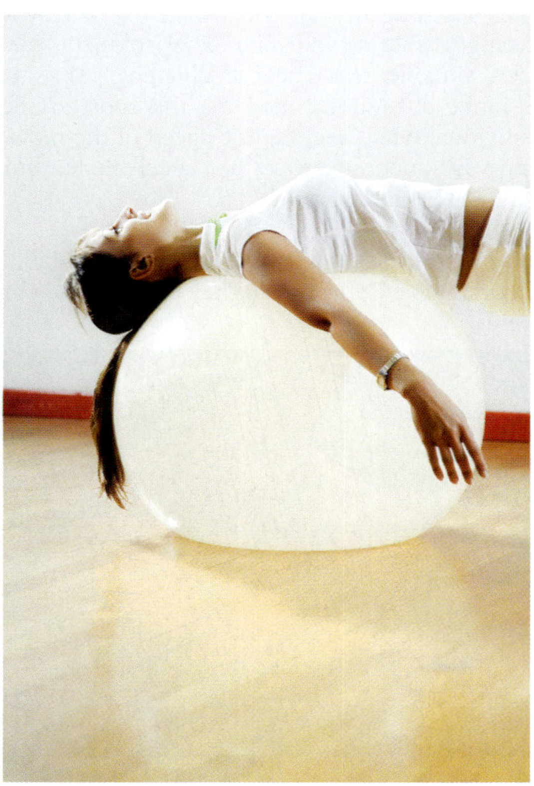

Proper fit is an important factor in choosing and using a stability ball.

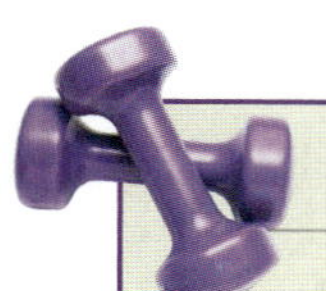

Fitness Tip

Think those resistance bands are just for beginners? Think again. Many serious weight trainers use elastic bands to provide variable resistance during large muscle lifts such as the squat and bench press. Bands might increase power, rate of force development, and speed.

resistance training devices, although some classes feature just mat or floor work. Pilates focuses on strengthening and stretching the core muscles in the back, abdomen, and buttocks to create a solid base of support for whole-body movement; the emphasis is on concentration, control, movement flow, and breathing. Mat exercises can be done at home, but because there are hundreds of Pilates exercises, some of them strenuous, it is best to begin with some qualified instruction. The Pilates Method Alliance (www.pilatesmethodalliance.org) offers advice on finding a qualified teacher.

Medicine Balls, Suspension Training, Stones, and Carrying Exercises Almost anything that provides resistance to movement will develop strength. Rubber medicine balls weigh up to 50 pounds and can be used for a variety of functional movements, such as squats and overhead throws. Suspension training uses body weight as the resistance and involves doing exercises with ropes or cords attached to a hook, bar, door jam, or sturdy tree branch. Stones can provide resistance to almost any movement, are free, and can be found in many shapes and sizes. Walking while carrying dumbbells, farmer's bars, or heavy stones is an easy and effective way to develop whole body strength.

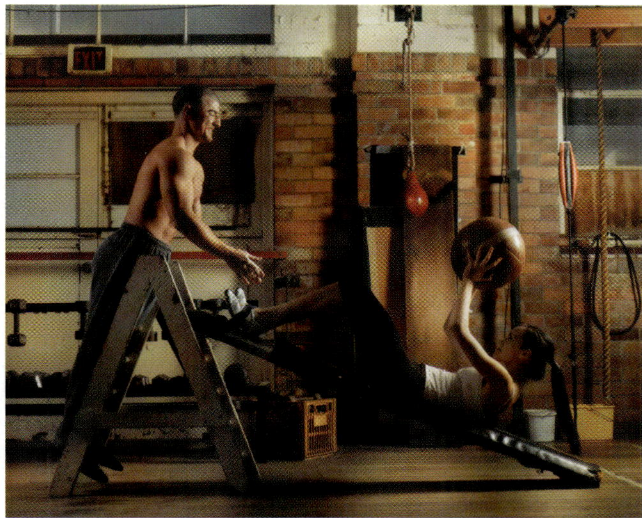

Medicine balls can be used in many ways to get an effective resistance workout.

No-Equipment Calisthenics You can use your own body weight as resistance for strength training. Exercises such as curl-ups, push-ups, squats, step-ups, heel raises, chair dips, and lunges can be done anywhere.

Applying the FITT Principle: Selecting Exercises and Putting Together a Program

A complete weight training program works all the major muscle groups. It usually takes about 8–10 different exercises to get a complete full-body workout. Use the FITT principle—frequency, intensity, time, and type—to set the parameters of your program.

Frequency of Exercise For general fitness, the American College of Sports Medicine (ACSM) recommends a frequency of at least 2 nonconsecutive days per week for weight training. Allow your muscles at least one day of rest between workouts; if you train too often, your muscles won't be able to work with enough intensity to improve their fitness, and soreness and injury are more likely to result. If you enjoy weight training and want to train more often, try working different muscle groups on alternate days—a training plan called a *split routine*. For example, work your arms and upper body one day, work your lower body the next day, and then return to upper-body exercises on the third day.

Intensity of Exercise: Amount of Resistance The amount of weight (resistance) you lift in weight training exercises is equivalent to intensity in cardiorespiratory endurance training. It determines how your body will adapt to weight training and how quickly these adaptations will occur.

Choose weights based on your current level of muscular fitness and your fitness goals. Choose a weight heavy enough to fatigue your muscles but light enough for you to complete the repetitions with good form. (For tips on perfecting your form, see the box "Improving Your Technique with Video.") To build strength rapidly, you should lift weights as heavy as 80% of your maximum capacity (1 RM). If you're more interested in building endurance, choose a lighter weight (perhaps 40–60% of 1 RM), and do more repetitions.

For example, if your maximum capacity for the leg press is 160 pounds, you might lift 130 pounds to build strength and 80 pounds to build endurance. For a general fitness program to develop both strength and endurance, choose a weight in the middle of this range, perhaps 70% of 1 RM. Or you can create a program that includes

spotter A person who assists with a weight training exercise done with free weights.

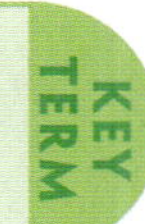

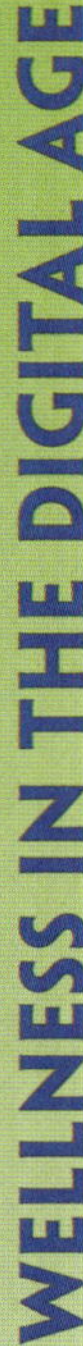

Improving Your Technique with Video

Want to get stronger? Then you need to focus on developing your skills at least as much as you focus on lifting more weight. Improving skill is the best way to increase strength during movements such as hitting a tennis ball or baseball, performing a bench press, driving a golf ball, skiing down a slope, or carrying a bag of groceries up a flight of stairs. In the world of weight training, skill means lifting weights with proper form; the better your form, the better your results.

The brain develops precise neural pathways as you learn a skill. As you improve, the pathways conduct nervous impulses faster and more precisely until the movement almost becomes reflexive. The best way to learn a skill is through focused practice that involves identifying mistakes, correcting them, and practicing the refined movement many times. However, simply practicing the skill is not enough if you want to improve and perform more powerful movements. You must perform the movements correctly instead of practicing mistakes or poor form over and over again.

Here's where technology can help. Watch videos of people performing weight-training movements correctly. You may be able to borrow videos from your instructor, purchase low-cost training videos through magazines and sporting goods stores, or find them on the Internet. If you watch training videos online, however, make sure they were produced by an authoritative source on weight training. Otherwise, you may be learning someone else's mistakes.

Film your movements using a phone camera or inexpensive video camera. Compare your movements with those of a more skilled person performing them correctly. Make a note of poor movement patterns and try to change your technique to make it more mechanically correct. Share your videos with your instructor or a certified personal trainer, who can help you identify poor form and teach you ways to correct your form.

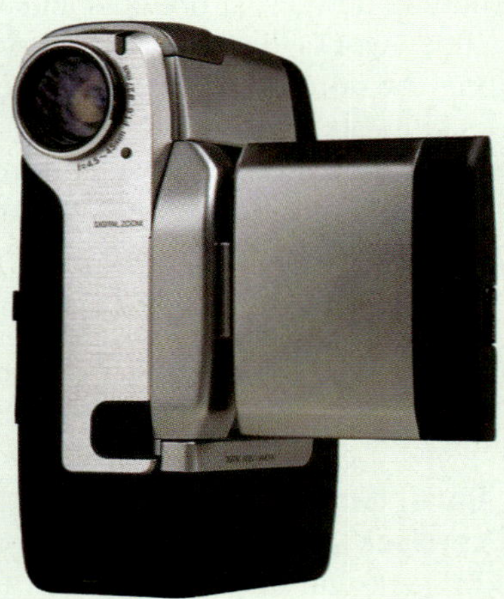

both higher-intensity exercise (80% of 1 RM for 8–10 repetitions) and lower-intensity exercise (60% of 1 RM for 15–20 repetitions); this routine will develop both fast-twitch and slow-twitch muscle fibers.

Because it can be tedious and time-consuming to continually reassess your maximum capacity for each exercise, you might find it easier to choose a weight based on the number of repetitions of an exercise you can perform with a given resistance.

Time of Exercise: Repetitions and Sets To improve fitness, you must do enough repetitions of each exercise to fatigue your muscles. The number of repetitions needed to cause fatigue depends on the amount of resistance: The heavier the weight, the fewer repetitions to reach fatigue. In general, a heavy weight and a low number of repetitions (1–5) build strength and overload primarily fast-twitch fibers, whereas a light weight and a high number of repetitions (15–20) build endurance and overload primarily slow-twitch fibers.

For a general fitness program to build both strength and endurance, try to do about 8–12 repetitions of each exercise; a few exercises, such as abdominal crunches and calf raises, may require more. To avoid injury, older (approximately age 50–60 and above) and frailer people should perform more repetitions (10–15) using a lighter weight.

In weight training, a **set** refers to a group of repetitions of an exercise followed by a rest period. To develop strength and endurance for general fitness, you can make gains doing a single set of each exercise, provided you use enough resistance to fatigue your muscles. (You should just barely be able to complete the 8–12 repetitions—using good form—for each exercise.) Doing more than one set of each exercise will increase strength development, and most serious weight trainers do at least three sets of each exercise (see the section "More Advanced Strength Training Programs" for guidelines on more advanced programs).

If you perform more than one set of an exercise, you need to rest long enough between sets to allow your muscles to work with enough intensity to increase fitness. The length of the rest interval depends on the amount of resistance. In a program to develop a combination of strength and endurance for wellness, a rest period of 1–3 minutes between sets is appropriate. If you are lifting heavier loads to build strength, rest 3–5 minutes between sets. You can save time in your workouts by alternating sets of different exercises. One muscle group can rest between sets while you work on another group.

Training volume is one method of quantifying the total load lifted during weight training. Use this formula to calculate the training volume for a workout:

repetitions × weight × sets

For example, if you did three sets of 10 repetitions for biceps curls using 50 pounds, the training volume for the exercise would be 1500 pounds ($3 \times 10 \times 50 = 1500$). Do the same calculation for every exercise in your program and add the results together to determine the total training volume for the entire workout.

Overtraining—doing more exercise than your body can recover from—can occur in response to heavy resistance training. Possible signs of overtraining include lack of progress or decreased performance, chronic fatigue, decreased coordination, and chronic muscle soreness. The best remedy for overtraining is rest; add more days of recovery between workouts. With extra rest, chances are you'll be refreshed and ready to train again. Adding variety to your program, as discussed later in the chapter, can also help you avoid overtraining with resistance exercise.

Type or Mode of Exercise For overall fitness, you need to include exercises for your neck, upper back, shoulders, arms, chest, abdomen, lower back, thighs, buttocks, and calves—about 8–10 exercises in all. If you are also training for a particular sport, include exercises to strengthen the muscles important for optimal performance *and* the muscles most likely to be injured. Weight training exercises for general fitness are presented later in this chapter, on pp. 238–246.

It is important to balance exercises between **agonist** and **antagonist** muscle groups. When a muscle contracts, it is known as the agonist; the opposing muscle, which must relax and stretch to allow contraction by the agonist, is known as the antagonist. Whenever you do an exercise that moves a joint in one direction, also select an exercise that works the joint in the opposite direction. For example, if you do knee extensions to develop the muscles on the front of your thighs, also do leg curls to develop the antagonist muscles on the back of your thighs.

The order of exercises can also be important. Do exercises for large-muscle groups or for more than one joint before you do exercises that use small-muscle groups or single joints. This allows for more effective overload of the larger, more powerful muscle groups. Small-muscle groups fatigue more easily than larger ones, and small-muscle fatigue limits your capacity to overload large-muscle groups. For example, lateral raises, which work the shoulder muscles, should be performed after bench presses, which work the chest and arms in addition to the shoulders. If you fatigue your shoulder muscles by doing lateral raises first, you won't be able to lift as much weight and effectively fatigue all the key muscle groups used during the bench press.

Also, order exercises so that you work agonist and antagonist muscle groups in sequence, one after the other. For example, follow biceps curls, which work the biceps, with triceps extensions, which exercise the triceps—the antagonist muscle to the biceps.

Wellness Tip

A standard push-up is equivalent to bench-pressing 60% of your body weight. A set of 12 push-ups is a quick, effective upper-body workout. No gym required!

The Warm-Up and Cool-Down

As with cardiorespiratory endurance exercise, you should warm up before every weight training session and cool down afterward (Figure 8.2). You should do both a general warm-up—several minutes of walking or easy jogging—and a warm-up for the weight training exercises you plan

Warm-up 5–10 minutes	Strength training exercises for major muscle groups (8–10 exercises)		Cool-down 5–10 minutes
	Sample program		
	Exercise	*Muscle group(s) developed*	
	Bench press	Chest, shoulders, triceps	
	Pull-ups	Lats, biceps	
	Shoulder press	Shoulders, trapezius, triceps	
	Upright rowing	Deltoids, trapezius	
	Biceps curls	Biceps	
	Lateral raises	Shoulders	
	Squats	Gluteals, quadriceps	
	Heel raises	Calves	
	Abdominal curls	Abdominals	
	Spine extensions	Low- and mid-back spine extensors	
Start	Side bridges	Obliques, quadratus lumborum	*Stop*

Frequency: 2–3 nonconsecutive days per week

Intensity/Resistance: Weights heavy enough to cause muscle fatigue when exercises are performed with good form for the selected number of repetitions

Time: Repetitions: 8–12 of each exercise (10–15 with a lower weight for people over age 50–60); **Sets:** 1 (doing more than 1 set per exercise may result in faster and greater strength gains); rest 1–2 minutes between exercises.

Type of activity: 8–10 strength training exercises that focus on major muscle groups

FIGURE 8.2 The FITT principle for a strength training workout.

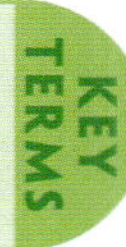

set A group of repetitions followed by a rest period.

agonist A muscle in a state of contraction, opposed by the action of another muscle, its *antagonist*.

antagonist A muscle that opposes the action of a contracting muscle, its *agonist*.

to perform. For example, if you plan to do one or more sets of 10 repetitions of bench presses with 125 pounds, you might do one set of 10 repetitions with 50 pounds as a warm-up. Do similar warm-up exercises for each exercise in your program.

To cool down after weight training, relax for 5–10 minutes after your workout. Although this is controversial, a few studies have suggested that including a period of postexercise stretching may help prevent muscle soreness; warmed-up muscles and joints make this a particularly good time to work on flexibility.

Getting Started and Making Progress

The first few sessions of weight training should be devoted to learning the movements and allowing your nervous system to practice communicating with your muscles so you can develop strength effectively. To start, choose a weight that you can move easily through 8–12 repetitions, do only one set of each exercise, and rest 1–2 minutes between exercises. Gradually add weight and (if you want) sets to your program over the first few weeks until you are doing one to three sets of 8–12 repetitions of each exercise.

As you progress, add weight according to the "two-for-two" rule: When you can perform two additional repetitions with a given weight on two consecutive training sessions, increase the load. For example, if your target is to perform 8–10 repetitions per exercise, and you performed 12 repetitions in your previous two workouts, it would be appropriate to increase your load. If adding weight means you can do only 7 or 8 repetitions, stay with that weight until you can again complete 12 repetitions per set. If you can do only 4–6 repetitions after adding weight, or if you can't maintain good form, you've added too much and should take some off.

You can add more resistance in large-muscle exercises, such as squats and bench presses, than you can in small-muscle exercises, such as curls. For example, when you can complete 12 repetitions of squats with good form, you may be able to add 10–20 pounds of additional resistance; for curls, on the other hand, you might add only 3–5 pounds. As a general guideline, try increases of approximately 5%, which is half a pound of additional weight for each 10 pounds you are currently lifting.

You can expect to improve rapidly during the first 6–10 weeks of training—a 10–30% increase in the amount of weight lifted. Gains will then come more slowly. Your rate of improvement will depend on how hard you work and how your body responds to resistance training. Factors such as age, gender, motivation, and heredity also will affect your progress.

After you achieve the level of strength and muscularity you want, you can maintain your gains by training 2–3 days per week. You can monitor the progress of your program by recording the amount of resistance and the number of repetitions and sets you perform on a workout card like the one shown in Figure 8.3.

WORKOUT CARD FOR Sara Lopez

Exercise/Date		9/14	9/16	9/18	9/21	9/23	9/25	9/28	9/30	10/2
Bench press	Wt.	45	45	45	50	50	50	60	60	60
	Sets	1	1	1	1	1	1	1	1	1
	Reps.	10	12	12	10	12	12	10	9	12
Pull-ups (assisted)	Wt.	–	–	–	–	–	–	–	–	–
	Sets	1	1	1	1	1	1	1	1	1
	Reps.	5	5	5	6	6	6	7	7	7
Shoulder press	Wt.	20	20	20	25	25	25	30	30	30
	Sets	1	1	1	1	1	1	1	1	1
	Reps.	10	12	12	10	12	12	8	10	9
Upright rowing	Wt.	5	5	10	10	10	10	12	12	12
	Sets	1	1	1	1	1	1	1	1	1
	Reps.	12	12	8	10	11	12	9	10	12
Biceps curls	Wt.	15	15	15	20	20	20	25	25	25
	Sets	1	1	1	1	1	1	1	1	1
	Reps.	10	10	10	10	12	12	8	10	10
Lateral raise	Wt.	5	5	5	5	5	5	7.5	7.5	7.5
	Sets	1	1	1	1	1	1	1	1	1
	Reps.	8	8	10	10	12	12	8	10	10
Squats	Wt.	–	–	–	45	45	45	55	55	55
	Sets	1	1	1	1	1	1	1	1	1
	Reps.	10	12	15	8	12	12	8	12	12
Heel raises	Wt.	–	–	–	45	45	45	55	55	55
	Sets	1	1	1	1	1	1	1	1	1
	Reps.	15	15	15	8	12	12	10	12	12
Abdominal curls	Wt.	–	–	–	–	–	–	–	–	–
	Sets	1	1	1	1	1	1	1	1	1
	Reps.	20	20	20	20	20	20	25	25	25
Spine extensions	Wt.	–	–	–	–	–	–	–	–	–
	Sets	1	1	1	1	1	1	1	1	1
	Reps.	5	5	5	8	8	8	10	10	10
Side bridge	Wt.	–	–	–	–	–	–	–	–	–
	Sets	1	1	1	1	1	1	1	1	1
	Seconds	60	60	60	65	65	70	70	70	70

FIGURE 8.3 A sample workout card for a general fitness strength training program.

More Advanced Strength Training Programs

The program just described is sufficient to develop and maintain muscular strength and endurance for general fitness. Performing more sets and fewer repetitions with a heavier load will cause greater increases in strength. Such a program might include three to five sets of 4–6 repetitions each; the load should be heavy enough to cause fatigue with the smaller number of repetitions. Rest long enough after a set (3–5 minutes) to allow your muscles to recover and work intensely during the next set.

Experienced weight trainers often practice some form of cycle training, also called *periodization,* in which the exercises, number of sets and repetitions, and intensity vary within a workout and/or between workouts. For example, you might do a particular exercise more intensely during some sets or on some days than others. You might also vary the exercises you perform for particular muscle groups. For more detailed information on these more advanced training techniques, consult a strength coach certified by the National Strength and Conditioning Association or

Safe Weight Training

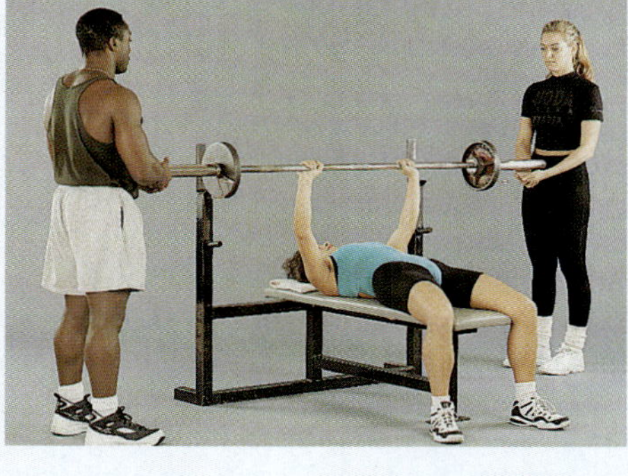

connect ACTIVITY DO IT ONLINE

TAKE CHARGE

General Guidelines

- When beginning a program or trying new exercises or equipment, ask a qualified trainer or instructor to show you how to do exercises safely and correctly.
- Lift weights from a stabilized body position; keep weights as close to your body as possible.
- Protect your back by maintaining control of your spine and avoiding dangerous positions. Don't twist your body while lifting.
- Observe proper lifting techniques and good form at all times. Don't lift beyond the limits of your strength.
- Don't hold your breath while doing weight training exercises. Doing so causes a decrease in blood returning to the heart and can make you become dizzy and faint. It can also increase blood pressure to dangerous levels. Exhale when exerting the greatest force, and inhale when moving the weight into position for the active phase of the lift. Breathe smoothly and steadily.
- Don't use defective equipment. Be aware of broken collars or bolts, frayed cables, broken chains, or loose cushions.
- Don't exercise if you're ill, injured, or overtrained. Do not try to work through the pain.

Free Weights

- Make sure the bar is loaded evenly on both sides and that weights are secured with collars or spring clips.
- When you pick a weight up from the ground, keep your back straight and your head level. Don't bend at the waist with straight legs.
- Lift weights smoothly; don't jerk them. Control the weight through the entire range of motion.
- Do most of your lifting with your legs. Keep your hips and buttocks back. When doing standing lifts, maintain a good posture so that you protect your back. Bend at the hips, not with the spine. Feet should be shoulder-width apart, heels and balls of the feet in contact with the floor, and knees slightly bent.
- Don't bounce weights against your body during an exercise.

Spotting

- Use spotters for free weights exercises in which the bar crosses the face or head (e.g., the bench press), is placed on the back (e.g., squats), or is racked in front of the chest (e.g., overhead press from the rack).
- If one spotter is used, the spotter should stand behind the lifter; if two spotters are used, one spotter should stand at each end of the barbell.
- For squats with heavy resistance, use at least three spotters—one behind the lifter (hands near lifter's hips, waist, or torso) and one at each end of the bar. Squatting in a power rack will increase safety during this exercise.
- Spot dumbbell exercises at the forearms, as close to the weights as possible.
- For over-the-face and over-the-head lifts, the spotter should hold the bar with an alternate grip (one palm up and one palm down) inside the lifter's grip.
- Ensure good communication between spotter and lifter by agreeing on verbal signals before the exercise.

another reliable source. If you decide to adopt a more advanced training regimen, start off slowly to give your body a chance to adjust and to minimize the risk of injury.

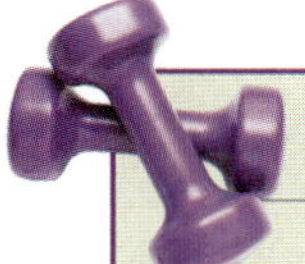

Fitness Tip

Doing three sets of resistance exercise is more anabolic than one set, meaning that doing multiple sets enhances muscle protein synthesis. If you're serious about strength training, do multiple sets of exercises to maximize muscle protein synthesis and muscle growth.

Weight Training Safety

Injuries happen in weight training. Maximum physical effort, elaborate machinery, rapid movements, and heavy weights can combine to make the weight room a dangerous place if proper precautions aren't taken. To help ensure that your workouts are safe and productive, follow the guidelines in the box "Safe Weight Training" and the following suggestions.

Use Proper Lifting Technique Every exercise has a proper technique that is important for obtaining maximum benefits and preventing injury. Your instructor or weight room attendant can help explain the specific techniques for different exercises and weight machines.

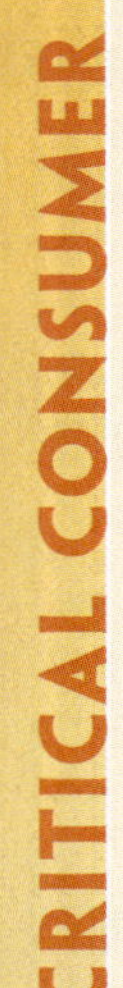

Dietary Supplements: A Consumer Dilemma

Wading through manufacturers' claims can be tricky when you are considering taking a dietary supplement. Although drugs and food products undergo stringent government testing, dietary supplements can be freely marketed without testing for safety or effectiveness. There is no guarantee that advertisements about dietary supplements are accurate or true.

What's the difference between a drug—which must be approved by the Food and Drug Administration (FDA)—and a dietary supplement? In some cases, the only real difference is in how the product is marketed. Some dietary supplements are as potentially dangerous as potent prescription drugs. But because dietary supplements have a different classification, manufacturers do not have to prove they are safe and effective before being sold; the FDA can, however, take action against any unsafe supplement product after it reaches the market.

Supplement manufacturers often make glowing claims about their products, such as "Builds lean muscle fast" or "Burns fat and gives you energy." With all the hype, how can you determine if a particular supplement might be helpful? Ask yourself the following questions:

- ***Do you really need a supplement at all?*** Nutritional authorities agree that most athletes and young adults can obtain all the necessary ingredients for health and top athletic performance by eating a well-balanced diet and training appropriately. No dietary supplement outperforms wholesome food and a good training regimen.

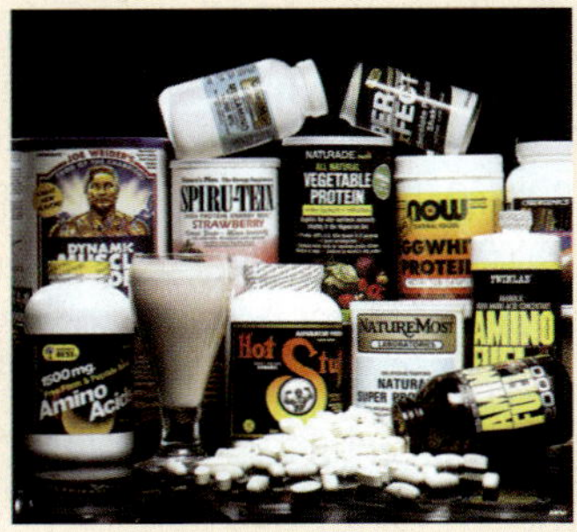

- ***Is the product safe and effective?*** The fact that a dietary supplement is available in your local store is no guarantee of safety. As described earlier, the FDA doesn't regulate supplements in the same way as drugs. The only way to determine if a supplement really works is to perform carefully controlled research on human subjects. Testimonials from individuals who claim to have benefited from the product don't count. Few dietary supplements have undergone careful human testing, so it is difficult to tell which of them may actually work.

- ***Can you be sure that the product is of high quality?*** There is no official agency that ensures the quality of dietary supplements. There is no guarantee that a supplement contains the desired ingredient, that dosages are appropriate, that potency is standardized, or that the product is free from contaminants. (See Chapter 3 for more information on dietary supplement labeling.)

Perform exercises smoothly and with good form. Lift or push the weight forcefully during the active phase of the lift and then lower it with control. Perform all lifts through the full range of motion and strive to maintain a neutral spine position during each exercise.

Use Spotters and Collars with Free Weights Spotters are necessary when an exercise has potential for danger; a weight that is out of control or falls can cause a serious injury. A spotter can assist you if you cannot complete a lift or if the weight tilts. A spotter can also help you move a weight into position before a lift and provide help or additional resistance during a lift. Spotting requires practice and coordination between the lifter and the spotter(s).

Collars are devices that secure weights to a barbell or dumbbell. Although people lift weights without collars, doing so is dangerous. It is easy to lose your balance or to raise one side of the weight faster than the other. Without collars, the weights can slip off and crash to the floor.

Be Alert for Injuries Report any obvious muscle or joint injuries to your instructor or physician, and stop exercising the affected area. Training with an injured joint or muscle can lead to a more serious injury. Make sure you get the necessary first aid. Even minor injuries heal faster if you use the R-I-C-E principle of treating injuries described in Chapter 4.

Consult a physician if you have any unusual symptoms during exercise or if you're uncertain whether weight training is a proper activity for you. Conditions such as heart disease and high blood pressure can be aggravated during weight training. Immediately report symptoms such as headaches; dizziness; labored breathing; numbness; vision disturbances; and chest, neck, or arm pain.

A Caution About Supplements and Drugs

Many active people use nutritional supplements and drugs in the quest for improved performance and appearance. Table 8.2 lists a selective summary of "performance aids" along with their potential side effects. Most of these substances are ineffective and expensive, and many are dangerous (see the box "Dietary Supplements: A Consumer Dilemma"). A balanced diet should be your primary nutritional strategy.

Table 8.2 Performance Aids Marketed to Weight Trainers

SUBSTANCE	SUPPOSED EFFECTS	ACTUAL EFFECTS	SELECTED POTENTIAL SIDE EFFECTS
Adrenal androgens, such as dehydroepiandrosterone (DHEA), androstenedione	Increased testosterone, muscle mass, and strength; decreased body fat	Increased testosterone, strength, and fat-free mass; decreased fat in older subjects (more studies needed in younger people)	Gonadal suppression, prostate hypertrophy, breast development in males, masculinization in women and children; long-term effects unknown
Amino acids	Increased muscle mass	No effects if dietary protein intake is adequate; consuming before or after training may improve performance	Minimal side effects; unbalanced amino acid intake can cause problems with protein metabolism
Amphetamines	Prevention of fatigue; increased confidence and training intensity	Increased arousal, wakefulness, and confidence; feeling of enhanced decision-making ability	Depression and fatigue (after drug wears off), extreme confusion; neural and psychological effects including aggressiveness, paranoia, hallucinations, compulsive behavior, restlessness, irritability, heart arrhythmia, high blood pressure, and chest pain
Anabolic steroids	Increased muscle mass, strength, power, psychological aggressiveness, and endurance	Increased strength, power, fat-free mass, and aggression; no effects on endurance	Liver damage and tumors, decrease in high-density lipoprotein (good cholesterol), depressed sperm and testosterone production, high blood pressure, depressed immune function, problems with sugar metabolism, psychological disturbances, gonadal suppression, liver disease, acne, breast development in males, masculinization in women and children, heart disease, thicker blood, and increased risk of cancer; steroids are controlled substances*
Beta-agonists, such as clenbuterol, salmeterol, terbutaline	Enhanced performance; prevention of muscle atrophy; increased fat-free weight; decreased body fat	Used to treat asthma, including exercise-induced asthma	Insomnia, heart arrhythmia, anxiety, anorexia, nausea, heart enlargement, heart attack (particularly if used with steroids), and heart failure
Chromium picolinate	Increased muscle mass, decreased body fat; improved blood sugar control	Well-controlled studies show no significant effect on fat-free mass or body fat	Moderate doses (50–200 μg) appear safe; higher doses may cause DNA damage and other serious effects; long-term effects unknown
Creatine monohydrate	Increased creatine phosphate levels in muscles, muscle mass, and capacity for high-intensity exercise	Increased muscle mass and performance in some types of high-intensity exercise	Minimal side effects; long-term effects unknown
Diuretics	Promote loss of body fluid	Promote loss of body fluid to accentuate muscle definition; often taken with potassium supplements and very-low-calorie diets	Muscle cell destruction, low blood pressure, blood chemistry abnormalities, and heart problems
Energy drinks	Increased energy, strength, power	Increased training volume	Insomnia, increased blood pressure, heart palpitations
Ephedra	Decreased body fat; increased training intensity due to stimulant effect	Decreased appetite, particularly when taken with caffeine; some evidence for increased training intensity	Abnormal heart rhythms, nervousness, headache, gastrointestinal distress, and heatstroke; banned by the FDA
Erythropoietin, darbepoetin	Enhanced performance during endurance events	Stimulated growth of red blood cells; enhanced oxygen uptake and endurance	Increased blood viscosity (thickness); can cause potentially fatal blood clots

(Continued)

Table 8.2 Performance Aids Marketed to Weight Trainers (*continued*)

SUBSTANCE	SUPPOSED EFFECTS	ACTUAL EFFECTS	SELECTED POTENTIAL SIDE EFFECTS
Ginseng	Decreased effects of physical and emotional stress; increased oxygen consumption	Most well-controlled studies show no effect on performance	No serious side effects; high doses can cause high blood pressure, nervousness, and insomnia
Green tea extract	Decreased body fat	Some studies show decreases in body fat	Insomnia, headache, nausea, heart palpitations
Growth hormone	Increased muscle mass, strength, and power; decreased body fat	Increased muscle mass and strength; decreased fat mass; studies show no effect on muscle or exercise performance	Elevated blood sugar, high insulin levels, and carpal tunnel syndrome; enlargement of the heart and other organs; acromegaly (disease characterized by increased growth of bones in hands and face); diseases of the heart, nerves, bones, and joints; an extremely expensive controlled substance*
Human chorionic gonadotrophin (HCG)	Increased testosterone production; prevention of muscle atrophy during steroid withdrawal	Increased testosterone production	Interferes with normal testosterone regulation; banned in most sports
Beta-hydroxy beta-methylbutyrate (HMB)	Increased strength and muscle mass; decreased body fat	Some studies show increased fat-free mass and decreased fat; more research needed	No reported side effects; long-term effects unknown
Insulin	Increased muscle mass	Effectiveness in stimulating muscle growth unknown	Insulin shock (characterized by extremely low blood sugar), which can lead to unconsciousness and death
Insulin-like growth factor (IGF)	Increased muscle mass; improved cellular function	Actual effects in healthy, active people unknown	Similar to side effects of growth hormone; long-term use promotes cancer
"Metabolic-optimizing" meals for athletes	Increased muscle mass and energy supply; decreased body fat	No proven effects beyond those of balanced meals	No reported side effets, extremely expensive
Over-the-counter stimulants, such as caffeine, phenylpropanolamine (PPA)	Weight loss; improved endurance; stimulant effect	Can be used for weight control; may improve endurance; does not appear to enhance short-term maximal exercise capacity	Increased risk of heart attack and stroke in some people (in high doses); increased incidence of abnormal heart rhythm and insomnia; caffeine is addictive
Prescription appetite suppressants, such as diethylproprion, phentermine, sibutramine, rimonabant	Weight control, weight loss	Weight loss; typically prescribed only for short-term use	Restlessness, anxiety, dizziness, depression, tremors, increased urination, diarrhea, constipation, vomiting, high blood pressure, swelling of legs or ankles, insomnia, seizures, fast or irregular heartbeat, heart palpitations, blurred vision, rashes, and difficulty breathing; can be habit-forming
Protein, amino acids, polypeptide supplements	Increased muscle mass and growth hormone release; accelerated muscle development; decreased body fat	No effects if dietary protein intake is adequate; may promote protein synthesis if taken immediately before or after weight training	Can be dangerous for people with liver or kidney disease; substituting amino acid or polypeptide supplements for protein-rich food can cause nutrient deficiencies

*Possession of a controlled substance is illegal without a prescription, and physicians are not allowed to prescribe controlled substances for the improvement of athletic performance. In addition, the use of anabolic steroids, growth hormone, or any of several other substances listed in this table is banned for athletic competition.

SOURCES: Brooks, G. A., et al. 2005. *Exercise Physiology: Human Bioenergetics and Its Applications,* 4th ed. New York: McGraw-Hill. Sports-supplement dangers. 2001. *Consumer Reports,* June. U.S. National Library of Medicine, National Institutes of Health. *MedlinePlus Medical Encyclopedia* (http://www.nlm.nih.gov/medlineplus/encyclopedia.html; retrieved).

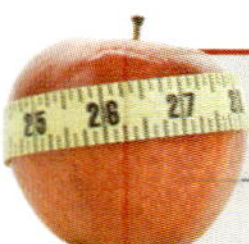

Wellness Tip

The FDA has issued several consumer warnings about dietary supplements—particularly the kinds that are marketed to people who want to build muscle and lose fat. A number of products have been pulled off store shelves after the FDA found they were not safe. Talk to your doctor before considering any dietary supplement.

Ask Yourself

QUESTIONS FOR CRITICAL THINKING AND REFLECTION

Do you think athletes should be allowed to use drugs and supplements to improve their sports performance? Would you be tempted to use a banned performance-enhancing drug if you thought you could get away with it?

WEIGHT TRAINING EXERCISES

A general book on fitness and wellness cannot include a detailed description of all weight training exercises. The following pages present a basic program for developing muscular strength and endurance for general fitness using free weights and weight machines. Instructions for each exercise are accompanied by photographs and a listing of the muscles being trained. See pages T4-2 and T4-3 of the color transparency insert "Touring the Musculoskeletal System" in this chapter for a clear illustration of the deep and superficial muscles referenced in the exercises.

Labs 8.2 and 8.3 will help you assess your current level of muscular endurance and design your own weight training program. If you want to develop strength for a particular activity, your program should contain exercises for general fitness, exercises for the muscle groups most important for the activity, and exercises for muscle groups most often injured. Regardless of the goals of your program or the type of equipment you use, your program should be structured so that you obtain maximum results without risking injury.

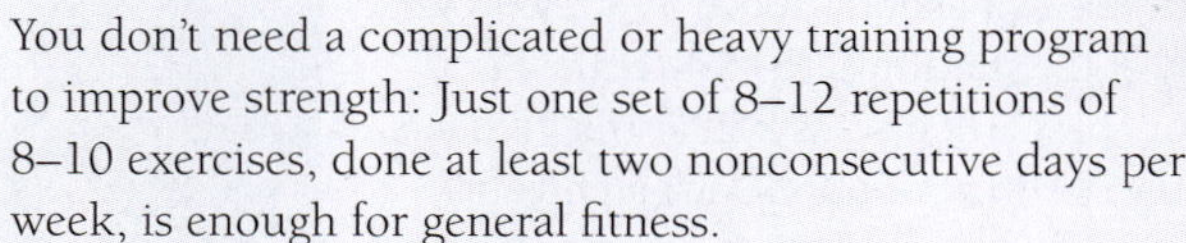

TIPS FOR TODAY AND THE FUTURE

You don't need a complicated or heavy training program to improve strength: Just one set of 8–12 repetitions of 8–10 exercises, done at least two nonconsecutive days per week, is enough for general fitness.

RIGHT NOW YOU CAN

- Do a set of static (isometric) exercises. If you're sitting, try tightening your abdominal muscles as you press your lower back into the seat, or work your arms by placing the palms of your hands on top of your thighs and pressing down. Hold the contraction for 6 seconds and do 5–10 repetitions; don't hold your breath.
- Think of three things you've done in the past 24 hours that would have been easier or more enjoyable if you increased your level of muscular strength and endurance. Visualize improvements in your quality of life that could come from increased muscular strength and endurance.

IN THE FUTURE YOU CAN

- Make an appointment with a trainer at your campus or neighborhood fitness facility. A trainer can help you put together an appropriate weight training program and introduce you to the equipment at the facility.
- Invest in an inexpensive set of free weights, kettlebells, a stability ball, or a resistance band. Then make a regular appointment with yourself to use your new equipment.

WEIGHT TRAINING EXERCISES Free Weights

EXERCISE 1 Bench Press

Instructions: **(a)** Lying on a bench on your back with your feet on the floor, grasp the bar with palms upward and hands shoulder-width apart. If the weight is on a rack, move the bar carefully from the supports to a point over the middle of your chest or slightly above it (at the lower part of the sternum). **(b)** Lower the bar to your chest. Then press it in a straight line to the starting position. Don't arch your back or bounce the bar off your chest. You can also do this exercise with dumbbells.

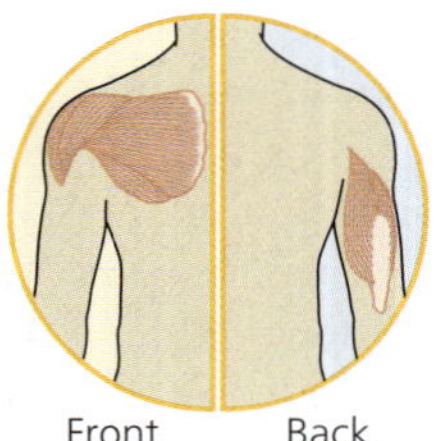

Muscles developed: Pectoralis major, triceps, deltoids

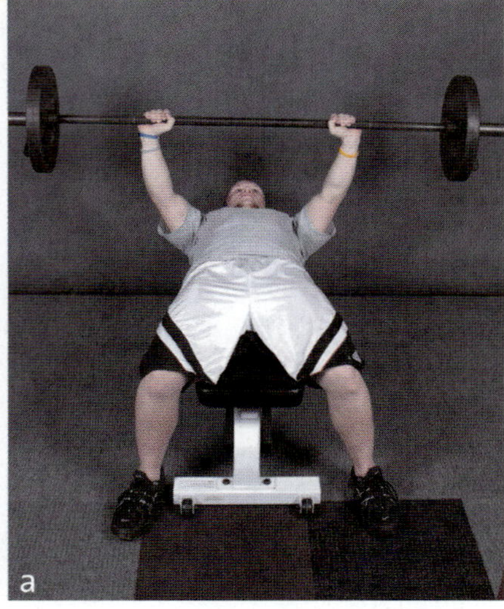

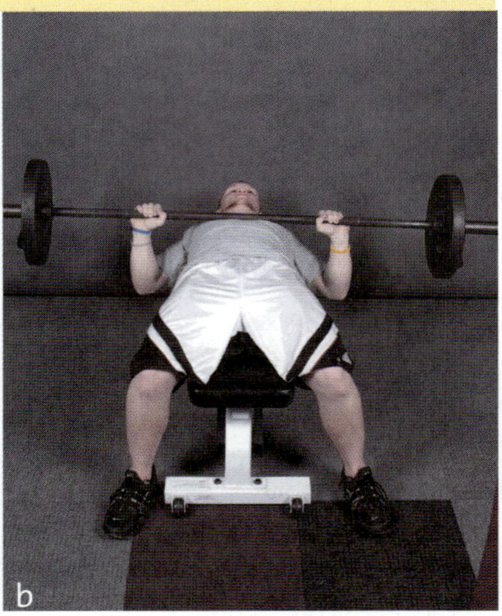

Note: *To allow an optimal view of exercise technique, a spotter does not appear in these demonstration photographs; however, spotters should be used for most exercises with free weights.*

EXERCISE 2 Pull-Up

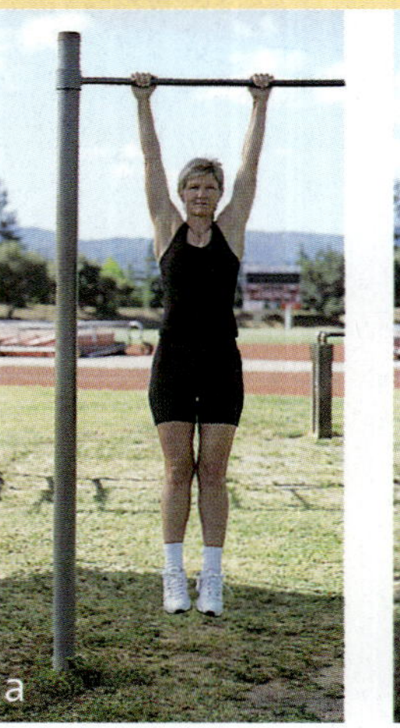

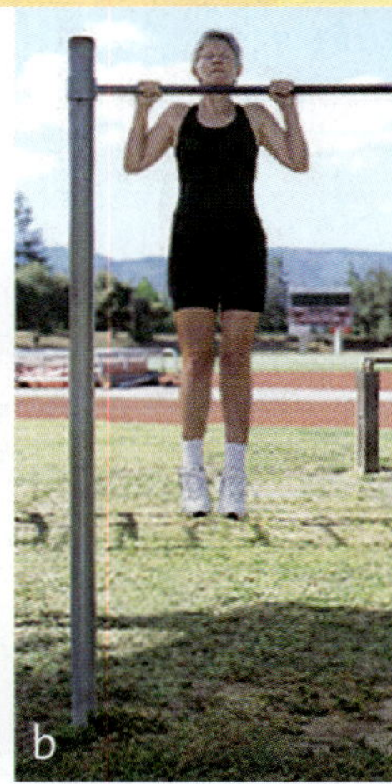

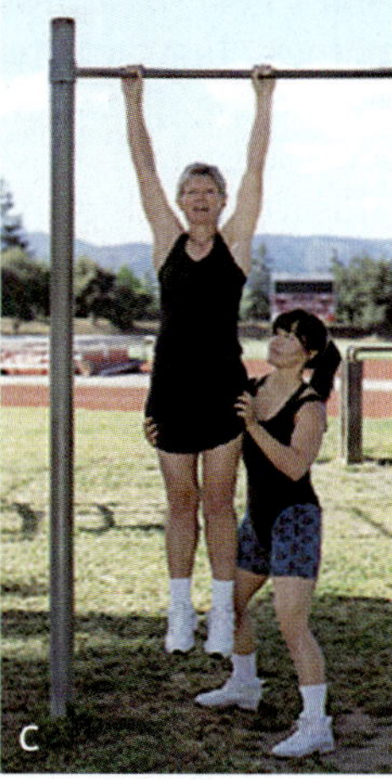

Assisted pull-up: **(c)** This is done as described for a pull-up, except that a spotter assists the person by pushing upward at the waist, hips, or legs during the exercise.

Instructions: **(a)** Begin by grasping the pull-up bar with both hands, palms facing forward and elbows extended fully. **(b)** Pull yourself upward until your chin goes above the bar. Then return to the starting position.

Muscles developed: Latissimus dorsi, biceps

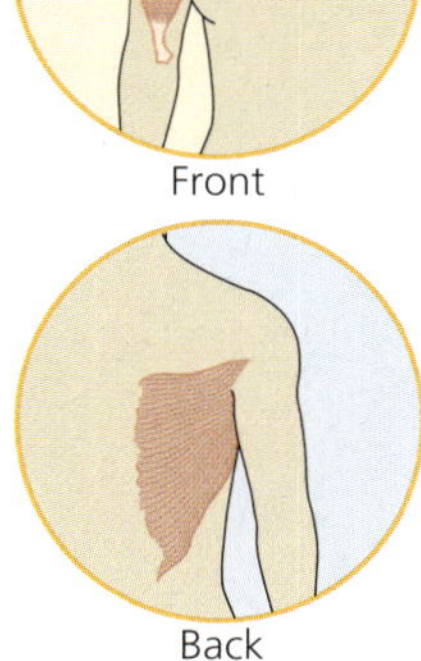

EXERCISE 3 Shoulder Press (Overhead or Military Press)

Instructions: This exercise can be done standing or seated, with dumbbells or a barbell. The shoulder press begins with the weight at your chest, preferably on a rack. **(a)** Grasp the weight with your palms facing away from you. **(b)** Push the weight overhead until your arms are extended. Then return to the starting position (weight at chest). Be careful not to arch your back excessively.

If you are a more advanced weight trainer, you can "clean" the weight (lift it from the floor to your chest). The clean should be attempted only after instruction from a knowledgeable coach; otherwise, it can lead to injury.

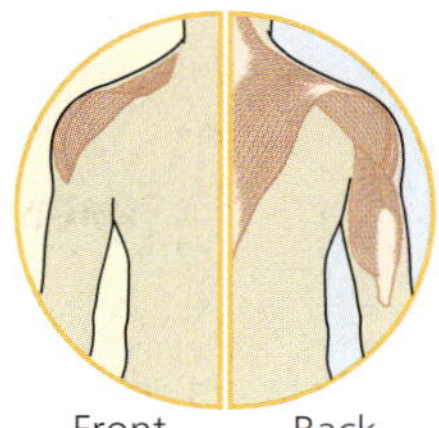

Muscles developed: Deltoids, triceps, trapezius

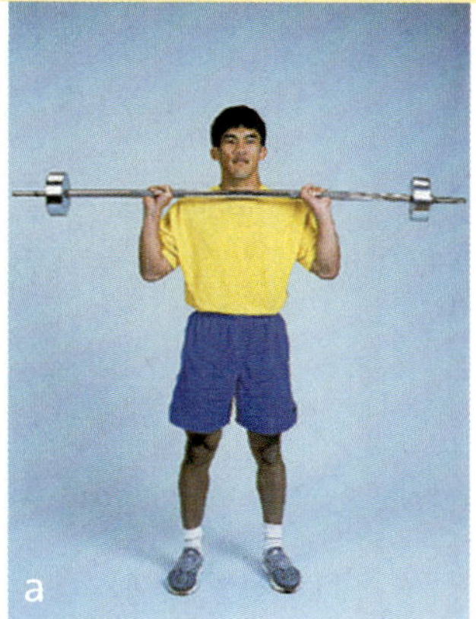

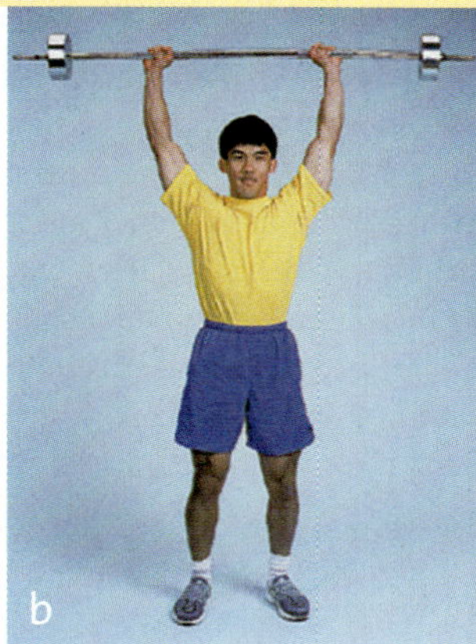

EXERCISE 4 Upright Rowing

Instructions: From a standing position with arms extended fully, grasp a barbell with a close grip (hands about 6–12 inches apart) and palms facing the body. Raise the bar to about the level of your collarbone, keeping your elbows above bar level at all times. Return to the starting position.

This exercise can be done using dumbbells, a weighted bar (shown), or a barbell.

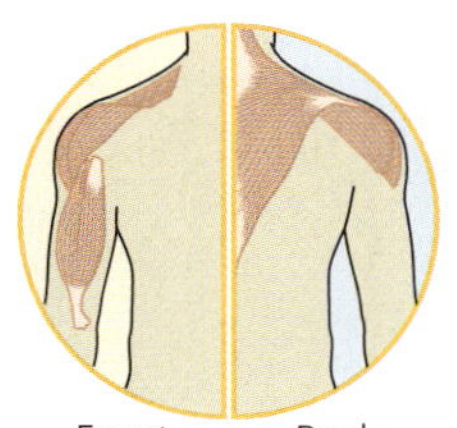

Muscles developed: Trapezius, deltoids, biceps

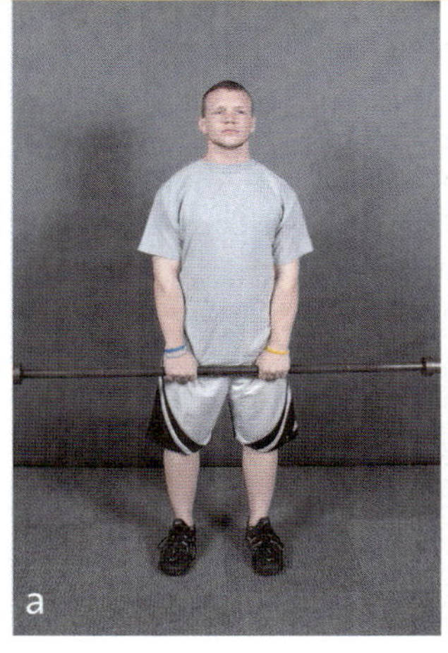

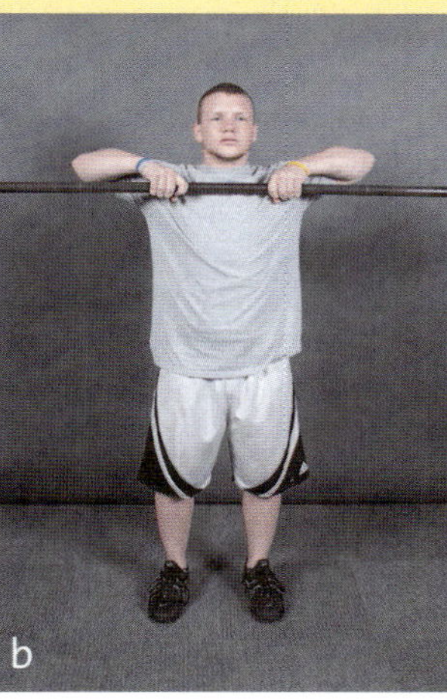

EXERCISE 5 Biceps Curl

Instructions: **(a)** From a standing position, grasp the bar with your palms facing away from you and your hands shoulder-width apart. **(b)** Keeping your upper body rigid, flex (bend) your elbows until the bar reaches a level slightly below the collarbone. Return the bar to the starting position.

This exercise can be done using dumbbells, a curl bar (shown), or a barbell; some people find that using a curl bar places less stress on the wrists.

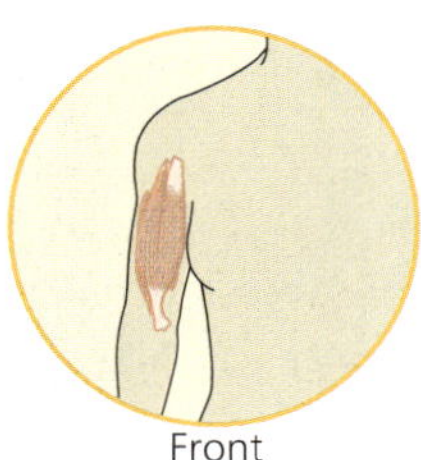

Muscles developed: Biceps, brachialis

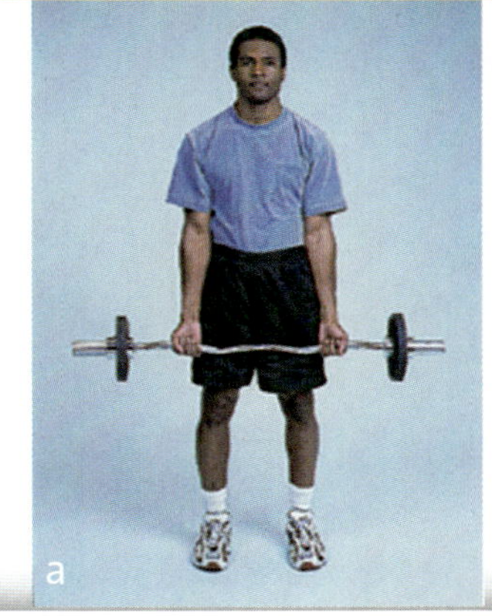

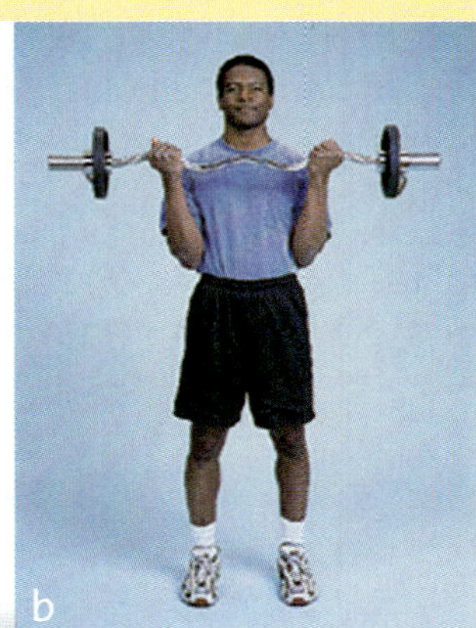

EXERCISE 6 Lateral Raise

Instructions: **(a)** Stand with feet shoulder-width apart and a dumbbell in each hand. Hold the dumbbells in front of you and parallel to each other. **(b)** With elbows slightly bent, slowly lift both weights until they reach shoulder level. Keep your wrists in a neutral position, in line with your forearms. Return to the starting position.

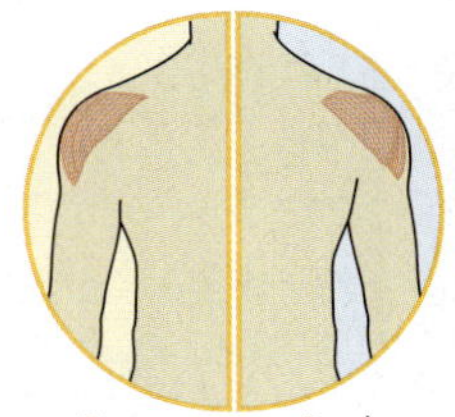

Muscles developed: Deltoids

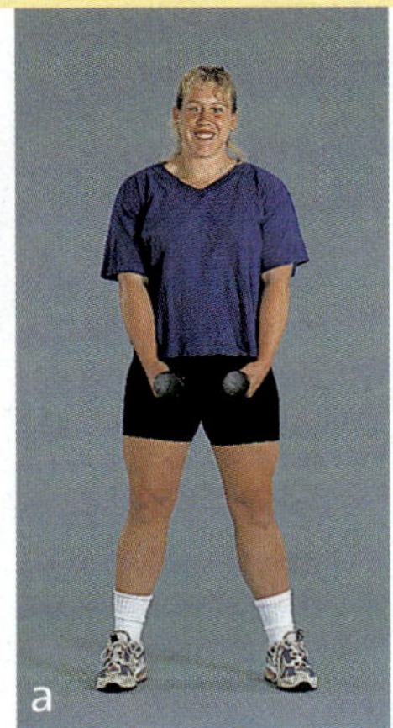

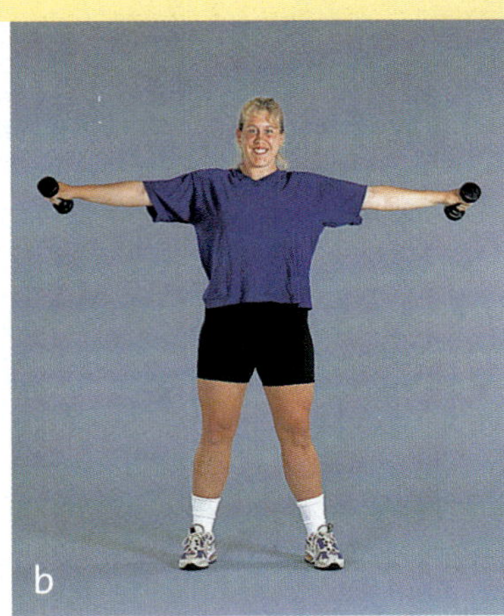

EXERCISE 7 Squat

Instructions: If the bar is racked, place the bar on the fleshy part of your upper back and grasp the bar at shoulder width. Keeping your back straight and head level, remove the bar from the rack and take a step back. Stand with feet slightly more than shoulder-width apart and toes pointed slightly outward. **(a)** Rest the bar on the back of your shoulders, holding it there with palms facing forward. **(b)** Keeping your head level and lower back straight and pelvis back, squat down until your thighs are below parallel with the floor. Let your thighs move laterally (outward) so that you "squat between your legs." This will help keep your back straight and keep your heels on the floor. Drive upward toward the starting position, hinging at the hips and keeping your back in a fixed position throughout the exercise.

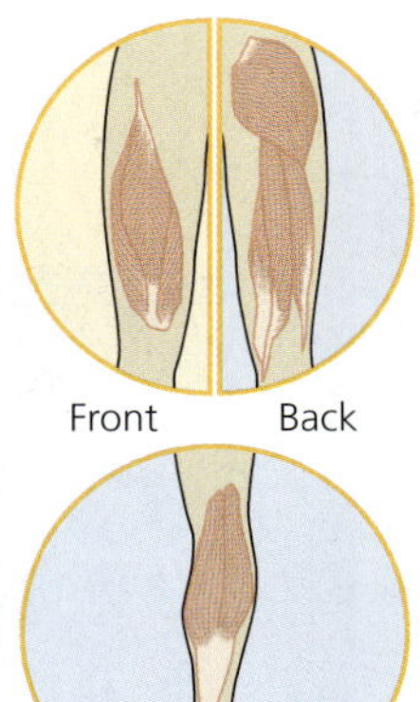

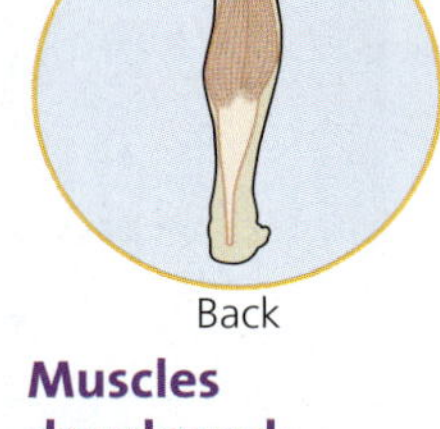

Muscles developed: Quadriceps, gluteus maximus, hamstrings, gastrocnemius

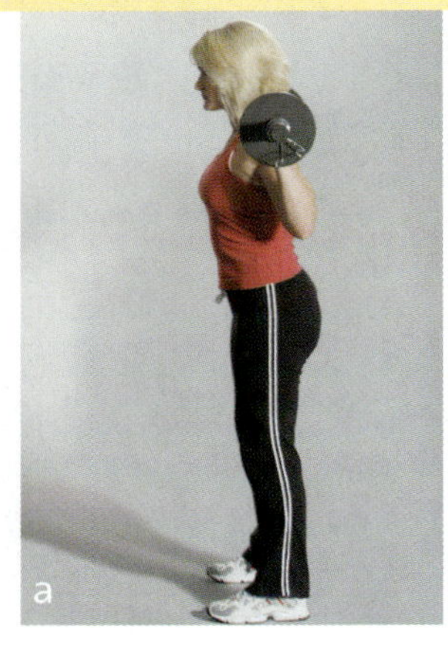

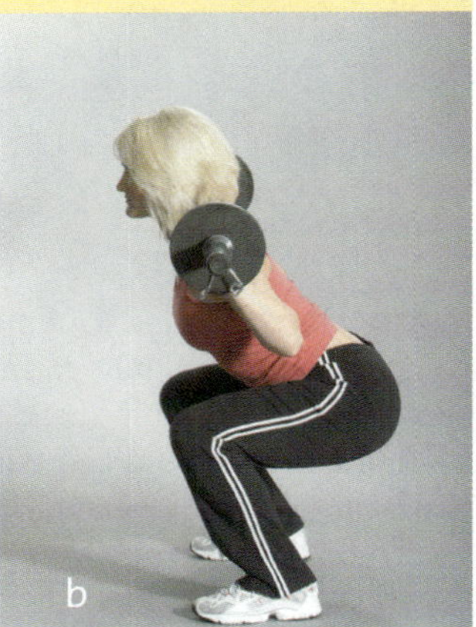

EXERCISE 8 Heel Raise

Instructions: Stand with feet shoulder-width apart and toes pointed straight ahead. **(a)** Rest the bar on the back of your shoulders, holding it there with palms facing forward. **(b)** Press down with your toes while lifting your heels. Return to the starting position.

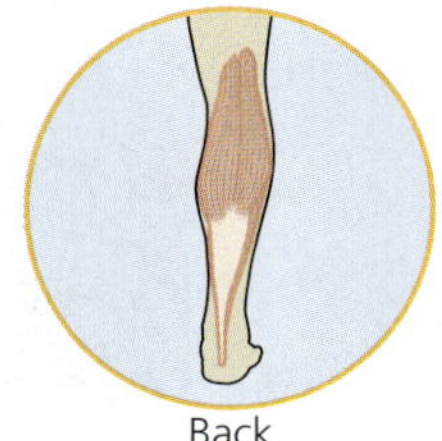

Muscles developed: Gastrocnemius, soleus

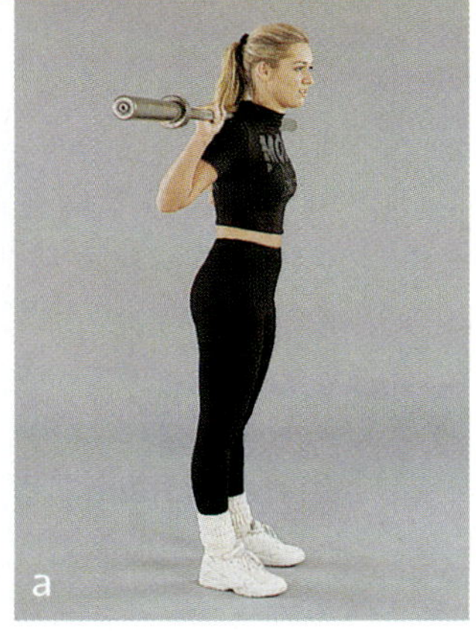

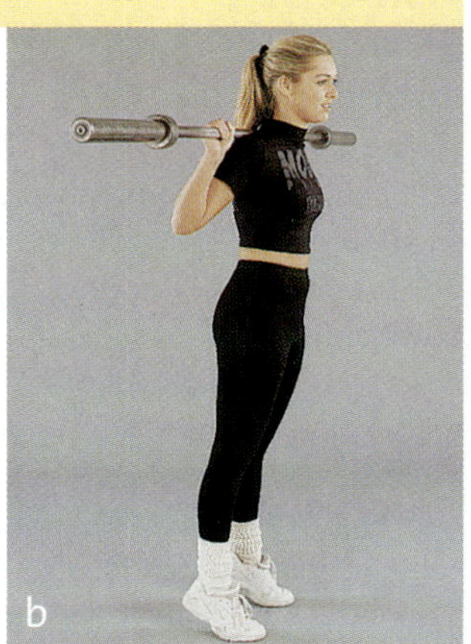

Touring the Musculoskeletal System

The Muscular System: Anterior View

The Muscular System: Posterior View

Muscle Hypertrophy: Gaining Muscle Through Strength Training

The Knee: Supporting and Maintaining Joint Stability

GOALS OF THE TOUR

5. **The Muscular System, Anterior View.** You will be able to use the illustration as a reference point for identifying the deep and superficial muscles of the front of the body in the context of understanding and performing strength training exercises.
6. **The Muscular System, Posterior View.** You will be able to use the illustration as a reference point for identifying the deep and superficial muscles of the back of the body in the context of understanding and performing strength training exercises.
7. **Muscle Hypertrophy.** You will be able to identify the components of skeletal muscle tissue and describe the process of muscle hypertrophy.
8. **The Knee.** You will be able to identify the muscles that support and stabilize the knee and describe the exercises that strengthen and stretch these muscles.

The Musculoskeletal System: Anterior View

5 Become familiar with and use the illustration as a reference point for identifying the deep and superficial muscles of the front of the body in the context of understanding and performing strength training exercises.

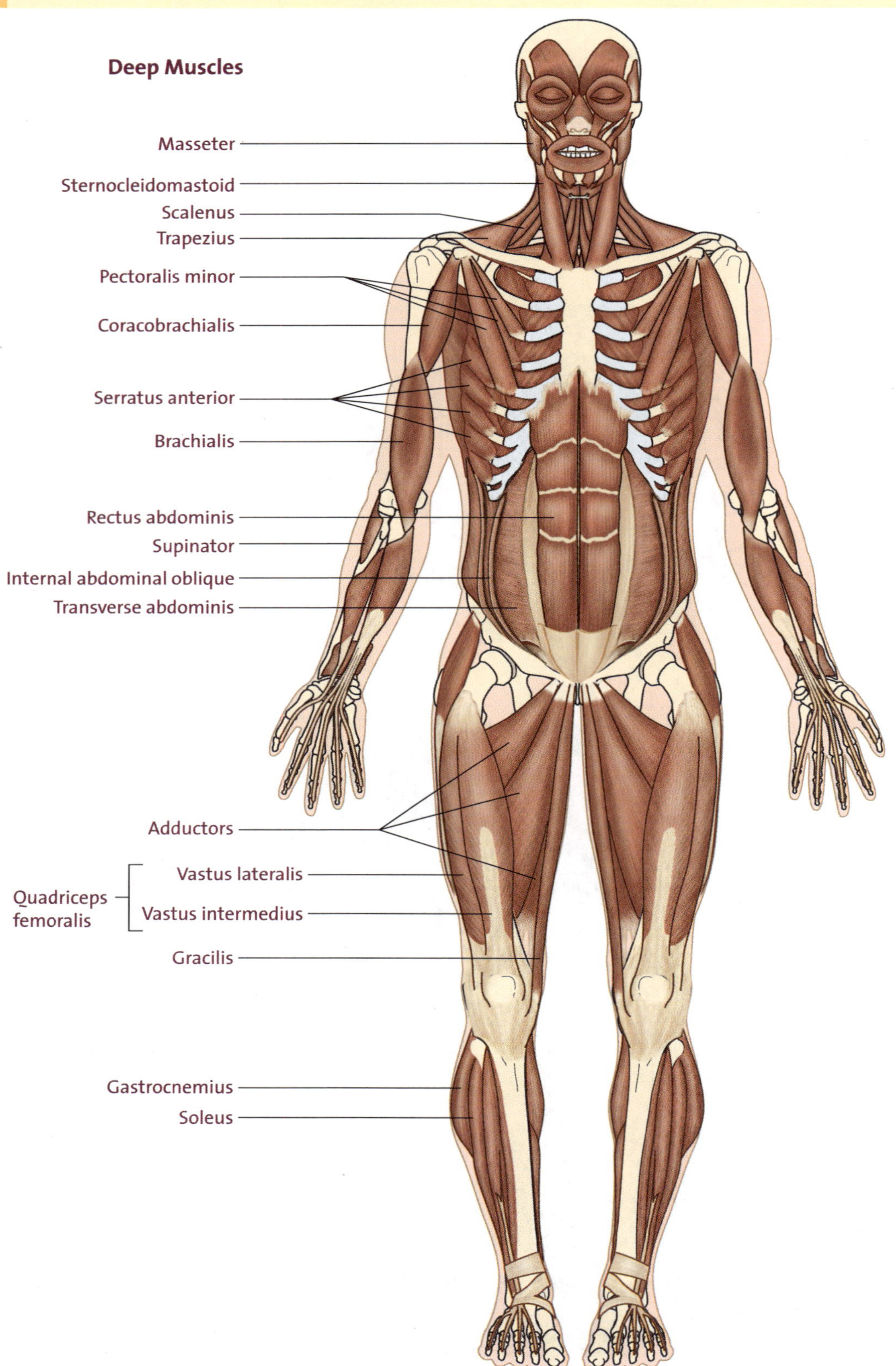

The Muscular System: Posterior View

Become familiar with and use the illustration as a reference point for identifying the deep and superficial muscles of the back of the body in the context of understanding and performing strength training exercises.

Deep Muscles

Semispinalis capitis
Splenius capitis
Levator scapulae
Supraspinatus
Rhomboids – Rhomboideus minor
Rhomboids – Rhomboideus major
Infraspinatus
External abdominal obliques
Internal abdominal obliques
Erector spinae
Quadratus lumborum (hidden by erector spinae)
Flexor carpi ulnaris
Gluteus minimus
Lateral rotators
Adductor magnus
Hamstrings – Semimembranosus
Hamstrings – Biceps femoris
Gastrocnemius *(cut)*
Soleus *(cut)*
Tibialis posterior

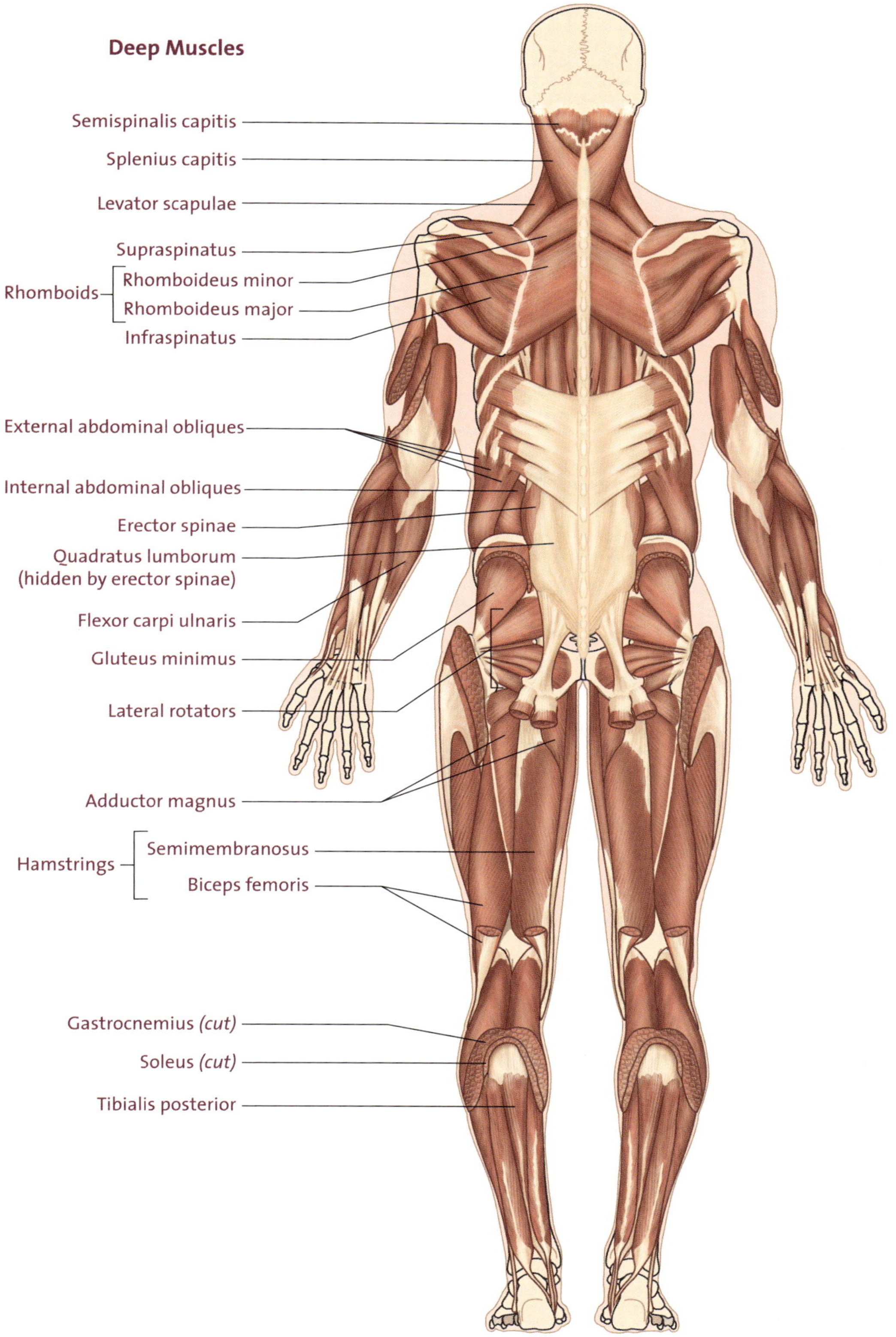

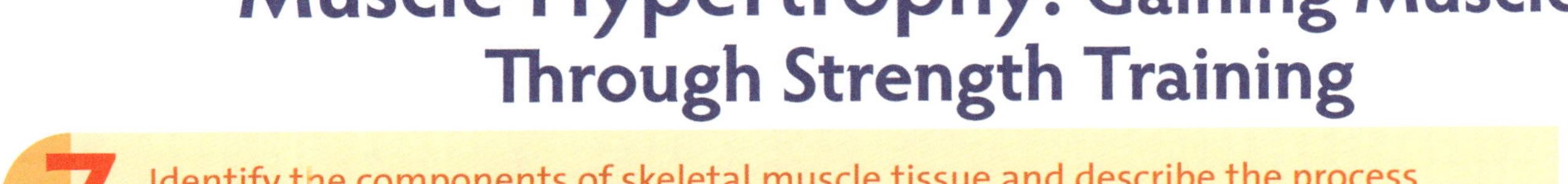

Muscle Hypertrophy: Gaining Muscle Through Strength Training

7 Identify the components of skeletal muscle tissue and describe the process of muscle hypertrophy.

Skeletal muscles are found throughout the body; they are attached to bones by tendons. Contraction of skeletal muscles allows the body to maintain posture and move. The number of muscle fibers a person has is set in childhood and does not change.

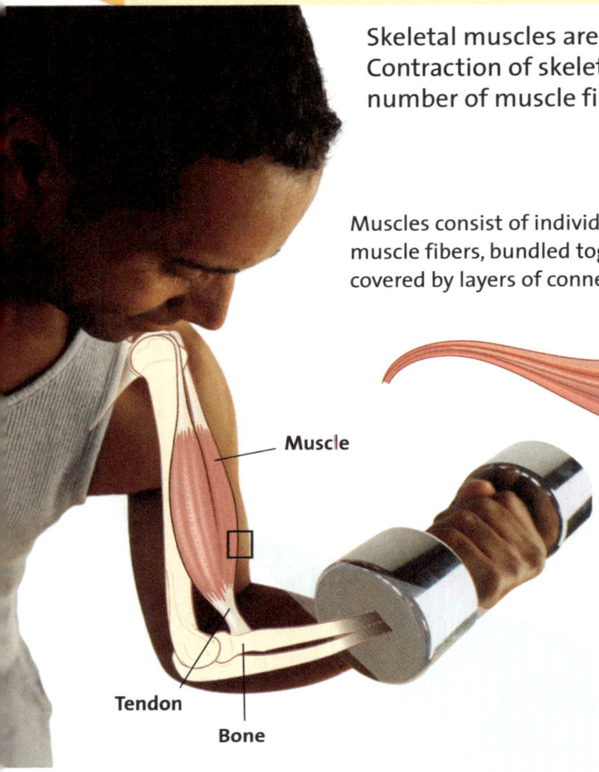

Muscle

Tendon

Bone

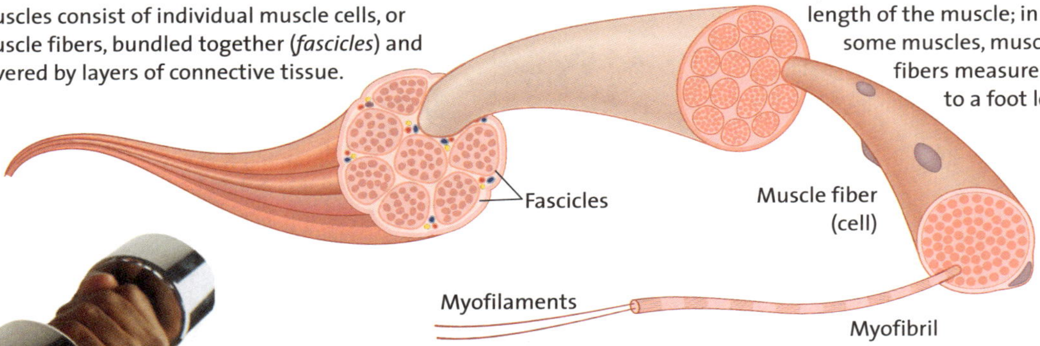

Muscles consist of individual muscle cells, or muscle fibers, bundled together (*fascicles*) and covered by layers of connective tissue.

A single muscle fiber is a cylindrical cell running the length of the muscle; in some muscles, muscle fibers measure up to a foot long.

Fascicles

Muscle fiber (cell)

Myofilaments

Myofibril

Muscle fibers are made up of smaller protein structures called myofibrils, which in turn are made up of even smaller structures called myofilaments.

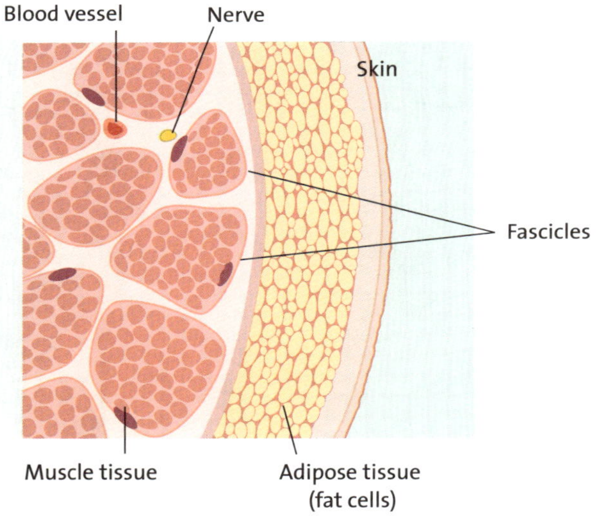

Blood vessel

Nerve

Skin

Fascicles

Muscle tissue

Adipose tissue (fat cells)

The Knee: Supporting and Maintaining Joint Stability

8 Identify the muscles that support and stabilize the knee, and describe the exercises that strengthen and stretch these muscles.

The knee is important both for weight bearing and for locomotion. Because of the stresses and strains placed on this joint, it is often subject to injury. Powerful muscles help provide support for the joint. The development of strength, endurance, and flexibility in these muscles is essential for injury prevention and maintenance of stability of the joint.

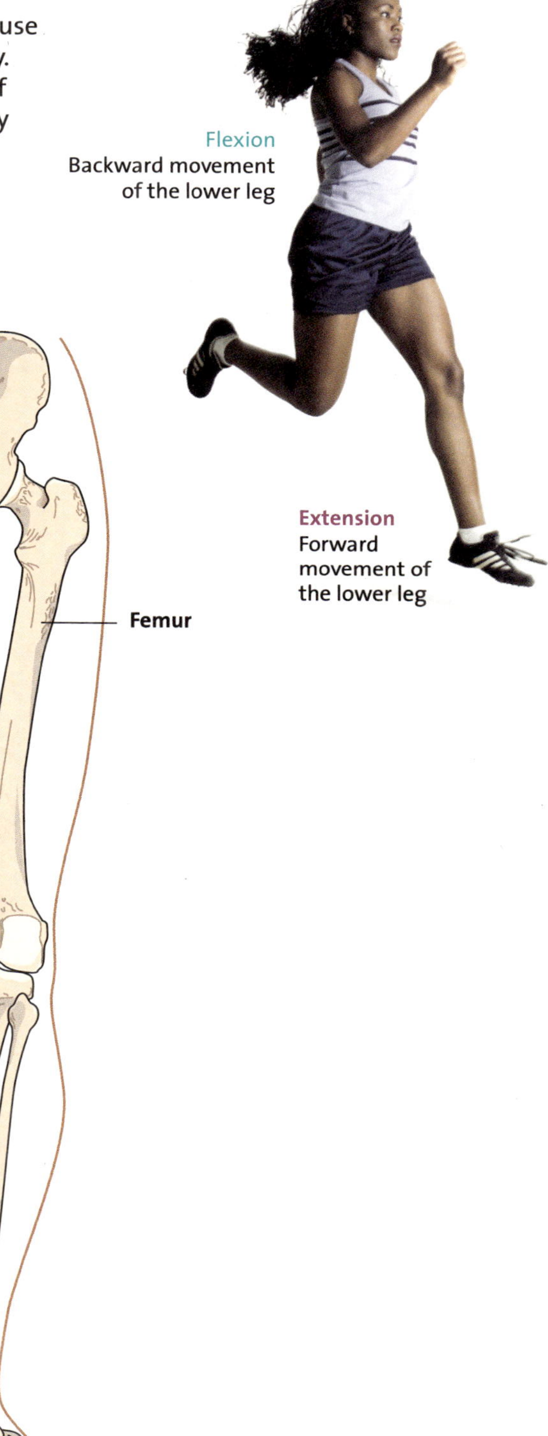

The knee is a hinge joint operating between the femur (thigh bone) and tibia (shin bone). Its primary movements are extension and flexion.

Cartilage
Flexible connective tissue lines the ends of the bones and protects them from wear.

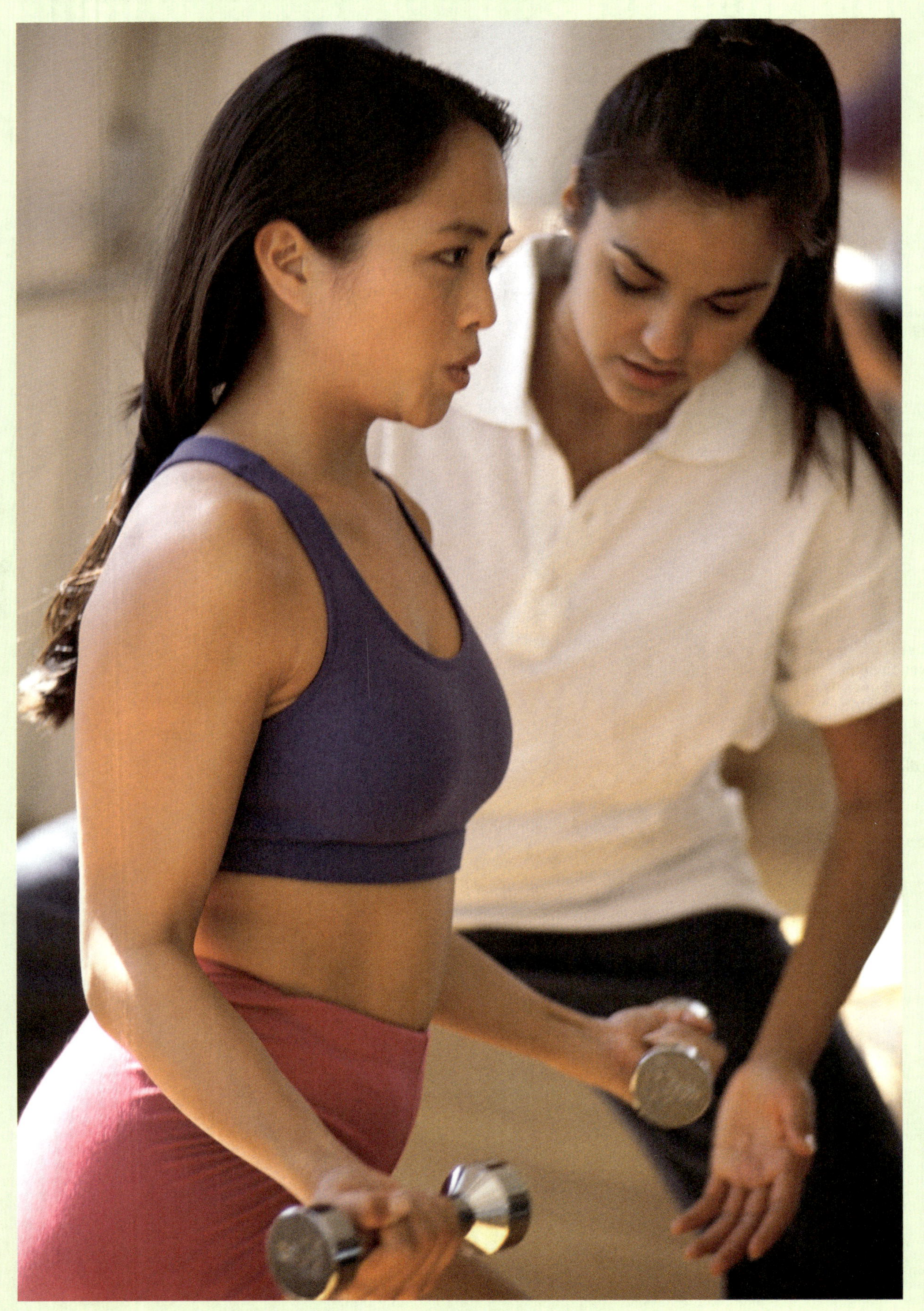

EXERCISE 9 — Curl-Up or Crunch

Instructions: **(a)** Lie on your back on the floor with your arms folded across your chest and your feet on the floor or on a bench. **(b)** Curl your trunk up, minimizing your head and shoulder movement. Lower to the starting position. Focus on using your abdominal muscles rather than the muscles in your shoulders, chest, and neck.

This exercise can also be done using an exercise ball (see p. 228).

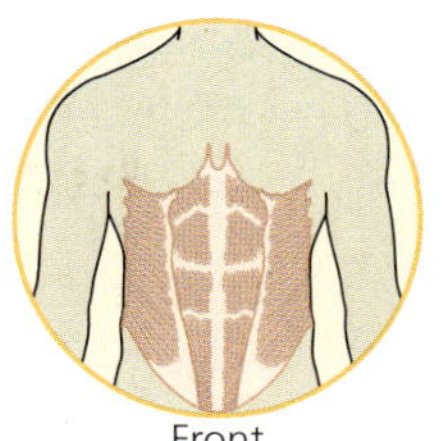
Front

Muscles developed: Rectus abdominis, obliques

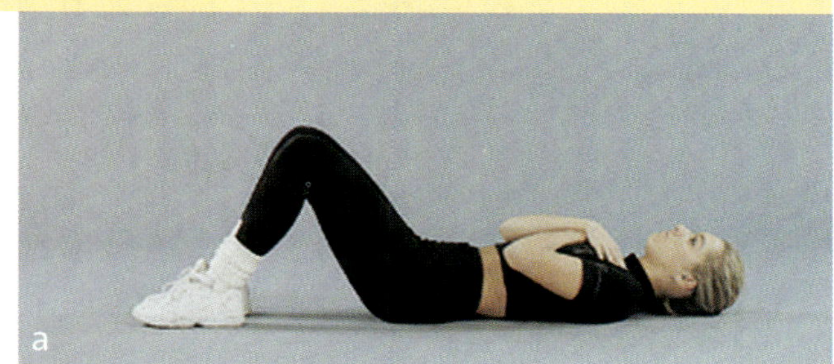
a

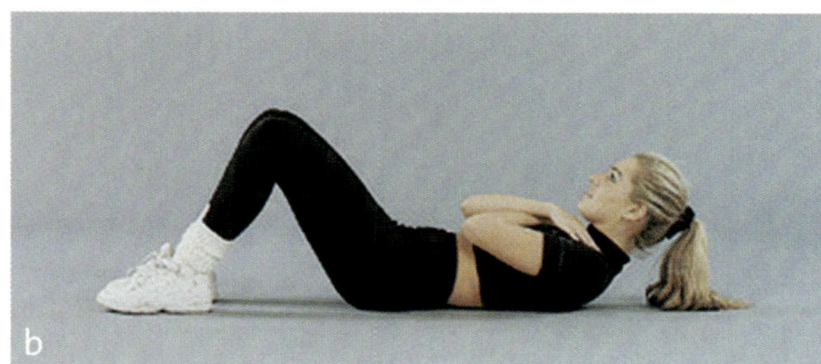
b

EXERCISE 10 — Spine Extension ("Bird Dog") (Isometric Exercise)

Instructions: Begin on all fours with your knees below your hips and your hands below your shoulders.

Unilateral spine extension:

(a) Extend your right leg to the rear and reach forward with your right arm. Keep your spine neutral and your raised arm and leg in line with your torso. Don't arch your back or let your hip or shoulder sag. Hold this position for 10–30 seconds. Repeat with your left leg and left arm.

Bilateral spine extension:

(b) Extend your left leg to the rear and reach forward with your right arm. Keep your spine neutral and your raised arm and leg in line with your torso. Don't arch your back or let your hip or shoulder sag. Hold this position for 10–30 seconds. Repeat with your right leg and left arm.

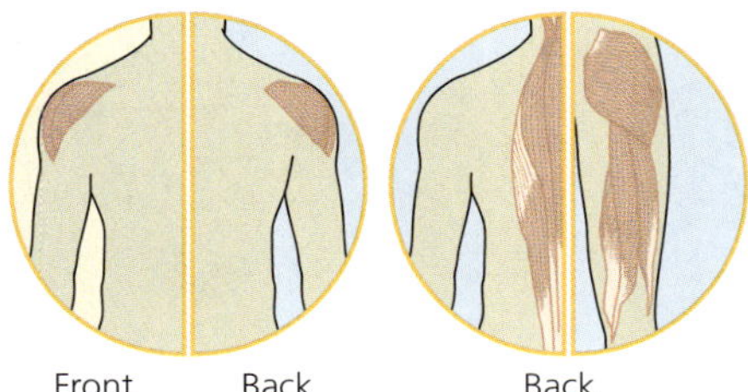
Front Back Back

Muscles developed: Erector spinae, gluteus maximus, hamstrings, deltoids

You can make this exercise more difficult by making box patterns with your arms and legs.

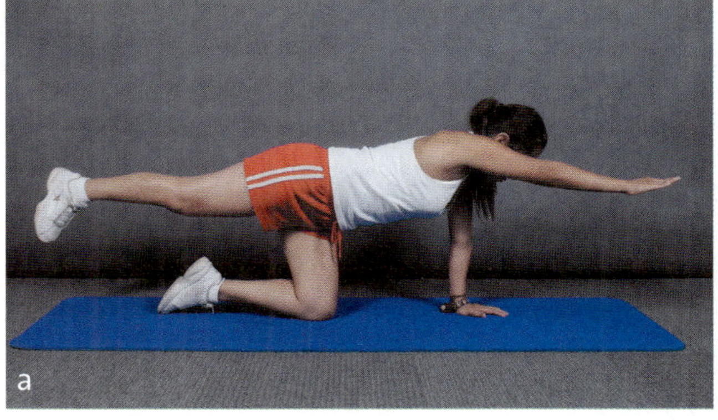
a

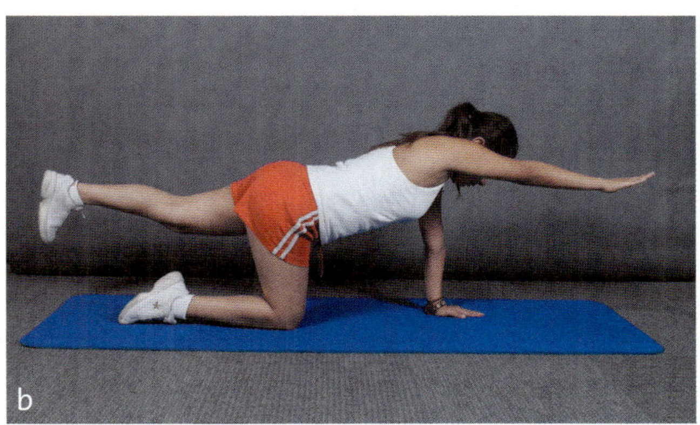
b

EXERCISE 11 Isometric Side Bridge

Instructions: Lie on the floor on your side with your knees bent and your top arm lying alongside your body. Lift and drive your hips forward so your weight is supported by your forearm and knee. Hold this position for 3–10 seconds, breathing normally. Repeat on the other side. Perform 3–10 repetitions on each side.

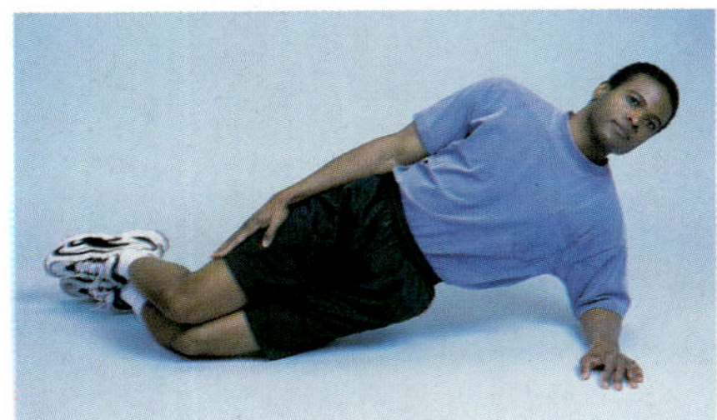

Variation: You can make the exercise more difficult by keeping your legs straight and supporting yourself with your feet and forearm (see Lab 9.3) or with your feet and hand (with elbow straight). You can also do this exercise on an exercise ball.

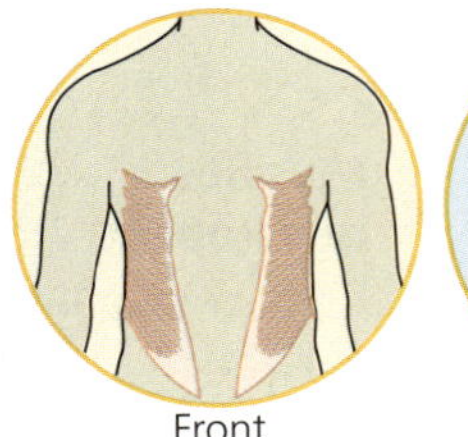

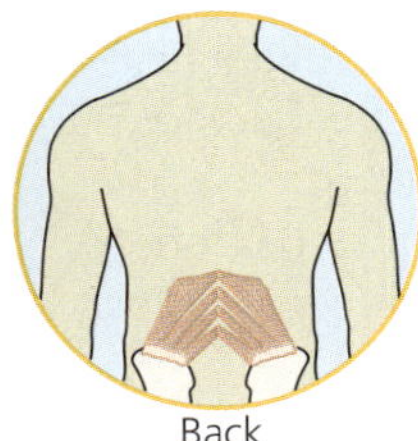

Muscles developed: Obliques, quadratus lumborum

WEIGHT TRAINING EXERCISES Weight Machines

EXERCISE 1 Bench Press (Chest or Vertical Press)

Instructions: Sit or lie on the seat or bench, depending on the type of machine and the manufacturer's instructions. Your back, hips, and buttocks should be pressed against the machine pads. Place your feet on the floor or the foot supports.

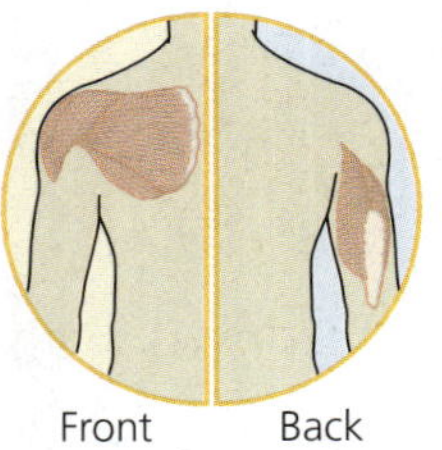

Muscles developed: Pectoralis major, anterior deltoids, triceps

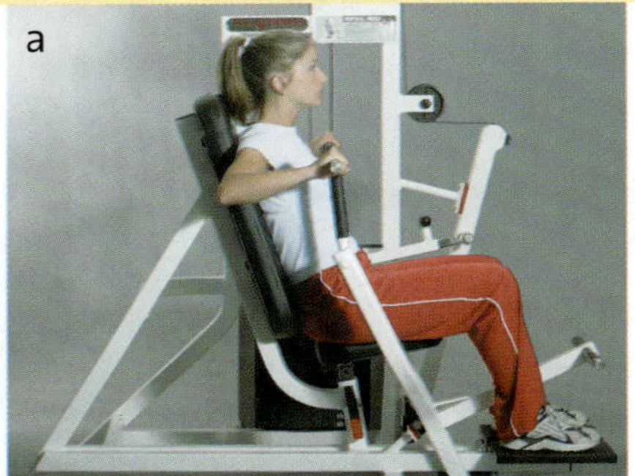

(a) Grasp the handles with your palms facing away from you; the handles should be aligned with your armpits.

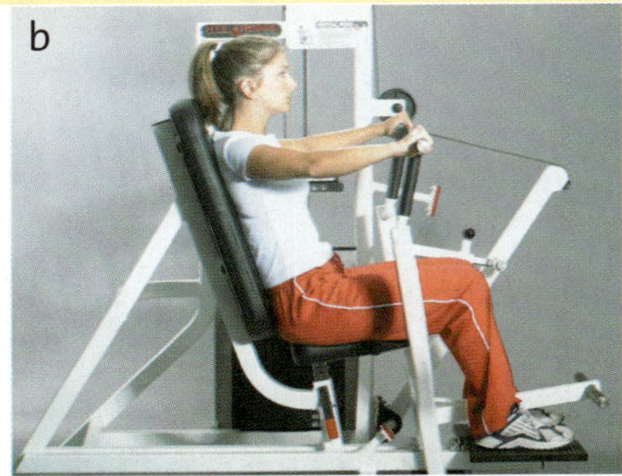

(b) Push the bars until your arms are fully extended, but don't lock your elbows. Return to the starting position.

EXERCISE 2 Lat Pull

Instructions: Begin in a seated or kneeling position, depending on the type of lat machine and the manufacturer's instructions.

Note: *This exercise focuses on the same major muscles as the assisted pull-up (Exercise 3); choose an appropriate exercise for your program based on your preferences and equipment availability.*

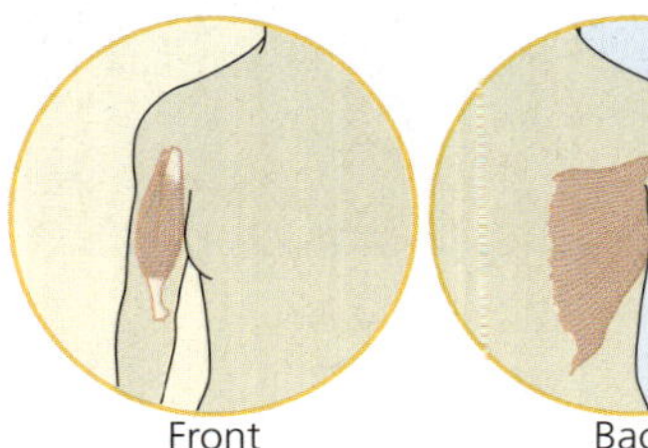

Muscles developed: Latissimus dorsi, biceps

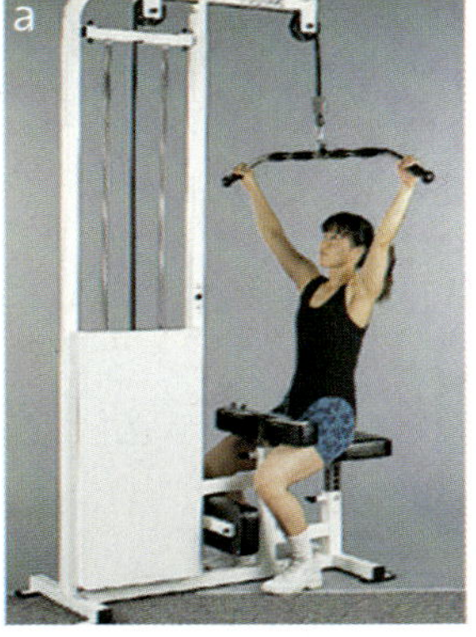

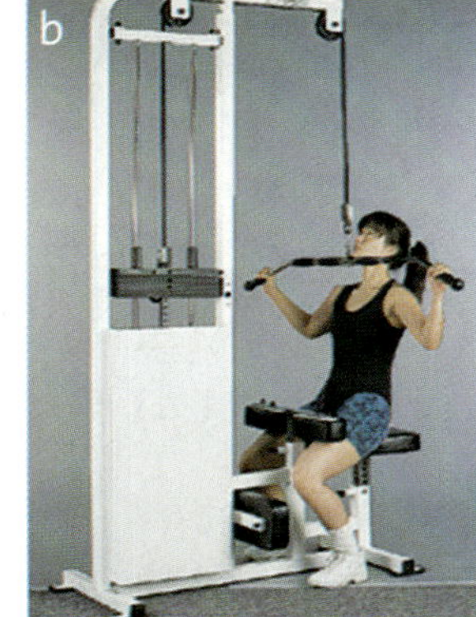

(a) Grasp the bar of the machine with arms fully extended. **(b)** Slowly pull the weight down until it reaches the top of your chest. Slowly return to the starting position.

EXERCISE 3 Assisted Pull-Up

Instructions: Set the weight according to the amount of assistance you need to complete a set of pull-ups—the heavier the weight, the more assistance provided.

(a) Stand or kneel on the assist platform, and grasp the pull-up bar with your elbows fully extended and your palms facing away. **(b)** Pull up until your chin goes above the bar, and then return to the starting position.

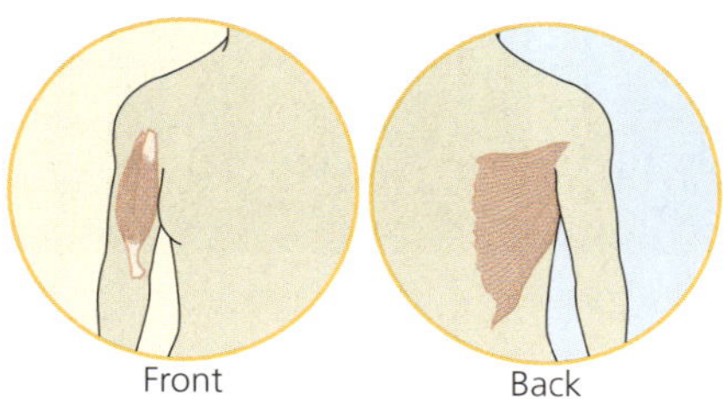

Muscles developed: Latissimus dorsi, biceps

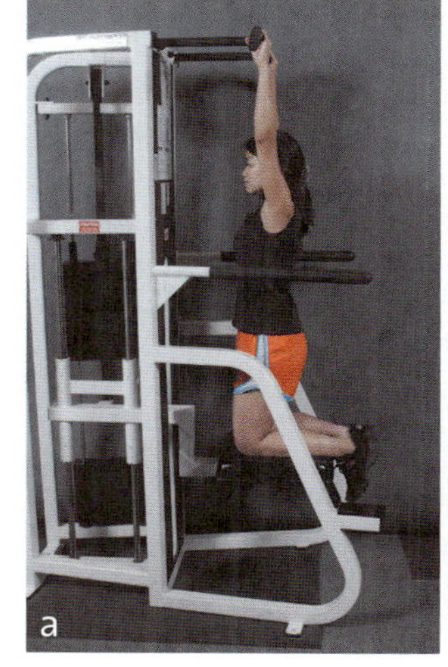

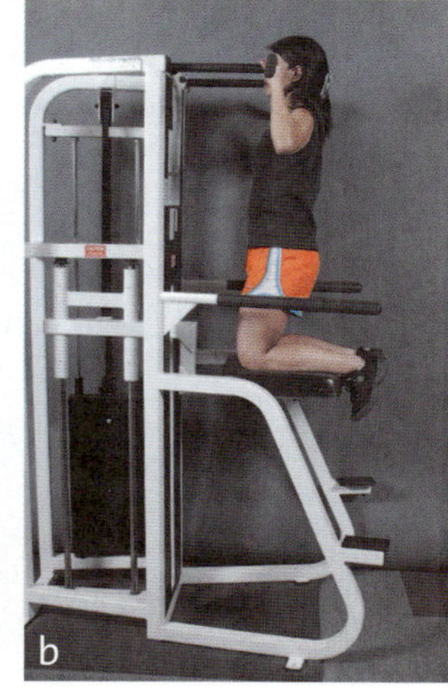

EXERCISE 4 Overhead Press (Shoulder Press)

Instructions: Adjust the seat so your feet are flat on the ground and the hand grips are slightly above your shoulders.

(a) Sit down, facing away from the machine, and grasp the hand grips with your palms facing forward. **(b)** Press the weight upward until your arms are extended. Return to the starting position.

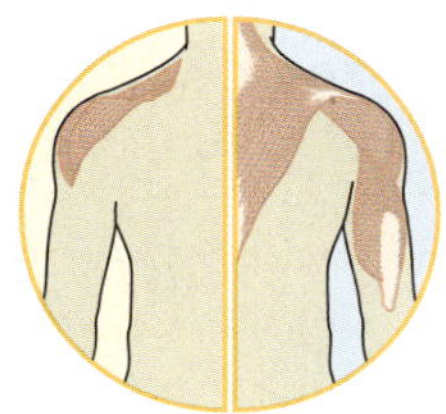

Muscles developed: Deltoids, trapezius, triceps

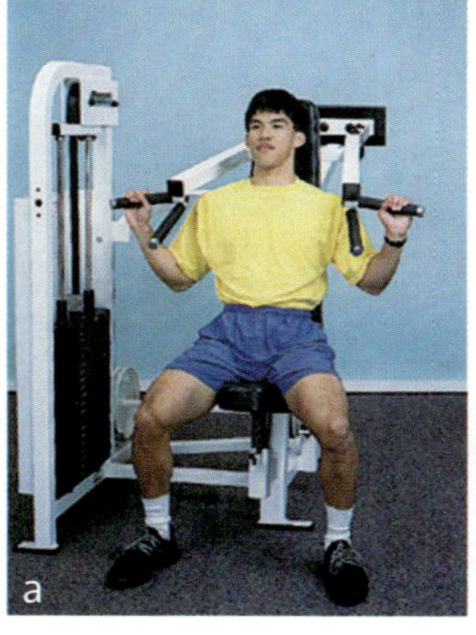

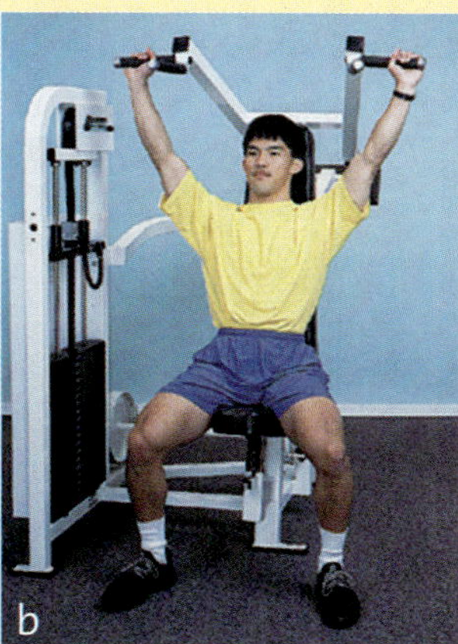

EXERCISE 5 Biceps Curl

Instructions: **(a)** Adjust the seat so that your back is straight and your arms rest comfortably against the top and side pads. Place your arms on the support cushions and grasp the hand grips with your palms facing up. **(b)** Keeping your upper body still, flex (bend) your elbows until the hand grips almost reach your collarbone. Return to the starting position.

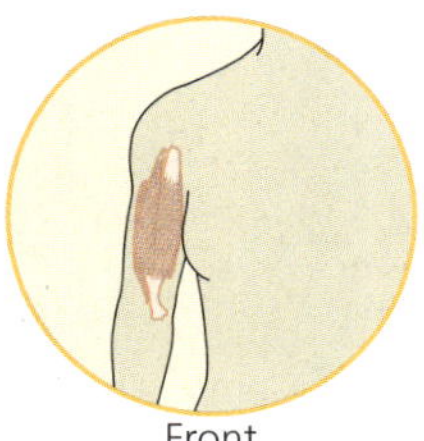

Muscles developed: Biceps, brachialis

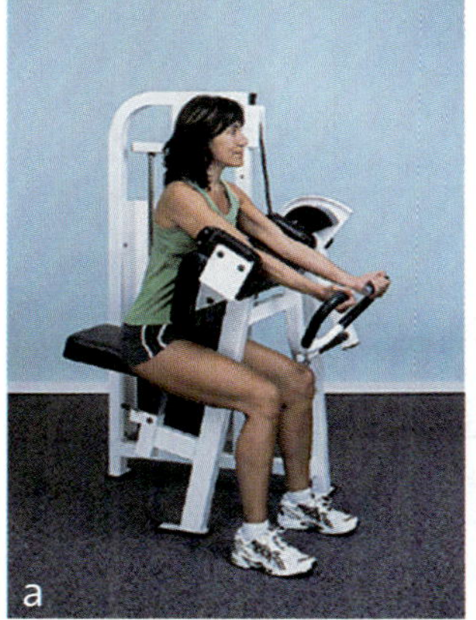

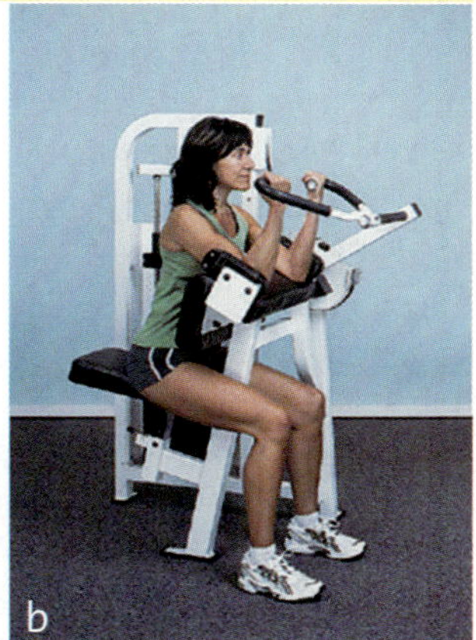

EXERCISE 6 Pullover

Instructions: Adjust the seat so your shoulders are aligned with the cams. Push down on the foot pads with your feet to bring the bar forward until you can place your elbows on the pads. Rest your hands lightly on the bar. If possible, place your feet flat on the floor. **(a)** To get into the starting position, let your arms go backward as far as possible. **(b)** Pull your elbows forward until the bar almost touches your abdomen. Return to the starting position.

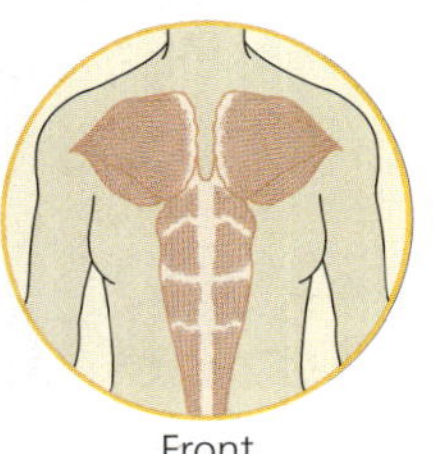
Front

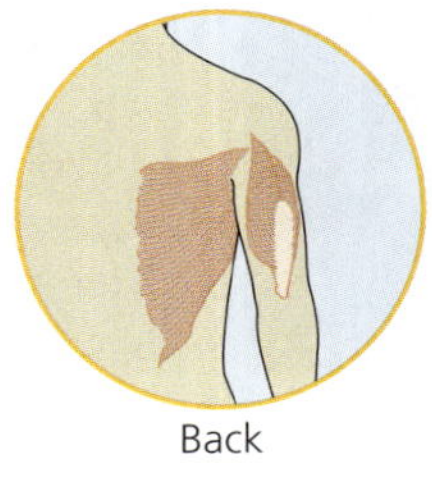
Back

Muscles developed: Latissimus dorsi, pectoralis major and minor, triceps, rectus abdominis

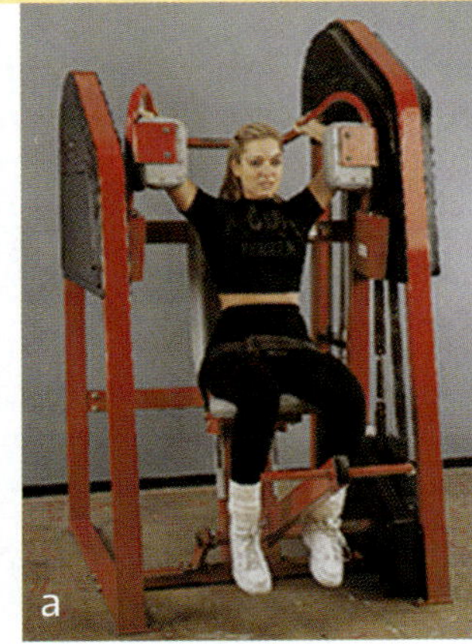
a

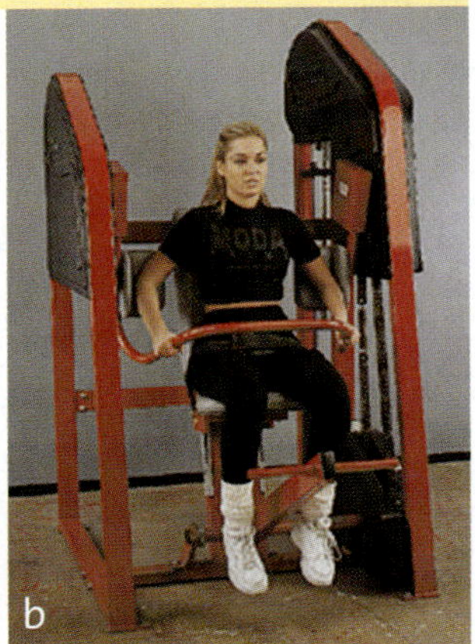
b

EXERCISE 7 Lateral Raise

Instructions: **(a)** Adjust the seat so the pads rest just above your elbows when your upper arms are at your sides, your elbows are bent, and your forearms are parallel to the floor. Lightly grasp the handles. **(b)** Push outward and up with your arms until the pads are at shoulder height. Lead with your elbows rather than trying to lift the bars with your hands. Return to the starting position.

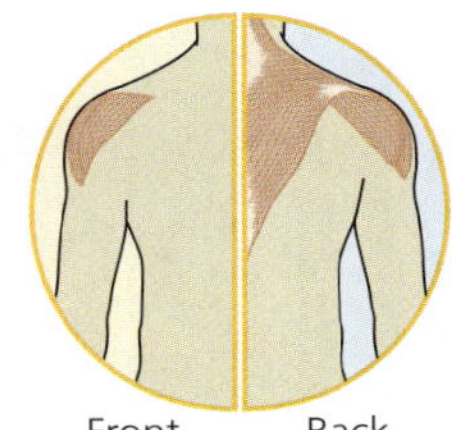
Front Back

Muscles developed: Deltoids, trapezius

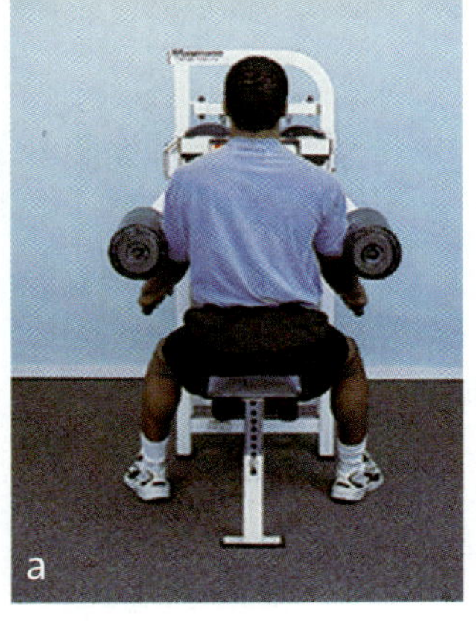
a

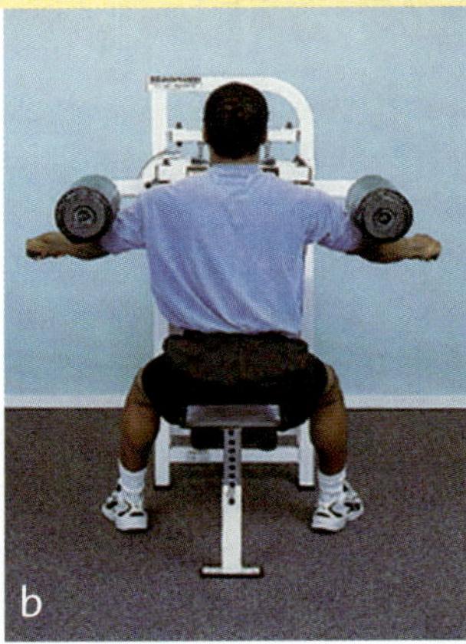
b

EXERCISE 8 Triceps Extension

Note: *This exercise focuses on some of the same muscles as the assisted dip (Exercise 9); choose an appropriate exercise for your program based on your preferences and equipment availability.*

Instructions: **(a)** Adjust the seat so your back is straight and your arms rest comfortably against the top and side pads. Place your arms on the support cushions and grasp the hand grips with palms facing inward. **(b)** Keeping your upper body still, extend your elbows as much as possible. Return to the starting position.

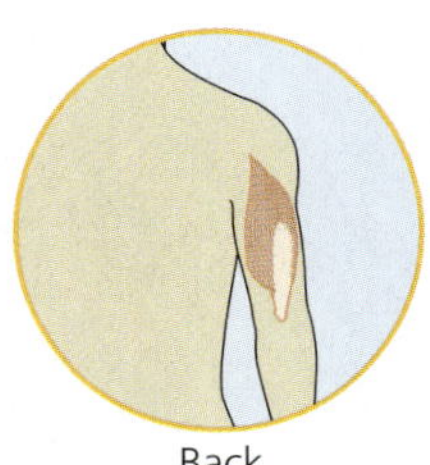
Back

Muscles developed: Triceps

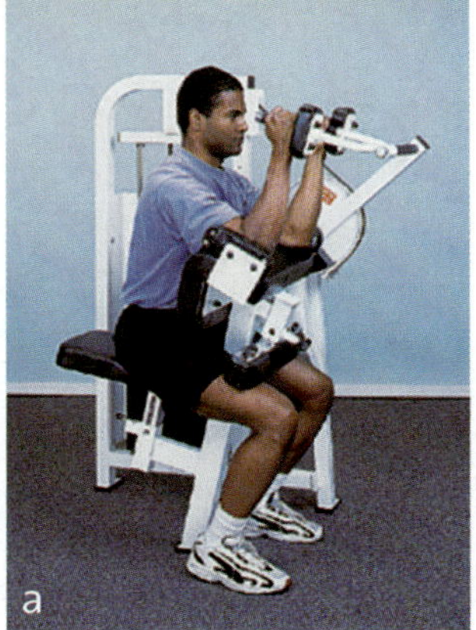
a

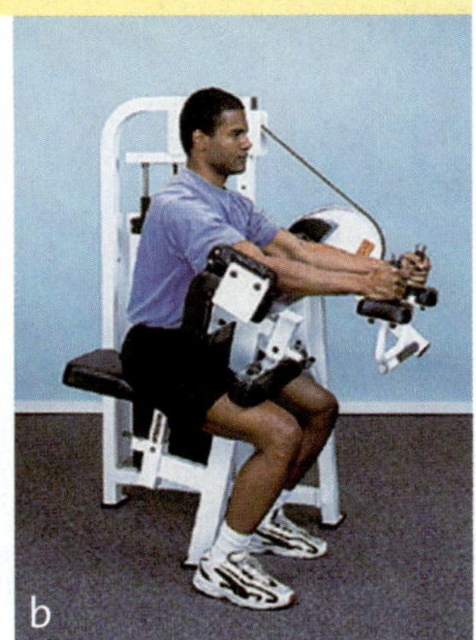
b

EXERCISE 9 Assisted Dip

Instructions: Set the weight according to the amount of assistance you need to complete a set of dips—the heavier the weight, the more assistance provided. **(a)** Stand or kneel on the assist platform with your body between the dip bars. With your elbows fully extended and palms facing your body, support your weight on your hands. **(b)** Lower your body until your upper arms are approximately parallel with the bars. Then push up until you reach the starting position.

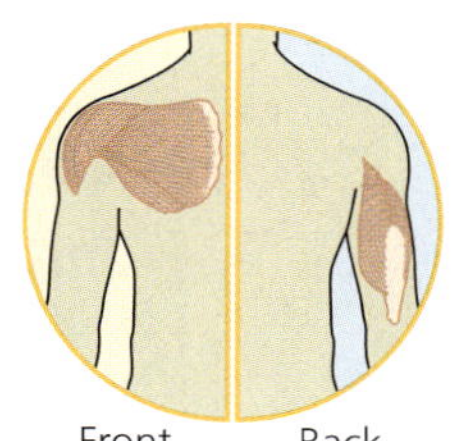

Muscles developed: Triceps, deltoids, pectoralis major

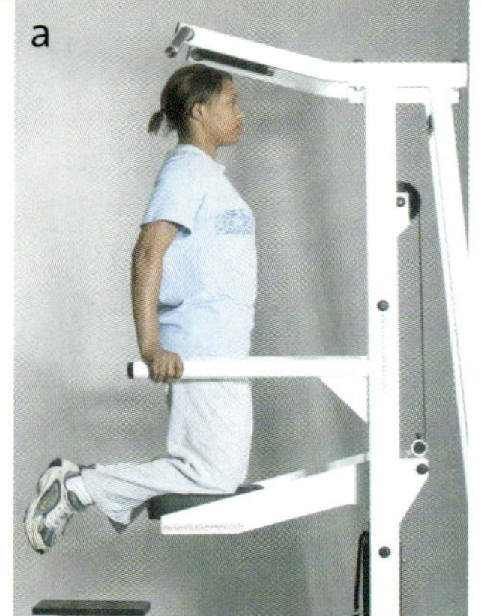

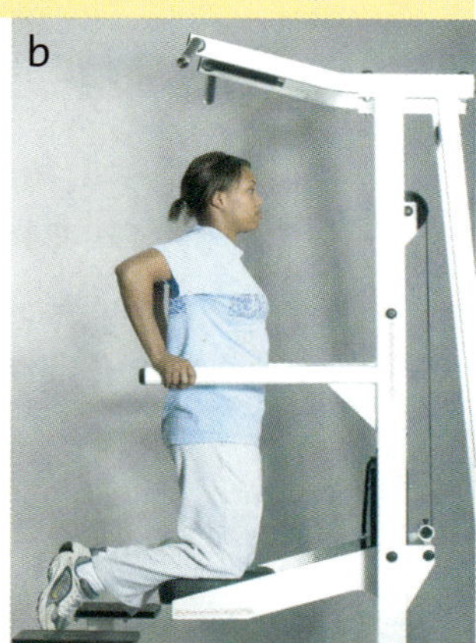

EXERCISE 10 Leg Press

Instructions: Sit or lie on the seat or bench, depending on the type of machine and the manufacturer's instructions. Your head, back, hips, and buttocks should be pressed against the machine pads. Loosely grasp the handles at the side of the machine. **(a)** Begin with your feet flat on the foot platform about shoulder-width apart. Extend your legs, but do not forcefully lock your knees. **(b)** Slowly lower the weight by bending your knees and flexing your hips until your knees are bent at about a 90-degree angle or your heels start to lift off the foot platform. Keep your lower back flat against the support pad. Then extend your knees and return to the starting position.

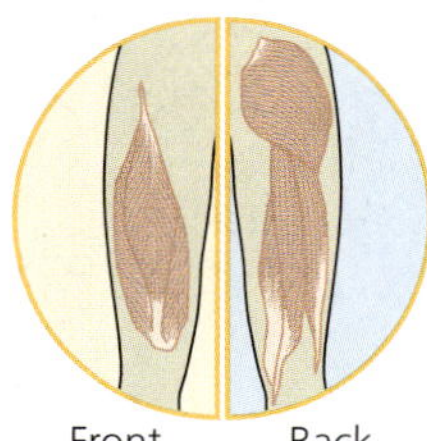

Muscles developed: Gluteus maximus, quadriceps, hamstrings

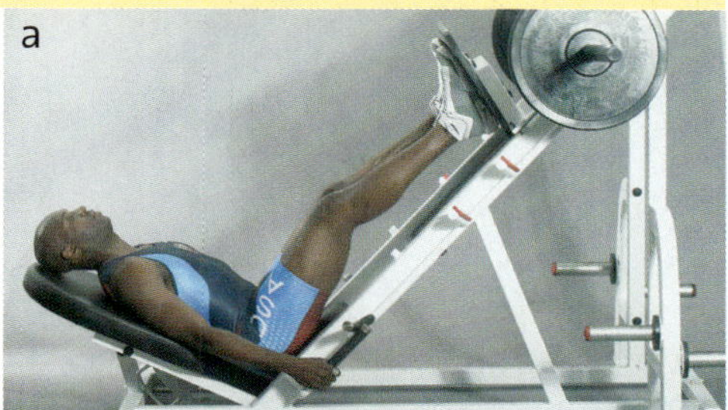

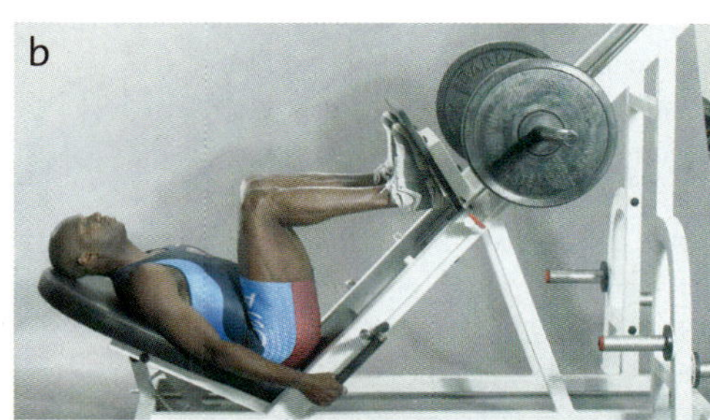

EXERCISE 11 Leg Extension (Knee Extension)

Instructions: **(a)** Adjust the seat so the pads rest comfortably on top of your lower shins. Loosely grasp the handles. **(b)** Extend your knees until they are almost straight. Return to the starting position.

Knee extensions cause kneecap pain in some people. If you have kneecap pain during this exercise, check with an orthopedic specialist before repeating it.

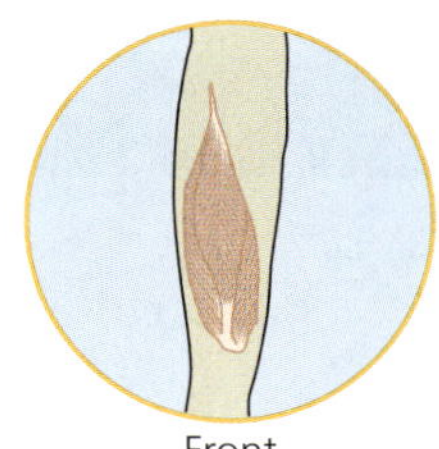

Muscles developed: Quadriceps

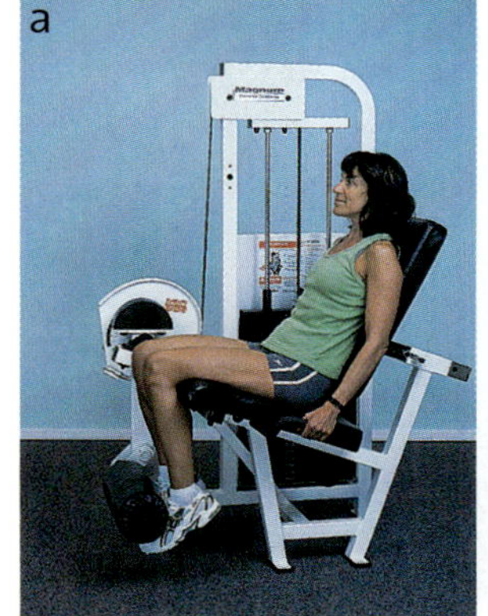

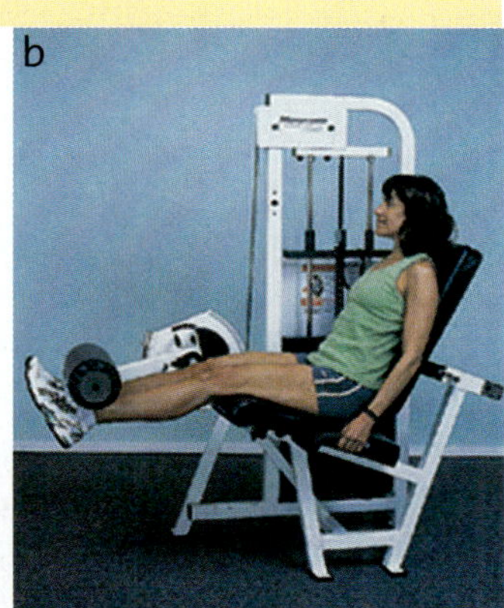

EXERCISE 12 Seated Leg Curl

Instructions: **(a)** Sit on the seat with your back against the back pad and the leg pad below your calf muscles. **(b)** Flex your knees until your lower and upper legs form a 90-degree angle. Return to the starting position.

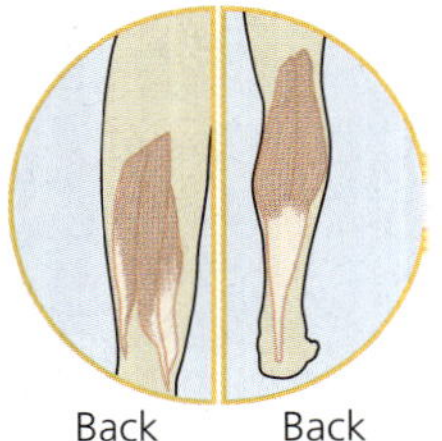

Muscles developed: Hamstrings, gastrocnemius

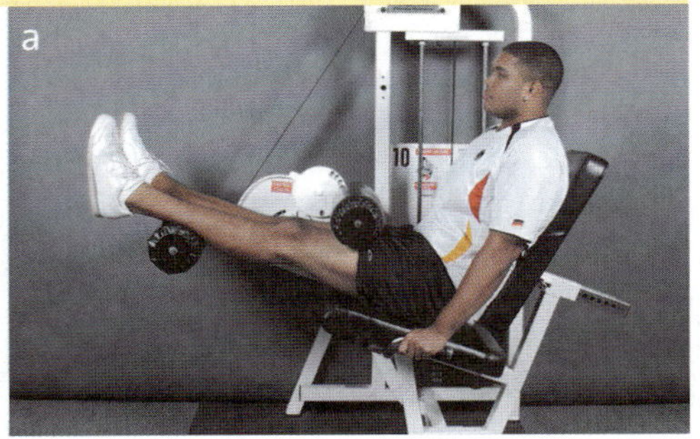

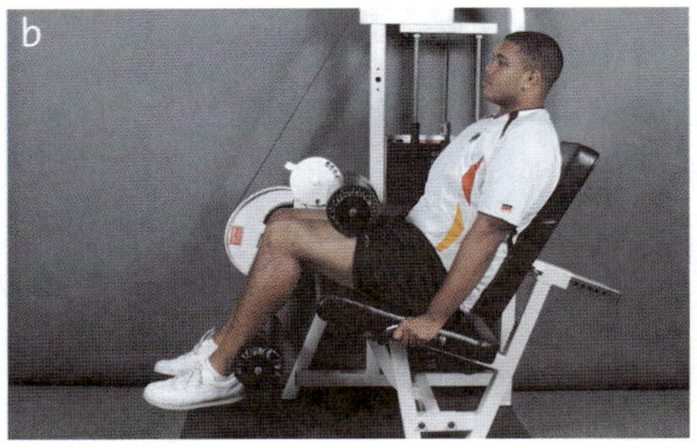

EXERCISE 13 Heel Raise

Instructions: **(a)** Stand with your head between the pads and one pad on each shoulder. The balls of your feet should be on the platform. Lightly grasp the handles. **(b)** Press down with your toes while lifting your heels. Return to the starting position. Changing the direction your feet are pointing (straight ahead, inward, and outward) will work different portions of your calf muscles.

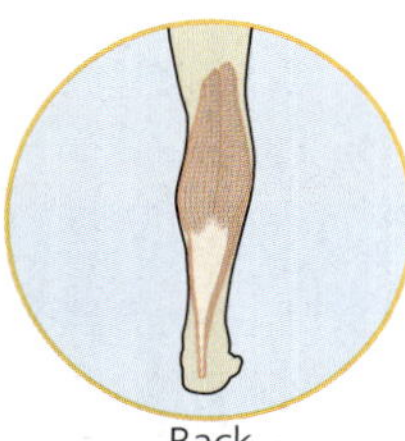

Muscles developed: Gastrocnemius, soleus

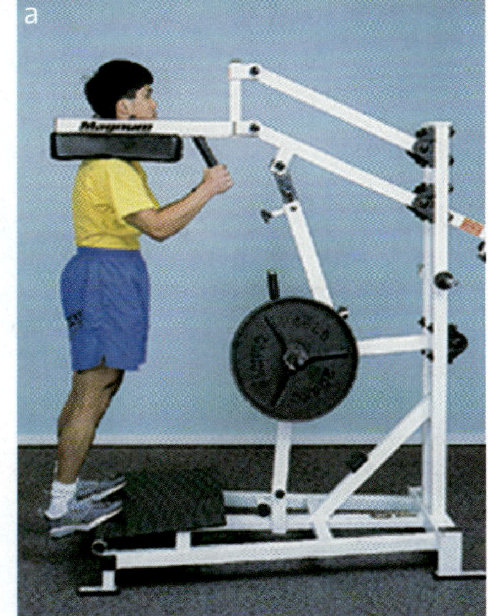

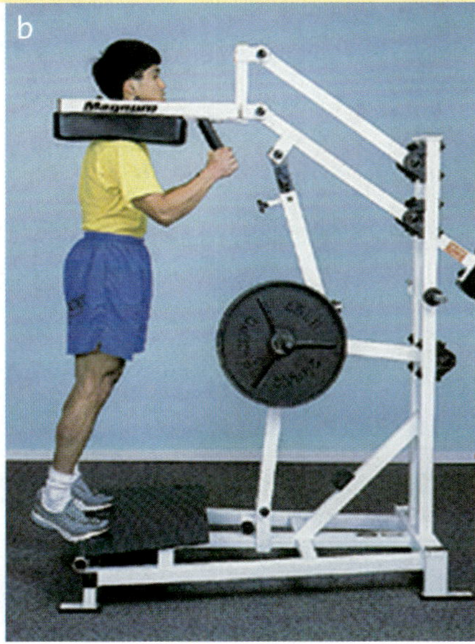

Note: *Abdominal machines, low-back machines, and trunk rotation machines are not recommended because of injury risk. Refer to the "Free Weights" exercise section for appropriate exercises to strengthen the abdominal and low-back muscles. For the rectus abdominus, obliques, and transvere abdominus, perform curl-ups (Exercise 9 in the "Free Weights" section), and for the erector spinae and quadratus lumborum, perform the spine extension and the isometric side bridge (Exercises 10 and 11 in the "Free Weights" section).*

Q Will I gain weight if I do resistance exercises?

A Your weight probably will not change significantly as a result of a general fitness program: one set of 8–12 repetitions of 8–10 exercises, performed on at least two nonconsecutive days per week. You will increase muscle mass and lose body fat, so your weight will stay about the same. You may notice a change in how your clothes fit, however, because muscle is denser than fat. Increased muscle mass will help you control body fat. Muscle increases your metabolism, which means you burn more calories every day. If you combine resistance exercises with endurance exercises, you will be on your way to developing a healthier body composition. Concentrate on fat loss rather than weight loss.

Q Do I need more protein in my diet when I train with weights?

A No. Although there is some evidence that power athletes involved in heavy training have a higher-than-normal protein requirement, there is no reason for most people to consume extra protein. Most Americans take in more protein than they need, so even if there is an increased protein need during heavy training, it is probably supplied by the average diet. Consuming a protein-rich snack before or after training may promote muscle hypertrophy.

Q What causes muscle soreness the day or two following a weight training workout?

A The muscle pain you feel a day or two after a heavy weight training workout is caused by injury to the muscle fibers and surrounding connective tissue. Contrary to popular belief, delayed-onset muscle soreness is not caused by lactic acid buildup. Scientists believe that injury to muscle fibers causes inflammation, which in turn causes the release of chemicals that break down part of the muscle tissue and cause pain. After a bout of intense exercise that causes muscle injury and delayed-onset muscle soreness, the muscles produce protective proteins that prevent soreness during future workouts. If you don't work out regularly, you lose these protective proteins and become susceptible to soreness again.

Q Will strength training improve my sports performance?

A Strength developed in the weight room does not automatically increase your power in sports such as skiing, tennis, or cycling. Hitting a forehand in tennis and making a turn on skis are precise skills that require coordination between your nervous system and muscles. For skilled people, movements become reflex; you don't think about them when you do them. Increasing strength can disturb this coordination. Only by simultaneously practicing a sport and improving fitness can you expect to become more powerful in the skill. Practice helps you integrate your new strength with your skills, which makes you more powerful. Consequently, you can hit the ball harder in tennis or make more graceful turns on the ski slopes. (Refer to Chapter 2 for more on the concept of specificity in physical training.)

Q Will I improve faster if I train every day?

A No. Your muscles need time to recover between training sessions. Doing resistance exercises every day will cause you to become overtrained, which will increase your chance of injury and impede your progress. If your strength training program reaches a plateau, try one of these strategies:

- Vary the number of sets. If you have been performing one set of each exercise, add sets.
- Train less frequently. If you are currently training the same muscle groups three or more times per week, you may not be allowing your muscles to fully recover from intense workouts.
- Change exercises. Using different exercises for the same muscle group may stimulate further strength development.
- Vary the load and number of repetitions. Try increasing or decreasing the loads you are using and changing the number of repetitions accordingly.
- If you are training alone, find a motivated training partner. A partner can encourage you and assist you with difficult lifts, forcing you to work harder.

Q If I stop training, will my muscles turn to fat?

A No. Fat and muscle are two different kinds of tissue, and one cannot turn into the other. Muscles that aren't used become smaller (atrophy), and body fat may increase if caloric intake exceeds calories burned. Although the result of inactivity may be smaller muscles and more fat, the change is caused by two separate processes.

Q Should I wear a weight belt when I lift?

A Until recently, most experts advised people to wear weight belts. However, several studies have shown that weight belts do not prevent back injuries and may, in fact, increase the risk of injury by encouraging people to lift more weight than they are capable of lifting with good form. Although wearing a belt may allow you to lift more weight in some lifts, you may not get the full benefit of your program because use of a weight belt reduces the effectiveness of the workout on the muscles that help support your spine.

For more Common Questions Answered about strength training, visit the Online Learning Center at www.mhhe.com/fahey.

SUMMARY

- Hypertrophy (increased muscle fiber size) occurs when weight training causes the size and number of myofibrils to increase, thereby increasing total muscle size. Strength also increases through muscle learning. Most women do not develop large muscles from weight training.

- Improvements in muscular strength and endurance lead to enhanced physical performance, protection against injury, improved body composition, better self-image, improved muscle and bone health with aging, reduced risk of chronic disease, and decreased risk of premature death.

- Muscular strength can be assessed by determining the amount of weight that can be lifted in one repetition of an exercise. Muscular endurance can be assessed by determining the number of repetitions of a particular exercise that can be performed.

- Static (isometric) exercises involve contraction without movement. They are most useful when a person is recovering from an injury or surgery or needs to overcome weak points in a range of motion.

- Dynamic (isotonic) exercises involve contraction that results in movement. The two most common types are constant resistance (free weights) and variable resistance (many weight machines).

- Free weights and weight machines have pluses and minuses for developing fitness, although machines tend to be safer.

- Lifting heavy weights for only a few repetitions helps develop strength. Lifting lighter weights for more repetitions helps develop muscular endurance.

- A strength training program for general fitness includes at least one set of 8–12 repetitions (enough to cause fatigue) of 8–10 exercises, along with warm-up and cool-down periods. The program should be carried out at least 2 nonconsecutive days per week.

- Safety guidelines for strength training include using proper technique, using spotters and collars when necessary, and taking care of injuries.

- Supplements or drugs that are promoted as instant or quick "cures" usually don't work and are either dangerous, expensive, or both.

FOR FURTHER EXPLORATION

BOOKS

Baechle, T., and R. W. Earl. 2008. National Strength and Conditioning Association's *Essentials of Strength and Conditioning.* Champaign, Ill.: Human Kinetics. *A textbook of strength and conditioning for fitness professionals*

Bjornlund, L. 2010. How Dangerous Are Performance-Enhancing Drugs? San Diego, Calif.: Referencepoint Press. *A discussion of the effects of performance-enhancing drugs on health, performance, and the integrity of sport. The author discusses the role of sports organizations in preventing drug use and whether they can be successful.*

Delavier, F. 2010. *Strength Training Anatomy,* 3rd ed. Champaign, Ill.: Human Kinetics. *Includes exercises for all major muscle groups as well as full anatomical pictures of the muscular system.* Women's Strength Training Anatomy, *a matching volume for women, was published in 2003.*

Fahey, T. D. 2011. *Basic Weight Training for Men and Women,* 8th ed. New York: McGraw-Hill. *A practical guide to developing training programs, using free weights, tailored to individual needs.*

Goldenberg, L., and P. Twist. 2007. *Strength Ball Training.* Champaign, Ill.: Human Kinetics. *A guide to incorporating exercise balls and medicine balls into a complete weight training program.*

Lethi, A., et al. 2007. *Free-Weight Training.* Berkeley, Calif.: Thunder Bay Press. *A complete guide to training with free weights, with special instructions for using weights with an exercise ball.*

Tsatsouline, P. 2010. *Enter the Kettlebell.* Minneapolis, Minn.: Dragon Door Publications. *A guide to basic strength training using kettlebells.*

ORGANIZATIONS AND WEB SITES

American College of Sports Medicine Position Stand: Progression Models in Resistance Training for Healthy Adults. Provides an in-depth look at strategies for setting up a strength training program and making progress based on individual program goals.
http://journals.lww.com/acsm-msse/Fulltext/2009/03000/Progression_Models_in_Resistance_Training_for.26.aspx

Dan John. An excellent Web site for people serious about improving strength and fitness, written by a world-class athlete and coach in track and field and Highland games.
http://danjohn.net

Georgia State University: Strength Training. Provides information about the benefits of strength training and ways to develop a safe and effective program; also includes illustrations of a variety of exercises.
http://www2.gsu.edu/~wwwfit/strength.html

Human Anatomy On-line. Provides text, illustrations, and animation about the muscular system, nerve-muscle connections, muscular contraction, and other topics.
http://www.innerbody.com/htm/body.html

Mayo Clinic: Weight Training: Improve Your Muscular Fitness. Provides a basic overview of weight training essentials along with links to many other articles on specific weight training-related topics.
http://www.mayoclinic.com/health/weight-training/HQ01627

National Strength and Conditioning Association. A professional organization that focuses on strength development for fitness and athletic performance.
http://www.nsca-lift.org

Pilates Method Alliance. Provides information about Pilates and about instructor certification; includes a directory of instructors.
http://www.pilatesmethodalliance.org

University of California, San Diego: Muscle Physiology Home Page. Provides an introduction to muscle physiology, including information about types of muscle fibers and energy cycles.
http://muscle.ucsd.edu/index.shtml

University of Michigan: Muscles in Action. Interactive descriptions of muscle movements.
http://www.med.umich.edu/lrc/Hypermuscle/Hyper.html

See also the listings in Chapter 2.

SELECTED BIBLIOGRAPHY

Ahtiainen, J. P., et al. 2011. Recovery after heavy resistance exercise and skeletal muscle androgen receptor and insulin-like growth factor-i isoform expression in strength trained men. *Journal of Strength and Conditioning Research* 25(3): 767–777.

American College of Sports Medicine. 2009. *ACSM's Guidelines for Exercise Testing and Prescription,* 8th ed. Philadelphia: Lippincott Williams and Wilkins.

American College of Sports Medicine. 2009. *ACSM's Resource Manual for Guidelines for Exercise Testing and Prescription,* 6th ed. Philadelphia: Lippincott Williams and Wilkins.

American College of Sports Medicine. 2009. American College of Sports Medicine position stand: Progression models in resistance training for healthy adults. *Medicine and Science in Sports and Exercise* 41(3): 687–708.

Arikawa, A. Y., et al. 2011. Adherence to a strength training intervention in adult women. *Journal of Physical Activity and Health* 8(1): 111–118.

Bellar, D. M., et al. 2011. The Effects of Combined Elastic- and Free-Weight Tension vs. Free-Weight Tension on One-Repetition Maximum Strength in the Bench Press. *Journal of Strength and Conditioning Research* 25(2): 459–463.

Blazevich, A. J., et al. 2007. Lack of human muscle architectural adaptation after short-term strength training. *Muscle and Nerve* 35(1): 78–86.

Bouchard, D. R., et al. 2011. Association between muscle mass, leg strength, and fat mass with physical function in older adults: Influence of age and sex. *Journal of Aging and Health* 23(2): 313–328.

Brentano, M. A., et al. 2011. A review on strength exercise-induced muscle damage: applications, adaptation mechanisms and limitations. *Journal of Sports Medicine and Physical Fitness* 51(1): 1–10.

Brooks, G. A., et al. 2005. *Exercise Physiology: Human Bioenergetics and Its Applications,* 4th ed. New York: McGraw-Hill.

Brooks, N., et al. 2006. Strength training improves muscle quality and insulin sensitivity in Hispanic older adults with type 2 diabetes. *International Journal of Medical Sciences* 4(1): 19–27.

Burt, J., et al. 2007. A comparison of once versus twice per week training on leg press strength in women. *Journal of Sports Medicine and Physical Fitness* 47(1): 13–17.

Cadore, E. L., et al. 2011. Effects of strength, endurance, and concurrent training on aerobic power and dynamic neuromuscular economy in elderly men. *Journal of Strength and Conditioning Research* 25(3): 758–766.

Carlsohn, A., et al. 2011. How much is too much? A case report of nutritional supplement use of a high-performance athlete. *British Journal Nutrition* 1–5.

Caserotti, P., et al. 2008. Explosive heavy-resistance training in old and very old adults: Changes in rapid muscle force, strength and power. *Scandinavian Journal of Medicine and Science in Sports* 18(6): 773–782.

Davis, W. J., et al. 2008. Concurrent training enhances athletes' strength, muscle endurance, and other measures. *Journal of Strength and Conditioning Research* 22(5): 1487–1502.

Dengel, D. R., et al. 2011. Gender differences in vascular function and insulin sensitivity in young adults. *Clinical Sciences* 120(4): 153–160.

Farrar, R. E., et al. 2010. Oxygen cost of kettlebell swings. *Journal of Strength and Conditioning Research* 24(4): 1034–1036.

Gee, T. I., et al. 2011. Strength and conditioning practices in rowing. *Journal of Strength and Conditioning Research* 25(3): 668–682.

Graham, M. R., et al. 2008. Anabolic steroid use: Patterns of use and detection of doping. *Sports Medicine* 38(6): 505–525.

Haskell, W. L., et al. 2007. Physical activity and public health: updated recommendation for adults from the American College of Sports Medicine and the American Heart Association. *Circulation* 116(9): 1081–1093.

Headley, S. A., et al. 2011. Effects of lifting tempo on one repetition maximum and hormonal responses to a bench press protocol. *Journal of Strength and Conditioning Research* 25(2): 406–413.

Heikkinen, A., et al. 2011. Use of dietary supplements in Olympic athletes is decreasing: A follow-up study between 2002 and 2009. *Journal of the International Society of Sports Nutrition* 8(1): 1.

Hoffman, J. R., et al. 2008. Nutritional supplementation and anabolic steroid use in adolescents. *Medicine and Science in Sports and Exercise* 40(1): 15–24.

Ikeda, E. R., et al. 2009. The valsalva maneuver revisited: The influence of voluntary breathing on isometric muscle strength. *Journal of Strength and Conditioning Research* 23(1): 127–132.

Jay, K., et al. 2010. Kettlebell training for musculoskeletal and cardiovascular health: A randomized controlled trial. *Scandinavian Journal of Work and Environmental Health.* Published online December 2010.

Kell, R. T. 2011. The influence of periodized resistance training on strength changes in men and women. *Journal of Strength and Conditioning Research* 25(3): 735–744.

Kirk, E. P., et al. 2007. Six months of supervised high-intensity low-volume resistance training improves strength independent of changes in muscle mass in young overweight men. *Journal of Strength and Conditioning Research* 21(1): 151–156.

Lindegaard, B., et al. 2008. The effect of strength and endurance training on insulin sensitivity and fat distribution in human immunodeficiency virus-infected patients with lipodystrophy. *Journal of Clinical Endocrinology and Metabolism* 93(10): 3860–3869.

Machado, M. V., et al. 2011. The dark side of sports: Using steroids may harm your liver. *Liver International* 31(3): 280–281.

Manore, M., et al. 2011. BJSM reviews: A-Z of nutritional supplements: dietary supplements, sports nutrition foods and ergogenic aids for health and performance—Part 16. *British Journal Sports Medicine* 45(1): 73–74.

Newsholme, P., et al. 2011. BJSM reviews: A to Z of nutritional supplements: dietary supplements, sports nutrition foods and ergogenic aids for health and performance—Part 18. *British Journal Sports Medicine* 45(3): 230–232.

Norrbrand, L., et al. 2008. Resistance training using eccentric overload induces early adaptations in skeletal muscle size. *European Journal of Applied Physiology* 102(3): 271–281.

Reitelseder, S., et al. 2011. Whey and casein labeled with L-[1-13C]leucine and muscle protein synthesis: Effect of resistance exercise and protein ingestion. *American Journal of Physiology, Endocrinology and Metabolism* 300(1): E231–242.

Ruiz, J. R., et al. 2008. Association between muscular strength and mortality in men: Prospective cohort study. *British Medical Journal* 337: a439, published online.

Saeterbakken, A. H., et al. 2011. A comparison of muscle activity and 1-RM strength of three chest-press exercises with different stability requirements. *Journal of Sports Science* 1–6.

Santos, E. J., et al. 2011. The effects of plyometric training followed by detraining and reduced training periods on explosive strength in adolescent male basketball players. *Journal of Strength and Conditioning Research* 25(2): 441–452.

Schick, E. E., et al. 2010. A comparison of muscle activation between a Smith machine and free weight bench press. *Journal of Strength and Conditioning Research* 24(3): 779–784.

Sedano, S., et al. 2011. Effects of plyometric training on explosive strength, acceleration capacity and kicking speed in young elite soccer players. *Journal of Sports Medicine and Physical Fitness* 51(1): 50–58.

Senchina, D. S., et al. 2011. BJSM reviews: A-Z of nutritional supplements: dietary supplements, sports nutrition foods and ergogenic aids for health and performance—Part 17. *British Journal Sports Medicine* 45(2): 150–151.

Wieser, M., and P. Haber. 2007. The effects of systematic resistance training in the elderly. *International Journal of Sports Medicine* 28(1): 59–65.

Winchester, J. B., et al. 2008. Eight weeks of ballistic exercise improves power independently of changes in strength and muscle fiber type expression. *Journal of Strength and Conditioning Research* 22(6): 1728–1734.

Young, W. B., et al. 2011. Enhancing foot velocity in football kicking: the role of strength training. *Journal of Strength and Conditioning Research* 25(2): 561–566.

Name ______________________ Section ______________ Date ____________

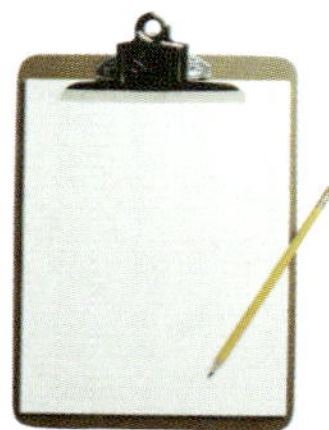

LAB 8.1 Assessing Your Current Level of Muscular Strength

For best results, don't do any strenuous weight training within 48 hours of any test. Use great caution when completing 1-RM tests; do not take the maximum bench press test if you have any injuries to your shoulders, elbows, back, hips, or knees. In addition, do not take these tests until you have had at least one month of weight training experience.

The Maximum Bench Press Test

Equipment

The free weights bench press test uses the following equipment

1. Flat bench (with or without racks)
2. Barbell
3. Assorted weight plates, with collars to hold them in place
4. One or two spotters
5. Weight scale

If a weight machine is preferred, use the following equipment:

1. Universal Gym Dynamic Variable Resistance Machine
2. Weight scale

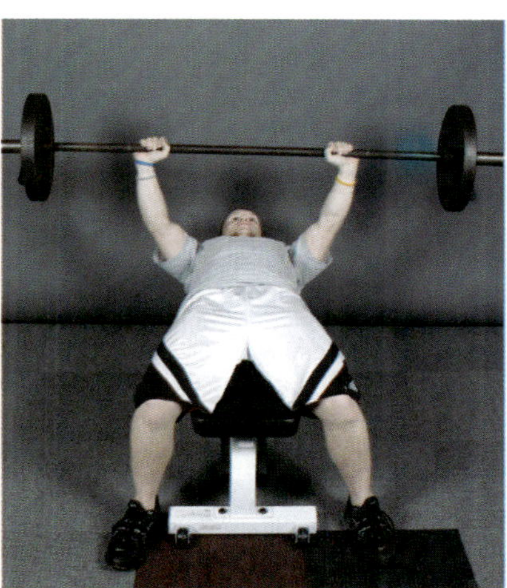

Maximum bench press test.

Preparation

Try a few bench presses with a small amount of weight so you can practice your technique, warm up your muscles, and, if you use free weights, coordinate your movements with those of your spotters. Weigh yourself and record the results.

Body weight: __________ lb

Instructions

1. Use a weight that is lower than the amount you believe you can lift. For free weights, men should begin with a weight about two-thirds of their body weight; women should begin with the weight of just the bar (45 lb).
2. Lie on the bench with your feet firmly on the floor. If you are using a weight machine, grasp the handles with palms away from you; the tops of the handles should be aligned with the tops of your armpits.

   If you are using free weights, grasp the bar slightly wider than shoulder width with your palms away from you. If you have one spotter, she or he should stand directly behind the bench; if you have two spotters, they should stand to the side, one at each end of the barbell. Signal to the spotter when you are ready to begin the test by saying "1, 2, 3." On "3," the spotter should help you lift the weight to a point over your midchest (nipple line).
3. Push the handles or barbell until your arms are fully extended. Exhale as you lift. If you are using free weights, the weight moves from a low point at the chest straight up. Keep your feet firmly on the floor, don't arch your back, and push the weight evenly with your right and left arms. Don't bounce the weight on your chest.
4. Rest for several minutes, then repeat the lift with a heavier weight. It will probably take several attempts to determine the maximum amount of weight you can lift (1 RM).

   1 RM: __________ lb Check one: __________ Free weights __________ Universal __________ Other
5. If you used free weights, convert your free weights bench press score to an estimated value for 1 RM on the Universal bench press using the appropriate formula:

   Males: Estimated Universal 1 RM = (1.016 × free weights 1 RM __________ lb) + 18.41 = __________ lb

   Females: Estimated Universal 1 RM = (0.848 × free weights 1 RM __________ lb) + 21.37 = __________ lb

Rating Your Bench Press Result

1. Divide your Universal 1-RM value by your body weight.

   1 RM ___________ lb ÷ body weight ___________ lb = ___________

2. Find this ratio in the table to determine your bench press strength rating. Record the rating here and in the chart at the end of this lab.

   Bench press strength rating: ___________

Strength Ratings for the Maximum Bench Press Test

	Pounds Lifted/Body Weight (lb)					
Men	*Very Poor*	*Poor*	*Fair*	*Good*	*Excellent*	*Superior*
Age: Under 20	Below 0.89	0.89–1.05	1.06–1.18	1.19–1.33	1.34–1.75	Above 1.75
20–29	Below 0.88	0.88–0.98	0.99–1.13	1.14–1.31	1.32–1.62	Above 1.62
30–39	Below 0.78	0.78–0.87	0.88–0.97	0.98–1.11	1.12–1.34	Above 1.34
40–49	Below 0.72	0.72–0.79	0.80–0.87	0.88–0.99	1.00–1.19	Above 1.19
50–59	Below 0.63	0.63–0.70	0.71–0.78	0.79–0.89	0.90–1.04	Above 1.04
60 and over	Below 0.57	0.57–0.65	0.66–0.71	0.72–0.81	0.82–0.93	Above 0.93
Women						
Age: Under 20	Below 0.53	0.53–0.57	0.58–0.64	0.65–0.76	0.77–0.87	Above 0.87
20–29	Below 0.51	0.51–0.58	0.59–0.69	0.70–0.79	0.80–1.00	Above 1.00
30–39	Below 0.47	0.47–0.52	0.53–0.59	0.60–0.69	0.70–0.81	Above 0.81
40–49	Below 0.43	0.43–0.49	0.50–0.53	0.54–0.61	0.62–0.76	Above 0.76
50–59	Below 0.39	0.39–0.43	0.44–0.47	0.48–0.54	0.55–0.67	Above 0.67
60 and over	Below 0.38	0.38–0.42	0.43–0.46	0.47–0.53	0.54–0.71	Above 0.71

SOURCE: Based on norms from The Cooper Institute of Aerobic Research, Dallas, Texas; from *The Physical Fitness Specialist Manual,* revised 2002. Used with permission.

Predicting 1 RM from Multiple-Repetition Lifts Using Free Weights

Instead of doing the 1-RM maximum strength bench press test, you can predict your 1 RM from multiple-repetition lifts.

Instructions

1. Choose a weight you think you can bench press five times.
2. Follow the instructions for lifting the weight given in the maximum bench press test.
3. Do as many repetitions of the bench press as you can. A repetition counts only if done correctly
4. Refer to the chart on p. 253, or calculate predicted 1 RM using the Brzycki equation:

   1 RM = *weight* ÷ (1.0278 − [0.0278 × *number of repetitions*])

   1 RM = ___________ lb ÷ (1.0278 − [0.0278 × ___________ repetitions]) =___________

5. Divide your predicted 1-RM value by your body weight.

   1 RM ___________ lb ÷ body weight ___________ lb = ___________

6. Find this ratio in the table above to determine your bench press strength rating. Record the rating here and in the chart at the end of the lab.

   Bench press strength rating: ___________

RMs from the Multiple-Repetitions Bench Press Test

	Repetitions											
Weight Lifted (lb)	*1*	*2*	*3*	*4*	*5*	*6*	*7*	*8*	*9*	*10*	*11*	*12*
66	66	68	70	72	74	77	79	82	85	88	91	95
77	77	79	82	84	87	89	92	96	99	103	107	111
88	88	91	93	96	99	102	106	109	113	117	122	127
99	99	102	105	108	111	115	119	123	127	132	137	143
110	110	113	116	120	124	128	132	137	141	147	152	158
121	121	124	128	132	136	141	145	150	156	161	168	174
132	132	136	140	144	149	153	158	164	170	176	183	190
143	143	147	151	156	161	166	172	178	184	191	198	206
154	154	158	163	168	173	179	185	191	198	205	213	222
165	165	170	175	180	186	192	198	205	212	220	229	238
176	176	181	186	192	198	204	211	219	226	235	244	254
187	187	192	198	204	210	217	224	232	240	249	259	269
198	198	204	210	216	223	230	238	246	255	264	274	285
209	209	215	221	228	235	243	251	259	269	279	289	301
220	220	226	233	240	248	256	264	273	283	293	305	317
231	231	238	245	252	260	268	277	287	297	308	320	333
242	242	249	256	264	272	281	290	300	311	323	335	349
253	253	260	268	276	285	294	304	314	325	337	350	364
264	264	272	280	288	297	307	317	328	340	352	366	380
275	275	283	291	300	309	319	330	341	354	367	381	396
286	286	294	303	312	322	332	343	355	368	381	396	412
297	297	305	314	324	334	345	356	369	382	396	411	428
308	308	317	326	336	347	358	370	382	396	411	427	444

SOURCE: Brzycki, M. 1993. Strength testing—predicting a one-rep max from reps to fatigue. *The Journal of Physical Education, Recreation and Dance* 64: 88–90. January 1993, a publication of the American Alliance for Health, Physical Education, Recreation and Dance, www.aahperd.org. Reprinted with permission.

Functional Leg Strength Tests

The following tests assess functional leg strength using squats. Most people do squats improperly increasing their risk of knee and back pain. Before you add weight-bearing squats to your weight training program, you should determine your functional leg strength, check your ability to squat properly, and give yourself a chance to master squatting movements. The following leg strength tests will help you in each of these areas.

These tests are progressively more difficult, so do not move to the next test until you have scored at least a 3 on the current test. On each test, give yourself a rating of 0, 1, 3, or 5, as described in the instructions that follow the last test.

1. Chair Squat

Instructions

1. Sit up straight in a chair with your back resting against the backrest and your arms at your sides. Your feet should be placed more than shoulder-width apart so that you can get them under the body.
2. Begin the motion of rising out of the chair by flexing (bending) at the hips—not the back. Then squat up using a hip hinge movement (no spine movement). Stand without rocking forward, bending your back, or using external support, and keep your head in a neutral position.

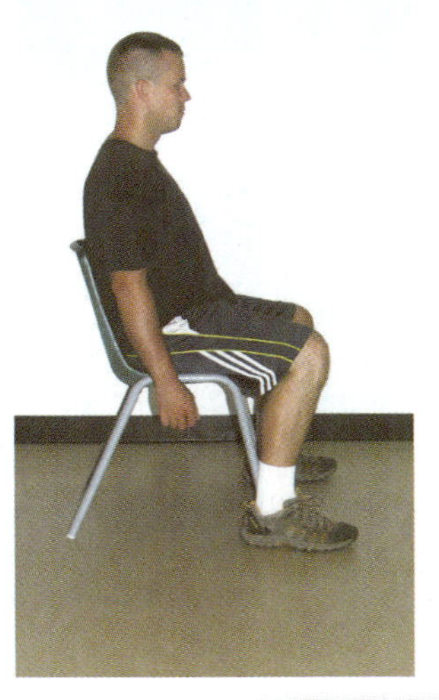

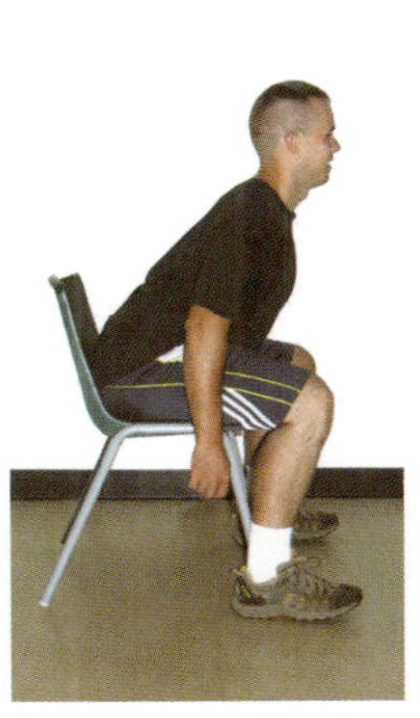

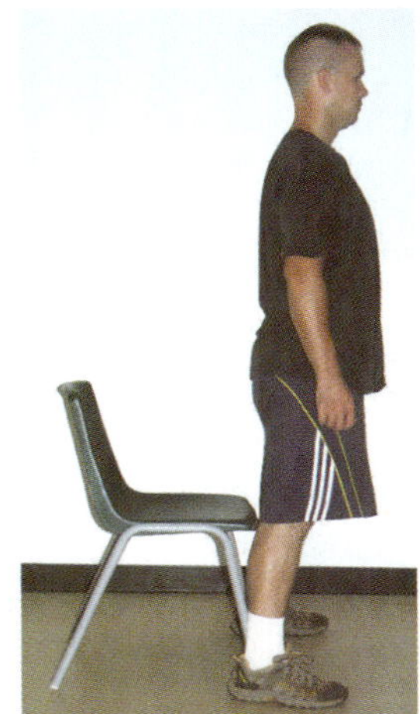

3. Return to the sitting position while maintaining a straight back and keeping your weight centered over your feet. Your thighs should abduct (spread) as you sit back in the chair. Use your rear hip and thigh muscles as much as possible as you sit.

Do five repetitions.

Your rating: ___________

(See rating instructions that follow.)

2. *Single-Leg Step-Up*

Instructions

1. Stand facing a bench, with your right foot placed on the middle of the bench, right knee bent at 90 degrees, and arms at your sides.
2. Step up on the bench until your right leg is straight, maximizing the use of the hip muscles.
3. Return to the starting position. Keep your hips stable, back straight, chest up, shoulders back, and head neutral during the entire movement.

Do five repetitions for each leg.

Your rating: ___________

(See rating instructions that follow.)

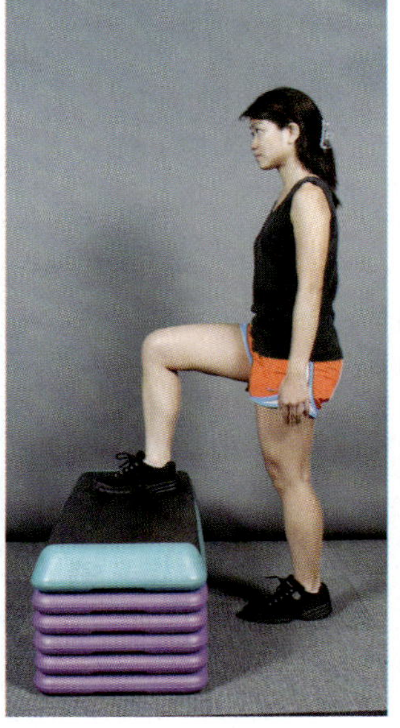

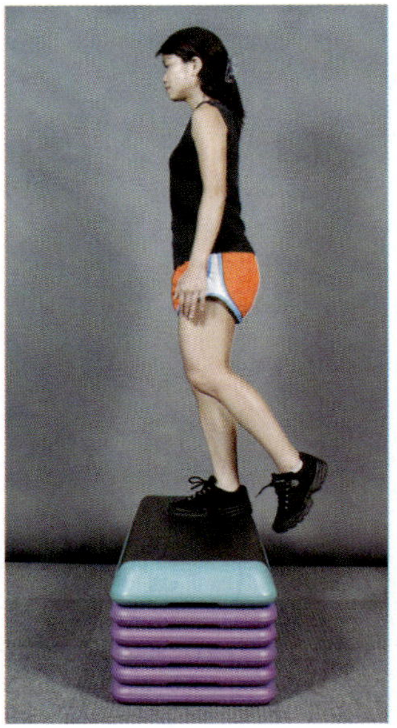

3. *Unweighted Squat*

Instructions

1. Stand with your feet placed slightly more than shoulder-width apart, toes pointed out slightly, hands on hips or across your chest, head neutral, and back straight. Center your weight over your arches or slightly behind.
2. Squat down, keeping your weight centered over your arches and actively flexing (bending) your hips until your legs break parallel. During the movement, keep your back straight, shoulders back, and chest out, and let your thighs part to the side so that you are "squatting between your legs."
3. Push back up to the starting position, hinging at the hips and not with the spine, maximizing the use of the rear hip and thigh muscles, and maintaining a straight back and neutral head position.

Do five repetitions.

Your rating: ___________

(See rating instructions that follow.)

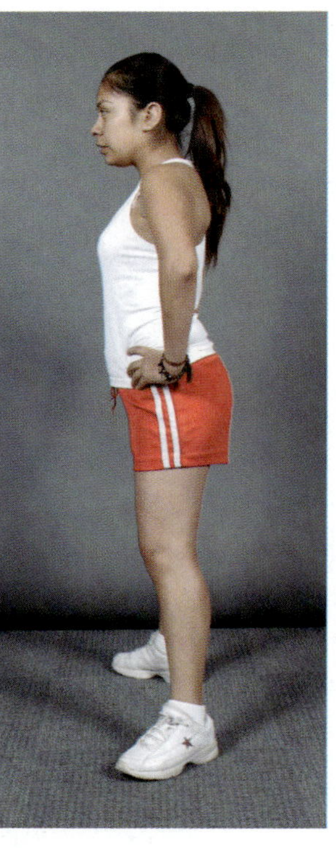

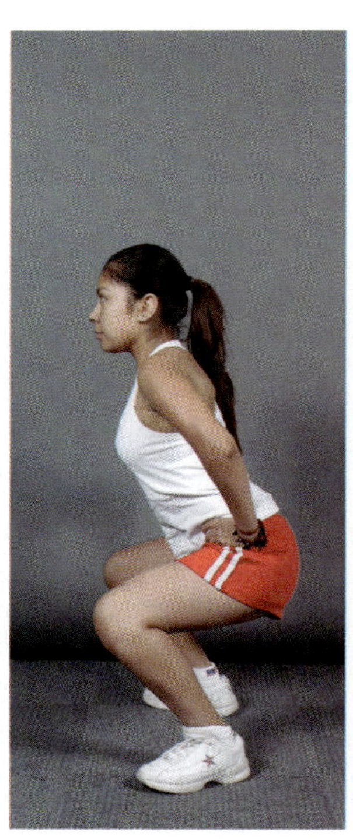

4. *Single-Leg Lunge-Squat with Rear-Foot Support*

Instructions

1. Stand about 3 feet in front of a bench (with your back to the bench).
2. Place the instep of your left foot on the bench, and put most of your weight on your right leg (your left leg should be bent), with your hands at your sides.
3. Squat on your right leg until your thigh is parallel with the floor. Keep your back straight, chest up, shoulders back, and head neutral.
4. Return to the starting position.

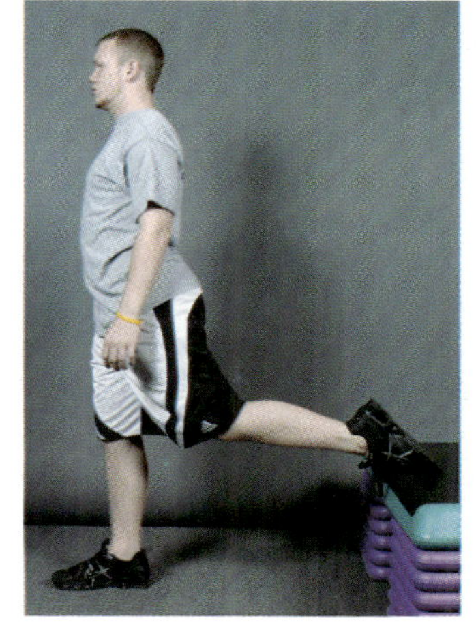

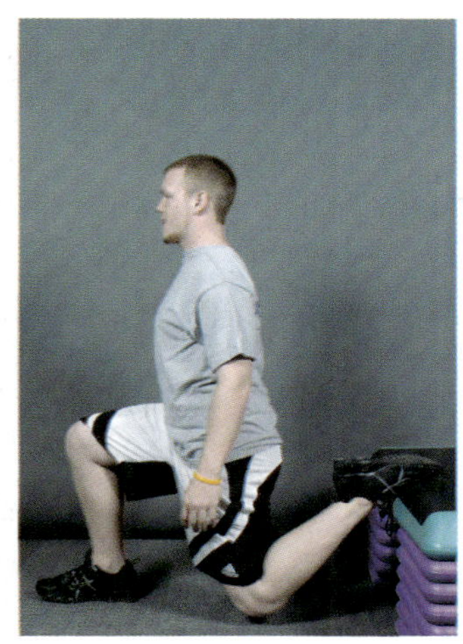

Do three repetitions for each leg.

Your rating: ___________

(See rating instructions that follow.)

Rating Your Functional Leg Strength Test Results

5 points: Performed the exercise properly with good back and thigh position, weight centered over the middle or rear of the foot, chest out, and shoulders back; good use of hip muscles on the way down and on the way up, with head in a neutral position throughout the movement; maintained good form during all repetitions; abducted (spread) the thighs on the way down during chair squats and double-leg squats; for single-leg exercises, showed good strength on both sides; for single-leg lunge-squat with rear-foot support, maintained straight back, and knees stayed behind toes.

3 points: Weight was forward on the toes, with some rounding of the back; used thigh muscles excessively, with little use of hip muscles; head and chest were too far forward; showed little abduction of the thighs during double-leg squats; when going down for single-leg exercises, one side was stronger than the other; form deteriorated with repetitions; for single-leg lunge-squat with rear-foot support, could not reach parallel (thigh parallel with floor).

1 point: Had difficulty performing the movement, rocking forward and rounding back badly; used thigh muscles excessively, with little use of hip muscles on the way up or on the way down; chest and head were forward; on unweighted squats, had difficulty reaching parallel and showed little abduction of the thighs; on single-leg exercises, one leg was markedly stronger than the other; could not perform multiple repetitions.

0 points: Could not perform the exercise.

Summary of Results

Maximum bench press test from either the 1-RM test or the multiple-repetition test: Weight pressed: ___________ lb Rating: ___________

Functional leg strength tests (0–5): Chair squat: ___________ Single-leg step-up: ___________ Unweighted squat: ___________

Single-leg lunge-squat with rear-foot support: ___________

Remember that muscular strength is specific: Your ratings may vary considerably for different parts of your body.

LABORATORY ACTIVITIES

Using Your Results

How did you score? Are you surprised by your ratings for muscular strength? Are you satisfied with your current ratings?

If you're not satisfied, set realistic goals for improvement:

Are you satisfied with your current level of muscular strength as evidenced in your daily life—for example, your ability to lift objects, climb stairs, and engage in sports and recreational activities?

If you're not satisfied, set realistic goals for improvement:

What should you do next? Enter the results of this lab in the Preprogram Assessment column in Appendix C. If you've set goals for improvement, begin planning your strength training program by completing the plan in Lab 8.3. After several weeks of your program, complete this lab again and enter the results in the Postprogram Assessment column of Appendix C. How do the results compare?

Name ______________________ Section ______________ Date ______________

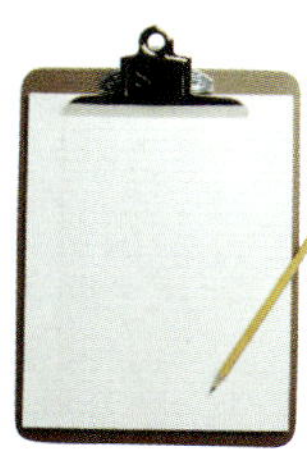

LAB 8.2 Assessing Your Current Level of Muscular Endurance

For best results, don't do any strenuous weight training within 48 hours of any test. To assess endurance of the abdominal muscles, perform the curl-up test. To assess endurance of muscles in the upper body, perform the push-up test. To assess endurance of the muscles in the lower body, perform the squat endurance test.

The Curl-Up Test

Equipment

1. Four 6-inch strips of self-stick Velcro or heavy tape
2. Ruler
3. Partner
4. Mat (optional)

Preparation

Affix the strips of Velcro or long strips of tape on the mat or testing surface. Place the strips 3 inches apart.

Instructions

1. Start by lying on your back on the floor or mat, arms straight and by your sides, shoulders relaxed, palms down and on the floor, and fingers straight. Adjust your position so that the longest fingertip of each hand touches the end of the near strip of Velcro or tape. Your knees should be bent about 90 degrees, with your feet about 12–18 inches from your buttocks.
2. To perform a curl-up, flex your spine while sliding your fingers across the floor until the fingertips of each hand reach the second strip of Velcro or tape. Then return to the starting position; the shoulders must be returned to touch the mat between curl-ups, but the head need not touch. Shoulders must remain relaxed throughout the curl-up, and feet and buttocks must stay on the floor. Breathe easily exhaling during the lift phase of the curl-up; do not hold your breath.
3. Once your partner says "go," perform as many curl-ups as you can at a steady pace with correct form. Your partner counts the curl-ups you perform and calls a stop to the test if she or he notices any incorrect form or drop in your pace.

   Number of curl-ups: ______________

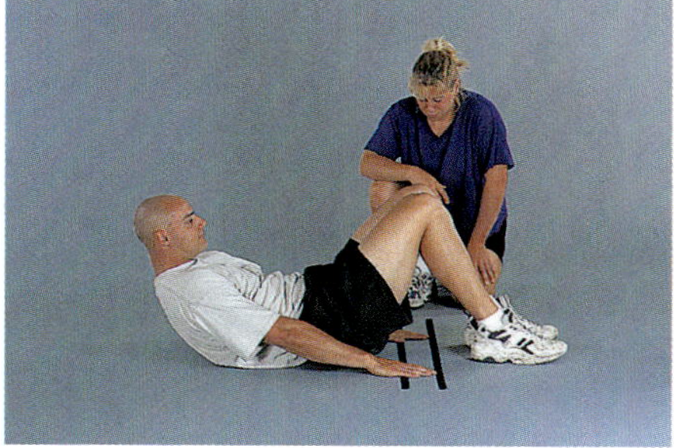

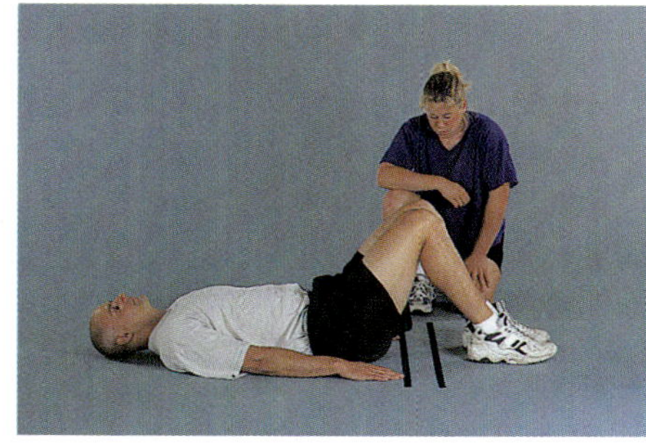

Rating Your Curl-Up Test Result

Your score is the number of completed curl-ups. Refer to the appropriate portion of the table for a rating of your abdominal muscular endurance. Record your rating below and in the summary at the end of this lab.

Rating: ______________

Ratings for the Curl-Up Test

	Number of Curl-Ups					
Men	*Very Poor*	*Poor*	*Average*	*Good*	*Excellent*	*Superior*
Age: 16–19	Below 48	48–57	58–64	65–74	75–93	Above 93
20–29	Below 46	46–54	55–63	64–74	75–93	Above 93
30–39	Below 40	40–47	48–55	56–64	65–81	Above 81
40–49	Below 38	38–45	46–53	54–62	63–79	Above 79
50–59	Below 36	36–43	44–51	52–60	61–77	Above 77
60–69	Below 33	33–40	41–48	49–57	58–74	Above 74
Women						
Age: 16–19	Below 42	42–50	51–58	59–67	68–84	Above 84
20–29	Below 41	41–51	52–57	58–66	67–83	Above 83
30–39	Below 38	38–47	48–56	57–66	67–85	Above 85
40–49	Below 36	36–45	46–54	55–64	65–83	Above 83
50–59	Below 34	34–43	44–52	53–62	63–81	Above 81
60–69	Below 31	31–40	41–49	50–59	60–78	Above 78

SOURCE: Ratings based on norms calculated from data collected by Robert Lualhati on 4545 college students, 16–80 years of age, at Skyline College, San Bruno, California. Used with permission.

The Push-Up Test

Equipment: Mat or towel (optional)

Preparation

In this test, you will perform either standard push-ups or modified push-ups, in which you support yourself with your knees. The Cooper Institute developed the ratings for this test with men performing push-ups and women performing modified push-ups. Biologically, males tend to be stronger than females; the modified technique reduces the need for upper-body strength in a test of muscular endurance. Therefore, for an accurate assessment of upper-body endurance, men should perform standard push-ups and women should perform modified push-ups. However, in using push-ups as part of a strength training program, individuals should choose the technique most appropriate for increasing their level of strength and endurance—regardless of gender.

Instructions

1. *For push-ups:* Start in the push-up position with your body supported by your hands and feet. *For modified push-ups:* Start in the modified push-up position with your body supported by your hands and knees. *For both positions*, keep your arms and your back straight and your fingers pointed forward.

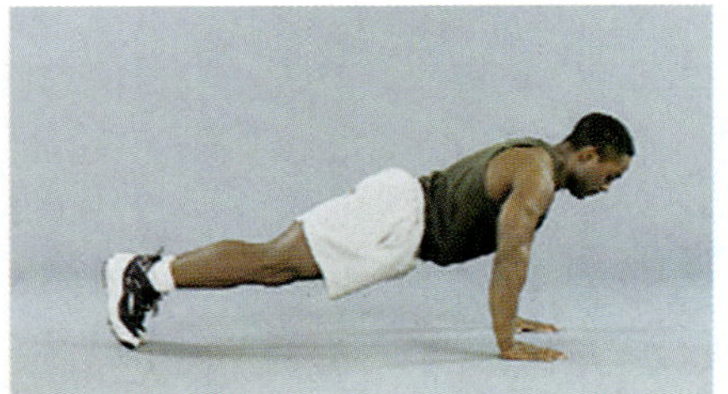

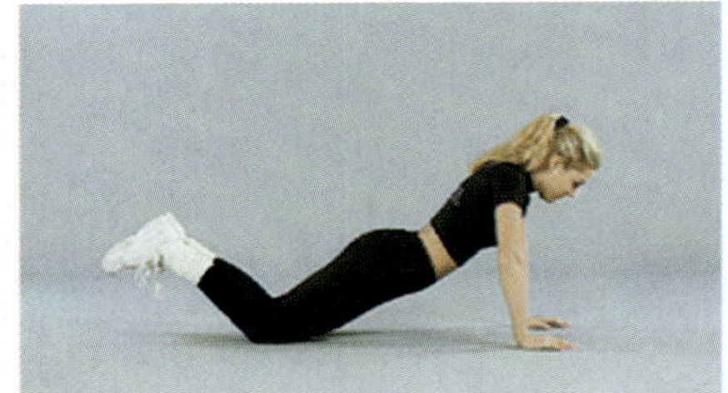

2. Lower your chest to the floor with your back straight, and then return to the starting position.
3. Perform as many push-ups or modified push-ups as you can without stopping.
   Number of push-ups: ____________ or number of modified push-ups: ____________

Rating Your Push-Up Test Result

Your score is the number of completed push-ups or modified push-ups. Refer to the appropriate portion of the table for a rating of your upper-body endurance. Record your rating below and in the summary at the end of this lab.

Rating: ____________

Ratings for the Push-Up and Modified Push-Up Tests

	Number of Push-Ups					
Men	*Very Poor*	*Poor*	*Fair*	*Good*	*Excellent*	*Superior*
Age: 18–29	Below 22	22–28	29–36	37–46	47–61	Above 61
30–39	Below 17	17–23	24–29	30–38	39–51	Above 51
40–49	Below 11	11–17	18–23	24–29	30–39	Above 39
50–59	Below 9	9–12	13–18	19–24	25–38	Above 38
60 and over	Below 6	6–9	10–17	18–22	23–27	Above 27
	Number of Modified Push-Ups					
Women	*Very Poor*	*Poor*	*Fair*	*Good*	*Excellent*	*Superior*
Age: 18–29	Below 17	17–22	23–29	30–35	36–44	Above 44
30–39	Below 11	11–18	19–23	24–30	31–38	Above 38
40–49	Below 6	6–12	13–17	18–23	24–32	Above 32
50–59	Below 6	6–11	12–16	17–20	21–27	Above 27
60 and over	Below 2	2–4	5–11	12–14	15–19	Above 19

SOURCE: Based on norms from The Cooper Institute of Aerobic Research, Dallas, Texas; from *The Physical Fitness Specialist Manual,* revised 2002. Used with permission.

The Squat Endurance Test

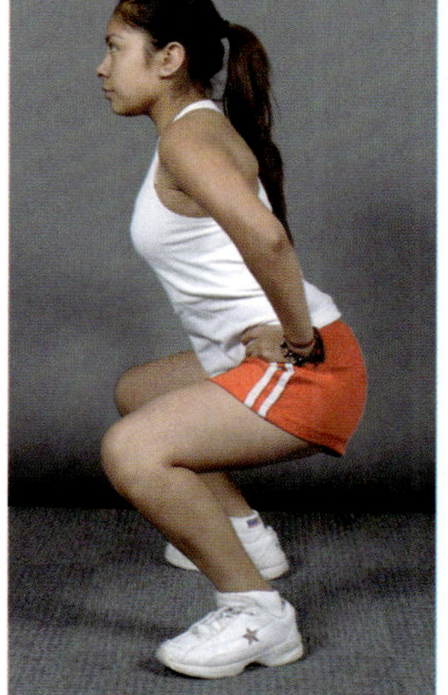

Instructions

1. Stand with your feet placed slightly more than shoulder width apart, toes pointed out slightly hands on hips or across your chest, head neutral, and back straight. Center your weight over your arches or slightly behind.
2. Squat down, keeping your weight centered over your arches, until your thighs are parallel with the floor. Push back up to the starting position, maintaining a straight back and neutral head position.
3. Perform as many squats as you can without stopping.

   Number of squats: ______________

Rating Your Squat Endurance Test Result

Your score is the number of completed squats. Refer to the appropriate portion of the table for a rating of your leg muscular endurance. Record your rating below and in the summary at the end of this lab.
Rating: ______________

Ratings for the Squat Endurance Test

	Number of Squats Performed						
Men	*Very Poor*	*Poor*	*Below Average*	*Average*	*Above Average*	*Good*	*Excellent*
Age: 18–25	<25	25–30	31–34	35–38	39–43	44–49	>49
26–35	<22	22–28	29–30	31–34	35–39	40–45	>45
36–45	<17	17–22	23–26	27–29	30–34	35–41	>41
46–55	<9	13–17	18–21	22–24	25–38	29–35	>35
56–65	<9	9–12	13–16	17–20	21–24	25–31	>31
65 +	<7	7–10	11–14	15–18	19–21	22–28	>28
Women	*Very Poor*	*Poor*	*Below Average*	*Average*	*Above Average*	*Good*	*Excellent*
Age: 18–25	<18	18–24	25–28	29–32	33–36	37–43	>43
26–35	<20	13–20	21–24	25–28	29–32	33–39	>39
36–45	<7	7–14	15–18	19–22	23–26	27–33	>33
46–55	<5	5–9	10–13	14–17	18–21	22–27	>27
56–65	<3	3–6	7–9	10–12	13–17	18–24	>24
65+	<2	2–4	5–10	11–13	14–16	17–23	>23

SOURCE: www.topendsports.com/testing/tests/home-squat.htm

Summary of Results

Curl-up test: Number of curl-ups: ____________ Rating: ____________

Push-up test: Number of push-ups: ____________ Rating: ____________

Squat endurance test: Number of squats: ____________ Rating: ____________

Remember that muscular endurance is specific: Your ratings may vary considerably for different parts of your body.

Using Your Results

How did you score? Are you surprised by your ratings for muscular endurance? Are you satisfied with your current ratings?

If you're not satisfied, set realistic goals for improvement:

Are you satisfied with your current level of muscular endurance as evidenced in your daily life—for example, your ability to carry groceries or your books, hike, and do yard work?

If you're not satisfied, set realistic goals for improvement:

What should you do next? Enter the results of this lab in the Preprogram Assessment column in Appendix C. If you've set goals for improvement, begin planning your strength training program by completing the plan in Lab 8.3. After several weeks of your program, complete this lab again and enter the results in the Postprogram Assessment column of Appendix C. How do the results compare?

Name ______________________ Section ____________ Date ____________

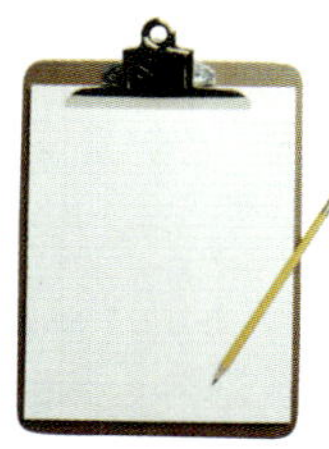

LAB 8.3 Designing and Monitoring a Strength Training Program

1. *Set goals.* List goals for your strength training program. Your goals can be specific or general, short or long term. In the first section, include specific, measurable goals that you can use to track the progress of your fitness program—for example, raising your upper-body muscular strength rating from fair to good or being able to complete 10 repetitions of a lat pull with 125 pounds of resistance. In the second section, include long-term and more qualitative goals, such as improving self-confidence and reducing your risk for back pain.

   Specific Goals: Current Status ______________________ Final Goals ______________________

   Other goals: ______________________

2. *Choose exercises.* Based on your goals, choose 8–10 exercises to perform during each weight training session. If your goal is general training for wellness, use the sample program in Figure 8.2 on p. 231. List your exercises and the muscles they develop in your program plan.
3. *Frequency: Choose the number of training sessions per week.* Work out at least 2 nonconsecutive days per week. Indicate the days you will train in your program plan; be sure to include days of rest to allow your body to recover.
4. *Intensity: Choose starting weights.* Experiment with different amounts of weight until you settle on a good starting weight, one that you can lift easily for 10–12 repetitions. As you progress in your program, add more weight. Fill in the starting weight for each exercise in your program plan.
5. *Time: Choose a starting number of sets and repetitions.* Include at least 1 set of 8–12 repetitions of each exercise. (When you add weight, you may have to decrease the number of repetitions slightly until your muscles adapt to the heavier load.) If your program is focusing on strength alone, your sets can contain fewer repetitions using a heavier load. If you are over approximately age 50–60, your sets should contain more repetitions (10–15) using a lighter load. Fill in the starting number of sets and repetitions of each exercise in your program plan.
6. *Monitor your progress.* Use the workout card on the next page to monitor your progress and keep track of exercises, weights, sets, and repetitions.

Program Plan for Weight Training

Exercise	Muscle(s) Developed	Frequency (check ✓)							Intensity: Weight (lb)	Time	
		M	T	W	Th	F	Sa	Su		Repetitions	Sets

WORKOUT CARD FOR ______________________

Exercise/Date																										
	Wt																									
	Sets																									
	Reps																									
	Wt																									
	Sets																									
	Reps																									
	Wt																									
	Sets																									
	Reps																									
	Wt																									
	Sets																									
	Reps																									
	Wt																									
	Sets																									
	Reps																									
	Wt																									
	Sets																									
	Reps																									
	Wt																									
	Sets																									
	Reps																									
	Wt																									
	Sets																									
	Reps																									
	Wt																									
	Sets																									
	Reps																									
	Wt																									
	Sets																									
	Reps																									
	Wt																									
	Sets																									
	Reps																									
	Wt																									
	Sets																									
	Reps																									

Flexibility and Low-Back Health

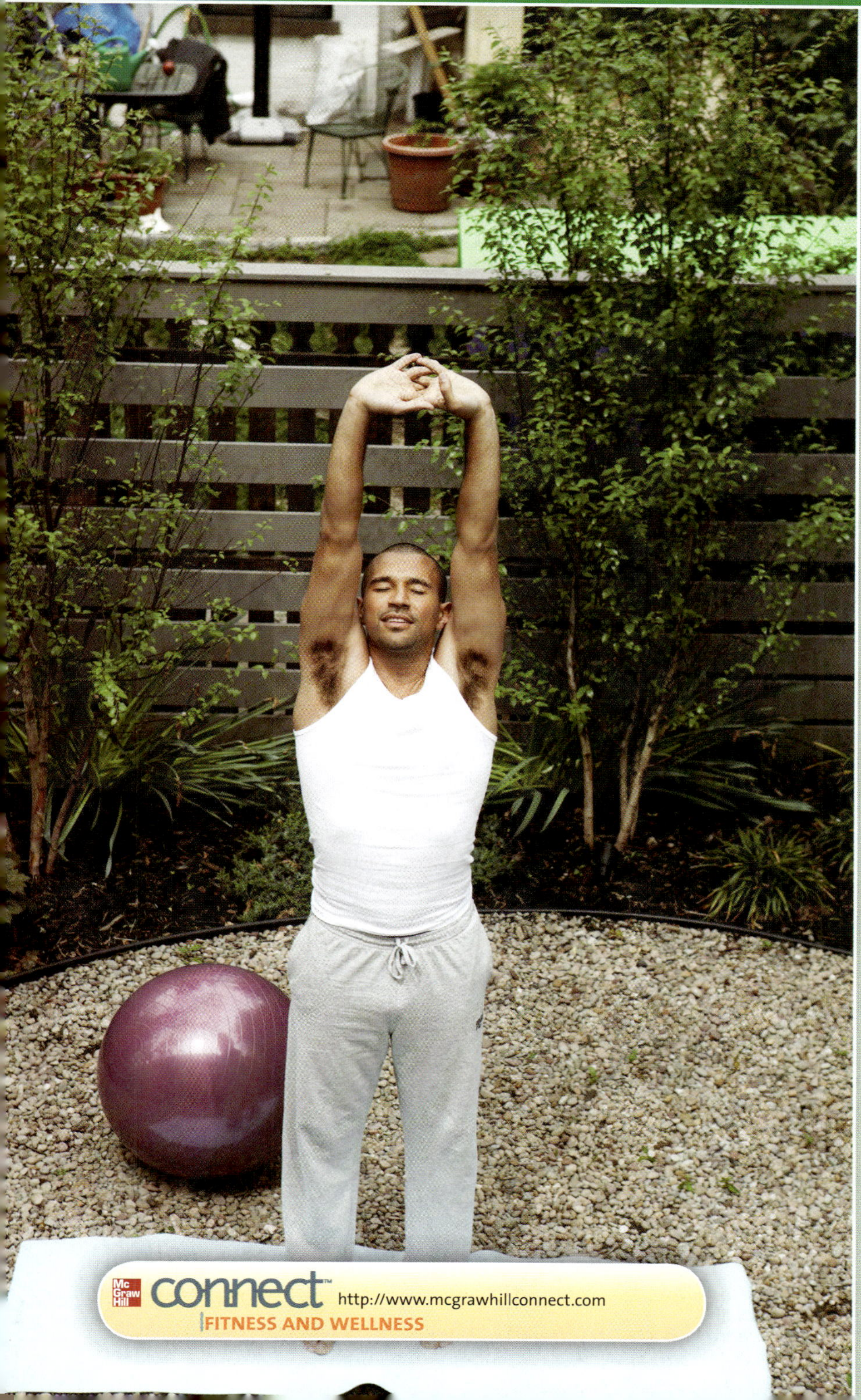

LOOKING AHEAD...

After reading this chapter, you should be able to:

- Identify the potential benefits of flexibility and stretching exercises
- List the factors that affect a joint's flexibility
- Describe the different types of stretching exercises and how they affect muscles
- Describe the intensity, duration, and frequency of stretching exercises that will develop the most flexibility with the lowest risk of injury
- List safe stretching exercises for major joints
- Explain how low-back pain can be prevented and managed

TEST YOUR KNOWLEDGE

1. Stretching exercises should be performed
   a. at the start of a warm-up.
   b. first thing in the morning.
   c. after endurance exercise or strength training.
2. If you injure your back, it's usually best to rest in bed until the pain is completely gone. True or false?
3. It is better to hold a stretch for a short time than to "bounce" while stretching. True or false?

Answers

1. **c.** It's best to do stretching exercises when your muscles are warm. Intensely stretching muscles before exercise may temporarily reduce their explosive strength and interfere with neuromuscular control.
2. **False.** Prolonged bed rest may actually worsen back pain. Limit bed rest to a day or less, treat pain and inflammation with cold and then heat, and begin moderate physical activity as soon as possible.
3. **True.** "Bouncing" during stretching can damage your muscles. This type of stretching, called ballistic stretching, should be used only by well-conditioned athletes for specific purposes. A person of average fitness should stretch slowly, holding each stretch for 10–30 seconds.

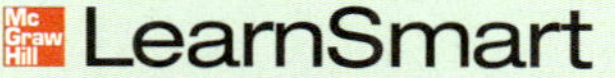

Flexibility—the ability of a joint to move through its normal, full **range of motion**—is important for general fitness and wellness. Flexibility is a highly adaptable physical fitness component. It increases in response to a regular program of stretching exercises and decreases with inactivity. Flexibility is also specific: Good flexibility in one joint doesn't necessarily mean good flexibility in another. You can increase your flexibility by doing regular stretching exercises for all your major joints.

This chapter describes the factors that affect flexibility and the benefits of maintaining good flexibility. It provides guidelines for assessing your current level of flexibility and putting together a successful stretching program. It also examines the common problem of low-back pain.

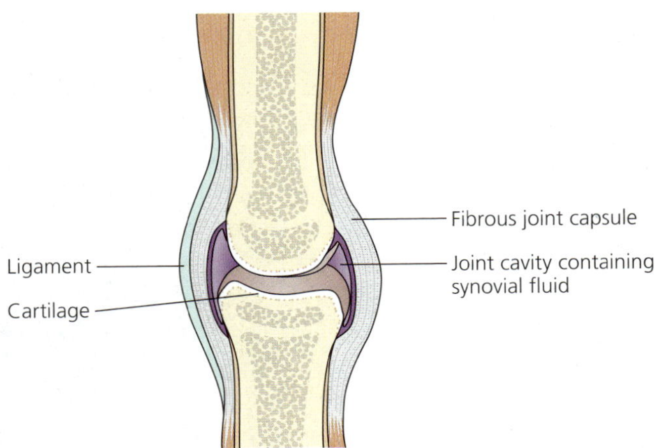

FIGURE 9.1 Basic joint structure.

TYPES OF FLEXIBILITY

There are two types of flexibility:

- *Static flexibility* is the ability to hold an extended position at one end or point in a joint's range of motion. For example, static flexibility determines how far you can extend your arm across the front of your body or out to the side. Static flexibility depends on your ability to tolerate stretched muscles; the structure of your joints; and the tightness of muscles, tendons, and ligaments.
- *Dynamic flexibility* is the ability to move a joint through its range of motion with little resistance. For example, dynamic flexibility affects your ability to pitch a ball or swing a golf club. Dynamic flexibility depends on static flexibility, but it also involves strength, coordination, and resistance to movement.

Dynamic flexibility is important for daily activities and sports. Because static flexibility is easier to measure and better researched, however, most assessment tests and stretching programs target that type of flexibility.

WHAT DETERMINES FLEXIBILITY?

The flexibility of a joint is affected by its structure, by muscle elasticity and length, and by nervous system regulation. Some factors, such as joint structure, can't be changed. Other factors, such as the length of resting muscle fibers, can be changed through exercise; these factors should be the focus of a program to develop flexibility.

Joint Structure

The amount of flexibility in a joint is determined in part by the nature and structure of the joint (Figure 9.1). Hinge joints such as those in your fingers and knees allow only limited forward and backward movement; they lock when fully extended. Ball-and-socket joints like the hip enable movement in many different directions and provide for a greater range of motion. Major joints are surrounded by **joint capsules**, semielastic structures that give joints strength and stability but limit movement. The bone surfaces within the joint are lined with cartilage and separated by a joint cavity containing ***synovial fluid***, which cushions the bones and reduces friction as the joint moves. Ligaments, both inside and outside the joint capsule, strengthen and reinforce the joint. For an illustration of the knee joint and more about its function, see page T4-5 of the color transparency insert "Touring the Musculoskeletal System," in Chapter 8.

Heredity plays a part in joint structure and flexibility. For example, although everyone has a broad range of motion in the hip joint, not everyone can do a split. Gender may also play a role. Some studies have found that women have greater flexibility in certain joints.

Muscle Elasticity and Length

Soft tissues—including skin, muscles, tendons, and ligaments—also limit the flexibility of a joint. Muscle tissue is the key to developing flexibility because it can be lengthened if it is stretched regularly. The most important component of muscle tissue related to flexibility is the connective tissue that surrounds and envelops every part of muscle tissue, from individual muscle fibers to entire muscles. Connective tissue provides structure, elasticity, and bulk and makes up about 30% of muscle mass. Two principal types of connective tissue are **collagen**—white fibers that provide structure and support—and **elastin**—yellow fibers that are elastic and flexible. Muscles contain both collagen and elastin, closely intertwined, so muscle tissue exhibits the properties of both types of fibers. A recently discovered structural protein in muscles called ***titin*** also has elastic properties and contributes to flexibility.

When a muscle is stretched, the wavelike elastin fibers straighten; when the stretch is relieved, they rapidly snap back to their resting position. This temporary lengthening

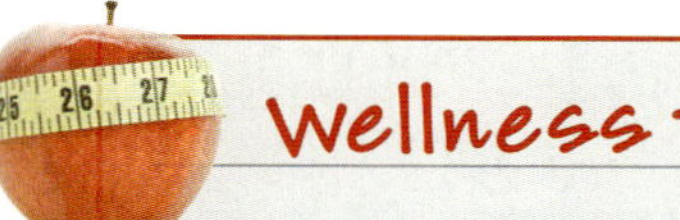

Wellness Tip

Muscles shrink after injury or surgery. Rehabilitation exercises can help muscles grow again. One caution: Overuse of drugs like ibuprofen can slow the regrowth process. Use such drugs only as prescribed by your doctor.

is called **elastic elongation.** If stretched gently and regularly, connective tissues may lengthen and flexibility may improve. This long-term lengthening is called **plastic elongation.** Without regular stretching, the process reverses: These tissues shorten, resulting in decreased flexibility. Regular stretching may contribute to flexibility by lengthening muscle fibers through the addition of contractile units called *sarcomeres.*

The amount of stretch a muscle will tolerate is limited, and as the limits of its flexibility are reached, connective tissue becomes more brittle and may rupture if overstretched. A safe and effective program stretches muscles enough to slightly elongate the tissues but not so much that they are damaged. Research has shown that flexibility is improved best by stretching when muscles are warm (following exercise or the application of heat) and the stretch is applied gradually and conservatively. Sudden, high-stress stretching is less effective and can lead to muscle damage.

Nervous System Regulation

Proprioceptors are nerves that send information about the muscular and skeletal systems to the nervous system. When these nerves detect any change in the position or force of muscles, tendons, and joints, they send signals to the spine and brain, which send signals back to coordinate muscle action in ways that protect muscles and tendons from injury. They help control the speed, strength, and coordination of muscle contractions.

When a muscle is stretched (lengthened), proprioceptors detect the amount and rate of the change in muscle length. The nerves send a signal to the spinal cord, which then sends a signal back to the muscle, triggering a muscle contraction that resists the change in muscle length. Another signal is sent to the antagonist muscle, causing it to relax and facilitate contraction of the stretched muscle. These reflexes occur frequently in active muscles and allow for fine control of muscle length and movement.

Small movements that only slightly stimulate these nerves cause small reflex actions. Rapid, powerful, and sudden changes in muscle length strongly stimulate the receptors and can cause large and powerful reflex muscle contractions. Thus, stretches that involve rapid, bouncy movements can be dangerous and cause injury because each bounce causes a reflex contraction, and so a muscle might be stretching at the same time it is contracting. Performing a gradual stretch and then holding it allows the proprioceptors to adjust to the new muscle length and to reduce the signals sent to the spine, thereby allowing muscles to lengthen and, over time, improving flexibility.

The stretching technique called *proprioceptive neuromuscular facilitation (PNF),* described later, takes advantage of nerve activity to improve flexibility. For example, contracting a muscle prior to stretching it can help allow the muscle to stretch farther. The advanced strength training technique called plyometrics (Chapter 8) also takes advantage of the nervous system action in stretching and contracting muscles.

Modifying nervous control through movement and specific exercises is the best way to improve the functional range of motion. Regular stretching trains the proprioceptors to allow greater lengthening of the muscles. Proprioceptors adapt quickly to stretching (or lack of stretching), so frequent training is beneficial for developing flexibility. Stretching before exercising, however, can disturb proprioceptors and interfere with motor control during exercise. This is another good reason to stretch after exercising.

Ask Yourself

QUESTIONS FOR CRITICAL THINKING AND REFLECTION

Have you ever noticed that you are markedly more or less flexible than your friends or classmates? To what do you attribute these differences? Did you know that you could increase your flexibility with a regular stretching program? Would it be meaningful to you to do so?

BENEFITS OF FLEXIBILITY

Good flexibility provides benefits for the entire musculoskeletal system. It may also prevent injuries and soreness and improve performance in all physical activities.

KEY TERMS

range of motion The full motion possible in a joint.

joint capsules Semielastic structures, composed primarily of connective tissue, that surround major joints.

soft tissues Tissues of the human body that include skin, fat, linings of internal organs and blood vessels, connective tissues, tendons, ligaments, muscles, and nerves.

collagen White fibers that provide structure and support in connective tissue.

elastin Yellow fibers that make connective tissue flexible.

elastic elongation Temporary change in the length of muscles, tendons, and supporting connective tissues.

plastic elongation Long-term change in the length of muscles, tendons, and supporting connective tissues.

proprioceptor A nerve that sends information about the muscular and skeletal systems to the nervous system.

THE EVIDENCE FOR EXERCISE

Does Physical Activity Increase or Decrease the Risk of Bone and Joint Disease?

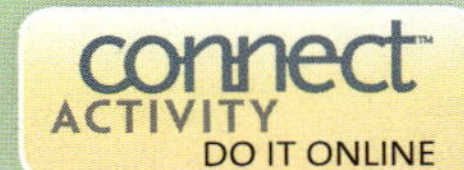

Most college students don't worry much about developing fall-related fractures or chronic bone-related illnesses such as osteoporosis—loss of bone mass—or osteoarthritis—degeneration of the cartilage lining the bones inside joints. Even so, bone health should be a concern throughout life. This is because girls amass 85% of their adult bone mass by age 18, and boys build the same amount by age 20, but most people begin losing bone mass around age 30. For many, bone loss is accelerated by poor diet and lack of exercise. According to the National Osteoporosis Foundation, 10 million Americans have osteoporosis. Meantime, 34 million Americans are at risk of disease because of low bone mass. Overall, osteoporosis is a health threat for about 55% of Americans aged 50 and older.

In addition to getting enough nutrients that are important for bone health (see Chapter 3), there is mounting evidence that exercise can preserve or improve bone health. For example, several studies have shown an inverse relationship between physical activity and the risk for bone fractures. That is, the more you exercise, the less likely you are to suffer fractures, especially of the upper leg and hip. Research has not determined conclusively how much exercise is required to reduce fracture risk, but reduced risk seems to become apparent when people walk at least 4 hours per week and devote at least 1 hour per week to other forms of physical activity. These findings seem to be consistent for women and men, but some studies disagree on this point, meaning that further research is needed on the sex-related response to exercise as it relates to bone fractures.

Both men and women can prevent fractures and osteoporosis by maintaining or increasing their bone mineral density throughout life, and physical activity plays a significant role in this. One way exercise helps is by increasing the mineral density of bones, or at least by decreasing the loss of mineral density over time. Several one-year-long studies found that exercise can increase bone mineral density by 1–2% per year, which is significant—especially considering that the same amount of bone mineral density can be lost every 1–4 years in older persons. Currently, the American College of Sports Medicine recommends that adults perform weight-bearing physical activities (such as walking) 3–5 days per week and strength training exercises 2–3 days per week to increase bone mass or avoid loss of mineral density. Exercise is particularly important in lactating (breastfeeding) women for preventing bone loss.

When it comes to exercise and osteoarthritis, the evidence is less conclusive but still fairly positive. All experts agree that regular, moderate-intensity exercise is necessary for joint health. However, they also warn that vigorous or too-frequent exercise may contribute to joint damage and encourage the onset of osteoarthritis. For this reason, experts try to strike a balance in their exercise recommendations, especially for persons with a family history of osteoarthritis. Research seems to support this cautious approach. Some studies have found that regular physical activity (as recommended for general health) does not increase osteoarthritis risk. Other studies show that moderate activity may provide some protection against the disease, but this evidence is limited.

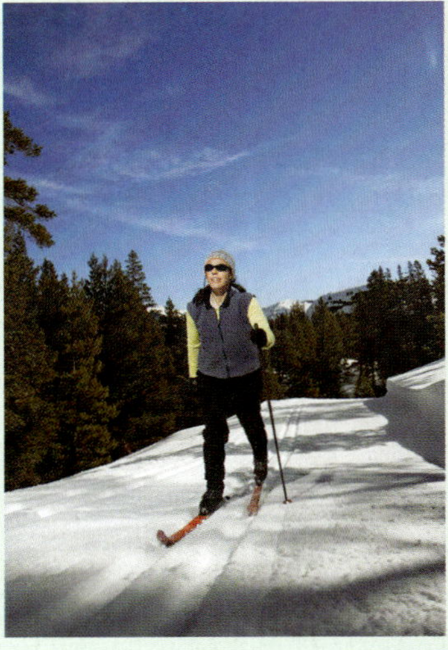

A few studies also reveal that the type of exercise you do may increase your risk. For example, competitive or strenuous sports such as ballet, orienteering, football, basketball, soccer, and tennis have been associated with the disease, whereas sports such as cross-country skiing, running, swimming, biking, and walking have not.

The bottom line is that the earlier in life you become physically active, the greater your protection against bone loss and bone-related diseases. However, if you have a family history of osteoporosis or osteoarthritis, or if you have already developed symptoms of one of these ailments, be sure to talk to your physician before beginning an exercise program.

SOURCES: Kemmler, W., and S. Stengel. 2011. Exercise and osteoporosis-related fractures: Perspectives and recommendations of the sports and exercise scientist. *Physician Sportsmedicine* 39(1): 142–157; Lovelady, et al. 2009. Effect of Exercise Training on Loss of Bone Mineral Density during Lactation. *Medicine and Science in Sports and Exercise* 41 (10): 1902–1907; American College of Sports Medicine. 2004. ACSM position stand: Physical activity and bone health. *Medicine and Science in Sports and Exercise* 36 (11): 1985–1996; National Osteoporosis Foundation. 2011. *Bone Basics: Fast Facts* (http://www.nof.org/node/40; retrieved March 23, 2011); Physical Activity Guidelines Advisory Committee. 2008. *Physical Activity Guidelines Advisory Committee Report, 2008*. Washington, D.C.: U.S. Department of Health and Human Services.

Joint Health

Good flexibility is essential to good joint health. When the muscles and other tissues that support a joint are tight, the joint is subject to abnormal stresses that can cause joint deterioration. For example, tight thigh muscles cause excessive pressure on the kneecap, leading to pain in the knee joint. Poor joint flexibility can also cause abnormalities in joint lubrication, leading to deterioration of the sensitive cartilage cells lining the joint; pain and further joint injury can result.

Improved flexibility can greatly improve your quality of life, particularly as you get older. People tend to exercise less as they age, leading to loss of joint mobility and increased incidence of joint pain. Aging also decreases the natural elasticity of muscles, tendons, and joints, resulting in stiffness. The problem is often compounded by arthritis (see the box "Does Physical Activity Increase or Decrease the Risk of Bone and Joint Disease?"). Good joint flexibility may prevent arthritis, and stretching may lessen pain in people who have the condition. Another benefit of good flexibility for older adults is that it increases balance and stability.

Prevention of Low-Back Pain and Injuries

Low-back pain can be related to poor spinal stability, which puts pressure on the nerves leading out from the spinal column. Strength and flexibility in the back, pelvis, and thighs may help prevent this type of back pain but may or may not improve back health or reduce the risk of injury. Good hip and knee flexibility protects the spine from excessive motion during the tasks of daily living.

Although scientific evidence is limited, people with either high or low flexibility seem to have an increased risk of injury. Extreme flexibility reduces joint stability, and poor flexibility limits a joint's range of motion. Persons of average fitness should try to attain normal flexibility in joints throughout the body, meaning each joint can move through its normal range of motion with no difficulty. Stretching programs are particularly important for older adults, people involved in high-power sports involving rapid changes in direction (such as football and tennis), workers involved in brief bouts of intense exertion (such as police officers and firefighters), and people who sit for prolonged periods (such as office workers and students).

However, stretching before a high-intensity activity (such as sprinting or basketball) may increase the risk of injury by interfering with neuromuscular control and reducing muscles' natural ability to stretch and contract. When injuries occur, flexibility exercises can be used in treatment: They reduce symptoms and help restore normal range of motion in affected joints.

Additional Potential Benefits

- ***Relief of aches and pains.*** Studying or working in one place for a long time can make your muscles tense. Stretching helps relieve tension and joint stiffness, so you can go back to work refreshed and effective. Stretching reduces the symptoms of exercise-induced muscle damage, and flexible muscles are less susceptible to the damage.
- ***Relief of muscle cramps.*** Recent research suggests that exercise-related muscle cramps are caused by increased electrical activity within the affected muscle. The best treatment for muscle cramps is gentle stretching, which reduces the electrical activity and allows the muscle to relax.
- ***Improved body position and strength for sports (and life).*** Good flexibility lets you assume more efficient body positions and exert force through a greater range of motion. For example, swimmers with more flexible shoulders have stronger strokes because they can pull their arms through the water in the optimal position. Some studies also suggest that flexibility training enhances strength development.

Fitness Tip

Many people have stopped stretching after hearing mixed results from research studies. This may be a mistake. Stretching after an intense workout can relieve soreness, in addition to providing all the other benefits listed here.

Ask Yourself

QUESTIONS FOR CRITICAL THINKING AND REFLECTION

When you think about the health-related components of fitness, how do you rank flexibility? Is it less important to you than cardiorespiratory endurance or muscular strength? If you place a low priority on flexibility, what can you do to increase your motivation to stretch?

- ***Maintenance of good posture and balance.*** Good flexibility also contributes to body symmetry and good posture. Bad posture can gradually change your body structures. Sitting in a slumped position, for example, can lead to tightness in the muscles in the front of your chest and overstretching and looseness in the upper spine, causing a rounding of the upper back. This condition, called ***kyphosis***, is common in older people. It may be prevented by stretching regularly.
- ***Relaxation.*** Flexibility exercises, particularly when practiced in combination with yoga or tai chi, reduce mental tension, slow your breathing rate, and reduce blood pressure.
- ***Improving impaired mobility.*** Stretching often decreases pain and improves functional capacity in people with arthritis, stroke, or muscle and nerve diseases and in people who are recovering from surgery or injury.

ASSESSING FLEXIBILITY

Because flexibility is specific to each joint, there are no tests of general flexibility. The most commonly used flexibility test is the sit-and-reach test, which rates the flexibility of the muscles in the lower back and hamstrings. To assess your flexibility and identify inflexible joints, complete Lab 9.1.

CREATING A SUCCESSFUL PROGRAM TO DEVELOP FLEXIBILITY

A successful program for developing flexibility includes safe exercises executed with the most effective techniques. Your goal should be to attain normal flexibility

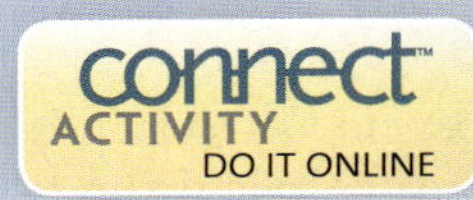

TAKE CHARGE

Safe Stretching

- Do stretching exercises statically. Stretch to the point of mild discomfort, hold the position for 10–30 seconds, rest for 30–60 seconds, and then repeat, trying to stretch a bit farther.
- Do not stretch to the point of pain. Any soreness after a stretching workout should be mild and last no more than 24 hours. If you are sore for a longer period, you stretched too intensely.
- Relax and breathe easily as you stretch. Inhale through the nose and exhale through pursed lips during the stretch. Try to relax the muscles being stretched.
- Perform all exercises on both sides of your body.
- Wear loose-fitting clothing that won't inhibit movement when you're stretching.
- To prevent falls, wear athletic shoes when stretching, or stretch on a no-slip surface.
- Increase intensity and duration gradually over time. Improved flexibility takes many months to develop.
- Stretch when your muscles are warm. Do gentle warm-up exercises such as easy jogging or calisthenics before doing a stretching routine.
- There are large individual differences in joint flexibility. Don't feel you have to compete with others during stretching workouts.
- Engage in a variety of physical activities to help you develop well-rounded functional physical fitness and allow you to perform all types of training more safely and effectively.

in the major joints. Balanced flexibility (not too much or too little) provides joint stability and facilitates smooth, economical movement patterns. You can achieve balanced flexibility by performing stretching exercises regularly and by using a variety of stretches and stretching techniques.

Applying the FITT Principle

As with other programs, the acronym FITT can be used to remember key components of a stretching program: Frequency, Intensity, Time, and Type of exercise.

Frequency The ACSM recommends that stretching exercises be performed at least 2–3 days per week, but more often is even better. It's best to stretch when your muscles are warm, so try incorporating stretching into your cool-down after cardiorespiratory endurance exercise or weight training.

Never stretch when your muscles are cold; doing so can increase your risk of injury as well as limit the amount of flexibility you can develop. Although stretching before exercise is a time-honored ritual practiced by athletes in many sports, many studies have found that preexercise stretching decreases muscle strength and performance and disturbs neuromuscular control. If your workout involves participation in a sport or high-performance activity, you may be better off stretching after your workout. For moderate-intensity activities like walking or cycling, stretching before your workout is unlikely to impair your performance.

Intensity and Time (Duration) For each exercise, slowly stretch your muscles to the point of slight tension or mild discomfort—but not to the point of pain. Hold the stretch for 10–30 seconds. As you hold the stretch, the feeling of slight tension should slowly subside; at that point, try to stretch a bit farther. Throughout the stretch, try to relax and breathe easily. Rest for about 30–60 seconds between each stretch, and do 2–4 repetitions of each stretch. A complete flexibility workout usually takes about 10–30 minutes (Figure 9.2).

Types of Stretching Techniques Stretching techniques vary from simply stretching the muscles during the course of normal activities to sophisticated methods based on patterns

Warm-up 5–10 minutes or following an endurance or strength training workout	Stretching exercises for major joints **Sample program**	
	Exercise	*Areas stretched*
	Head turns and tilts	Neck
	Towel stretch	Triceps, shoulders, chest
	Across-the-body and overhead stretches	Shoulders, upper back, back of arm
	Upper-back stretch	Upper back
	Lateral stretch	Trunk muscles
	Step stretch	Hip, front of thigh
	Side lunge	Inner thigh, hip, calf
	Inner-thigh stretch	Inner thigh, hip
	Hip and trunk stretch	Trunk, outer thigh, hip, buttocks, lower back
	Modified hurdler stretch	Back of thigh, lower back
	Alternate leg stretcher	Back of thigh, hip, knee, ankle, buttocks
	Lower-leg stretch	Calf, soleus, Achilles tendon

Frequency: 2–3 days per week (minimum); 5–7 days per week (ideal)

Intensity: Stretch to the point of mild discomfort, not pain

Time (duration): All stretches should be held for 15–30 seconds and performed 2–4 times

Type of activity: Stretching exercises that focus on major joints

FIGURE 9.2 The FITT principle for a flexibility program.

of muscle reflexes. Improper stretching can do more harm than good, so it's important to understand the different types of stretching exercises and how they affect the muscles (see the box "Safe Stretching"). Four common techniques are static stretches, ballistic stretches, dynamic stretches, and PNF. These techniques can be performed passively or actively.

STATIC STRETCHING In **static stretching**, each muscle is gradually stretched, and the stretch is held for 10–30 seconds. A slow stretch prompts less reaction from proprioceptors, and the muscles can safely stretch farther than usual. Static stretching is the type most often recommended by fitness experts because it is safe and effective.

The key to this technique is to stretch the muscles and joints to the point where a pull is felt, but not to the point of pain. (One note of caution: Excess static stretching can decrease joint stability and increase the risk of injury. This may be a particular concern for women, who naturally have joints that are less stable and more flexible than men.) The sample stretching program presented later in this chapter features static stretching exercises.

BALLISTIC STRETCHING In **ballistic stretching,** the muscles are stretched suddenly in a forceful bouncing movement. For example, touching the toes repeatedly in rapid succession is a ballistic stretch for the hamstrings. A problem with this technique is that the heightened activity of proprioceptors caused by the rapid stretches can continue for some time, possibly causing injuries during any physical activities that follow. Another concern is that triggering strong responses from the nerves can cause a reflex muscle contraction that makes it harder to stretch. For these reasons, ballistic stretching is usually not recommended, especially for people of average fitness.

Ballistic stretching trains the muscle dynamically, so it can be an appropriate stretching technique for some well-trained athletes. For example, tennis players stretch their hamstrings and quadriceps ballistically when they lunge for a ball during a tennis match. Because this movement is part of their sport, they might benefit from ballistic training of these muscle groups.

DYNAMIC (FUNCTIONAL) STRETCHING The emphasis in **dynamic stretching** is on functional movements. Dynamic stretching is similar to ballistic stretching in that it includes movement, but it differs in that it does not involve rapid bouncing. Instead, dynamic stretching involves moving the joints through the range of motion used in a specific exercise or sport in an exaggerated but controlled manner; movements are fluid rather than jerky. An example of a dynamic stretch is the lunge walk, in which a person takes slow steps with an exaggerated stride length and reaches a lunge stretch position with each step.

Slow dynamic stretches can lengthen the muscles in many directions without developing high tension in the tissues. These stretches elongate the tissues and train the neuromuscular system. Because dynamic stretches are based on sports movements or movements used in daily life, they develop functional flexibility that translates well into activities.

Dynamic stretches are more challenging than static stretches because they require balance and coordination and may carry a greater risk of muscle soreness and injury. People just beginning a flexibility program might want to start off with static stretches and try dynamic stretches only after they are comfortable with static stretching techniques and have improved their flexibility. It is also a good idea to seek expert advice on dynamic stretching technique and program development.

Serious athletes may use dynamic stretches as part of their warm-up before a competitive event or a high-intensity training session in order to move their joints through the range of motion required for the activity. Functional flexibility training can also be combined with functional strength training. For example, lunge curls, which combine dynamic lunges with free weights biceps curls, stretch the hip, thigh, and calf muscles; stabilize the core muscles in the trunk; and build strength in the arm muscles. Many activities build functional flexibility and strength at the same time, including yoga, Pilates, taijiquan, Olympic weight lifting, plyometrics, stability training (including Swiss and Bosu ball exercises), medicine ball exercises, and functional training machines (for example, Life Fitness and Cybex).

PROPRIOCEPTIVE NEUROMUSCULAR FACILITATION (PNF) PNF techniques use reflexes initiated by both muscle and joint nerves to cause greater training effects. The most popular PNF stretching technique is the contract-relax stretching method, in which a muscle is contracted before it is stretched. The contraction activates proprioceptors, causing relaxation in the muscle about to be stretched. For example, in a seated stretch of calf muscles, the first step in PNF is to contract the calf muscles. The individual or a partner can provide resistance for an isometric

Wellness Tip

You don't have to be at the gym to stretch. There are lots of simple, small-movement stretches you can do anywhere—even at your desk. For some examples, visit a good health Web site such as MayoClinic.com and search for "stretching exercises."

KEY TERMS

static stretching A technique in which a muscle is slowly and gently stretched and then held in the stretched position.

ballistic stretching A technique in which muscles are stretched by the force generated as a body part is repeatedly bounced, swung, or jerked.

dynamic stretching A technique in which muscles are stretched by moving joints slowly and fluidly through their range of motion in a controlled manner; also called *functional stretching*.

contraction. Following a brief period of relaxation, the next step is to stretch the calf muscles by pulling the tops of the feet toward the body. A duration of six seconds for the contraction and 10–30 seconds for the stretch is recommended. PNF appears to be most effective if the individual pushes hard during the isometric contraction.

Another example of a PNF stretch is the contract-relax-contract pattern. In this technique, begin by contracting the muscle to be stretched and then relaxing it. Next, contract the opposing muscle (the antagonist). Finally, stretch the first muscle. For example, using this technique to stretch the hamstrings (the muscles in the back of the thigh) would require the following steps: Contract the hamstrings, relax the hamstrings, contract the quadriceps (the muscles in the front of the thigh), then stretch the hamstrings.

PNF appears to allow more effective stretching and greater increases in flexibility than static stretching, but it tends to cause more muscle stiffness and soreness. It also usually requires a partner and takes more time.

PASSIVE VERSUS ACTIVE STRETCHING Stretches can be done either passively or actively. In **passive stretching,** an outside force or resistance provided by yourself, a partner, gravity, or a weight helps your joints move through their range of motion. For example, a seated stretch of the hamstring and back muscles can be done by reaching the hands toward the feet until a pull is felt in those muscles. You can achieve a greater range of motion (a more intense stretch) using passive stretching. However, because the stretch is not controlled by the muscles themselves, there is a greater risk of injury. Communication between partners in passive stretching is important to ensure that joints aren't forced outside their normal functional range of motion.

In **active stretching,** a muscle is stretched by a contraction of the opposing muscle (the muscle on the opposite side of the limb). For example, an active seated stretch of the calf muscles occurs when a person actively contracts the muscles on the top of the shin. The contraction of this opposing muscle produces a reflex that relaxes the muscles to be stretched. The muscle can be stretched farther with a low risk of injury.

The only disadvantage of active stretching is that a person may not be able to produce enough stress (enough stretch) to increase flexibility using only the contraction of opposing muscle groups. The safest and most convenient technique is active static stretching, with an occasional passive assist. For example, you might stretch your calves both by contracting the muscles on the top of your shin and by pulling your feet toward you. This way you combine the advantages of active stretching—safety and the relaxation reflex—with those of passive stretching—greater range of motion. People who are just beginning flexibility training may be better off doing active rather than passive stretches. For PNF techniques, it is particularly important to have a knowledgeable partner.

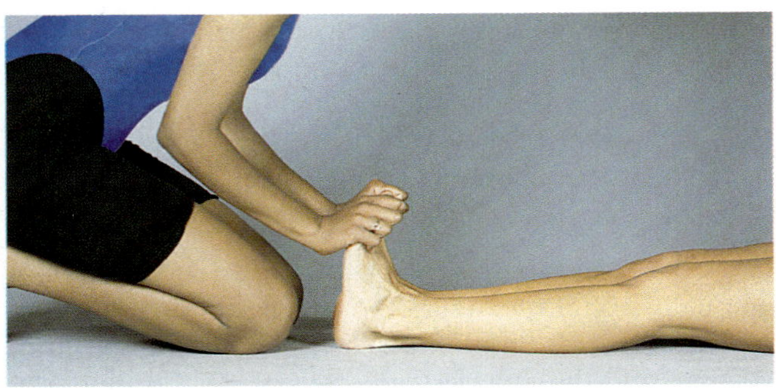

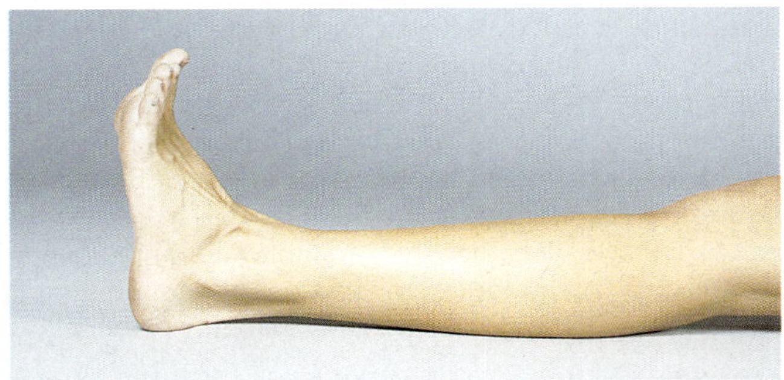

In passive stretching (top), an outside force—such as pressure exerted by another person—helps move the joint and stretch the muscles. In active stretching (bottom), the force to move the joint and stretch the muscles is provided by a contraction of the opposing muscles.

KEY TERMS

passive stretching A technique in which muscles are stretched by force applied by an outside source.

active stretching A technique in which muscles are stretched by the contraction of the opposing muscles.

Making Progress

As with any type of training, you will make progress and improve your flexibility if you stick with your program. Judge your progress by noting your body position while stretching. For example, note how far you can lean forward during a modified hurdler stretch. Repeat the assessment tests that appear in Lab 9.1 periodically and be sure to take the test at the same time of day each time. You will likely notice some improvement after only 2–3 weeks of stretching, but you may need at least 2 months to attain significant improvements. By then, you can expect flexibility increases of about 10–20% in many joints.

Exercises to Improve Flexibility: A Sample Program

There are hundreds of exercises that can improve flexibility. Your program should include exercises that work all the major joints of the body by stretching their associated muscle groups (refer back to Figure 9.2). The exercises illustrated here are simple to do and pose a minimum risk of injury. Use these exercises to create a well-rounded program for developing flexibility. Be sure to perform each stretch using the proper technique. Hold each position

FLEXIBILITY EXERCISES

EXERCISE 1 Head Turns and Tilts

Instructions:
Head turns: Turn your head to the right and hold the stretch. Repeat to the left.

Head tilts: Tilt your head to the right and hold the stretch. Repeat to the left.

Areas stretched: Neck

Variation: Place your right palm on your right cheek; try to turn your head to the right as you resist with your hand. Repeat on the left side.

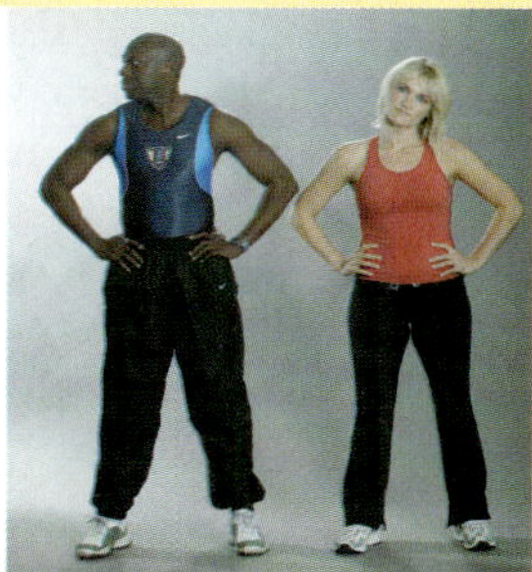

EXERCISE 2 Towel Stretch

Instructions: Roll up a towel and grasp it with both hands, palms down. With your arms straight, slowly lift the towel back over your head as far as possible. The closer together your hands are, the greater the stretch.

Areas stretched: Triceps, shoulders, chest

Variation: Repeat the stretch with your arms down and the towel behind your back. Grasp the towel with your palms forward and thumbs pointing out. Gently raise your arms behind your back. This exercise can also be done without a towel.

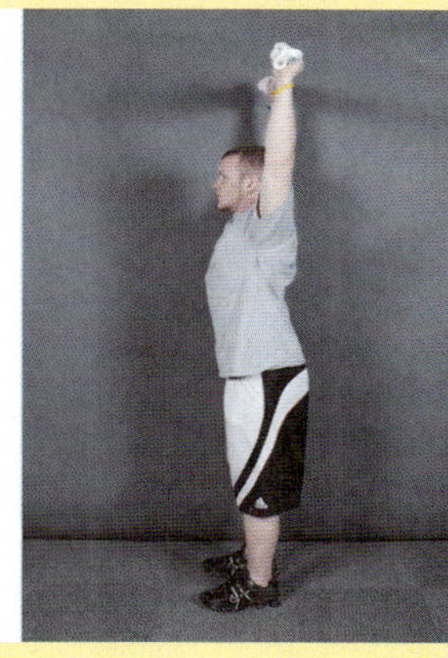

EXERCISE 3 Across-the-Body and Overhead Stretches

Instructions: (a) Keeping your back straight, cross your right arm in front of your body and grasp it with your left hand. Stretch your arm, shoulders, and back by gently pulling your arm as close to your body as possible. Hold.
(b) Bend your right arm over your head, placing your right elbow as close to your right ear as possible. Grasp your right elbow with your left hand over your head. Stretch the back of your arm by gently pulling your right elbow back and toward your head. Hold. Repeat both stretches on your left side.

Areas stretched: Shoulders, upper back, back of the arm (triceps)

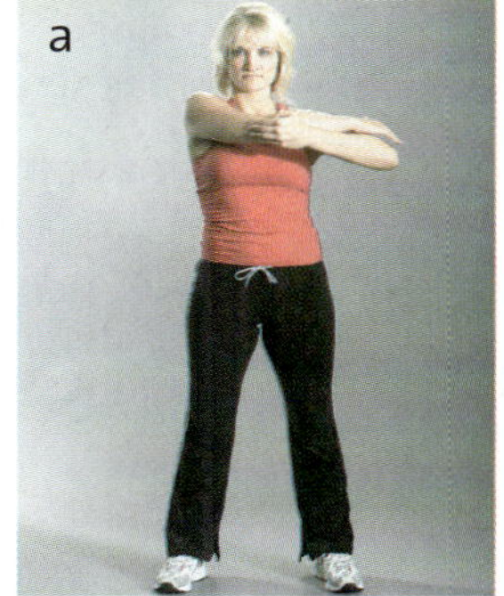
a

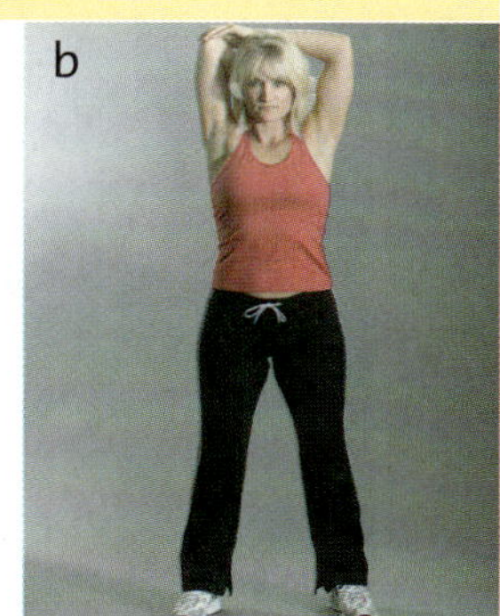
b

EXERCISE 4 Upper-Back Stretch

Instructions: Stand with your feet shoulder-width apart, knees slightly bent, and pelvis tucked under. Lace your fingers in front of your body and press your palms forward.

Areas stretched: Upper back

Variation: In the same position, wrap your arms around your body as if you were giving yourself a hug.

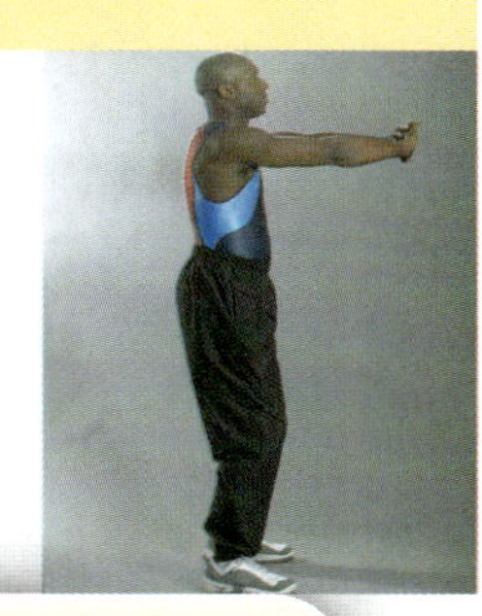

EXERCISE 5 Lateral Stretch

Instructions: Stand with your feet shoulder-width apart, knees slightly bent, and pelvis tucked under. Raise one arm over your head and bend sideways from the waist. Support your trunk by placing the hand or forearm of your other arm on your thigh or hip for support. Be sure you bend directly sideways and don't move your body below the waist. Repeat on the other side.

Areas stretched: Trunk muscles

Variation: Perform the same exercise in a seated position.

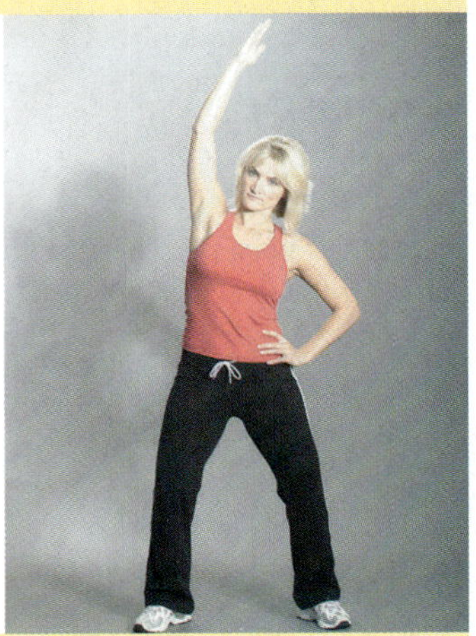

EXERCISE 6 Step Stretch

Instructions: Step forward and bend your forward knee, keeping it directly above your ankle. Stretch your other leg back so that your shin is parallel to the floor. Press your hips forward and down to stretch. Your arms can be at your sides, on top of your knee, or on the ground for balance. Repeat on the other side.

Areas stretched: Hip, front of thigh (quadriceps)

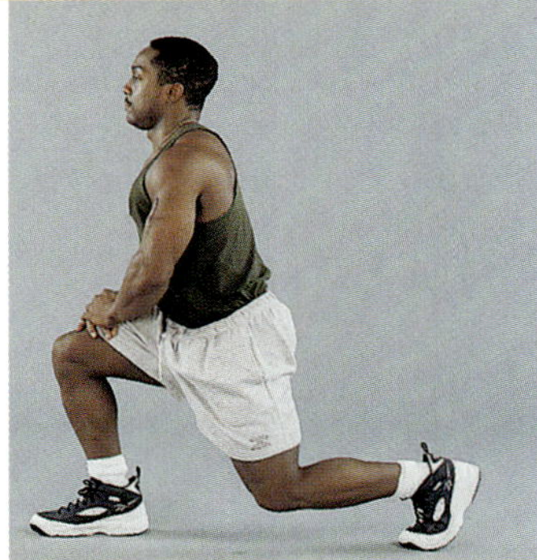

EXERCISE 7 Side Lunge

Instructions: Stand in a wide straddle with your legs turned out from your hip joints and your hands on your thighs. Lunge to one side by bending one knee and keeping the other leg straight. Keep your bent knee directly over your ankle; do not bend it more than 90 degrees. Repeat on the other side.

Areas stretched: Inner thigh, hip, calf

Variation: In the same position, lift the heel of the bent knee to provide additional stretch. The exercise may also be performed with your hands on the floor for balance.

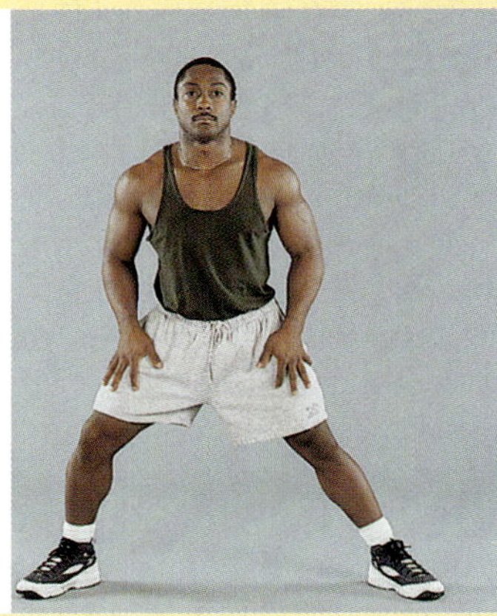

EXERCISE 8 Inner Thigh Stretch

Instructions: Sit with the soles of your feet together. Push your knees toward the floor using your hands or forearms.

Areas stretched: Inner thigh, hip

Variation: When you first begin to push your knees toward the floor, use your legs to resist the movement. Then relax and press your knees down as far as they will go.

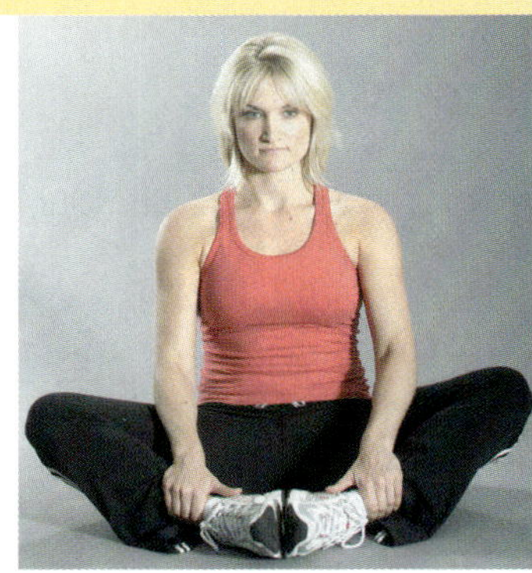

EXERCISE 9 Hip and Trunk Stretch

Instructions: Sit with your left leg straight, right leg bent and crossed over the left knee, and right hand on the floor next to your right hip. Turn your trunk as far as possible to the right by pushing against your right leg with your left forearm or elbow. Keep your right foot on the floor. Repeat on the other side.

Areas stretched: Trunk, outer thigh and hip, buttocks, lower back

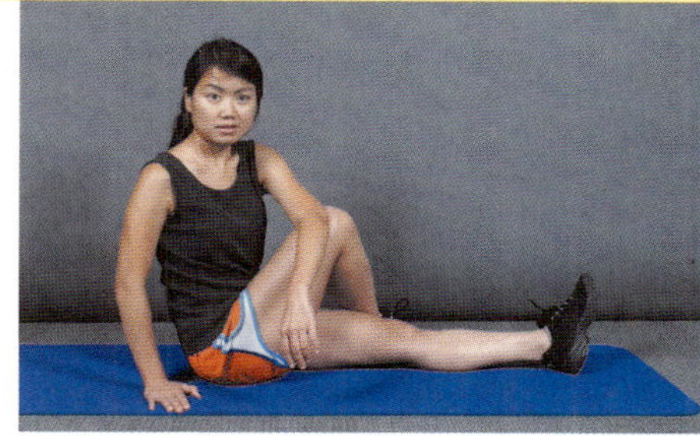

EXERCISE 10 Modified Hurdler Stretch (Seated Single-Leg Hamstring)

Instructions: Sit with your left leg straight and your right leg tucked close to your body. Reach toward your left ankle as far as possible. Repeat for the other leg.

Areas stretched: Back of the thigh (hamstring), lower back

Variation: As you stretch forward, alternately flex and point the foot of your extended leg.

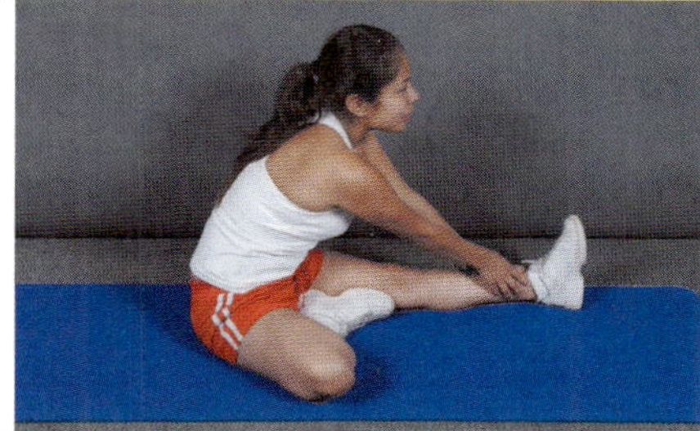

EXERCISE 11 Alternate Leg Stretcher

Instructions: Lie flat on your back with both legs straight. **(a)** Grasp your left leg behind the thigh, and pull it in to your chest. **(b)** Hold this position, and then extend your left leg toward the ceiling. **(c)** Hold this position, and then bring your left knee back to your chest and pull your toes toward your shin with your left hand. Stretch the back of the leg by attempting to straighten your knee. Repeat for the other leg.

Areas stretched: Back of the thigh (hamstring), hip, knee, ankle, buttocks

Variation: Perform the stretch on both legs at the same time.

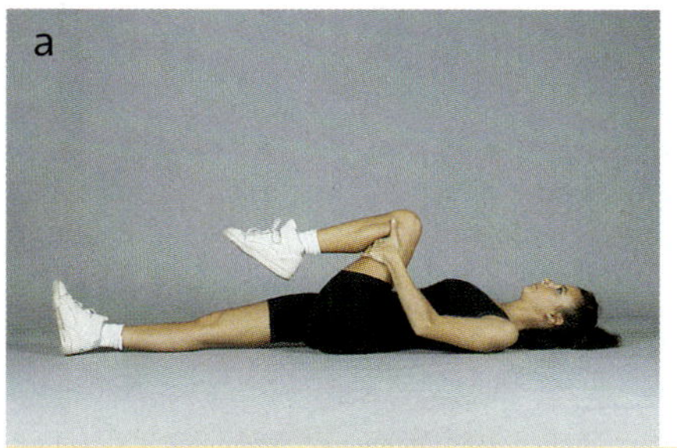
a

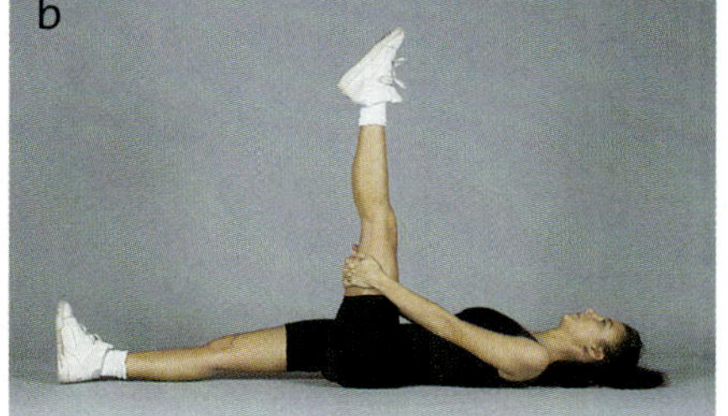
b

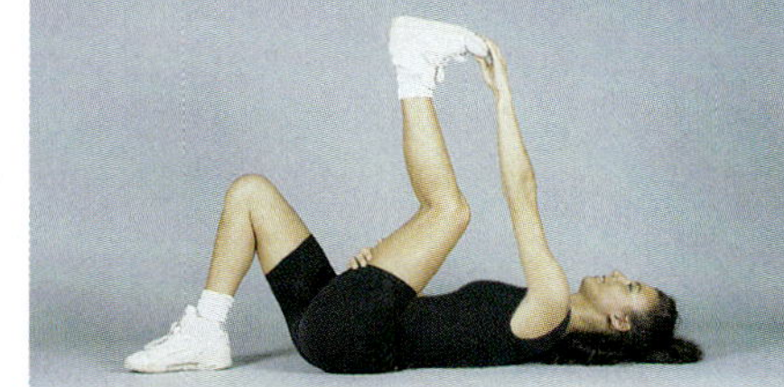
c

EXERCISE 12 Lower-Leg Stretch

Instructions: Stand with one foot about 1–2 feet in front of the other, with both feet pointing forward. **(a)** Keeping your back leg straight, lunge forward by bending your front knee and pushing your rear heel backward. Hold. **(b)** Then pull your back foot in slightly, and bend your back knee. Shift your weight to your back leg. Hold. Repeat on the other side.

Areas stretched: Back of the lower leg (calf, soleus, Achilles tendon)

Variation: Place your hands on a wall and extend one foot back, pressing your heel down to stretch, or stand with the balls of your feet on a step or bench and allow your heels to drop below the level of your toes.

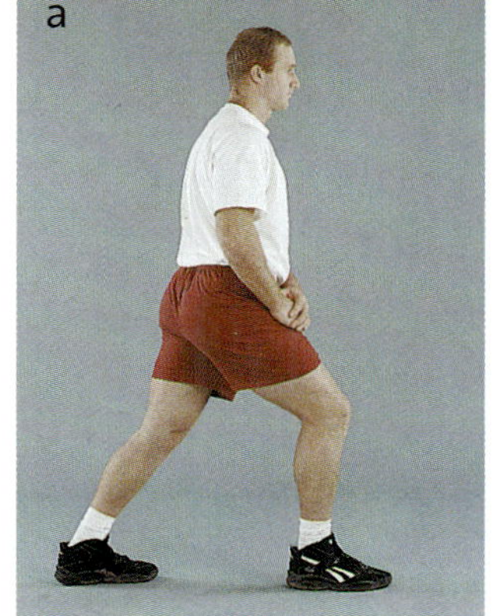
a

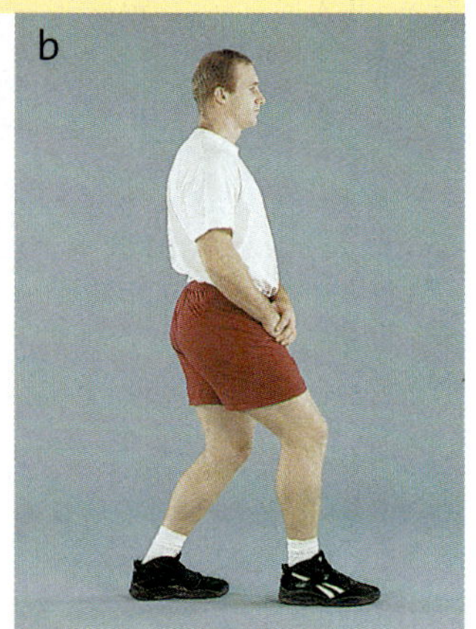
b

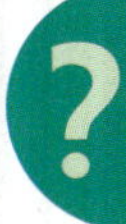

Ask yourself

QUESTIONS FOR CRITICAL THINKING AND REFLECTION

Why do you think improper stretching can do more harm than good? How can stretching cause injury? Of all the types of stretches described, which ones do you think would be safest for you? Which ones appeal to you most?

for 10–30 seconds and perform 2–4 repetitions of each exercise. Avoid exercises that put excessive pressure on your joints (see the box "Stretches to Avoid"). Complete Lab 9.2 when you're ready to start your program.

PREVENTING AND MANAGING LOW-BACK PAIN

More than 85% of Americans experience back pain by age 50. Low-back pain is the second most common ailment in the United States—headache tops the list—and the second most common reason for absences from work and visits to a physician. Low-back pain is estimated to cost as much as $50 billion a year in lost productivity, medical and legal fees, and disability insurance and compensation.

Back pain can result from sudden traumatic injuries, but it is more often the long-term result of weak and inflexible muscles, poor posture, or poor body mechanics during activities like lifting and carrying. Any abnormal strain on the back can result in pain. Most cases of low-back pain clear up within a few weeks or months, but some people have recurrences or suffer from chronic pain.

Function and Structure of the Spine

The spinal column performs many important functions in the body.

- It provides structural support for the body, especially the thorax (upper-body cavity).
- It surrounds and protects the spinal cord.
- It supports much of the body's weight and transmits it to the lower body.
- It serves as an attachment site for a large number of muscles, tendons, and ligaments.
- It allows movement of the neck and back in all directions.

The spinal column is made up of bones called **vertebrae** (Figure 9.3). The spine consists of 7 cervical vertebrae in the neck, 12 thoracic vertebrae in the upper

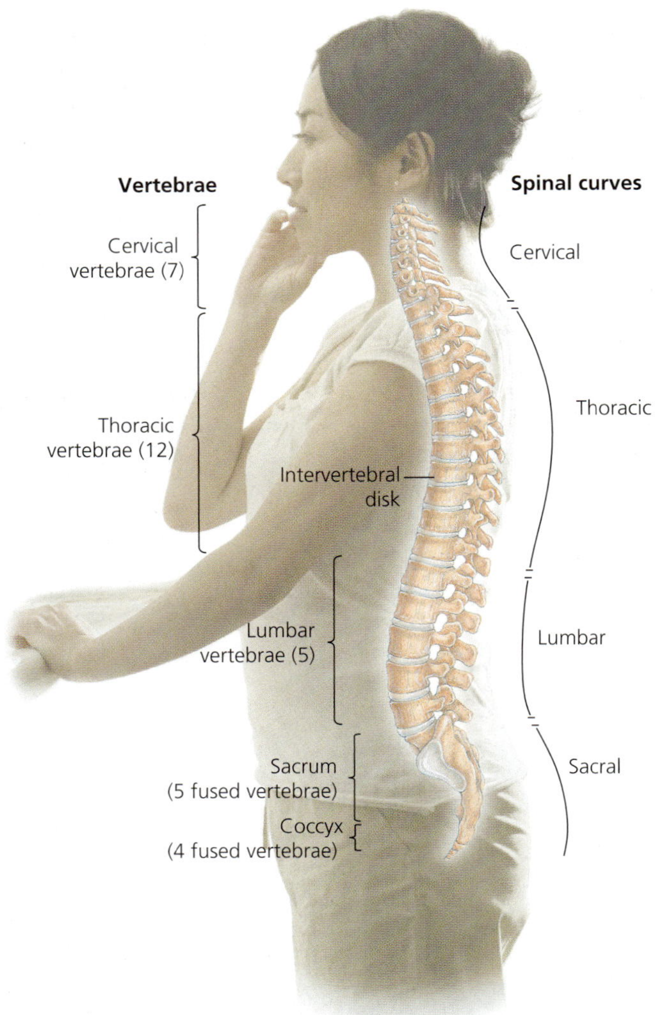

FIGURE 9.3 The spinal column.
The spine is made up of five separate regions and has four distinct curves. An intervertebral disk is located between adjoining vertebrae.

back, and 5 lumbar vertebrae in the lower back. The 9 vertebrae at the base of the spine are fused into two sections and form the sacrum and the coccyx (tailbone). The spine has four curves: the cervical, thoracic, lumbar, and sacral curves. These curves help bring the body weight supported by the spine in line with the axis of the body.

Although the structure of vertebrae depends on their location on the spine, the different types of vertebrae share common characteristics. Each consists of a body, an arch, and several bony processes (Figure 9.4). The vertebral body is cylindrical, with flattened surfaces where **intervertebral disks** are attached. The vertebral body is designed to carry the stress of body weight and physical activity. The vertebral arch surrounds and protects the spinal cord. The bony processes serve as joints for adjacent vertebrae and attachment sites for muscles and ligaments. **Nerve roots** from the spinal cord pass through notches in the vertebral arch.

Intervertebral disks, which absorb and disperse the stresses placed on the spine, separate vertebrae from each

Stretches to Avoid

TAKE CHARGE

The safe alternatives listed under each stretch are described and illustrated on pp. 271–273 as part of a complete program of safe flexibility exercises.

Standing Toe Touch

Problem: Puts excessive strain on the spine.

Alternatives: Modified hurdler stretch (Exercise 10), alternate leg stretcher (Exercise 11), and lower-leg stretch (Exercise 12).

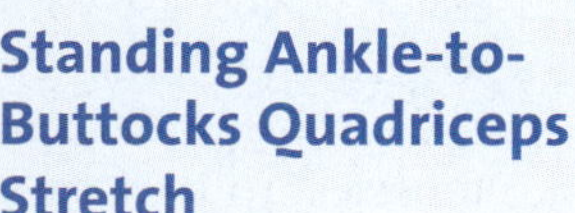

Standing Ankle-to-Buttocks Quadriceps Stretch

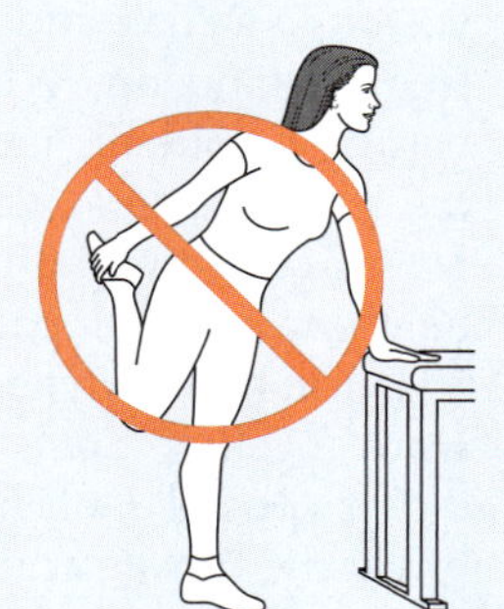

Problem: Puts excessive strain on the ligaments of the knee.

Alternative: Step stretch (Exercise 6).

Full Squat with Bent Back

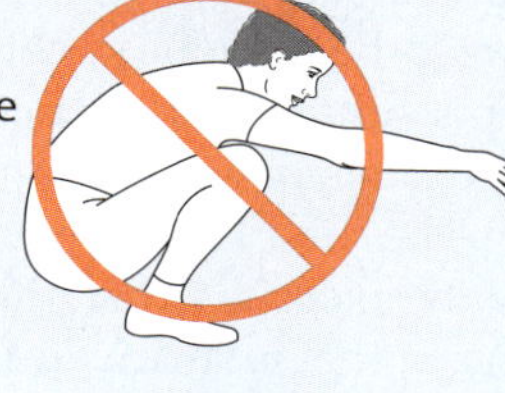

Problem: Puts excessive strain on the ankles, knees, and spine.

Alternatives: Alternate leg stretcher (Exercise 11) and lower-leg stretch (Exercise 12).

Prone Arch

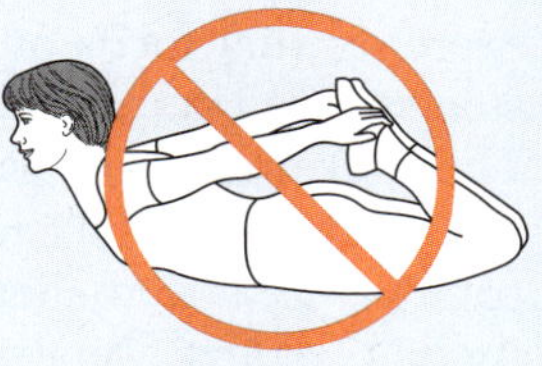

Problem: Puts excessive strain on the spine, knees, and shoulders.

Alternatives: Towel stretch (Exercise 2) and step stretch (Exercise 6).

Standing Hamstring Stretch

Problem: Puts excessive strain on the knee and lower back.

Alternatives: Modified hurdler stretch (Exercise 10) and alternate leg stretcher (Exercise 11).

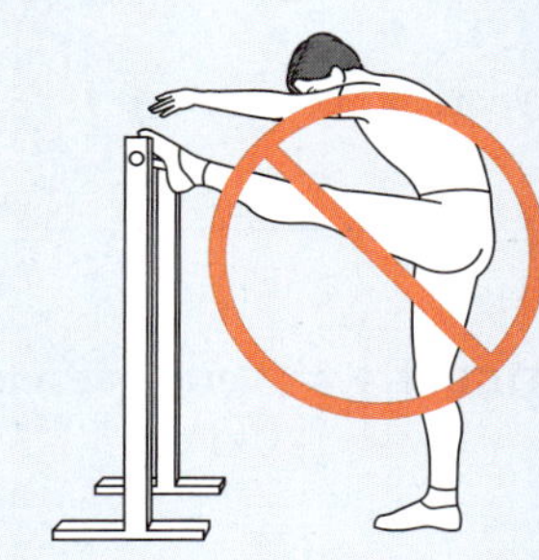

Yoga Plow

Problem: Puts excessive strain on the neck, shoulders, and back.

Alternatives: Head turns and tilts (Exercise 1), across-the-body and overhead stretches (Exercise 3), and upper-back stretch (Exercise 4).

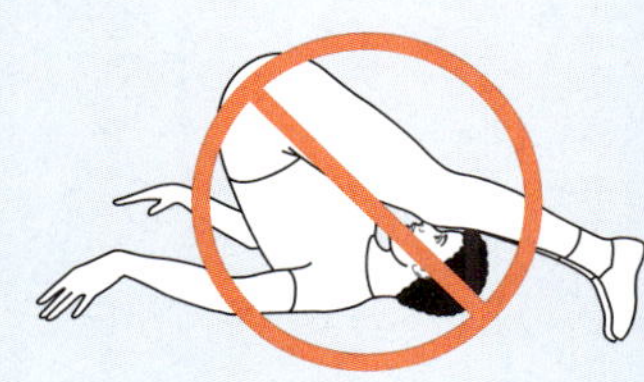

Hurdler Stretch

Problem: Turning out the bent leg can put excessive strain on the ligaments of the knee.

Alternative: Modified hurdler stretch (Exercise 10).

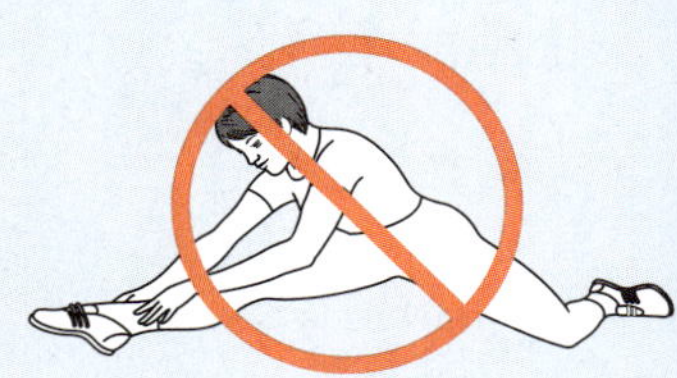

Neck Circles

Problem: Puts excessive strain on the neck and cervical disks.

Alternatives: Head turns and tilts (Exercise 1).

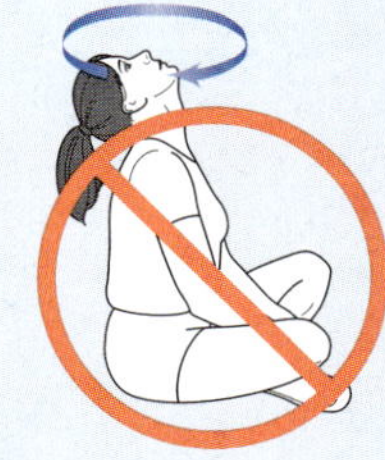

NOTE: Prone leg extensions, in which a person lifts both the chest and the legs while lying on the stomach but without grabbing the ankles, should also be avoided; spine extensions (p. 282) are a safe alternative.

other. Disks are made up of a gel- and water-filled nucleus surrounded by a series of fibrous rings. The liquid nucleus can change shape when it is compressed, allowing the disk to absorb shock. The intervertebral disks also help maintain the spaces between vertebrae where the spinal nerve roots are located.

Core Muscle Fitness

The **core muscles** include those in the abdomen, pelvic floor, sides of the trunk, back, buttocks, hip, and

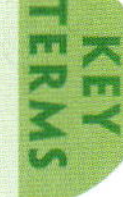

vertebrae Bony segments composing the spinal column that provide structural support for the body and protect the spinal cord.

intervertebral disk An elastic disk located between adjoining vertebrae, consisting of a gel- and water-filled nucleus surrounded by fibrous rings; serves as a shock absorber for the spinal column.

nerve root The base of each of the 31 pairs of spinal nerves that branch off the spinal cord through spaces between vertebrae.

core muscles The trunk muscles extending from the hips to the upper back.

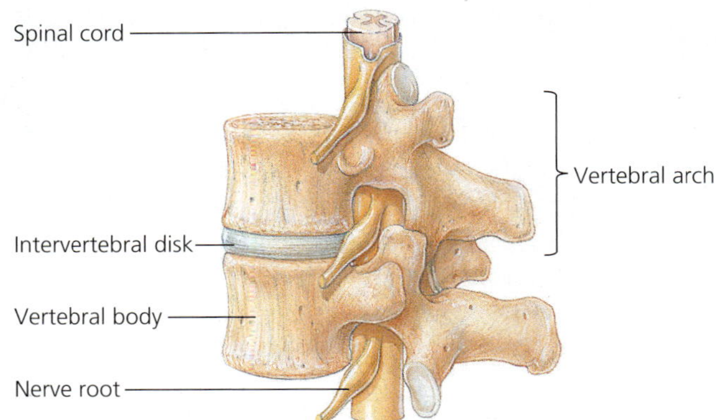

FIGURE 9.4 Vertebrae and an intervertebral disk.

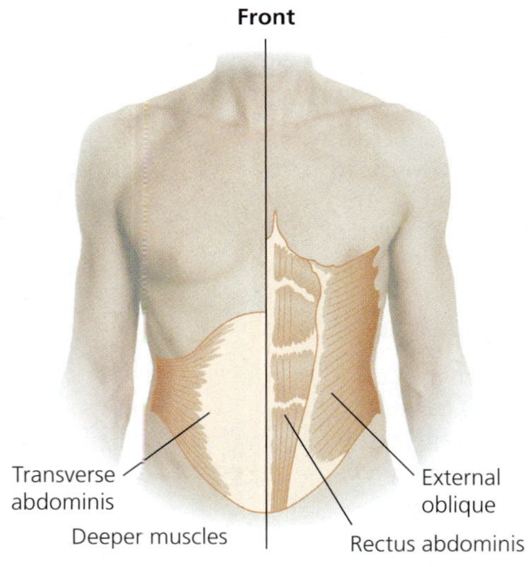

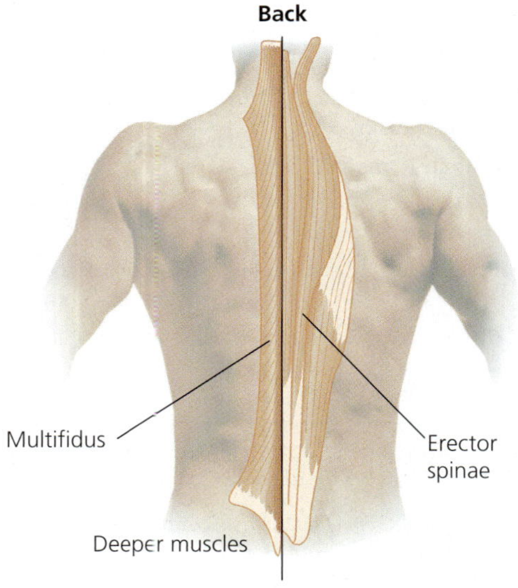

FIGURE 9.5 Major core muscles.

pelvis (Figure 9.5). There are 29 of these muscles, attaching to the ribs, hips, spinal column, and other bones in the trunk of the body. As described in Chapter 8, the core muscles stabilize the spine and help transfer force between the upper body and lower body. They stabilize the midsection when you sit, stand, reach, walk, jump, twist, squat, throw, or bend. The muscles on the front, back, and sides of your trunk support your spine when you sit in a chair and fix your midsection as you use your legs to stand up. When hitting a forehand in tennis or batting a softball, most of the force is transferred from the legs and hips, across the core muscles, to the arms. Strong core muscles make movements more forceful and help prevent back pain.

During any dynamic movement, the core muscles work together. Some shorten to cause movement, while others contract and hold to provide stability, lengthen to brake the movement, or send signals to the brain about the movements and positions of the muscles and bones (proprioception). When specific core muscles are weak or tired, the nervous system steps in and uses other muscles. This substitution causes abnormal stresses on the joints, decreases power, and increases the risk of injury.

The best exercises for low-back health are whole-body exercises that force the core muscles to stabilize the spine in many different directions. The low-back exercises presented later in this chapter include several exercises that focus on the core muscles, including the step stretch (lunge), side bridges, and spine extensions. These exercises are generally safe for beginning exercisers and, with physician approval, people with some back pain. More challenging core exercises utilize stability balls or free weights. Stability ball exercises require the core muscles to stabilize the ball (and the body) while performing nearly any type of exercise. Many traditional exercises with free weights can strengthen the core muscles if you do them in a standing position. Weight machines train muscles in isolation, while exercises with free weights done while standing help train the body for real-world movements—an essential principle of core training.

> **Fitness Tip**
>
> Swiss ball exercises are great for building core muscles. Swiss ball training increases trunk flexion and extension, strength, abdominal endurance, lower back flexibility, and balance.

Causes of Back Pain

Back pain can occur at any point along your spine. The lumbar area, because it bears the majority of your weight, is the most common site. Any movement that causes excessive stress on the spinal column can cause injury and pain. The spine is well equipped to bear body weight and the force or stress of body movements along its long axis. However, it is less capable of bearing loads at an angle to its long axis or when the trunk is flexed (bent). You do not have to carry a heavy load or participate in a vigorous contact sport to injure your back. Picking a pencil up from the floor while using poor body mechanics—reaching too far out in front of you or bending over with your knees straight, for example—can also result in back pain.

Risk factors associated with low-back pain include age greater than 34 years, degenerative diseases such as arthritis or osteoporosis, a family or personal history of back pain or trauma, a sedentary lifestyle, low job satisfaction, and low socioeconomic status. Smoking increases risk because smoking appears to hasten degenerative changes in the spine. Excess body weight also increases strain on the back, and psychological stress or depression can cause muscle tension and back pain. Occupations and activities associated with low-back pain are those involving physically hard work, such as frequent lifting, twisting, bending, standing up, or straining in forced positions; those requiring high concentration demands (such as computer programming); and those involving vibrations affecting the entire body (such as truck driving).

Underlying causes of back pain include poor muscle endurance and strength in the core muscles; excess body weight; poor posture or body position when standing, sitting, or sleeping; and poor body mechanics when performing actions like lifting and carrying, or sports movements. Strained muscles, tendons, or ligaments can cause pain and can, over time, lead to injuries to vertebrae, intervertebral disks, and surrounding muscles and ligaments.

Stress can cause disks to break down and lose some of their ability to absorb shock. A damaged disk may bulge out between vertebrae and put pressure on a nerve root, a condition commonly referred to as a *slipped disk*. Painful pressure on nerves can also occur if damage to a disk narrows the space between two vertebrae. With age, you lose fluid from the disks, making them more likely to bulge and put pressure on nerve roots. Depending on the amount of pressure on a nerve, symptoms may include numbness in the back, hip, leg, or foot; radiating pain; loss of muscle function; depressed reflexes; and muscle spasm. If the pressure is severe enough, loss of function can be permanent.

Preventing Low-Back Pain

Incorrect posture is responsible for many back injuries. Strategies for maintaining good posture are presented in the box "Good Posture and Low-Back Health." Follow the same guidelines when you engage in sports or recreational activities. Control your movements, and warm up thoroughly before you exercise. Take special care when lifting weights.

The role of exercise in preventing and treating back pain is still being investigated. However, many experts recommend exercise, especially for people who have already experienced an episode of low-back pain. Regular exercise aimed at increasing muscle endurance and strength in the back and abdomen is often recommended to prevent back pain, as is lifestyle physical activity such as walking. Movement helps lubricate your spinal joints and increases muscle fitness in your trunk and legs. Other lifestyle recommendations for preventing back pain include the following:

- Maintain a healthy weight. Excess fat contributes to poor posture, which can place harmful stresses on the spine.
- Stop smoking, and reduce stress.
- Avoid sitting, standing, or working in the same position for too long. Stand up every hour or half-hour and move around.
- Use a supportive seat and a medium-firm mattress.
- Use lumbar support when driving, particularly for long distances, to prevent muscle fatigue and pain.
- Warm up thoroughly before exercising.
- Progress gradually when attempting to improve strength or fitness.

Managing Acute Back Pain

Sudden (acute) back pain usually involves tissue injury. Symptoms may include pain, muscle spasms, stiffness, and inflammation. Many cases of acute back pain go away by themselves within a few days or weeks. You may be able to reduce pain and inflammation by applying cold and then heat (see Chapter 4). Apply ice several times a day; once inflammation and spasms subside, you can apply heat using a heating pad or a warm bath. If the pain is bothersome, an over-the-counter, nonsteroidal anti-inflammatory medication such as ibuprofen or naproxen may be helpful. Stronger pain medications and muscle relaxants are available by prescription.

Bed rest immediately following the onset of back pain may make you feel better, but it should be of very short duration. Prolonged bed rest—5 days or more—was once thought to be an effective treatment for back pain, but most physicians now advise against it because it may weaken muscles and actually worsen pain. Limit bed rest to one day and begin moderate physical activity as soon as possible. Exercise can increase muscular endurance and flexibility and protect disks from loss of fluid. Three of the back exercises discussed later in the chapter may be particularly helpful following an episode of acute back pain: curl-ups, side bridges, and spine extensions ("bird dogs").

See your physician if acute back pain doesn't resolve within a short time. Other warning signals of a more severe problem that requires a professional evaluation include severe pain, numbness, pain that radiates down one or both legs, problems with bladder or bowel control, fever, and rapid weight loss.

PERSONAL CHALLENGE

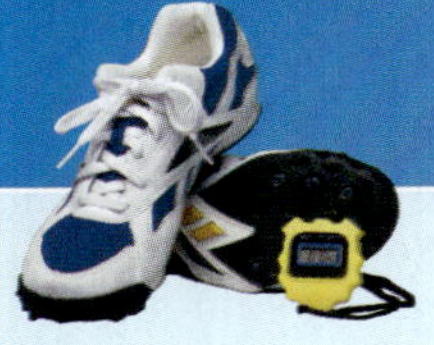

Keeping Your Back Pain-Free

About 85% of Americans suffer from back pain at some point in their lives. Back pain can be annoying and even disabling, and every day, many Americans miss school and work because of their pain. Luckily, you can minimize the risk of back problems by doing a few simple exercises every day. Keep a personal back pain prevention journal and do the following exercises on as many days of the week as possible.

EXERCISE	MON.	TUES.	WEDS.	THUR.	FRI.	SAT.	SUN.
Curl-ups: one set of 10 reps	✓		✓		✓		✓
Side bridge: five sets, 3-second hold, each side	✓		✓		✓		✓
Bird dog: five sets, 3-second hold, each side	✓		✓		✓		✓
Walking: 15-60 minutes		✓	✓		✓		✓
Kettlebell swings: one set 20 repetitions	✓				✓	✓	✓

Make a chart like the one shown above, and place a new copy in your training log each week. Enter a check mark every time you do the exercise. Try to enter a check mark for each exercise as often as you can during the week. In this one-week example, the person didn't do all the exercises every day, but she tried to do something on as many days a week as she could. Regularity is the key; if you miss a day, try not to miss the next one.

Managing Chronic Back Pain

Low-back pain is considered chronic if it persists for more than 3 months. Symptoms vary—some people experience stabbing or shooting pain, and others a steady ache accompanied by stiffness. Sometimes pain is localized; in other cases, it radiates to another part of the body. Underlying causes of chronic back pain include injuries, infection, muscle or ligament strains, and disk herniations.

Because symptoms and causes are so varied, different people benefit from different treatment strategies, and researchers have found that many treatments have only limited benefits. Potential treatments include over-the-counter or prescription medications; exercise; physical therapy, massage, yoga, or chiropractic care; acupuncture; percutaneous electrical nerve stimulation (PENS), in which acupuncture-like needles are used to deliver an electrical current; education and advice about posture, exercise, and body mechanics; and surgery (see the box "Yoga for Relaxation and Pain Relief").

Psychological therapy may also be beneficial in some cases. Reducing emotional stress that causes muscle tension can provide direct benefits, and other therapies can help people deal better with chronic pain and its effects on their daily lives. Support groups and expressive writing are beneficial for people with chronic pain and other conditions.

Exercises for the Prevention and Management of Low-Back Pain

The tests in Lab 9.3 can help you assess low-back muscular endurance. The exercises that follow are designed to help you maintain a healthy back by stretching and strengthening the major muscle groups that affect the back—the abdominal muscles, the muscles along your spine and sides, and the muscles of your hips and thighs. If you have back problems, check with your physician before beginning any exercise program. Perform the exercises slowly and progress very gradually. Stop and consult your physician if any exercise causes back pain. General guidelines for back exercise programs include the following:

- Do low-back exercises at least 3 days per week. Most experts recommend daily back exercises.
- Emphasize muscular endurance rather than muscular strength—endurance is more protective.
- Don't do spine exercises involving a full range of motion early in the morning. Your disks have a high fluid content early in the day and injuries may result.
- Engage in regular endurance exercise such as cycling or walking in addition to performing exercises that specifically build muscular endurance and flexibility. Brisk walking with a vigorous arm swing may help relieve back pain. Start with fast walking if your core muscles are weak or you have back pain.
- Be patient and stick with your program. Increased back fitness and pain relief may require as long as 3 months of regular exercise.
- The adage "no pain, no gain" does not apply to back exercises. Always use good form and stop if you feel pain.

Good Posture and Low-Back Health

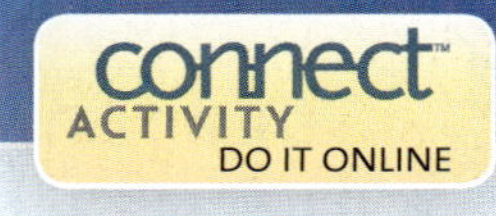

Changes in everyday posture and behavior can help prevent and alleviate low-back pain.

- ***Lying down.*** When resting or sleeping, lie on your side with your knees and hips bent. If you lie on your back, place a pillow under your knees. However, do not elevate your knees so much that the curve in your lower spine is flattened. Don't lie on your stomach. Use a medium-firm mattress.

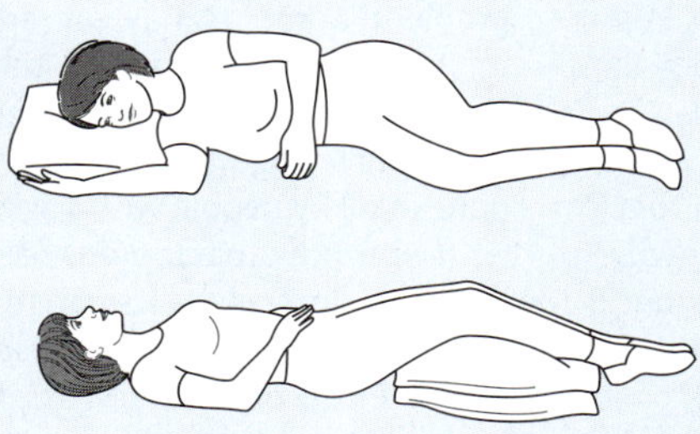

- ***Sitting at a computer.*** Sit in a slightly reclined position of 100–110 degrees, not an upright 90-degree position. Adjust your chair so your knees are slightly lower than your hips. If your back flattens as you sit, try using a lumbar roll to maintain your back's natural curvature. Place your feet flat on the floor or on a footrest. Place the monitor directly in front of you and adjust it so your eyes are level with the top of the screen; you should be looking slightly downward at the middle of the screen. Adjust the keyboard and mouse so your forearms and wrists are in a neutral position, parallel with the floor.

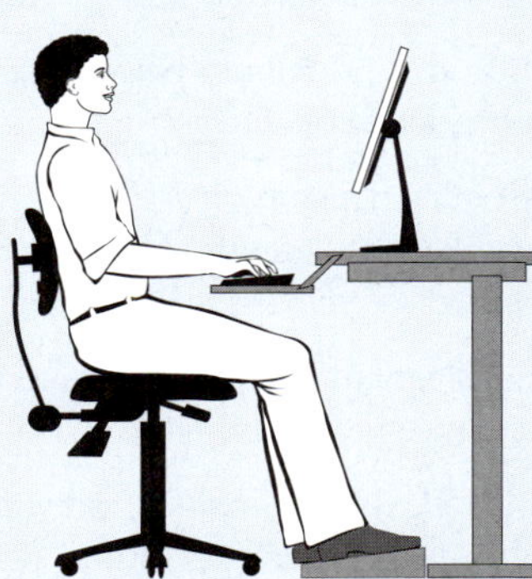

- ***Lifting.*** If you need to lower yourself to grasp an object, bend at the knees and hips rather than at the waist. Your feet should be about shoulder-width apart. Lift gradually, keeping your arms straight, by standing up or by pushing with your leg muscles. Keep the object close to your body. Don't twist; if you have to turn with the object, change the position of your feet.

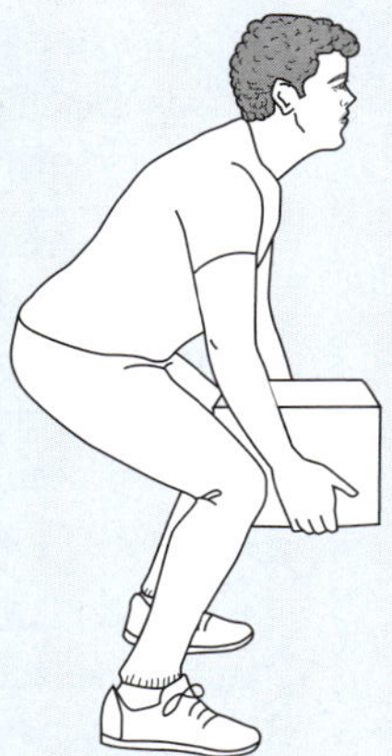

- ***Standing.*** When you are standing, a straight line should run from the top of your ear through the center of your shoulder, the center of your hip, the back of your kneecap, and the front of your ankle bone. Support your weight mainly on your heels, with one or both knees slightly bent. Don't let your pelvis tip forward or your back arch. Shift your weight back and forth from foot to foot. Avoid prolonged standing.

  To check your posture, stand normally with your back to a wall. Your upper back and buttocks should touch the wall; your heels may be a few inches away. Slide one hand into the space between your lower back and the wall. It should slide in easily but should almost touch both your back and the wall. Adjust your posture as needed, and try to hold this position as you walk away from the wall.

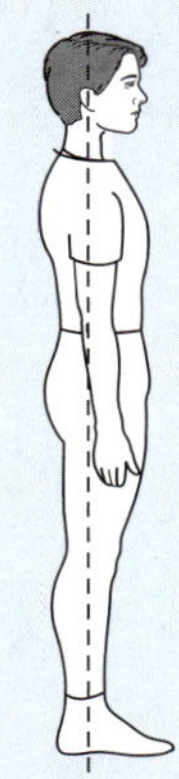

- ***Walking.*** Walk with your toes pointed straight ahead. Keep your back flat, head up and centered over your body, and chin in. Swing your arms freely. Don't wear tight or high-heeled shoes. Walking briskly is better for back health than walking slowly.

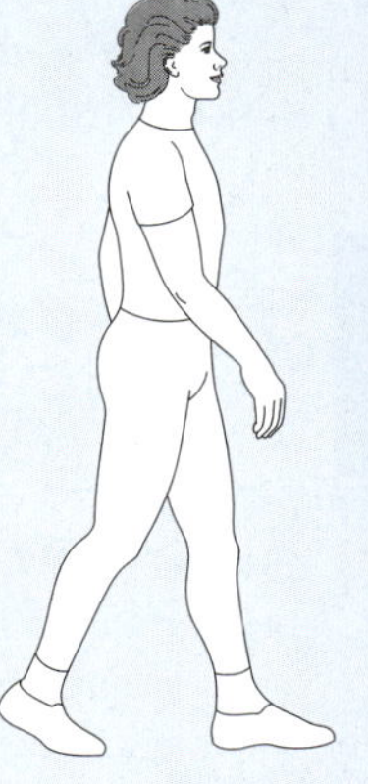

TAKE CHARGE

IN FOCUS

Yoga for Relaxation and Pain Relief

Certain types of exercise can provide relief from back pain, depending on the pain's underlying cause. Effective exercises stretch the muscles and connective tissue in the hips, stabilize the spine, and strengthen and build endurance in the core muscles of the back and abdomen.

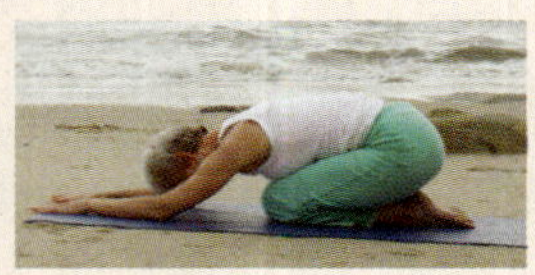

Yoga may be an option for many back pain sufferers because it offers a variety of exercises that target the spine and the core muscles. Yoga is an ancient practice involving slow, gentle movements performed with controlled breathing and focused attention. Yoga practitioners slowly move into a specific posture (called an *asana*) and hold the posture for up to 60 seconds. There are hundreds of asanas, many of which are easy to do and provide good stretches.

Yoga also involves simple breathing exercises that gently stretch the muscles of the upper back while helping the practitioner focus. Yoga experts say that breathing exercises not only encourage relaxation but also clear the mind and can help relieve mild to moderate pain. Yoga enthusiasts end their workouts energized and refreshed but calm and relaxed.

Many medical professionals now recommend yoga for patients with back pain, particularly postures that involve arching and gently stretching the back, such as the cat pose (similar to the cat stretch shown on p. 281) and the child pose (shown here). These are basic asanas that most people can perform repeatedly and hold for a relatively long time.

Because asanas must be performed correctly to be beneficial, qualified instruction is recommended. For those with back pain, physicians advise choosing an instructor who is not only accomplished in yoga but also knowledgeable about back pain and its causes. Such instructors can steer students away from exercises that do more harm than good. It is especially important to choose postures that will benefit the back without worsening the underlying problem. Some asanas can aggravate an injured or painful back if they are performed incorrectly or too aggressively. In fact, a few yoga postures should not be done at all by people with back pain.

If you have back pain, see your physician to determine its cause before beginning any type of exercise program. Even gentle exercise or stretching can be bad for an already injured back, especially if the spinal disks or nerves are involved. For some back conditions, rest or therapy may be better options than exercise, at least in the short term.

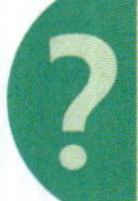

Ask Yourself

QUESTIONS FOR CRITICAL THINKING AND REFLECTION

Do you know anyone who suffers from chronic back pain? If so, how has it affected that person's life? Have you ever had back pain? Do you have any of the risk factors listed in the text? If so, what can you do to lower your risk and avoid developing chronic back problems?

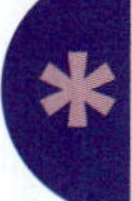

TIPS FOR TODAY AND THE FUTURE

To improve and maintain your flexibility, perform stretches that work the major joints at least twice a week.

RIGHT NOW YOU CAN

- Stand up and stretch—do either the upper-back stretch or the across-the-body stretch shown in the chapter.
- Practice the recommended sitting and standing postures described in the chapter. If needed, adjust your chair or find something to use as a footrest.

IN THE FUTURE YOU CAN

- Build up your flexibility by incorporating more sophisticated stretching exercises into your routine.
- Increase the frequency of your flexibility workouts to 5 or more days per week.
- Increase the efficiency of your workouts by adding stretching exercises to the cool-down period of your endurance or strength workouts.

SUMMARY

- Flexibility, the ability of joints to move through their full range of motion, is highly adaptable and specific to each joint.
- Range of motion can be limited by joint structure, muscle inelasticity, and proprioceptor activity.
- Developing flexibility depends on stretching the elastic tissues within muscles regularly and gently until they lengthen. Overstretching can make connective tissue brittle and lead to rupture.
- Signals sent between muscle and tendon nerves and the spinal cord can enhance flexibility.
- The benefits of flexibility include preventing abnormal stresses that lead to joint deterioration and possibly reducing the risk of injuries.
- Stretches should be held for 10–30 seconds; perform 2–4 repetitions. Flexibility training should be done a minimum of 2–3 days per week, preferably following activity, when muscles are warm.
- Static stretching is done slowly and held to the point of mild tension; ballistic stretching consists of bouncing stretches and can lead to injury. Dynamic stretching involves moving joints slowly and fluidly through their range of motion. Proprioceptive neuromuscular facilitation uses muscle receptors in contracting and relaxing a muscle.
- Passive stretching, using an outside force in moving muscles and joints, achieves a greater range of motion (and has a higher injury risk) than active stretching, which uses opposing muscles to initiate a stretch.

LOW-BACK EXERCISES

EXERCISE 1 Cat Stretch

Instructions: Begin on all fours with your knees below your hips and your hands below your shoulders. Slowly and deliberately move through a cycle of extension and flexion of your spine. **(a)** Begin by slowly pushing your back up and dropping your head slightly until your spine is extended (rounded). **(b)** Then slowly lower your back and lift your chin slightly until your spine is flexed (relaxed and slightly arched). *Do not press at the ends of the range of motion*. Stop if you feel pain. Do 10 slow, continuous cycles of the movement.

Target: Improved flexibility, relaxation, and reduced stiffness in the spine

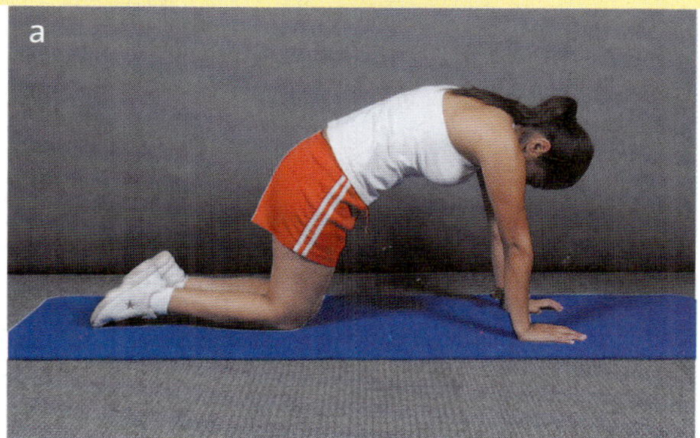
a

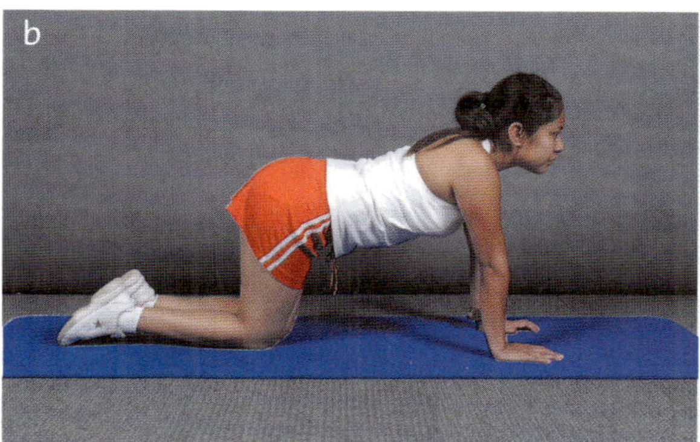
b

EXERCISE 2 Step Stretch *(See Exercise 6 in the flexibility program, p. 272)*

Instructions: Hold each stretch for 10–30 seconds and do 2–4 repetitions on each side.

Target: Improved flexibility, strength, and endurance in the muscles of the hip and the front of the thigh

EXERCISE 3 Alternate Leg Stretcher *(See Exercise 11 in the flexibility program, p. 273)*

Instructions: Hold each stretch for 10–30 seconds and do 2–4 repetitions on each side.

Target: Improved flexibility in the back of the thigh, hip, knee, and buttocks

EXERCISE 4 Trunk Twist

Instructions: Lie on your side with top knee bent, lower leg straight, lower arm extended in front of you on the floor, and upper arm at your side. Push down with your upper knee while you twist your trunk backward. Try to get your shoulders and upper body flat on the floor, turning your head as well. Return to the starting position, and then repeat on the other side. Hold the stretch for 10–30 seconds and do 2–4 repetitions on each side.

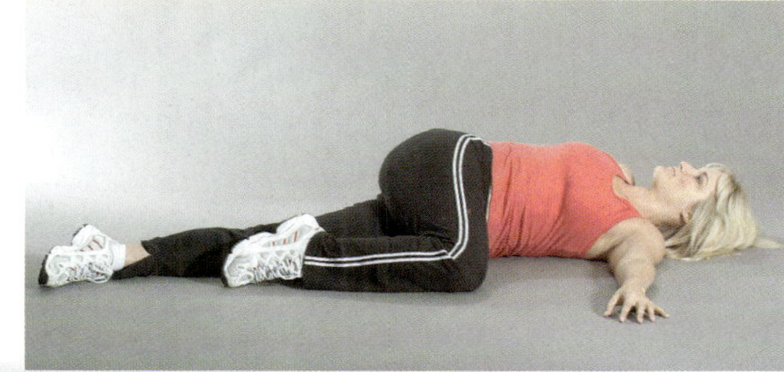

Target: Improved flexibility in the lower back and sides

EXERCISE 5 Curl-Up

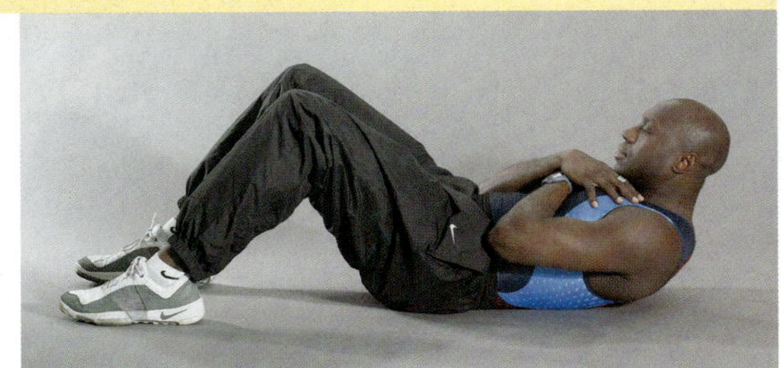

Instructions: Lie on your back with one or both knees bent and arms crossed on your chest or hands under your lower back. Maintain a neutral spine. Tuck your chin in and slowly curl up, one vertebra at a time, as you use your abdominal muscles to lift your head first and then your shoulders. Stop when you can see your knees and hold for 5–10 seconds before returning to the starting position. Do 10 or more repetitions.

Target: Improved strength and endurance in the abdomen

Variation: Add a twist to develop other abdominal muscles. When you have curled up so that your shoulder blades are off the floor, twist your upper body so that one shoulder is higher than the other; reach past your knee with your upper arm. Hold and then return to the starting position. Repeat on the opposite side. Curl-ups can also be done using an exercise ball.

EXERCISE 6 Isometric Side Bridge *(See Exercise 11 in the free weights program in Chapter 8, p. 242)*

Instructions: Hold the bridge position for 10 seconds, breathing normally. Work up to a 60-second hold. Perform one or more repetitions on each side.

Target: Increased strength and endurance in the muscles along the sides of the abdomen

Variation: You can make the exercise more difficult by keeping your legs straight and supporting yourself with your feet and forearm (see Lab 9.3) or with your feet and hand (with elbow straight).

EXERCISE 7 Spine Extensions *("Bird dogs"; see Exercise 10 in the free weights program in Chapter 8, p. 241)*

Instructions: Hold each position for 10–30 seconds. Begin with one repetition on each side, and work up to several repetitions.

Target: Increased strength and endurance in the back, buttocks, and back of the thighs

Variation: If you have experienced back pain in the past or if this exercise is difficult for you, do the exercise with both hands on the ground rather than with one arm lifted. You can make this exercise more difficult by doing it balancing on an exercise ball. Find a balance point on your chest while lying face down on the ball with one arm and the opposite leg on the ground. Tense your abdominal muscles while reaching and extending with one arm and reaching and extending with the opposite leg. Repeat this exercise using the other arm and leg.

EXERCISE 8 Wall Squat (Phantom Chair)

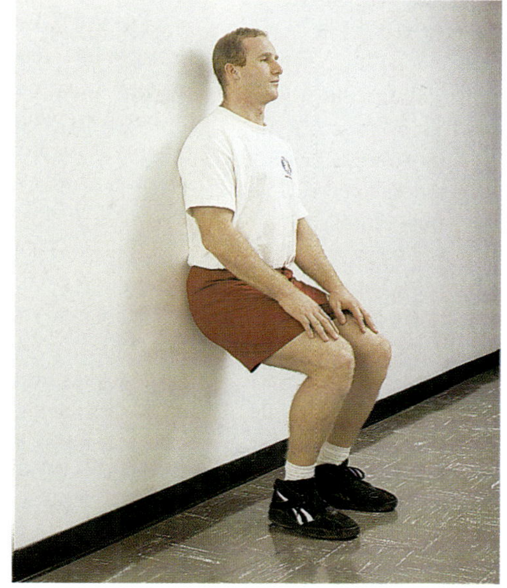

Instructions: Lean against a wall and bend your knees as though you are sitting in a chair. Support your weight with your legs. Begin by holding the position for 5–10 seconds. Squeeze your gluteal muscles together as you do the exercise. Build up to 1 minute or more. Perform one or more repetitions.

Target: Increased strength and endurance in the lower back, thighs, and abdomen

EXERCISE 9 Pelvic Tilt

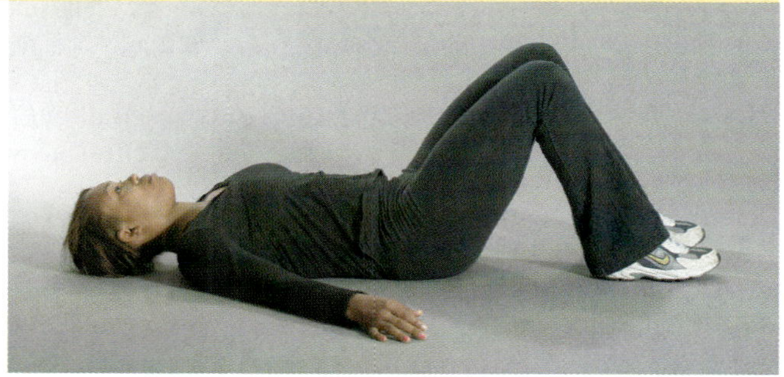

Instructions: Lie on your back with knees bent and arms extended to the side. Tilt your pelvis under and try to flatten your lower back against the floor. Tighten your buttock and abdominal muscles while you hold this position for 5–10 seconds. Don't hold your breath. Work up to 10 repetitions of the exercise. Pelvic tilts can also be done standing or leaning against a wall.

Note: *Although this is a popular exercise with many therapists, some experts question the safety of pelvic tilts. Stop if you feel pain in your back at any time during the exercise.*

Target: Increased strength and endurance in the abdomen and buttocks

EXERCISE 10 Back Bridge

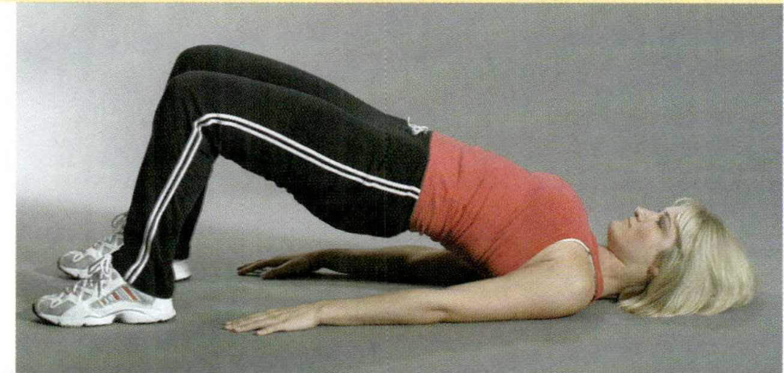

Instructions: Lie on your back with knees bent and arms extended to the side. Tuck your pelvis under, contract your gluteal muscles, and then lift your tailbone, buttocks, and lower back from the floor. Hold this position for 5–10 seconds with your weight resting on your feet, arms, and shoulders, and then return to the starting position. Work up to 10 repetitions of the exercise.

Target: Increased strength and endurance in the hips and buttocks

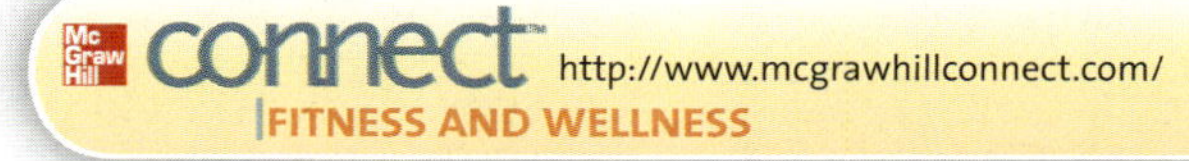

COMMON QUESTIONS ANSWERED

Q Is stretching the same as warming up?

A No. They are two distinct activities. A warm-up is light exercise that involves moving the joints through the same motions used during a more intense activity; it increases body temperature so your metabolism works better when you're exercising at high intensity. Stretching increases the movement capability of your joints, so you can move more easily with less risk of injury. It is best to stretch at the end of your aerobic or weight training workout, when your muscles are warm. Warmed muscles stretch better than cold ones and are less prone to injury.

Q How much flexibility do I need?

A This question is not always easy to answer. If you're involved in a sport such as gymnastics, figure skating, or ballet, you are often required to reach extreme joint motions to achieve success. However, nonathletes do not need to reach these extreme joint positions. In fact, too much flexibility may, in some cases, create joint instability and increase your risk of injury. As with other types of fitness, moderation is the key. You should regularly stretch your major joints and muscle groups but not aspire to reach extreme flexibility.

Q Can I stretch too far?

A Yes. As muscle tissue is progressively stretched, it reaches a point where it becomes damaged and may rupture. The greatest danger occurs during passive stretching when a partner is doing the stretching for you. It is critical that your stretching partner not force your joint outside its normal functional range of motion.

Q Can physical training limit flexibility?

A Weight training, jogging, or any physical activity will decrease flexibility if the exercises are not performed through a full range of motion. When done properly, weight training increases flexibility. However, because of the limited range of motion used during the running stride, jogging tends to compromise flexibility. It is important for runners to do flexibility exercises for the hamstrings and quadriceps regularly.

Q Does stretching affect muscular strength?

A Flexibility training increases muscle strength over time, but preexercise stretching can cause short-term decreases in strength and power. Several recent studies have found that stretching decreases strength, power, and motor control following the stretch. This is one reason some experts suggest that people not stretch as part of their exercise warm-up. It is important to warm up before any workout by engaging in 5–10 minutes of light exercise such as walking or slow jogging.

For more Common Questions Answered about flexibility and low-back health, visit the Online Learning Center at www.mhhe.com/fahey.

- The spinal column consists of vertebrae separated by intervertebral disks. It provides structure and support for the body and protects the spinal cord. The core muscles stabilize the spine and transfer force between the upper and lower body.
- Acute back pain can be treated as a soft tissue injury, with cold treatment followed by application of heat (once swelling subsides); prolonged bed rest is not recommended. A variety of treatments have been suggested for chronic back pain, including regular exercise, physical therapy, acupuncture, education, and psychological therapy.
- In addition to good posture, proper body mechanics, and regular physical activity, a program for preventing low-back pain includes exercises that develop flexibility, strength, and endurance in the muscle groups that affect the lower back.

FOR FURTHER EXPLORATION

BOOKS

Anderson, B., and J. Anderson. 2010. *Stretching,* 30th anniv. ed. Bolinas, Calif.: Shelter Publications. *A best-selling exercise book, updated with more than 200 stretches for 60 sports and activities.*

Armiger, P., and M. A. Martyn. 2010. *Stretching for Functional Flexibility.* Philadelphia: Lippincott Williams & Wilkins. *Presents stretching methods for fitness, athletics, and rehabilitation.*

Blahnik, J. 2011. *Full-Body Flexibility,* 2nd ed. Champaign, Ill.: Human Kinetics. *Presents a blend of stretching techniques derived from sports training, martial arts, yoga, and Pilates.*

McGill, S. 2007. *Low Back Disorders: Evidence-Based Prevention and Rehabilitation,* 2nd ed. Champaign, Ill.: Human Kinetics. *A comprehensive guide to the prevention, diagnosis, and treatment of back pain.*

McGill, S. 2009. *Ultimate Back Fitness and Performance,* 4th ed. Waterloo, Canada: Backfit Pro. *Written by one of the premier researchers in the world on back biomechanics and back pain; describes mechanisms of back pain and exercises and movement patterns for preventing it.*

McGill, S. 2010. *Ultimate Back: Enhancing Performance* (DVD). Waterloo, Canada: Backfit Pro. *A video by the authors of* Ultimate Back Fitness and Performance.

Nelson, A. G., et al. 2006. *Stretching Anatomy.* Champaign, Ill.: Human Kinetics. *A guide to stretching that features highly detailed illustrations of the muscles that are affected by each exercise.*

ORGANIZATIONS AND WEB SITES

American Academy of Orthopaedic Surgeons. Provides information about a variety of joint problems.
http://orthoinfo.aaos.org

Back Fit Pro. A Web site maintained by Dr. Stuart McGill, a professor of spine biomechanics at the University of Waterloo, which provides evidence-based information on preventing and treating back pain.

http://www.backfitpro.com

CUErgo: Cornell University Ergonomics Web Site. Provides information about how to arrange a computer workstation to prevent back pain and repetitive strain injuries, as well as other topics related to ergonomics.

http://ergo.human.cornell.edu

Georgia State University: Flexibility. Provides information about the benefits of stretching and ways to develop a safe and effective program; includes illustrations of stretches.

http://www2.gsu.edu/~wwwfit/flexibility.html

Mayo Clinic: Focus on Flexibility. Presents an easy-to-use program of basic stretching exercises for beginners, with a focus on the benefits of greater flexibility.

http://www.mayoclinic.com/health/stretching/HQ01447

NIH Back Pain Fact Sheet. Provides basic information on the prevention and treatment of back pain.

http://www.ninds.nih.gov/disorders/backpain/backpain.htm

Southern California Orthopedic Institute. Provides information on a variety of orthopedic problems, including back injuries; also has illustrations of spinal anatomy.

http://www.scoi.com

Stretching and Flexibility. Provides information on the physiology of stretching and different types of stretching exercises.

http://www.ifafitness.com/stretch/index.html

See also the listings for Chapters 2 and 8.

SELECTED BIBLIOGRAPHY

American College of Sports Medicine. 2009. *ACSM's Guidelines for Exercise Testing and Prescription,* 8th ed. Philadelphia: Lippincott Williams and Wilkins.

American College of Sports Medicine. 2009. *ACSM's Resource Manual for Guidelines for Exercise Testing and Prescription,* 6th ed. Philadelphia: Lippincott Williams and Wilkins.

Aquino, C. F., et al. 2010. Stretching versus strength training in lengthened position in subjects with tight hamstring muscles: a randomized controlled trial. *Manual Therapy* 15(1): 26–31.

Ayala, F., et al. 2010. Effect of active stretch on hip flexion range of motion in female professional futbal players. *The Journal of Sports Medicine and Physical Fitness* 50(4): 428–435.

Bacurau, R. F., et al. 2009. Acute effect of a ballistic and a static stretching exercise bout on flexibility and maximal strength. *Journal of Strength and Conditioning Research* 23(1): 304–308.

Bazett-Jones, D. M., et al. 2008. Sprint and vertical jump performances are not affected by six weeks of static hamstring stretching. *Journal of Strength and Conditioning Research* 22(1): 25–31.

Bogduk, N. 2010. A cure for back pain? *Pain* 149(1): 7–8.

Carpes, F. P., et al. 2008. Effects of a program for trunk strength and stability on pain, low back and pelvis kinematics, and body balance: A pilot study. *Journal of Bodywork and Movement Therapies* 12(1): 22–30.

Chen, C. H., et al. 2011. Effects of flexibility training on eccentric exercise-induced muscle damage. *Medicine and Science in Sports and Exercise* 43(3): 491–500.

Chen, K. M., et al. 2008. Physical fitness of older adults in senior activity centers after 24-week silver yoga exercises. *Journal of Clinical Nursing* 17(19): 2634–2646.

Christiansen, C. L. 2008. The effects of hip and ankle stretching on gait function of older people. *Archive of Physical Medicine and Rehabilitation* 89(8): 1421–1428.

Costa, P. B., et al. 2009. The acute effects of different durations of static stretching on dynamic balance performance. *Journal of Strength and Conditioning Research* 23(1): 141–147.

Davis, D. S., et al. 2008. Concurrent validity of four clinical tests used to measure hamstring flexibility. *Journal of Strength and Conditioning Research* 22(2): 583–588.

Deleget, A. 2010. Overview of thigh injuries in dance. *Journal of Dance Medicine and Science* 14(3): 97–102.

Duehring, M. D., et al. 2009. Strength and conditioning practices of United States high school strength and conditioning coaches. *Journal of Strength and Conditioning Research* 23(8): 2188–2203.

Duque, I., et al. 2011. Maximal aerobic power in patients with chronic low back pain: A comparison with healthy subjects. *European Spine Journal* 20(1): 87–93.

Fasen, J. M., et al. 2009. A randomized controlled trial of hamstring stretching: comparison of four techniques. *Journal of Strength and Conditioning Research.* 23(2): 660–667.

Favero, J. P., et al. 2009. Effects of an acute bout of static stretching on 40 m sprint performance: Influence of baseline flexibility. *Research in Sports Medicine* 17(1): 50–60.

Feland, J. B., et al. 2010. Whole body vibration as an adjunct to static stretching. *International Journal of Sports Medicine* 31(8): 584–589.

Fenwick, C. M., et al. 2009. Comparison of different rowing exercises: Trunk muscle activation and lumbar spine motion, load, and stiffness. *Journal of Strength and Conditioning Research* 23(5): 1408–1417.

Field, T. 2011. Yoga clinical research review. *Complementary Therapies in Clinical Practice* 17(1): 1–8.

Garber, C. E., et al. 2011. Quantity and quality of exercise for developing and maintaining cardiorespiratory, musculoskeletal, and neuromotor fitness in apparently healthy adults: guidance for prescribing exercise. *Medicine and Science in Sports and Exercise* 43(7): 1334–1359.

Gergley, J. C. 2010. Latent effect of passive static stretching on driver clubhead speed, distance, accuracy, and consistent ball contact in young male competitive golfers. *Journal of Strength and Conditioning Research* 24(12): 3326–3333.

Guidetti, L., et al. 2009. Precompetition warm-up in elite and subelite rhythmic gymnastics. *Journal of Strength and Conditioning Research.* 23(6): 1877–1882.

Guillot, A., et al. 2010. Does motor imagery enhance stretching and flexibility? *Journal of Sports Sciences* 28(3): 291–298.

Gurjao, A. L., et al. 2009. Acute effect of static stretching on rate of force development and maximal voluntary contraction in older women. *Journal of Strength and Conditioning Research* 23(7): 2149–2154.

Henchoz, Y., and A. Kai-Lik So. 2008. Exercise and nonspecific low back pain: A literature review. *Joint Bone Spine* 75(5): 533–539.

Herman, S. L., et al. 2008. Four-week dynamic stretching warm-up intervention elicits longer-term performance benefits. *Journal of Strength and Conditioning Research* 22(4): 1286–1297.

Heuser, M., et al. 2010. The effects of stretching on knee flexor fatigue and perceived exertion. *Journal of Sports Sciences* 28(2): 219–226.

Higgs, F., et al. 2009. The effect of a four-week proprioceptive neuromuscular facilitation stretching program on isokinetic torque production. *Journal of Strength and Conditioning Research* 23(5): 1442–1447.

Jaggers, J. R., et al. 2008. The acute effects of dynamic and ballistic stretching on vertical jump height, force, and power. *Journal of Strength and Conditioning Research* 22(6): 1844–1849.

Jenkins, J., et al. 2010. Flexibility for runners. *Clinics in Sports Medicine* 29(3): 365–377.

Judge, L. W., et al. 2009. An examination of the stretching practices of Division I and Division III college football programs in the midwestern United States. *Journal of Strength and Conditioning Research* 23(4): 1091–1096.

Keller, A., et al. 2008. Predictors of change in trunk muscle strength for patients with chronic low back pain randomized to lumbar fusion or cognitive intervention and exercises. *Pain Medicine* 9(6): 680–687.

Kiecolt-Glaser, J. K., et al. 2010. Stress, inflammation, and yoga practice. *Psychosomatic Medicine* 72(2): 113–121.

Lariviere, C., et al. 2010. Poor back muscle endurance is related to pain catastrophizing in patients with chronic low back pain. *Spine* 35(22): E1178–1186.

LaRoche, D. P., et al. 2008. Chronic stretching and voluntary muscle force. *Journal of Strength and Conditioning Research* 22(2): 589–596.

McGill, S. M., et al. 2009. Comparison of different strongman events: trunk muscle activation and lumbar spine motion, load, and stiffness. *Journal of Strength and Conditioning Research* 23(4): 1148–1161.

McHugh, M. P., and M. Nesse. 2008. Effect of stretching on strength loss and pain after eccentric exercise. *Medicine and Science in Sports and Exercise* 40(3): 566–573.

Meroni, R., et al. 2010. Comparison of active stretching technique and static stretching technique on hamstring flexibility. *Clinical Journal of Sport Medicine* 20(1): 8–14

Molacek, Z. D., et al. 2010. Effects of low- and high-volume stretching on bench press performance in collegiate football players. *Journal of Strength and Conditioning Research* 24(3): 711–716.

Monteiro, W. D., et al. 2008. Influence of strength training on adult women's flexibility. *Journal of Strength and Conditioning Research* 22(3): 672–677.

Morse, C. I., et al. 2008. The acute effect of stretching on the passive stiffness of the human gastrocnemius muscle tendon unit. *Journal of Physiology* 586(1): 97–106.

Nieman, D. C. 2011. *Exercise Testing and Prescription: A Health-Related Approach*, 7th ed. New York: McGraw-Hill.

Purcell, L. 2009. Causes and prevention of low back pain in young athletes. *Paediatrics and Child Health* 14(8): 533–538.

Rancour, J., et al. 2009. The effects of intermittent stretching following a 4-week static stretching protocol: A randomized trial. *Journal of Strength and Conditioning Research* 23(8): 2217–2222.

Rasmussen-Barr, E., et al. 2009. Graded exercise for recurrent low-back pain: A randomized, controlled trial with 6-, 12-, and 36-month follow-ups. *Spine* 34(3): 221–228.

Ryan, E. D., et al. 2008. Do practical durations of stretching alter muscle strength? A dose-response study. *Medicine and Science in Sports and Exercise* 40(8): 1529–1537.

Saeed, S. A., et al. 2010. Exercise, yoga, and meditation for depressive and anxiety disorders. *American Family Physician* 81(8): 981–986.

Samuel, M. N., et al. 2008. Acute effects of static and ballistic stretching on measures of strength and power. *Journal of Strength and Conditioning Research* 22(5): 1422–1428.

Scannell, J. P., et al. 2009. Disc prolapse: Evidence of reversal with repeated extension. *Spine* 34(4): 344–350.

Small, K., et al. 2008. A systematic review into the efficacy of static stretching as part of a warm-up for the prevention of exercise-related injury. *Research in Sports Medicine* 16(3): 213–231.

Tekur, P., et al. 2008. Effect of short-term intensive yoga program on pain, functional disability and spinal flexibility in chronic low back pain: A randomized control study. *Journal of Alternative and Complementary Medicine* 14(6): 637–644.

Torres, E. M., et al. 2008. Effects of stretching on upper-body muscular performance. *Journal of Strength and Conditioning Research* 22(4): 1279–1285.

Verbunt, J. A., et al. 2010. Cause or effect? Deconditioning and chronic low back pain. *Pain* 149(3): 428–430.

Weil, R. 2008. Exercising the aging body. Part 2: Flexibility, balance, and diabetes control. *Diabetes Self-Management* 25(1): 42–52.

Werner, G. 2010. Strength and conditioning techniques in the rehabilitation of sports injury. *Clinics in Sports Medicine* 29(1): 177–191.

Winchester, J. B., et al. 2008. Static stretching impairs sprint performance in collegiate track and field athletes. *Journal of Strength and Conditioning Research* 22(1): 13–19.

Winke, M. R., et al. 2010. Moderate static stretching and torque production of the knee flexors. *Journal of Strength and Conditioning Research* 24(3): 706–710.

Ylinen, J., et al. 2009. Effect of stretching on hamstring muscle compliance. *Journal of Rehabilitation Medicine* 41(1): 80–84.

Name ______________________ Section ______________ Date ____________

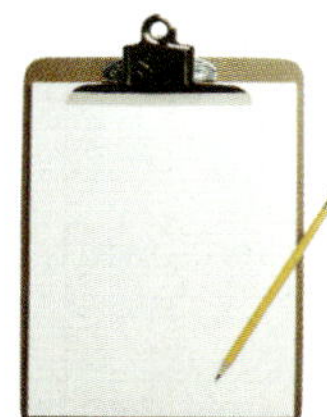

LAB 9.1 Assessing Your Current Level of Flexibility

Part I Sit-and-Reach Test

Equipment

Use a modified Wells and Dillon flexometer or construct your own measuring device using a firm box or two pieces of wood about 30 centimeters (12 inches) high attached at right angles to each other. Attach a metric ruler to measure the extent of reach. With the low numbers of the ruler toward the person being tested, set the 26-centimeter mark of the ruler at the footline of the box. Individuals who cannot reach as far as the footline will have scores below 26 centimeters; those who can reach past their feet will have scores above 26 centimeters. Most studies show no relationship between performance on the sit-and-reach test and the incidence of back pain.

Preparation

Warm up your muscles with a low-intensity activity such as walking or easy jogging. Then perform slow stretching movements.

Instructions

1. Remove your shoes and sit facing the flexibility measuring device with your knees fully extended and your feet flat against the device about 10 centimeters (4 inches) apart.
2. Reach as far forward as you can, with palms down, arms evenly stretched, and knees fully extended; hold the position of maximum reach for about 2 seconds.
3. Perform the stretch 2 times, recording the distance of maximum reach to the nearest 0.5 centimeters: __________ cm

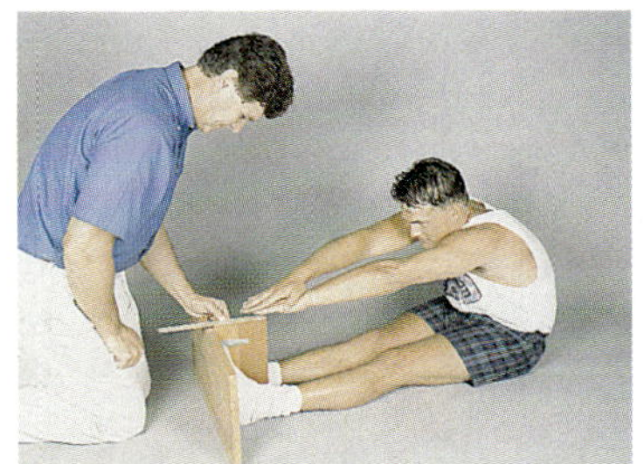

Rating Your Flexibility

Find the score in the table below to determine your flexibility rating. Record it here and on the final page of this lab.

Rating: 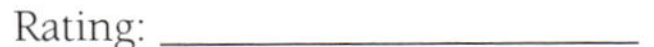

Ratings for Sit-and-Reach Test

	Rating/Score (cm)*				
Men	*Needs Improvement*	*Fair*	*Good*	*Very Good*	*Excellent*
Age: 15–19	Below 24	24–28	29–33	34–38	Above 38
20–29	Below 25	25–29	30–33	34–39	Above 39
30–39	Below 23	23–27	28–32	33–37	Above 37
40–49	Below 18	18–23	24–28	29–34	Above 34
50–59	Below 16	16–23	24–27	28–34	Above 34
60–69	Below 15	15–19	20–24	25–32	Above 32
Women					
Age: 15–19	Below 29	29–33	34–37	38–42	Above 42
20–29	Below 28	28–32	33–36	37–40	Above 40
30–39	Below 27	27–31	32–35	36–40	Above 40
40–49	Below 25	25–29	30–33	34–37	Above 37
50–59	Below 25	25–29	30–32	33–38	Above 38
60–69	Below 23	23–26	27–30	31–34	Above 34

*Footline is set at 26 cm.

SOURCE: *The Canadian Physical Activity, Fitness & Lifestyle Approach: CSEP-Health & Fitness Program's Health-Related Appraisal and Counselling Strategy,* 3rd edition, 2003. Adapted with permission from the Canadian Society for Exercise Physiology.

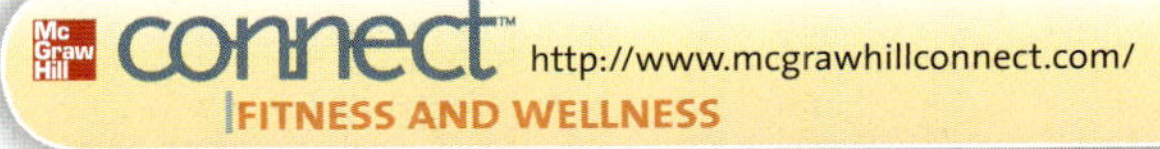

Part II Range-of-Motion Assessment

This portion of the lab can be completed by doing visual comparisons or by measuring joint range of motion with a goniometer or other instrument.

Equipment

1. A partner to do visual comparisons or to measure the range of motion of your joints. (You can also use a mirror to perform your own visual comparisons.)
2. For the measurement method, you need a goniometer, flexometer, or other instrument to measure range of motion.

Preparation

Warm up your muscles with some low-intensity activity such as walking or easy jogging.

Instructions

On the following pages, the average range of motion is illustrated and listed quantitatively for some of the major joints. Visually assess the range of motion in your joints, and compare it to that shown in the illustrations. For each joint, note (with a check mark) whether your range of motion is above average, average, or below average and in need of improvement. Average values for range of motion are given in degrees for each joint in the assessment. You can also complete the assessment by measuring your range of motion with a goniometer, flexometer, or other instrument. If you are using this measurement method, identify your rating (above average, average, or below average) and record your range of motion in degrees next to the appropriate category. Although the measurement method is more time-consuming, it allows you to track the progress of your stretching program more precisely and to note changes within the broader ratings categories (below average, above average).

Record your ratings on the following pages and on the chart on the final page of this lab. (Ratings were derived from several published sources.)

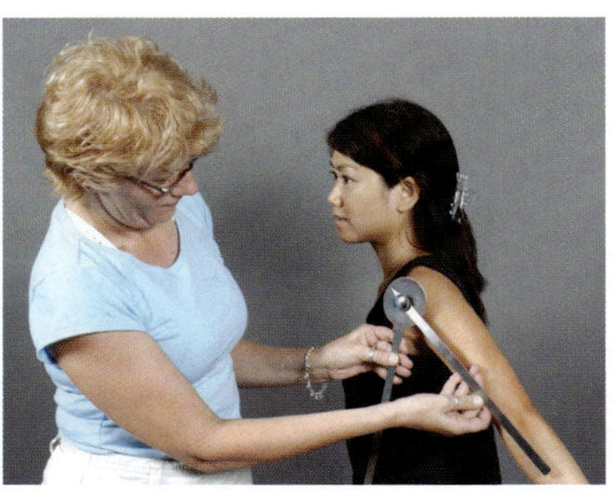

Assessment of range of motion using a goniometer

1. Shoulder Abduction and Adduction

For each position and arm, check one of the following; fill in degrees if using the measurement method.

Shoulder abduction—raise arm up to the side.

Right	*Left*	
________	________	Below average/needs improvement
________	________	Average (92–95°)
________	________	Above average

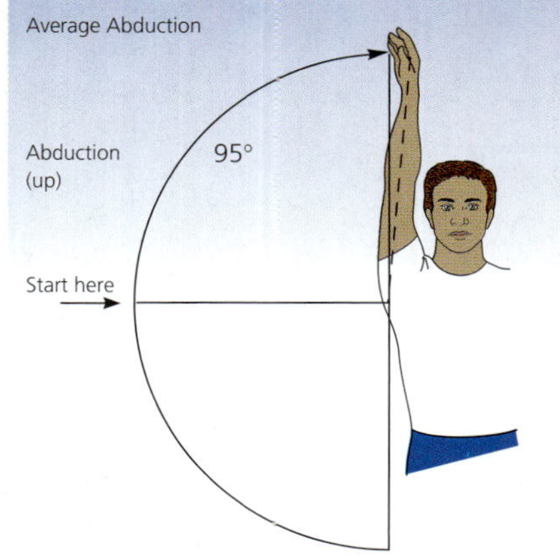

Shoulder abduction—move arm down and in front of body.

Right	*Left*	
________	________	Below average/needs improvement
________	________	Average (124–127°)
________	________	Above average.

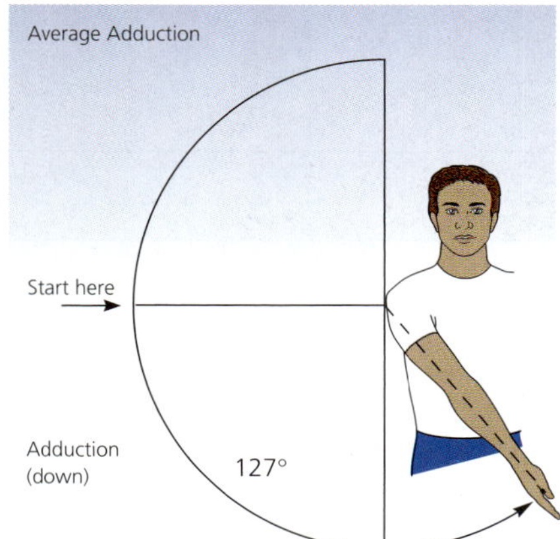

2. Shoulder Flexion and Extension

For each position and arm, check one of the following; fill in degrees if using the measurement method.

Shoulder flexion—raise arm up in front of the body.

Right	*Left*	
________	________	Below average/needs improvement
________	________	Average (92–95°)
________	________	Above average

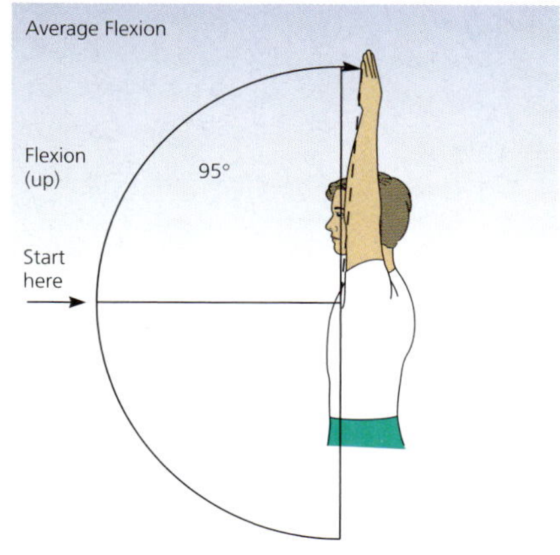

Shoulder extension—move arm down and behind the body.

Right	*Left*	
________	________	Below average/needs improvement
________	________	Average (145–150°)
________	________	Above average

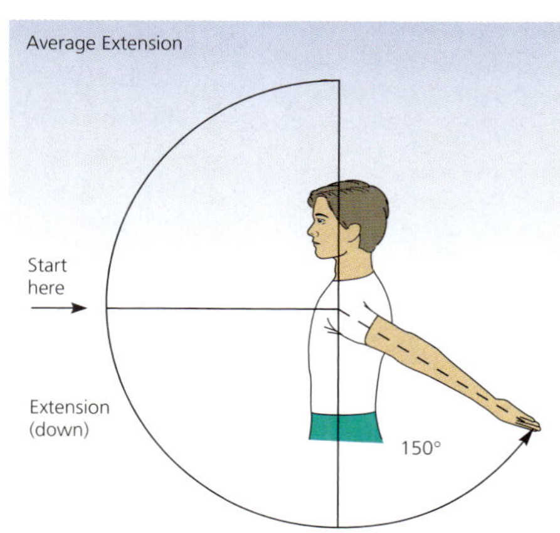

3. Trunk/Low-Back Lateral Flexion

Bend directly sideways at your waist. To prevent injury, keep your knees slightly bent, and support your trunk by placing your hand or forearm on your thigh. Check one of the following for each side; fill in degrees if using the measurement method.

Right	*Left*	
________	________	Below average/needs improvement
________	________	Average (36–40°)
________	________	Above average

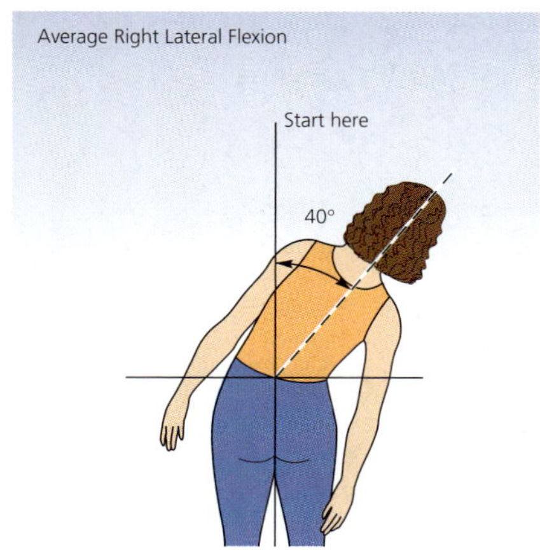

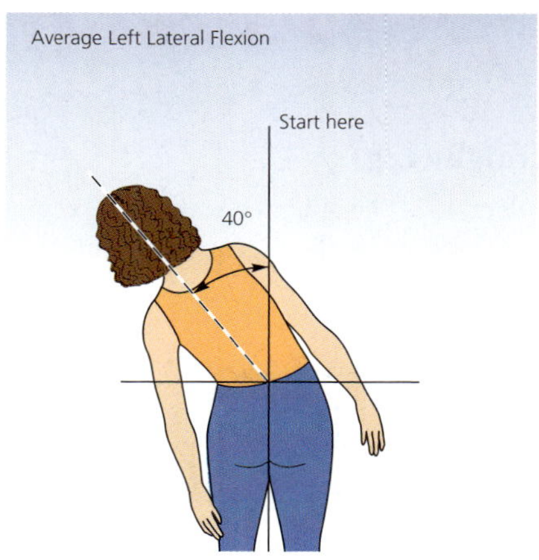

4. Hip Abduction

Raise your leg to the side at the hip. Check one of the following for each leg; fill in degrees if using the measurement method.

Right	*Left*	
________	________	Below average/needs improvement
________	________	Average (40–45°)
________	________	Above average

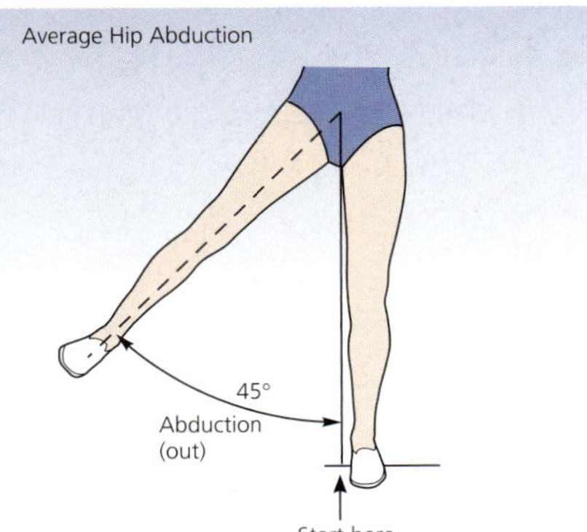

5. Hip Flexion (Bent Knee)

With one leg flat on the floor, bend the other knee and lift the leg up at the hip. Check one of the following for each leg; fill in degrees if using the measurement method.

Right	*Left*	
________	________	Below average/needs improvement
________	________	Average (121–125°)
________	________	Above average

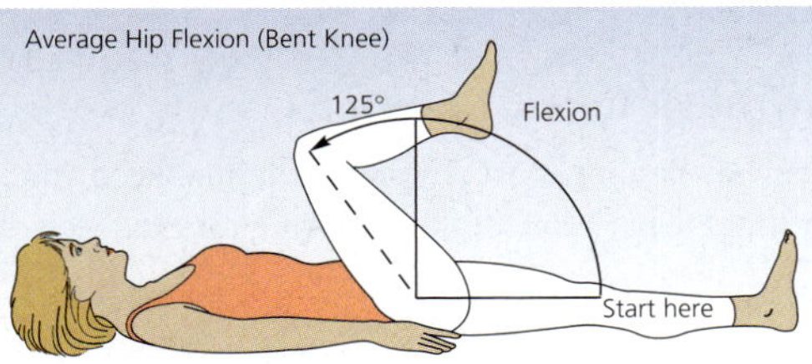

6. Hip Flexion (Straight Leg)

With one leg flat on the floor, raise the other leg at the hip, keeping both legs straight. Take care not to put excess strain on your back. Check one of the following for each leg; fill in degrees if using the measurement method.

Right	*Left*	
________	________	Below average/needs improvement
________	________	Average (79–81°)
________	________	Above average

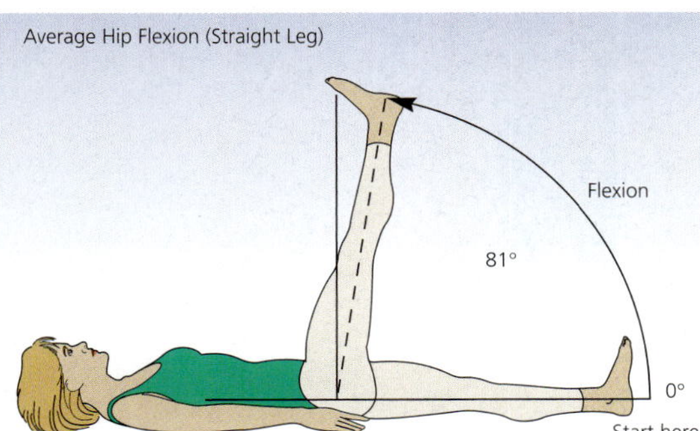

7. Ankle Dorsiflexion and Plantar Flexion

For each position and foot, check one of the following; fill in degrees if using the measurement method.

Ankle dorsiflexion—pull your toes toward your shin.

Right	*Left*	
________	________	Below average/needs improvement
________	________	Average (9–13°)
________	________	Above average

Plantar flexion—point your toes.

Right	*Left*	
________	________	Below average/needs improvement
________	________	Average (50–55°)
________	________	Above average

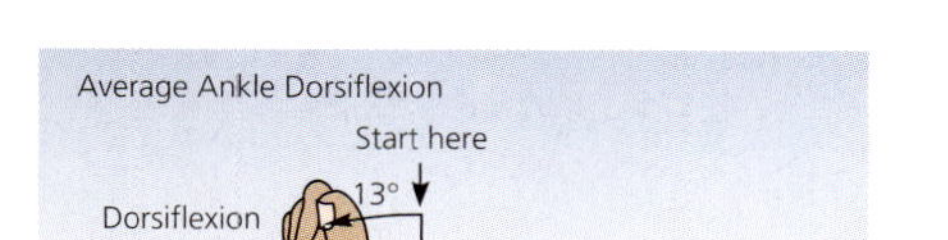

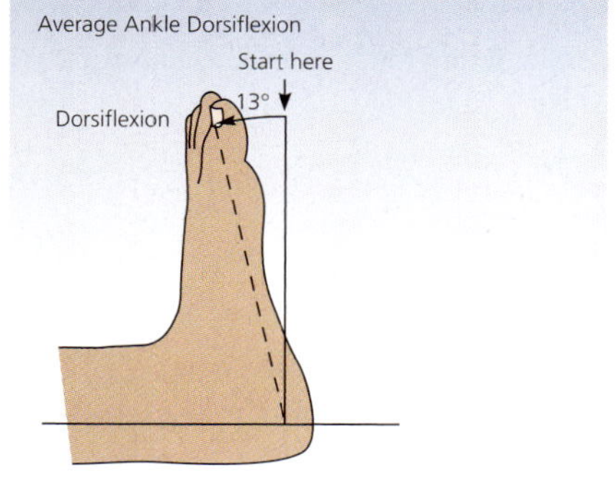

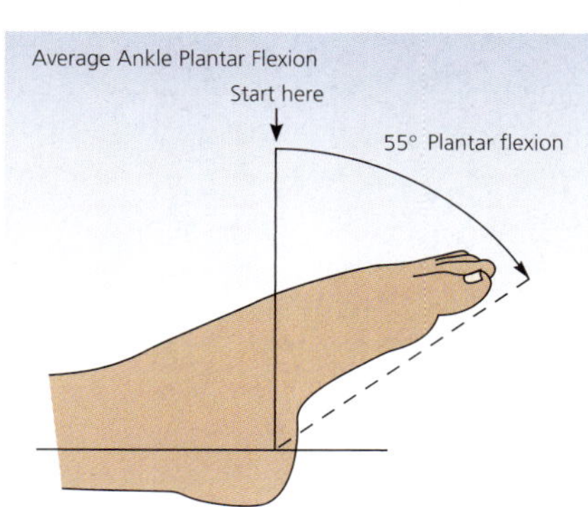

Rating Your Flexibility

Sit-and-reach test: Score: ______________ cm Rating: ______________

Range-of-Motion Assessment

Identify your rating for each joint on each side of the body. If you used the comparison method, put check marks in the appropriate categories; if you measured range of motion, enter the degrees for each joint in the appropriate category.

		Right			Left		
Joint/Assessment		Below Average	Average	Above Average	Below Average	Average	Above Average
1. Shoulder abduction and adduction	Abduction						
	Adduction						
2. Shoulder flexion and extension	Flexion						
	Extension						
3. Trunk/low-back lateral flexion	Flexion						
4. Hip abduction	Abduction						
5. Hip flexion (bent knee)	Flexion						
6. Hip flexion (straight leg)	Flexion						
7. Ankle dorsiflexion and plantar flexion	Dorsiflexion						
	Plantar flexion						

Using Your Results

How did you score? Are you surprised by your ratings for flexibility? Are you satisfied with your current ratings?

If you're not satisfied, set a realistic goal for improvement.

Are you satisfied with your current level of flexibility as expressed in your daily life—for example, your ability to maintain good posture and move easily and without pain?

If you're not satisfied, set some realistic goals for improvement:

What should you do next? Enter the results of this lab in the Preprogram Assessment column in Appendix C. If you've set goals for improvement, begin planning your flexibility program by completing the plan in Lab 9.2. After several weeks of your program, complete this lab again and enter the results in the Postprogram Assessment column of Appendix C. How do the results compare?

Name ______________________ Section ______________ Date ____________

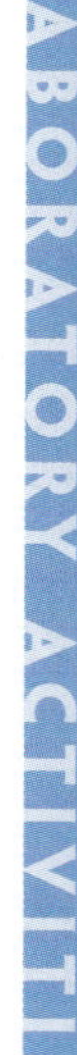

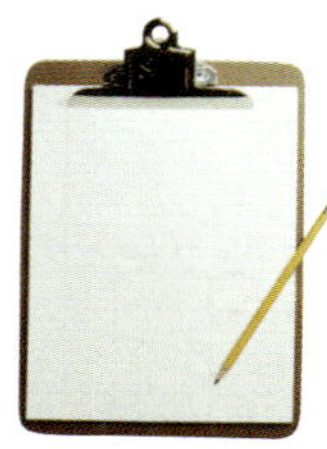

LAB 9.2 Creating a Personalized Program for Developing Flexibility

1. *Goals.* List goals for your flexibility program. On the left, include specific, measurable goals that you can use to track the progress of your fitness program. These goals might be things like raising your sit-and-reach score from fair to good or your bent-leg hip flexion rating from below average to average. On the right, include long-term and more qualitative goals, such as reducing your risk for back pain.

   Specific Goals: Current Status ______________________ Final Goals ______________________

   ______________________ ______________________

   ______________________ ______________________

   Other Goals: ______________________

   ____

2. *Exercises.* The exercises in the program plan below are from the general stretching program presented in Chapter 9. You can add or delete exercises depending on your needs, goals, and preferences. For any exercises you add, fill in the areas of the body affected.
3. *Frequency.* A minimum frequency of 2–3 days per week is recommended; 5–7 days per week is ideal. You may want to do your stretching exercises the same days you plan to do cardiorespiratory endurance exercise or weight training, because muscles stretch better following exercise, when they are warm.
4. *Intensity.* All stretches should be done to the point of mild discomfort, not pain.
5. *Time/duration.* All stretches should be held for 15–30 seconds. (PNF techniques should include a 6-second contraction followed by a 10–30-second assisted stretch.) All stretches should be performed 2–4 times.

Program Plan for Flexibility

Exercise	Areas Stretched	Frequency (check ✓)						
		M	T	W	Th	F	Sa	Su
Head turns and tilts	Neck							
Towel stretch	Triceps, shoulders, chest							
Across-the-body and overhead stretches	Shoulders, upper back, back of the arm							
Upper-back stretch	Upper back							
Lateral stretch	Trunk muscles							
Step stretch	Hip, front of thigh							
Side lunge	Inner thigh, hip, calf							
Inner-thigh stretch	Inner thigh, hip							
Trunk rotation	Trunk, outer thigh and hip, lower back							
Modified hurdler stretch	Back of the thigh, lower back							
Alternate leg stretcher	Back of the thigh, hip, knee, ankle, buttocks							
Lower-leg stretch	Back of the lower leg							

You can monitor your program using a chart like the one on the next page.

Flexibility Program Chart

Fill in the dates you perform each stretch, the number of seconds you hold each stretch (should be 15–30), and the number of repetitions of each (should be 2–4). For an easy check on the duration of your stretches, count "one thousand one, one thousand two," and so on. You will probably find that over time you'll be able to hold each stretch longer (in addition to being able to stretch farther).

Exercise/Date																				
	Duration																			
	Reps																			
	Duration																			
	Reps																			
	Duration																			
	Reps																			
	Duration																			
	Reps																			
	Duration																			
	Reps																			
	Duration																			
	Reps																			
	Duration																			
	Reps																			
	Duration																			
	Reps																			
	Duration																			
	Reps																			
	Duration																			
	Reps																			
	Duration																			
	Reps																			
	Duration																			
	Reps																			
	Duration																			
	Reps																			
	Duration																			
	Reps																			
	Duration																			
	Reps																			
	Duration																			
	Reps																			
	Duration																			
	Reps																			
	Duration																			
	Reps																			

Name ______________________________ Section ______________ Date ____________

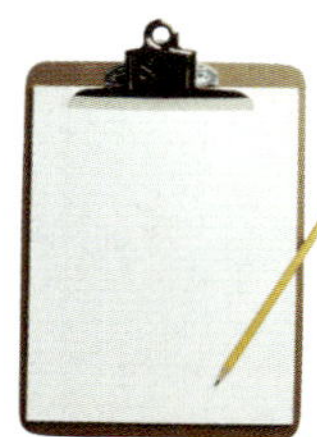

LAB 9.3 Assessing Muscular Endurance for Low-Back Health

The three tests in this lab evaluate the muscular endurance of major spine-stabilizing muscles.

Side Bridge Endurance Test

Equipment

1. Stopwatch or clock with a second hand
2. Exercise mat
3. Partner

Preparation

Warm up your muscles with some low-intensity activity such as walking or easy jogging. Practice assuming the side bridge position described below.

Instructions

1. Lie on the mat on your side with your legs extended. Place your top foot in front of your lower foot for support. Lift your hips off the mat so that you are supporting yourself on one elbow and your feet (see photo). Your body should maintain a straight line. Breathe normally; don't hold your breath.
2. Hold the position as long as possible. Your partner should keep track of the time and make sure that you maintain the correct position. Your final score is the total time you are able to hold the side bridge with correct form—from the time you lift your hips until your hips return to the mat.
3. Rest for 5 minutes and then repeat the test on the other side. Record your times here and on the chart at the end of the lab. Right side bridge time: ______________ sec   Left side bridge time: ______________ sec

Trunk Flexors Endurance Test

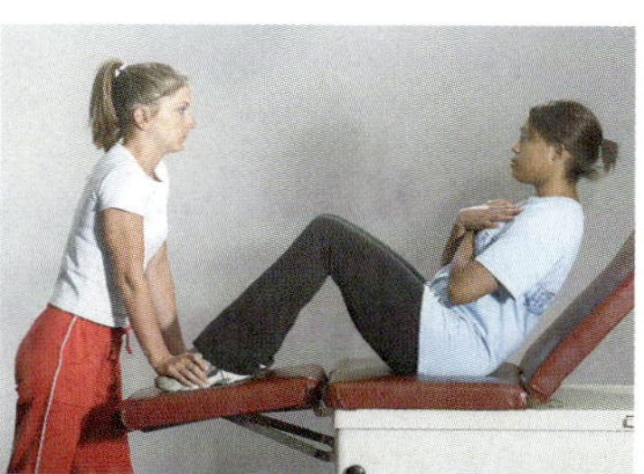

Equipment

1. Stopwatch or clock with a second hand
2. Exercise mat or padded exercise table
3. Two helpers
4. Jig angled at 60 degrees from the floor or padded bench (optional)

Preparation

Warm up with some low-intensity activity such as walking or easy jogging.

Instructions

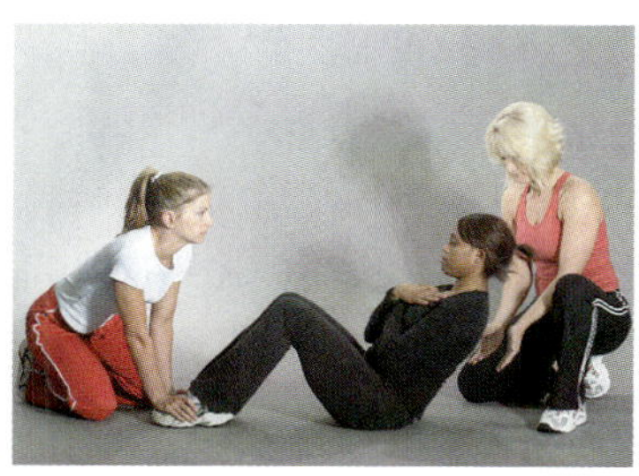

1. To start, assume a sit-up posture with your back supported at an angle of 60 degrees from the floor; support can be provided by a jig, a padded bench, or a spotter (see photos). Your knees and hips should both be flexed at 90 degrees, and your arms should be folded across your chest with your hands placed on the opposite shoulders. Your toes should be secured under a toe strap or held by a partner.
2. Your goal is to hold the starting position (isometric contraction) as long as possible after the support is pulled away. To begin the test, a helper should pull the jig or other support back about 10 centimeters (4 inches). The helper should keep track of the time; if a spotter is acting as your support, she or he should be ready to support your weight as soon as your torso begins to move back. Your final score is the total time you are able to hold the contraction—from the time the support is removed until any part of your back touches the support. Remember to breathe normally throughout the test.
3. Record your time here and on the chart at the end of the lab. Trunk flexors endurance time: ______________ sec

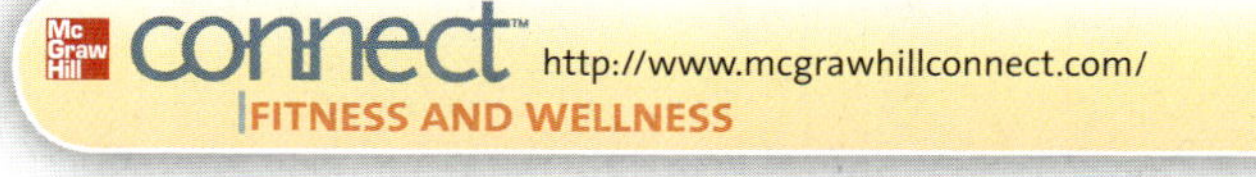

Back Extensors Endurance Test

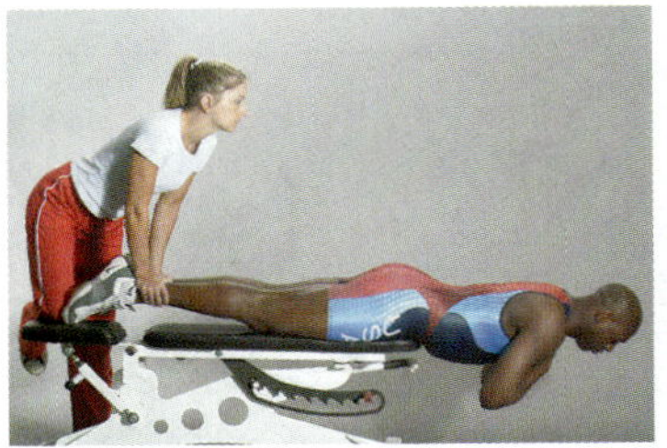

Equipment

1. Stopwatch or clock with a second hand
2. Extension bench with padded ankle support or any padded bench
3. Partner

Preparation

Warm up with some low-intensity activity such as walking or easy jogging.

Instructions

1. Lie face down on the test bench with your upper body extending out over the end of the bench and your pelvis, hips, and knees flat on the bench. Your arms should be folded across your chest with your hands placed on the opposite shoulders. Your feet should be secured under a padded strap or held by a partner.
2. Your goal is to hold your upper body in a straight horizontal line with your lower body as long as possible. Keep your neck straight and neutral; don't raise your head and don't arch your back. Breathe normally. Your partner should keep track of the time and watch your form. Your final score is the total time you are able to hold the horizontal position—from the time you assume the position until your upper body drops from the horizontal position.
3. Record your time here and on the chart below. Back extensors endurance time: ________________ sec

Rating Your Test Results for Muscular Endurance for Low-Back Health

The table below shows mean endurance test times for healthy young college students with a mean age of 21 years. Compare your scores with the times shown in the table. (If you are older or have suffered from low-back pain in the past, these ratings are less accurate; however, your time scores can be used as a point of comparison.)

Mean Endurance Times (sec)

	Right side bridge	Left side bridge	Trunk flexors	Back extensors
Men	95	99	136	161
Women	75	78	134	185

SOURCE: Adapted with permission from S. M. McGill, 2007, *Low Back Disorders: Evidence-Based Prevention and Rehabilitation*, 2nd ed., p. 211. Champaign, IL: Human Kinetics.

Right side bridge: ________________ sec   Rating (above mean, at mean, below mean): ________________
Left side bridge: ________________ sec   Rating (above mean, at mean, below mean): ________________
Trunk flexors: ________________ sec   Rating (above mean, at mean, below mean): ________________
Back extensors: ________________ sec   Rating (above mean, at mean, below mean): ________________

Using Your Results

How did you score? Are you surprised by your scores for the low-back tests? Are you satisfied with your current ratings?

If you're not satisfied, set a realistic goal for improvement. The norms in this lab are based on healthy young adults, so a score above the mean may or may not be realistic for you. Instead, you may want to set a specific goal based on time rather than rating; for example, set a goal of improving your time by 10%. Imbalances in muscular endurance have been linked with back problems, so if your rating is significantly lower for one of the three tests, you should focus particular attention on that area of your body.
Goal:

What should you do next? Enter the results of this lab in the Preprogram Assessment column in Appendix C. If you've set a goal for improvement, begin a program of low-back exercises such as that suggested in this chapter. After several weeks of your program, complete this lab again and enter the results in the Postprogram Assessment column of Appendix C. How do the results compare?

CHAPTER 10

Stress

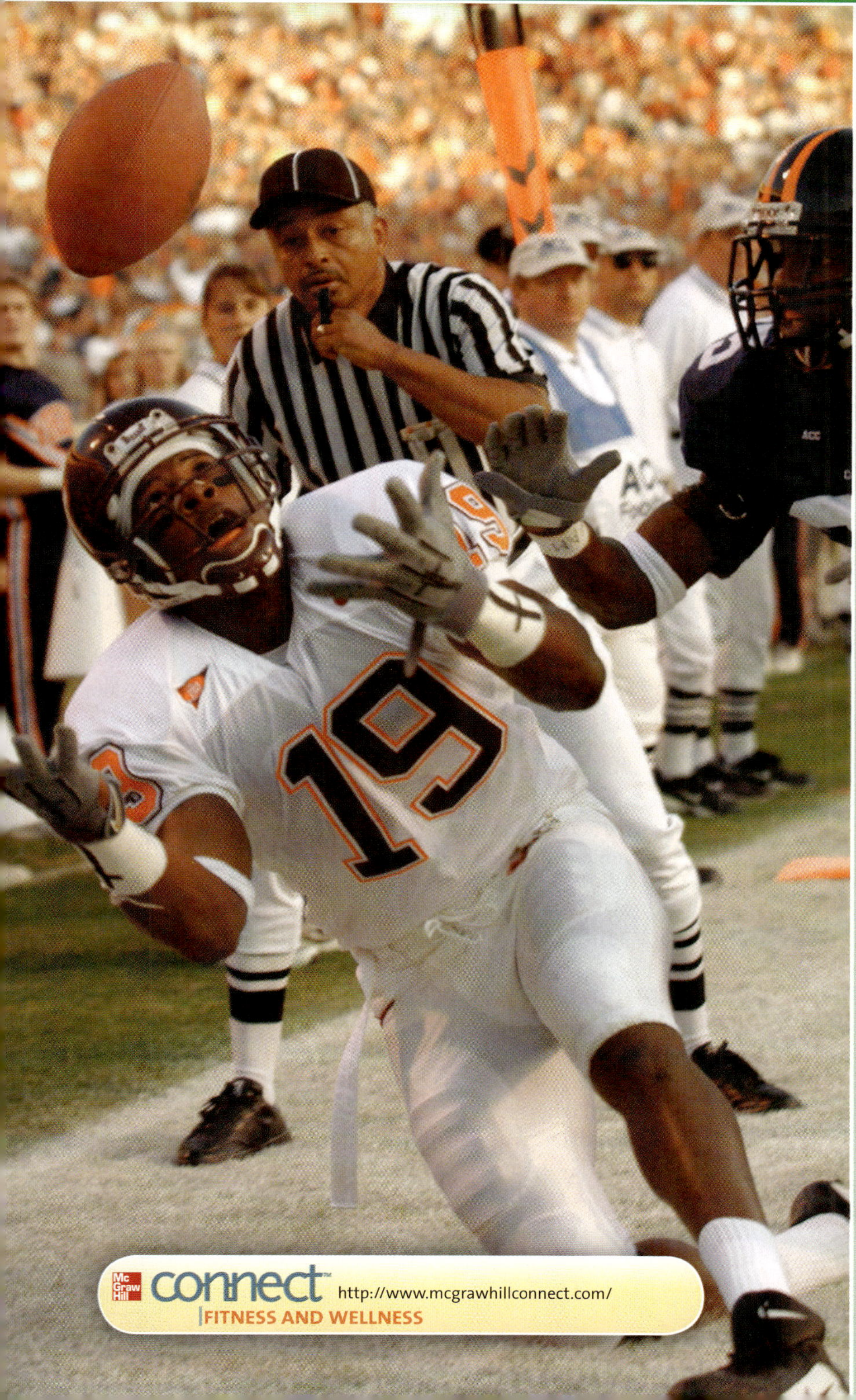

LOOKING AHEAD...

After reading this chapter, you should be able to:

- Explain what stress is and how people react to it—physically, emotionally, and behaviorally
- Describe the relationship between stress and disease
- List common sources of stress
- Describe techniques for preventing and managing stress
- Put together a plan for successfully managing the stress in your life

TEST YOUR KNOWLEDGE

1. Which of the following events can cause stress?
   a. taking out a loan
   b. failing a test
   c. graduating from college
2. Exercise stimulates which of the following?
   a. analgesia (pain relief)
   b. birth of new brain cells
   c. relaxation
3. Which of the following can be a result of chronic stress?
   a. violence
   b. heart attack
   c. stroke

Answers

1. **All three.** Stress-producing factors can be pleasant or unpleasant and can include physical challenges, goal achievement, and events that are perceived as negative.
2. **All three.** Regular exercise is linked to improvements in many dimensions of wellness.
3. **All three.** Chronic—or ongoing— stress can last for years. People who suffer from long-term stress may ultimately become violent toward themselves or others. They also run a greater-than-normal risk for certain ailments, especially cardiovascular disease.

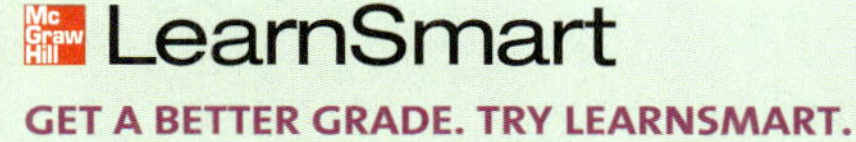

Like the term *fitness, stress* is a word many people use without really understanding its precise meaning. Stress is popularly viewed as an uncomfortable response to a negative event, which probably describes *nervous tension* more than the cluster of physical and psychological responses that actually constitute stress. In fact, stress is not limited to negative situations; it is also a response to pleasurable physical challenges and the achievement of personal goals.

Whether stress is experienced as pleasant or unpleasant depends largely on the situation and the individual. Because learning effective responses to stress can enhance psychological health and help prevent a number of serious diseases, stress management can be an important part of daily life.

This chapter explains the physiological and psychological reactions that make up the stress response and describes how these reactions can be risks to good health. The chapter also presents methods of managing stress.

WHAT IS STRESS?

In common usage, the term *stress* refers to two different things: situations that trigger physical and emotional reactions *and* the reactions themselves. This text uses the more precise term **stressor** for a situation that triggers physical and emotional reactions and the term **stress response** for those reactions. A first date and a final exam are examples of stressors; sweaty palms and a pounding heart are symptoms of the stress response. We'll use the term **stress** to describe the general physical and emotional state that accompanies the stress response. So, a person taking a final exam experiences stress.

KEY TERMS

stressor Any physical or psychological event or condition that produces physical and emotional reactions.

stress response The physical and emotional reactions to a stressor.

stress The general physical and emotional state that accompanies the stress response.

autonomic nervous system The branch of the nervous system that controls basic body processes; consists of the sympathetic and parasympathetic divisions.

parasympathetic division A division of the autonomic nervous system that moderates the excitatory effect of the sympathetic division, slowing metabolism and restoring energy supplies.

sympathetic division A division of the autonomic nervous system that reacts to danger or other challenges by almost instantly accelerating body processes.

norepinephrine A neurotransmitter released by the sympathetic nervous system onto specific tissues to increase their function in the face of increased activity; when released by the brain, causes arousal (increased attention, awareness, and alertness); also called *noradrenaline.*

Physical Responses to Stressors

Imagine a near miss: As you step off the curb, a car speeds toward you. With just a fraction of a second to spare, you leap safely out of harm's way. In that split second of danger and in the moments following it, you experience a predictable series of physical reactions. Your body goes from a relaxed state to one prepared for physical action to cope with a threat to your life.

Two systems in your body are responsible for your physical response to stressors: the nervous system and the endocrine system. Through rapid chemical reactions affecting almost every part of your body, you are primed to act quickly and appropriately in time of danger.

Actions of the Nervous System The nervous system consists of the brain, spinal cord, and nerves. Part of the nervous system is under voluntary control, as when you tell your arm to reach for a chocolate. The part that is not under conscious supervision—for example, the part that controls the digestion of the chocolate—is the **autonomic nervous system.** In addition to digestion, it controls your heart rate, breathing, blood pressure, and hundreds of other involuntary functions.

The autonomic nervous system consists of two divisions:

- The **parasympathetic division** is in control when you are relaxed. It aids in digesting food, storing energy, and promoting growth.
- The **sympathetic division** is activated during times of arousal, including exercise, and when there is an emergency, such as severe pain, anger, or fear.

Sympathetic nerves use the neurotransmitter **norepinephrine** (or *noradrenaline*) to exert their actions on nearly every organ, sweat gland, blood vessel, and muscle to enable your body to handle an emergency. In general, the sympathetic division commands your body to stop storing energy and to use it in response to a crisis.

Actions of the Endocrine System During stress, the sympathetic nervous system triggers the **endocrine system.** This system of glands, tissues, and cells helps control body functions by releasing **hormones** and other chemical messengers into the bloodstream to influence metabolism and other body processes. These chemicals act on a variety of targets throughout the body. Along with the nervous system, the endocrine system prepares the body to respond to a stressor.

The Two Systems Together How do both systems work together in an emergency? Let's go back to your near-collision with a car. Both reflexes and higher cognitive (thinking) areas in your brain quickly make the decision that you are facing a threat, and your body prepares to meet the danger. Chemical messages and actions of sympathetic nerves cause the release of key hormones,

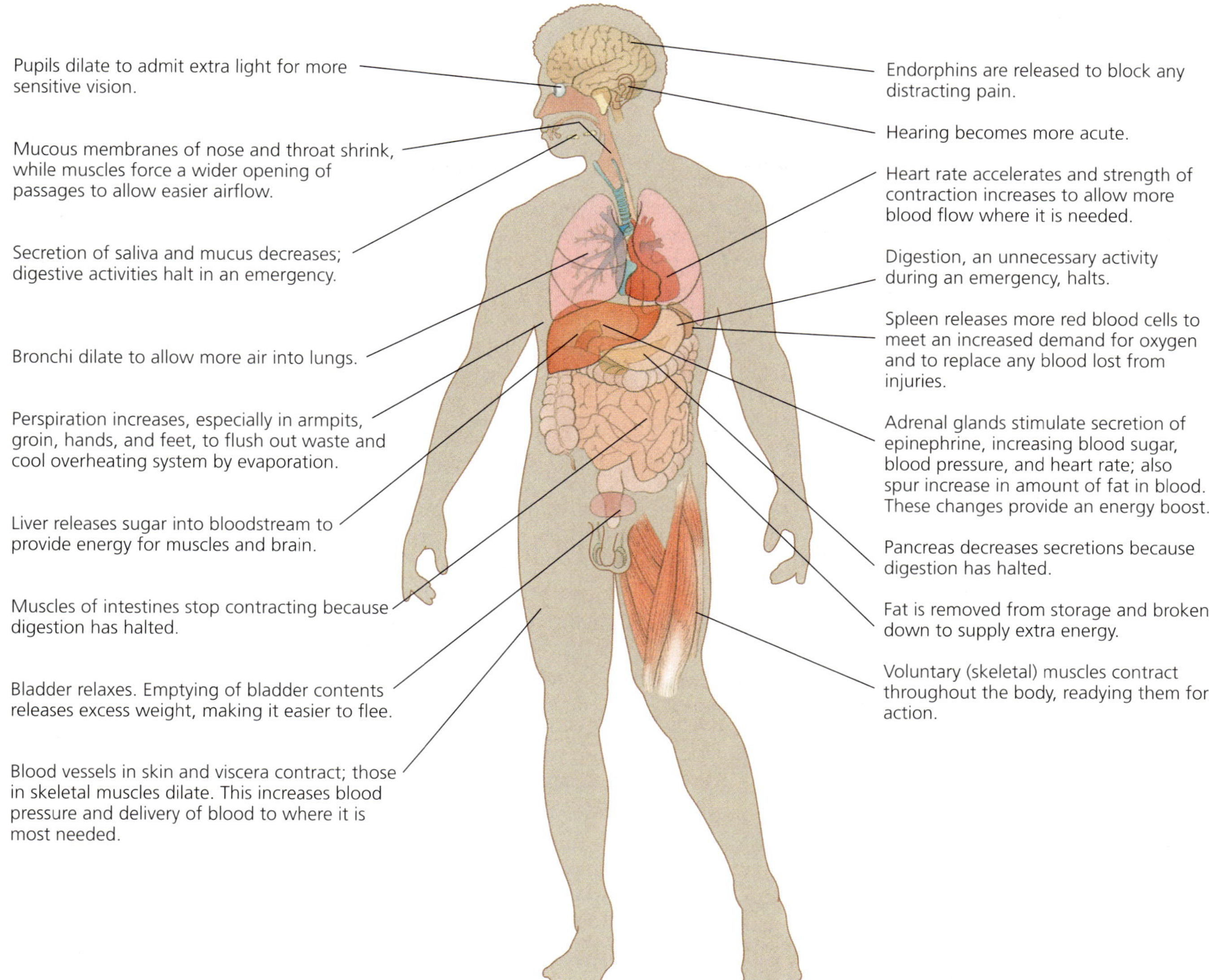

FIGURE 10.1 The fight-or-flight reaction.

including **cortisol** and **epinephrine.** These hormones trigger the physiological changes shown in Figure 10.1, including these:

- Heart and respiration rates accelerate to speed oxygen through the body.
- Hearing and vision become more acute.
- The liver releases extra sugar into the bloodstream to boost energy.
- Perspiration increases to cool the skin.
- The brain releases **endorphins**—chemicals that can inhibit or block sensations of pain—in case you are injured.

Taken together, these almost-instantaneous physical changes are called the **fight-or-flight reaction.** They give you the heightened reflexes and strength you need to

KEY TERMS

endocrine system The system of glands, tissues, and cells that secretes hormones into the bloodstream to influence metabolism and other body processes.

hormone A chemical messenger produced in the body and transported in the bloodstream to targeted cells or organs for specific regulation of their activities.

cortisol A steroid hormone secreted by the cortex (outer layer) of the adrenal gland; also called *hydrocortisone*.

epinephrine A hormone secreted by the medulla (inner core) of the adrenal gland that affects the functioning of organs involved in responding to a stressor; also called *adrenaline*.

endorphins Brain secretions that have pain-inhibiting effects.

fight-or-flight reaction A defense reaction that prepares a person for conflict or escape by triggering hormonal, cardiovascular, metabolic, and other changes.

dodge the car or deal with other stressors. Although these physical changes may vary in intensity, the same basic set of physical reactions occurs in response to any type of stressor—positive or negative, physical or psychological.

The Return to Homeostasis Once a stressful situation ends, the parasympathetic division of your autonomic nervous system takes command and halts the stress response. It restores **homeostasis**, a state in which your body maintains blood pressure, heart rate, hormone levels, and other vital functions within a narrow range of normal. Your parasympathetic nervous system calms your body down, slowing a rapid heartbeat, drying sweaty palms, and returning breathing to normal. Gradually, your body resumes its normal "housekeeping" functions, such as digestion and temperature regulation. Damage that may have been sustained during the fight-or-flight reaction is repaired. The day after you narrowly dodge the car, you wake up feeling fine. In this way, your body can grow, repair itself, and build energy reserves. When the next crisis comes, you'll be ready to respond again.

The Fight-or-Flight Reaction in Modern Life The fight-or-flight reaction is a part of our biological heritage, and it's a survival mechanism that has served both humans and animals well. In modern life, however, it is often absurdly inappropriate. Many stressors we face in everyday life—such as an exam, a mess left by a roommate, or a stop light—do not require a physical response. The fight-or-flight reaction prepares the body for physical action regardless of whether such action is a necessary or appropriate response to a particular stressor.

Emotional and Behavioral Responses to Stressors

We all experience a similar set of physical responses to stressors, which make up the fight-or-flight reaction. These responses, however, vary from person to person and from one situation to another. People's perceptions of potential stressors—and their reactions to such stressors—also vary greatly. For example, you may feel confident about taking exams but be nervous about talking to people you don't know, while your roommate may love challenging social situations but be nervous about taking tests. Many factors, some external and some internal, help explain these differences.

Your cognitive appraisal of a potential stressor strongly influences how you respond to it. Two factors that can reduce the magnitude of the stress response are successful prediction and the perception of control. For instance, receiving course syllabi at the beginning of the term allows you to predict the timing of major deadlines and exams. Having this predictive knowledge also allows you to exert some control over your study plans and can help reduce the stress caused by exams.

Cognitive appraisal is highly individual and strongly related to emotions. The facts of a situation—Who? What? Where? When?—typically are evaluated fairly consistently from person to person. Evaluation with respect to personal outcome, however, varies: What does this mean for me? Can I do anything about it? Will it improve or worsen? If an individual perceives a situation as exceeding her or his ability to cope, the result can be negative emotions and an inappropriate stress response. If, on the other hand, a person perceives a situation as a challenge that is within her or his ability to manage, more positive and appropriate responses are likely. A moderate level of stress, if coped with appropriately, can help promote optimal performance (Figure 10.2).

Effective and Ineffective Responses Common emotional responses to stressors include anxiety, depression, and fear. Although emotional responses are determined in part by inborn personality or temperament, we often can moderate or learn to control them. Coping techniques are discussed later in the chapter.

Wellness Tip

Chronic stress not only harms your health, it can make you age faster. A study of women who were long-term caregivers to very sick children revealed that, over time, the women's bodies lost their ability to create new red blood cells. On average, these women were physically 10 years older than their actual chronological age. This is one reason it pays to learn to manage stress, especially when you're young!

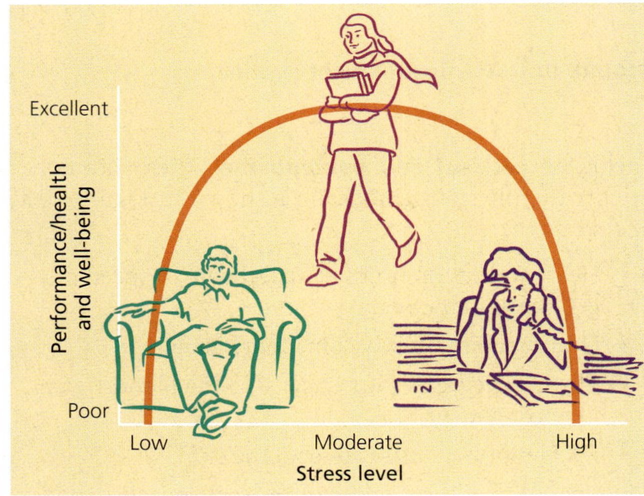

FIGURE 10.2 Stress level, performance, and well-being. A moderate level of stress challenges individuals in a way that promotes optimal performance and well-being. Too little stress, and people are not challenged enough to improve; too much stress, and the challenges become stressors that can impair physical and emotional health.

Behavioral responses to stressors—controlled by the **somatic nervous system**, which manages our conscious actions—are entirely under our control. Effective behavioral responses such as talking, laughing, exercising, meditating, learning time-management skills, and becoming more assertive can promote wellness and enable us to function at our best. Ineffective behavioral responses to stressors include overeating, expressing hostility, and using tobacco, alcohol, or other drugs.

Personality and Stress Some people seem to be nervous, irritable, and easily upset by minor annoyances; others are calm and composed even in difficult situations. Scientists remain unsure just why this is or how the brain's complex emotional mechanisms work. But **personality**—the sum of behavioral, cognitive, and emotional tendencies—clearly affects how people perceive and react to stressors. To investigate the links among personality, stress, and wellness, researchers have looked at different clusters of characteristics, or "personality types."

- ***Type A.*** People with Type A personality are described as ultracompetitive, controlling, impatient, aggressive, and even hostile. Type A people have a higher perceived stress level and more problems coping with stress. They react explosively to stressors and are upset by events that others would consider only annoyances. Studies indicate that certain characteristics of the Type A pattern—anger, cynicism, and hostility—increase the risk of heart disease.
- ***Type B.*** The Type B personality is relaxed and contemplative. Type B people are less frustrated by daily events and more tolerant of the behavior of others.
- ***Type C.*** The Type C personality is characterized by anger suppression, difficulty expressing emotions, feelings of hopelessness and despair, and an exaggerated response to minor stressors. This heightened response may impair immune functions.

Studies of Type A and C personalities suggest that expressing your emotions is beneficial but that habitually expressing exaggerated stress responses or hostility is unhealthy.

Researchers have also looked for personality traits that enable people to deal more successfully with stress. One such trait is *hardiness*, a particular form of optimism. People with a hardy personality view potential stressors as challenges and opportunities for growth and learning, rather than as burdens. Hardy people perceive fewer situations as stressful, and their reaction to stressors tends to be less intense. They are committed to their activities, have a sense of inner purpose and an inner locus of control, and feel at least partly in control of their lives.

You probably can't change your basic personality, but you can change your typical behaviors and patterns of thinking, and you can use positive stress-management techniques like those described later in the chapter.

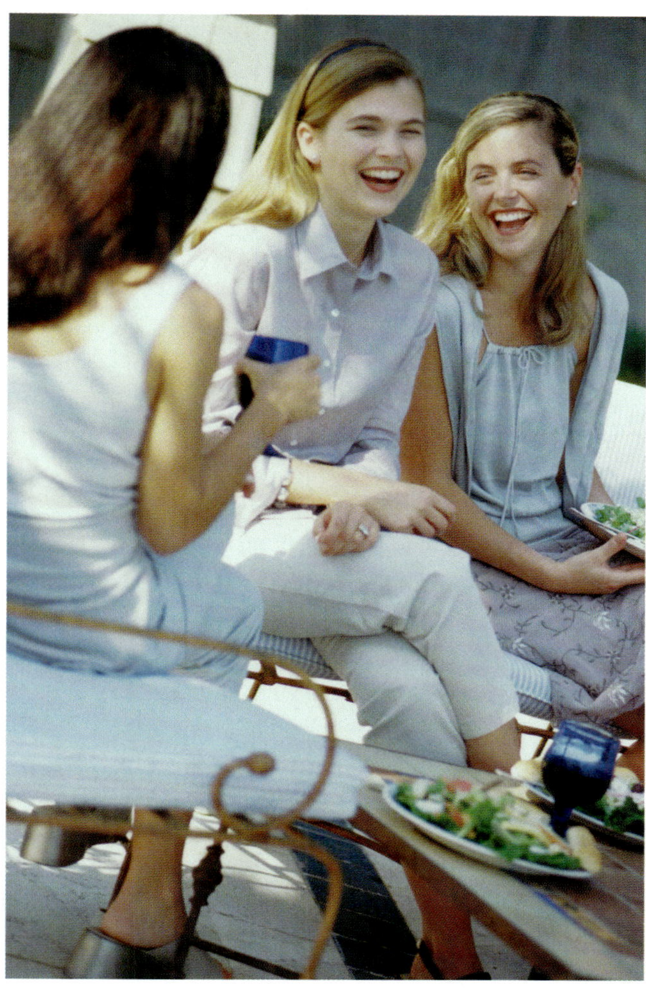

A person's emotional and behavioral responses to stressors depend on many different factors, including personality, gender, and cultural background. Research suggests that women are more likely than men to respond to stressors by seeking social contact and support.

Gender and Stress Our gender role—the activities, abilities, and behaviors our culture expects of us based on our sex—can affect our experience of stress. Some behavioral responses to stressors, such as crying or openly expressing anger, may be deemed more appropriate for one gender than the other.

Strict adherence to gender roles can limit one's response to stress and can itself become a source of stress. Adherence

KEY TERMS

homeostasis A state of stability and consistency in a person's physiological functioning.

somatic nervous system The branch of the peripheral nervous system that governs motor functions and sensory information, largely under conscious control.

personality The sum of behavioral, cognitive, and emotional tendencies.

Table 10.1 Symptoms of Excess Stress

PHYSICAL SYMPTOMS	EMOTIONAL SYMPTOMS	BEHAVIORAL SYMPTOMS
Dry mouth	Anxiety	Crying
Excessive perspiration	Depression	Disrupted eating habits
Frequent illnesses	Edginess	Disrupted sleeping habits
Gastrointestinal problems	Fatigue	Harsh treatment of others
Grinding of teeth	Hypervigilance	Problems communicating
Headaches	Impulsiveness	Sexual problems
High blood pressure	Inability to concentrate	Social isolation
Pounding heart	Irritability	Increased use of tobacco, alcohol, or other drugs
Stiff neck or aching lower back	Trouble remembering things	

Ask yourself

QUESTIONS FOR CRITICAL THINKING AND REFLECTION

Think of the last time you faced a significant stressor. How did you respond? List the physical, emotional, and behavioral reactions you felt. Did these responses help you deal with the stress, or did they interfere with your efforts to handle it?

to traditional gender roles can also affect the perception of a stressor. For example, if a man derives most of his sense of self-worth from his work, retirement may be a more stressful life change for him than for a woman whose self-image is based on several different roles.

Although both men and women experience the fight-or-flight response to stress, women are more likely to respond with a behavioral pattern known as "tend-and-befriend"—nurturing friends and family and seeking social support and social contacts. Rather than becoming aggressive or withdrawing from difficult situations, women are more likely to create or enhance their social networks in ways that reduce stress.

Experience Past experiences can profoundly influence the way you evaluate a potential stressor. Someone who has had a bad experience giving a speech in the past is much more likely to perceive an upcoming speech as stressful than someone who has had positive public speaking experiences. Effective behavioral responses, such as preparing carefully and visualizing success, can help overcome the effects of negative past experiences.

The Stress Experience as a Whole

As Table 10.1 shows, the physical, emotional, and behavioral symptoms of excess negative stress are distinct. But they are also intimately interrelated. The more intense the emotional response, the stronger the physical response. Effective behavioral responses can lessen stress; ineffective ones only worsen it. Sometimes people have such intense responses to stressors or such ineffective coping techniques that they need professional help to overcome the stress in their lives. More often, however, people can learn to handle stressors on their own.

STRESS AND WELLNESS

According to the American Psychological Association, 43% of adult Americans suffer from stress-related health problems. The role of stress in health is complex, but evidence suggests that stress can increase vulnerability to many ailments. Several theories have been proposed to explain the relationship between stress and disease.

The General Adaptation Syndrome

Biologist Hans Selye was one of the first scientists to develop a comprehensive theory of stress and disease. Based on his work in the 1930s and 1940s, Selye coined the term **general adaptation syndrome (GAS)** to describe what he believed to be a universal and predictable response pattern to all stressors. Some stressors are pleasant, such as attending a party, or unpleasant, such as a bad grade. In the GAS theory, stress triggered by a pleasant stressor is called **eustress;** stress triggered by an unpleasant stressor is called **distress.** The sequence of physical responses associated with GAS (Figure 10.3) is the same for both eustress and distress and occurs in three stages:

- ***Alarm.*** The alarm stage includes the complex sequence of events brought on by the fight-or-flight reaction. At this stage, the body is more susceptible to disease or injury because it is geared up to deal with a crisis. Someone in this phase may experience headaches, indigestion, anxiety, and disrupted sleeping and eating patterns.
- ***Resistance.*** With continued stress, the body develops a new level of homeostasis in which it is more

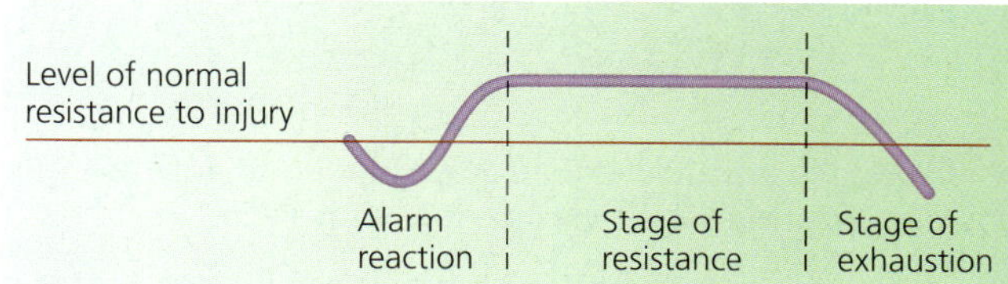

FIGURE 10.3 The general adaptation syndrome. During the alarm stage, a lower resistance to injury is evident. With continued stress, resistance to injury is actually enhanced. With prolonged exposure to repeated stressors, exhaustion sets in, with a return of low resistance levels seen during acute stress.

resistant to disease and injury than normal. In this stage, a person can cope with normal life and added stress.

- *Exhaustion.* The first two stages of GAS require a great deal of energy. If a stressor persists, or if several stressors occur in succession, general exhaustion results. This is not the sort of exhaustion you feel after a long, busy day. Rather, it's a life-threatening type of physiological exhaustion.

Allostatic Load

Although GAS is still viewed as a key conceptual contribution to the understanding of stress, some aspects of it are considered outdated. For example, increased susceptibility to disease after repeated or prolonged stress is now thought to be due to the effects of the stress response itself rather than to a depletion of resources (the exhaustion stage). In particular, long-term overexposure to stress hormones such as cortisol has been linked with health problems. Further, although physical stress reactions promote homeostasis (resistance stage), they also have negative effects on the body.

The long-term wear and tear of the stress response is called the **allostatic load.** A person's allostatic load depends on many factors, including genetics, life experiences, and emotional and behavioral responses to stressors. A high allostatic load may be due to frequent stressors, poor adaptation to common stressors, an inability to shut down the stress response, or imbalances in the stress responses of different body systems. High allostatic load is linked to heart disease, hypertension, obesity, and reduced brain and immune system functioning. In other words, when your allostatic load exceeds your ability to cope, you are more likely to get sick.

Psychoneuroimmunology

One of the most fruitful areas of current research into the relationship between stress and disease is **psychoneuroimmunology (PNI).** PNI is the study of the interactions among the nervous system, the endocrine system, and the immune system. The underlying premise of PNI is that stress, through the actions of the nervous and endocrine systems, impairs the immune system and thereby affects health.

A complex network of nerve and chemical connections exists between the nervous, endocrine, and immune systems. In general, increased levels of stress hormones are linked to a decreased number of immune system cells, or lymphocytes. Epinephrine appears to promote the release of lymphocytes but at the same time reduces their efficiency. Scientists have identified hormone-like substances called *neuropeptides* that appear to translate emotions into biochemical events, some of which impact the immune system, providing a physical link between emotions and immune function.

Different types of stress may affect immunity in different ways. For example, during acute stress (typically lasting less than 100 minutes), white blood cells move into the skin, where they enhance the immune response. During a stressful sequence of events, such as a personal trauma and the events that follow, however, there are typically no overall significant immune changes. Chronic (ongoing) stressors such as unemployment have negative effects on almost all functional measures of immunity. Chronic stress may cause prolonged secretion of cortisol and may accelerate the course of diseases that involve inflammation, including multiple sclerosis, heart disease, and type 2 diabetes.

Mood, personality, behavior, and immune functioning are intertwined. For example, people who are generally pessimistic may neglect the basics of health care, become

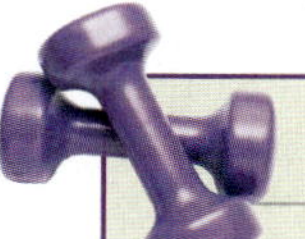

Fitness Tip

Stressed out? Then walk away—literally. Walking is a proven countermeasure against stress, and it contributes to your health in many other ways. A brisk, 10-minute walk may be enough to help you put things in perspective and get back to your normal routine. If not, just keep walking until you feel better. As you walk, try not to think too much about anything specific; the idea is to clear your head!

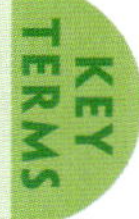

general adaptation syndrome (GAS) A pattern of stress responses consisting of three stages: alarm, resistance, and exhaustion.

eustress Stress resulting from a pleasant stressor.

distress Stress resulting from an unpleasant stressor.

allostatic load The long-term negative impact of the stress response on the body.

psychoneuroimmunology (PNI) The study of the interactions among the nervous, endocrine, and immune systems.

Overcoming Insomnia

TAKE CHARGE

Most people can overcome insomnia by discovering the cause of poor sleep and taking steps to remedy it. Insomnia that lasts for more than 6 months and interferes with daytime functioning requires consultation with a physician. Sleeping pills are not recommended for chronic insomnia because they can be habit-forming; they also lose their effectiveness over time.

If you're bothered by insomnia, try the following:

- Determine how much sleep you need to feel refreshed the next day, and don't sleep longer than that.
- Go to bed at the same time every night, and, more important, get up at the same time every morning, 7 days a week, regardless of how much sleep you got.
- Don't nap more than 30 minutes per day.
- Exercise regularly, but not too close to bedtime. Your metabolism needs at least 6 hours to slow down after exercise.
- Avoid tobacco and caffeine late in the day, and alcohol before bedtime (it causes disturbed, fragmented sleep).
- If you take any medications (prescription or not), ask your doctor or pharmacist if they interfere with sleep.
- Have a light snack before bedtime; you'll sleep better if you're not hungry.
- Use your bed only for sleep. Don't eat, read, study, or watch television in bed.
- Establish a relaxing bedtime routine that helps you unwind and lets your brain know it's time to go to sleep. Read, listen to music, or practice a relaxation technique. Don't lie down in bed until you're sleepy.
- If you don't fall asleep in 15–20 minutes, or if you wake up and can't fall asleep again, get out of bed, leave the room if possible, and do something monotonous until you feel sleepy. Try distracting yourself with imagery instead of counting sheep; imagine yourself on a pleasant vacation or enjoying some beautiful scenery.
- If sleep problems persist, ask your doctor for a referral to a sleep specialist in your area. You may be a candidate for a sleep study—an overnight evaluation of your sleep pattern that can uncover many sleep-related disorders.

Ask Yourself

QUESTIONS FOR CRITICAL THINKING AND REFLECTION

Have you ever been so stressed that you felt ill in some way? If so, what were your symptoms? How did you handle them? Did the experience affect the way you reacted to other stressful events?

passive when ill, and fail to engage in health-promoting behaviors. People who are depressed may reduce physical activity and social interaction, which may in turn affect the immune system and the cognitive appraisal of a stressor. Optimism, successful coping, and positive problem solving, on the other hand, may positively influence immunity.

Links Between Stress and Specific Conditions

Although much remains to be learned, it is clear that people who have unresolved chronic stress in their lives or who handle stressors poorly are at risk for a wide range of health problems. In the short term, the problem might just be a cold, a stiff neck, or a stomachache. Over the long term, the problems can be more severe, such as cardiovascular disease or impairment of the immune system.

Cardiovascular Disease The stress response profoundly affects the cardiovascular system. During the stress response, heart rate increases and blood vessels constrict, causing blood pressure to rise. Chronic high blood pressure is a major cause of *atherosclerosis*, a disease in which the lining of the blood vessels becomes damaged and caked with fatty deposits. These deposits can block arteries, causing heart attacks and strokes (see Chapter 5).

Certain types of emotional responses increase a person's risk of cardiovascular disease. People who exhibit extreme increases in heart rate and blood pressure in response to emotional stressors may face an increased risk of cardiovascular problems.

Altered Immune Function PNI research helps explain how stress affects the immune system. Some of the health problems linked to stress-related changes in immune function include vulnerability to colds and other infections, asthma and allergy attacks, susceptibility to cancer, and flare-ups of chronic diseases such as genital herpes and HIV infection.

Other Health Problems Many other health problems may be caused or worsened by excessive stress, including the following:

- Digestive problems such as stomachaches, diarrhea, constipation, irritable bowel syndrome, and ulcers
- Tension headaches and migraines

- Insomnia and fatigue (see the box "Overcoming Insomnia")
- Injuries, including on-the-job injuries caused by repetitive strain
- Menstrual irregularities, impotence, and pregnancy complications
- Psychological problems, including depression, anxiety, panic attacks, eating disorders, and post-traumatic stress disorder (PTSD), which afflicts people who have suffered or witnessed severe trauma

COMMON SOURCES OF STRESS

Recognizing potential sources of stress is an important step in successfully managing the stress in your life.

Major Life Changes

Any major change in your life that requires adjustment and accommodation can be a source of stress. Early adulthood and the college years are associated with many significant changes, such as moving out of the family home. Even changes typically thought of as positive—such as graduation, job promotion, or marriage—can be stressful.

Clusters of life changes, particularly those that are perceived negatively, may be linked to health problems in some people. Personality and coping skills, however, are important moderating influences. People with a strong support network and a stress-resistant personality are less likely to become ill in response to life changes than people with fewer resources.

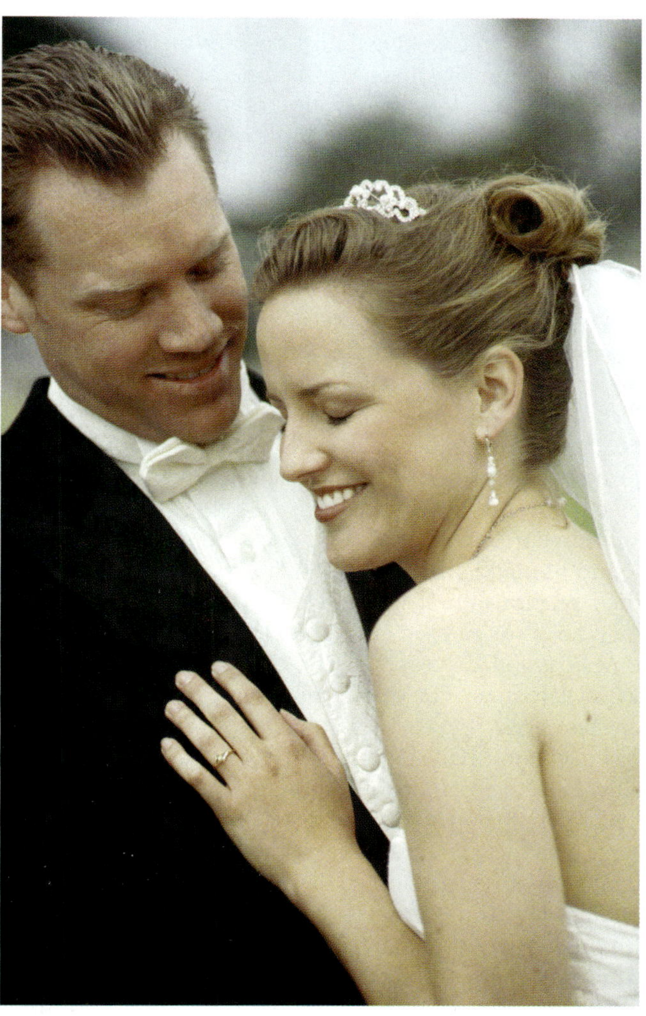

Even a joyful occasion can be a source of stress, especially if it involves a major life change.

Daily Hassles

Although major life changes are undoubtedly stressful, they seldom occur regularly. Researchers have proposed that minor problems—life's daily hassles, such as losing your keys or wallet—can be an even greater source of stress because they occur much more often.

People who perceive hassles negatively are likely to experience a moderate stress response every time they are faced with one. Over time, this can take a significant toll on health. Studies indicate that for some people, daily hassles contribute to a general decrease in overall wellness.

College Stressors

College is a time of major changes and minor hassles. For many students, college means being away from home and family for the first time. Nearly all students share stresses like the following:

- ***Academic stress.*** Exams, grades, and an endless workload await every college student but can be especially troublesome for young students just out of high school.
- ***Interpersonal stress.*** Most students are more than just students; they are also friends, children, employees, spouses, parents, and so on. Managing relationships while juggling the rigors of college life can be daunting, especially if some friends or family are less than supportive.
- ***Time pressures.*** Class schedules, assignments, and deadlines are an inescapable part of college life. But these time pressures can be drastically compounded for students who also have a job and/or family responsibilities.
- ***Financial concerns.*** The majority of college students need financial aid not just to cover the cost of tuition but to survive from day to day while in school. For many, college life isn't possible without a job, and the pressure to stay afloat financially competes with academic and other stressors.
- ***Worries about the future.*** As college life comes to an end, students face the reality of life after college. This means thinking about a career, choosing a place to live, and leaving the friends and routines of school behind.

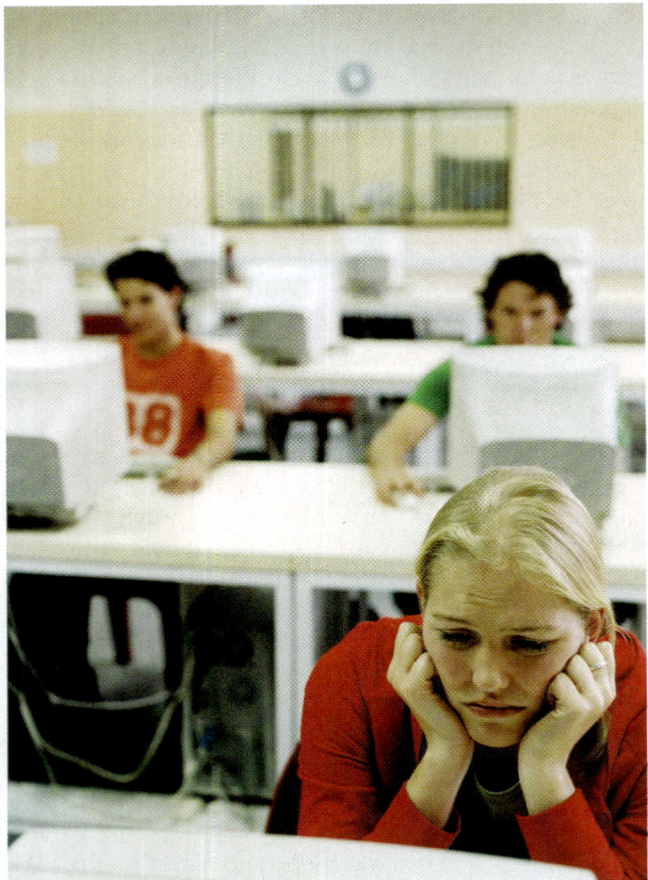

College students face a host of stressors, not the least of which is the pressure to perform academically.

Job-Related Stressors

Americans rate their jobs as a key source of stress in their lives. According to the 2010 *Stress in America* survey, 70% of working Americans say their job is a key source of stress in their life. Tight schedules and overtime leave less time for exercising, socializing, and other stress-proofing activities. Worries about job performance, salary, job security, and interactions with others can contribute to stress. High levels of job stress are also common for people who are left out of important decisions relating to their jobs. When workers are given the opportunity to shape their job descriptions and responsibilities, job satisfaction goes up and stress levels go down.

If job-related (or college-related) stress is severe or chronic, the result can be *burnout,* a state of physical, mental, and emotional exhaustion. Burnout occurs most often in highly motivated and driven individuals who come to feel that their work is not recognized or that they are not accomplishing their goals. People in the helping professions—teachers, social workers, caregivers, police officers, and so on—are also prone to burnout. For some people who suffer from burnout, a vacation or leave of absence may be appropriate. For others, a reduced work schedule, better communication with superiors, or a change in job goals may be necessary. Improving time-management skills can also help.

> **Wellness Tip**
>
> If you worry about money, you definitely aren't alone. In the American Psychological Association's 2010 *Stress in America* survey, 76% of Americans cited money as a key source of stress in their lives. If money is a constant cause of worry for you, see the advice on financial wellness in Chapter 1, and get help from a financial planner. It's never too early to have a solid financial plan in place.

Relationships and Stress

Human beings need social relationships; we cannot thrive as solitary creatures. Simply put, people need people. Even so, our interpersonal relationships—even our deepest, most intimate ones—can be one of the most significant sources of stress in our life.

The first relationships we form outside the family are friendships. With members of either the same or the other sex, friendships give people the opportunity to share themselves and discover others. Friendships are often more stable and longer lasting than intimate partnerships. Friends are often more accepting and less critical than lovers, probably because their expectations are different. Friendships provide people with emotional support and buffer them from stress. Friendships tend to weather conflict and stressful events better than intimate relationships do. During times of stress, in fact, many people initially turn to their friends for comfort, rather than family members or lovers.

Intimate love relationships are among the most profound human experiences. When two people fall in love, their relationship at first is likely to be characterized by high levels of passion and rapidly increasing intimacy. In time, passion decreases as the partners become familiar with each other. The diminishing of passionate love often creates stress between partners (usually affecting one partner more than the other) and can be experienced as a crisis in the relationship. If a quieter, more lasting love fails to emerge, the relationship will likely break up, and each person will search for another who will once again ignite his or her passion.

The key to developing and maintaining any type of friendship or intimate relationship is good communication. Miscommunication creates frustration and distances us from our friends and partners. (For more information, see the section "Communication" later in this chapter.)

Counterproductive Strategies for Coping with Stress

IN FOCUS

College students develop a variety of habits in response to stress—some of them ineffective and even unhealthy. Here are a few unhealthy coping techniques to avoid:

- ***Alcohol.*** A few drinks might make you feel at ease, and getting drunk may help you forget the stress in your life—but any relief alcohol provides is temporary. Binge drinking and excessive alcohol consumption are not effective ways to handle stress, and using alcohol to deal with stress puts you at risk for all the short- and long-term problems associated with alcohol abuse.
- ***Tobacco.*** The nicotine in cigarettes and other tobacco products can make you feel relaxed and may even increase your ability to concentrate. Tobacco, however, is highly addictive, and smoking causes cancer, heart disease, sexual problems, and many other health problems. Tobacco use is the leading preventable cause of death in the United States.
- ***Other drugs.*** Altering your body chemistry to cope with stress is a strategy with many pitfalls. Caffeine, for example, raises cortisol levels and blood pressure and can disrupt sleep. Marijuana can elicit panic attacks with repeated use, and some research suggests that it heightens the body's stress response.
- ***Binge eating.*** Eating can induce relaxation, which reduces stress. Eating as a means of coping with stress, however, may lead to weight gain and to binge eating, a risky behavior associated with eating disorders.

There is one other problem with these methods of fighting stress: None of them addresses the actual cause of the stress in your life. To combat stress in a healthy way, learn some of the stress-management techniques described in this chapter.

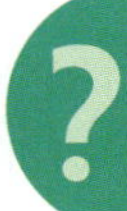

Ask Yourself

QUESTIONS FOR CRITICAL THINKING AND REFLECTION

What are the top two or three stressors in your life right now? Are they new to your life—as part of your college experience—or are they stressors you've experienced in the past? Do they include both positive and negative experiences (eustress and distress)?

Other Stressors

Environmental stressors—external conditions or events that cause stress—include loud noises, unpleasant smells, industrial accidents, violence, and natural disasters. (See Appendix A for preparation and coping strategies for large-scale disasters.) Internal stressors are found within ourselves. We put pressure on ourselves to reach personal goals and then evaluate our progress and performance. Physical and emotional states such as illness and exhaustion are also internal stressors.

MANAGING STRESS

What can you do about all this stress? A great deal. By pursuing a wellness lifestyle—being physically active, eating well, getting enough sleep, and so on—and by learning simple ways to identify and moderate individual stressors, you can control the stress in your life. (There are also some stress-management practices you should avoid; see the box "Counterproductive Strategies for Coping with Stress.")

Exercise

Researchers have found that people who exercise regularly react with milder physical stress responses before, during, and after exposure to stressors and that their overall sense of well-being increases as well (see the box "Does Exercise Improve Mental Health?"). Although even light exercise can have a beneficial effect, an integrated fitness program can have a significant impact on stress.

For some people, however, exercise can become just one more stressor in an already-stressful life. People who exercise compulsively risk overtraining, a condition characterized by fatigue, irritability, depression, and diminished athletic performance. An overly strenuous exercise program can even make a person sick by compromising immune function.

Nutrition

A healthy, balanced diet can help you cope with stress. In addition, eating wisely will enhance your feelings of self-control and self-esteem. Avoiding or limiting caffeine is also important in stress management. Although one or two cups of coffee a day probably won't hurt you, caffeine is a mildly addictive stimulant that leaves some people jittery, irritable, and unable to sleep. Consuming caffeine during stressful situations can raise blood pressure and increase levels of cortisol. (For more on sound nutrition and for advice on evaluating dietary supplements, many of which are marketed for stress, see Chapter 3.)

THE EVIDENCE FOR EXERCISE

Does Exercise Improve Mental Health?

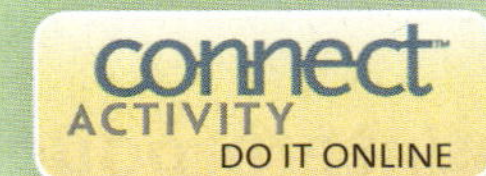

Since 1995, more than 30 major population-based studies (involving 175,000 Americans) have been published on the association between physical activity and mental health. The overall conclusion is that exercise—even modest activity such as taking a daily walk—can help combat a variety of mental health problems. For example, studies found that regular physical activity protects against depression and the onset of major depressive disorder; it can also reduce symptoms of depression in otherwise healthy people. Other studies found that physical activity protects against anxiety and the onset of anxiety disorders (such as specific phobia, social phobia, generalized anxiety, and panic disorder); it also helps reduce symptoms in people affected with anxiety disorders.

Physical activity can enhance feelings of well-being in some people, which may provide some protection against psychological distress. Overall, physically active people are about 25–30% less likely to feel distressed than inactive people. Regardless of the number, age, or health status of the people being studied, those who were active managed stress better than their inactive counterparts.

Researchers have also looked at specific aspects of the activity-stress association. For example, one study found that taking a long walk can be effective at reducing anxiety and blood pressure. Another showed that a brisk walk of as little as 10 minutes' duration can leave people feeling more relaxed and energetic for up to 2 hours. People who took three brisk 45-minute walks each week for 3 months reported that they perceived fewer daily hassles and had a greater sense of general wellness.

The findings are not surprising. The stress response mobilizes energy resources and readies the body for physical emergencies. If you experience stress and do not exert yourself physically, you are not completing the energy cycle. You may not be able to exercise while your daily stressors are occurring, but you can be active later in the day. Such activity allows you to expend the nervous energy you have built up and trains your body to return more readily to homeostasis after stressful situations.

Physical activity also helps you sleep better, and consistently sound sleep is critical to managing stress. According to the National Sleep Foundation, about two-thirds of Americans have trouble sleeping at least a few nights a week, and about 40% say they have difficulty sleeping virtually every night. There are about 70 known sleep disorders, and disordered sleep is associated with a variety of physical and neurological problems, including health problems relating to stress. Although only a few small-scale studies have been done on the relationship between physical activity and sleep, most experts have concluded that regular activity promotes better sleep and provides some protection against sleep interruptions such as insomnia and sleep apnea. Consistent, restful sleep is now regarded as a protective factor in disorders such as depression, anxiety, obesity, and heart disease.

SOURCES: Physical Activity Guidelines Advisory Committee. 2008. *Physical Activity Guidelines Advisory Committee Report, 2008*. Washington, D.C.: U.S. Department of Health and Human Services. National Sleep Foundation. 2011. *2011 Sleep in America Poll: Summary of Findings*. Washington, D.C.: National Sleep Foundation.

Sleep

Most adults need 7–9 hours of sleep every night to stay healthy and perform their best. Getting enough sleep isn't just good for you physically; adequate sleep also improves mood, fosters feelings of competence and self-worth, enhances mental functioning, and supports emotional functioning.

Sleep and Stress Stress hormone levels in the bloodstream vary throughout the day and are related to sleep patterns. Peak concentrations of these hormones occur in the early morning, followed by a slow decline during the day and evening. Concentrations return to peak levels during the final stages of sleep and in the early morning hours.

Even though stress hormones are released during sleep, it is the lack of sleep that has the greatest impact on stress. In someone who is suffering from sleep deprivation (not getting enough sleep over time), mental and physical processes deteriorate steadily. A sleep-deprived person experiences headaches, feels irritable, is unable to concentrate, and is more prone to forgetfulness. Poor-quality sleep has long been associated with stress and depression. A small 2008 study of female college students further associated sleep deprivation with an increased risk of suicide.

Acute sleep deprivation slows the daytime decline in stress hormones, so evening levels are higher than normal. A decrease in total sleep time also causes an increase in the level of stress hormones. Together, these changes may cause an increase in stress hormone levels throughout the day and may contribute to physical and mental exhaustion. Extreme sleep deprivation can lead to hallucinations and other psychotic symptoms, as well as to a significant increase in heart attack risk.

Sleep Disorders According to the National Sleep Foundation's 2011 *Sleep in America Poll,* adults sleep just under 7 hours per night during the week, on average. (Compare this to the recommended 7–9 hours per night.) Many Americans cope with lack of sleep by trying to get extra sleep on the weekends, by napping, and by consuming lots of caffeine during the day. As many as 70 million Americans suffer from chronic sleep disorders—medical conditions that prevent them from sleeping well.

Building Social Support

TAKE CHARGE

Meaningful connections with others can play a key role in stress management and overall wellness. A sense of isolation can lead to chronic stress, which in turn can increase one's susceptibility to temporary illnesses like colds and to chronic illnesses like heart disease. Although the mechanism isn't clear, social isolation can be as significant to mortality rates as factors like smoking, high blood pressure, and obesity.

There is no single best pattern of social support that works for everyone. However, research suggests that having a variety of types of relationships may be important for wellness. Here are some tips for strengthening your social ties:

- ***Foster friendships.*** Keep in regular contact with your friends. Offer respect, trust, and acceptance, and provide help and support in times of need. Express appreciation for your friends.
- ***Keep your family ties strong.*** Stay in touch with the family members you feel close to. If your family doesn't function well as a support system for its members, create a second "family" of people with whom you have built meaningful ties.
- ***Get involved with a group.*** Do volunteer work, take a class, attend a lecture series, or join a religious group. These types of activities can give you a sense of security, a place to talk about your feelings or concerns, and a way to build new friendships. Choose activities that are meaningful to you and that include direct involvement with other people.
- ***Build your communication skills.*** The more you share your feelings with others, the closer the bonds between you will become. When others are speaking, be a considerate and attentive listener.

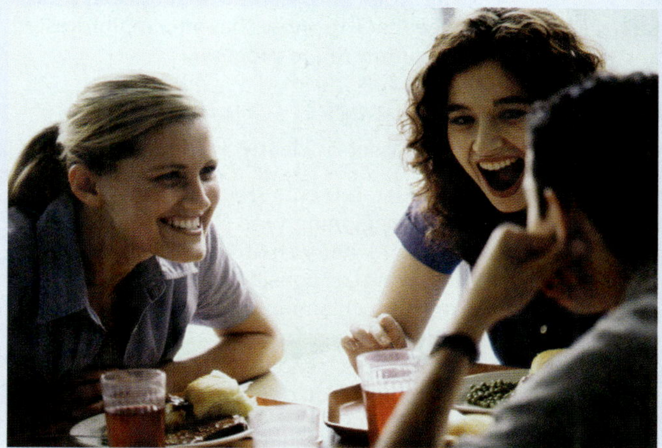

SOURCE: Friends Can Be Good Medicine. 1998. As found in the *Mind/Body Newsletter* 7(1): 3–6.

According to the Institute of Medicine, more than 50% of adults suffer from *insomnia*—trouble falling asleep or staying asleep. The most common causes of insomnia are lifestyle factors, such as high caffeine or alcohol intake before bedtime; medical problems, such as a breathing disorder; and stress. About 75% of people who suffer from chronic insomnia report some stressful life event at the onset of their sleeping problems.

Another type of chronic sleep problem, called *sleep apnea*, occurs when a person stops breathing while asleep (Figure 10.4). Apnea can be caused by a number of factors, but it typically results when the soft tissue at the back of the mouth (such as the tongue or soft palate) "collapses" during sleep, blocking the airway. When breathing is interrupted, so is sleep, as the sleeper awakens repeatedly throughout the night to begin breathing again. In most cases, this occurs without the sleeper even being aware of it. However, the disruption to sleep can be significant, and over time acute sleep deprivation can result from apnea. There are several treatments for apnea, including medications, special devices that help keep the airway open during sleep, and surgery.

Social Support

Sharing fears, frustrations, and joys makes life richer and seems to contribute to the well-being of body and mind. One study of college students living in overcrowded apartments, for example, found that those with a strong social support system were less distressed by their cramped quarters than were the loners who navigated life's challenges on their own. Other studies have shown that married people live longer than single people and have lower death rates from a wide range of conditions. And people infected with HIV remain symptom-free longer if they have a strong social support network. For more on developing and maintaining your social network, see the box "Building Social Support."

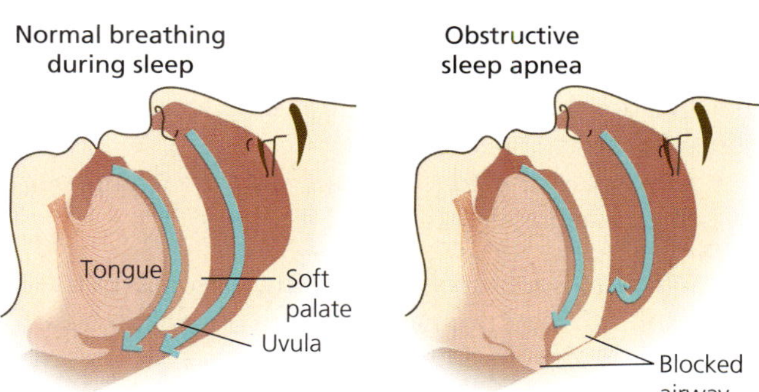

FIGURE 10.4 Sleep apnea.
Sleep apnea occurs when soft tissues surrounding the airway relax, "collapsing" the airway and restricting airflow.

TAKE CHARGE

Guidelines for Effective Communication

Getting Started

- When you want to have a serious discussion with your partner, choose an appropriate time and place. Find a private place and a time when you will not be interrupted.
- Face your partner and maintain eye contact. Use nonverbal feedback to show that you are interested and involved in the communication process.

Being an Effective Speaker

- State your concern or issue as clearly as you can.
- Use "I" statements—statements about how *you* feel—rather than statements beginning with "You," which tell another person how you think he or she feels. When you use "I" statements, you are taking responsibility for your feelings. "You" statements are often blaming or accusatory and will probably get a defensive or resentful response. The statement "I feel unloved," for example, sends a clearer, less blaming message than the statement "You don't love me."
- Focus on a specific behavior rather than on the whole person. Be specific about the behavior you like or don't like. Avoid generalizations beginning with "You always" or "You never." Such statements make people feel defensive.
- Make constructive requests. Opening your request with "I would like" keeps the focus on your needs rather than your partner's supposed deficiencies.
- Avoid blaming, accusing, and belittling. Even if you are right, you have little to gain by putting your partner down. Studies have shown that when people feel criticized or attacked, they are less able to think rationally or solve problems constructively.
- Ask for action ahead of time. Tell your partner what you would like to have happen in the future; don't wait for him or her to blow it and then express anger or disappointment.

Being an Effective Listener

- Provide appropriate nonverbal feedback (nodding, smiling, and so on).
- Don't interrupt.
- Develop the skill of reflective listening. Don't judge, evaluate, analyze, or offer solutions (unless asked to do so). Your partner may just need to have you there in order to sort out feelings. By jumping in right away to "fix" the problem, you may be cutting off communication.
- Don't give unsolicited advice. Giving advice implies that you know more about what a person needs to do than he or she does; therefore, it often evokes anger or resentment.
- Clarify your understanding of what your partner is saying by restating it in your own words and asking if your understanding is correct.
- Be sure you are really listening, not off somewhere in your mind rehearsing your reply. Try to tune in to your partner's feelings as well as the words.
- Let your partner know that you value what she or he is saying and want to understand. Respect for the other person is the cornerstone of effective communication.

Communication

Good communication skills can help everyone form and maintain healthy relationships. Communicating in an assertive way that respects the rights of others—as well as your own—can prevent potentially stressful situations from getting out of control. When friends or partners communicate effectively, they can reduce the stresses in their relationship and spend more time focusing on the positive aspects of being together.

Three keys to good communication in relationships are self-disclosure, listening, and feedback.

- ***Self-disclosure*** involves revealing personal information that we ordinarily wouldn't reveal because of the risk involved. It usually increases feelings of closeness and moves the relationship to a deeper level of intimacy.
- ***Listening*** is a rare skill. Good listening skills require that we spend more time and energy trying to fully understand another person's "story" and less time judging, evaluating, blaming, advising, analyzing, or trying to control. Empathy, warmth, respect, and genuineness are qualities of skillful listeners. Attentive listening encourages friends or partners to share more and, in turn, to be attentive listeners. To connect with other people and develop real emotional intimacy, listening is essential.
- ***Feedback,*** a constructive response to another's self-disclosure, is the third key to good communication. Giving positive feedback means acknowledging that the friend's or partner's feelings are valid—no matter how upsetting or troubling—and offering self-disclosure in response. Self-disclosure and feedback can open the door to change, whereas other responses block communication and change.

For tips on improving your skills, see the box "Guidelines for Effective Communication."

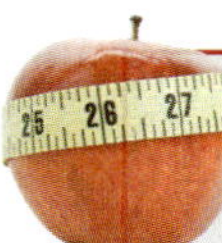

Wellness Tip

In a stressful situation, do you ever stop and count to 10? If not, you should. It works! In the few seconds it takes to count to 10, you can calm your mind, get your breathing under control, slow your heart rate, and lower your blood pressure. In effect, that quick 10-count can offset the stress reaction and help you avoid making things worse.

Some people have trouble either telling others what they need or saying no to the needs of others. They may suppress their feelings of anger, frustration, and resentment, and they may end up feeling taken advantage of or suffering in unhealthy relationships. At the other extreme are people who express anger openly and directly by being verbally or physically aggressive or indirectly by making critical, hurtful comments to others. Their abusive behavior pushes other people away, so they also have problems with relationships.

If you typically suppress your feelings, you might want to take an assertiveness training course that can help you identify and change your patterns of communication. If you have trouble controlling your anger, you can benefit from learning anger management strategies; see the box "Dealing with Anger."

Conflict Resolution

Conflict is natural in any relationship, and it can become a key source of stress for friends, coworkers, family members, and intimate partners. No matter how close two people become, they still remain separate individuals with their own needs, desires, past experiences, and ways of seeing the world. Conflict itself isn't dangerous to a relationship; it may simply indicate that the relationship is growing. But if it isn't handled in a constructive way, conflict can damage—and ultimately destroy—a relationship.

Conflict is often accompanied by anger—a natural emotion, but one that can be difficult to handle. When angry, both parties should back off until they calm down and then come back to the issue later and try to resolve it rationally. Negotiation will help dissipate the anger so the conflict can be resolved. Some basic strategies are useful in successfully negotiating with a friend, family member, colleague, or intimate partner:

1. ***Clarify the issue.*** Take responsibility for thinking through your feelings and discovering what's really bothering you. Agree that one of you will speak first and have the chance to speak fully while the other listens. Then reverse the roles. Try to understand the other person's position fully by repeating what you've heard and asking questions to clarify or elicit more information.
2. ***Find out what each person wants.*** Ask the other person to express her or his desires. Don't assume you already know what those desires are, and don't try to speak for your friend or partner.
3. ***Determine how you both can get what you want.*** Brainstorm to generate a variety of options.
4. ***Decide how to negotiate.*** Work out a plan for change. For example, agree that one of you will do one task and the other will do another task or that one of you will do a task in exchange for something she or he wants.
5. ***Solidify the agreements.*** Go over the plan verbally and write it down, if necessary, to ensure that you both understand and agree to it.
6. ***Review and renegotiate.*** Decide on a time frame for trying out the new plan and set a time to discuss how it's working. Make adjustments as needed.

Striving for Spiritual Wellness

Spiritual wellness is associated with greater coping skills and higher levels of overall wellness. It is a very personal wellness component, and there are many ways to develop it. Researchers have linked spiritual wellness to longer life expectancy, reduced risk of disease, faster recovery, and improved emotional health. Although spirituality is difficult to study, and researchers aren't sure how or why spirituality seems to improve health, several explanations have been offered. Lab 10.3 includes exercises designed to help you build spiritual wellness.

Confiding in Yourself Through Writing

Keeping a diary is like confiding in someone else, except that you are confiding in yourself. This form of coping with severe stress may be especially helpful for those who are shy or introverted and find it difficult to open up to others. Although writing about traumatic and stressful events may have a short-term negative effect on mood, over the long term, stress is reduced and positive changes in health occur. A key to promoting health and well-being through journaling is to write about your emotional responses to stressful events. Set aside a special time each day or week to write down your feelings about stressful events in your life.

Time Management

Learning to manage your time can be crucial to coping with everyday stressors. Overcommitment, procrastination, and even boredom are significant stressors for many people. Along with gaining control of nutrition and exercise to maintain a healthy energy balance, time management is an

TAKE CHARGE

Dealing with Anger

Anger is a natural response to something we perceive as an injustice, a betrayal, an insult, or some other wrong—whether real or imagined. We may respond physically with faster heart and breathing rates, muscle tension, trembling, a knot in the stomach or a red face. When anger alerts us that something is wrong, it is a useful emotion that can lead to constructive change. When anger leads to loss of control and to aggression, it causes problems.

According to current popular wisdom, it's healthy to express your feelings, including anger. However, research has shown that people who are overtly hostile are at higher risk for heart disease and heart attacks than calmer people. In addition, expressing anger in thoughtless or out-of-control ways can damage personal and professional relationships.

People who experience rage or explosive anger are particularly at risk for negative repercussions. Some of these people may have *intermittent explosive disorder,* characterized by aggressiveness that is impulsive and out of proportion to the stimulus. Explosive anger renders people temporarily unable to think straight or act in their own best interests. Counseling can help very angry people learn how to manage their anger.

In dealing with anger, it is important to distinguish between a reasonable degree of self-assertiveness and a gratuitous expression of aggression. When you are *assertive,* you stand up for your own rights at the same time that you respect the rights of others. When you are *aggressive,* you violate the rights of others.

Managing Your Own Anger

What are the best ways to handle anger? If you find yourself in a situation where you are getting angry, answer these questions:

- Is the situation important enough to get angry about?
- Are you truly justified in getting angry?
- Is expressing your anger going to make a positive difference?

If the answer to all these questions is yes, then calm, assertive communication may be appropriate. Use "I" statements to express your feelings ("I would like . . . ," "I feel . . ."), and listen respectfully to the other person's point of view. Don't attack verbally or make demands; try to negotiate a constructive, mutually satisfying solution.

If you answer no to any of the questions, try to calm yourself. First, reframe the situation by thinking about it differently. Try these strategies:

- Don't take it personally—maybe the driver who cut you off simply didn't see you.
- Look for mitigating factors—maybe the classmate who didn't say hello was preoccupied with money concerns.
- Practice empathy—try to see the situation from the other person's point of view.
- Ask questions—clarify the situation by asking what the other person meant. Avoid defensiveness.
- Focus on the present—don't let this situation trigger thoughts of past incidents that you perceive as similar.

Second, calm your body down.

- Use the old trick of counting to 10 before you respond.
- Concentrate on your breathing, and take long, slow breaths.
- Imagine yourself in a beautiful, peaceful place.
- If needed, take a longer cooling-off period by leaving the situation until your anger has subsided.

Dealing with Other People's Anger

If someone you are with becomes very angry, try these strategies:

- Respond asymmetrically—remain calm. Don't get angry in response.
- Apologize if you think you are to blame. (Don't apologize if you don't think you are to blame.)
- Validate the other person by acknowledging that he or she has some reason to be angry. However, don't accept verbal abuse.
- Focus on the problem and ask what can be done to alleviate the situation.
- If the person cannot be calmed, disengage from the situation, at least temporarily. After a time-out, attempts at rational problem solving may be more successful.

Warning Signs of Violence

Violence is never acceptable. The following behaviors over a period of time suggest the potential for violence:

- A history of making threats and engaging in aggressive behavior
- Drug or alcohol abuse
- Gang membership
- Access to or fascination with weapons
- Feelings of rejection or aloneness; the feeling of constantly being disrespected; victimization by bullies
- Withdrawal from usual activities and friends; poor school performance
- Failure to acknowledge the rights of others

The following are immediate warning signs of violence:

- Daily loss of temper or frequent physical fighting
- Significant vandalism or property damage
- Increased risk-taking behavior; increased drug or alcohol abuse
- Threats or detailed plans to commit acts of violence
- Pleasure in hurting animals
- The presence of weapons

Don't spend time with someone who shows these warning signs of violence. Don't carry a weapon or resort to violence to protect yourself. Ask someone in authority or an experienced professional for help.

important element in a wellness program. Try these strategies for improving your time-management skills:

- ***Set priorities.*** Divide your tasks into three groups: essential, important, and trivial. Focus on the first two, and ignore the third.
- ***Schedule tasks for peak efficiency.*** You probably know that you're most productive at certain times of the day (or night). Schedule as many of your tasks for those hours as you can, and stick to your schedule.
- ***Set realistic goals and write them down.*** Attainable goals spur you on. Impossible goals, by definition, cause frustration and failure. Fully commit yourself to achieving your goals by putting them in writing.
- ***Budget enough time.*** For each project you undertake, calculate how much time you will need to finish it. Then tack on another 10–15%, or even 25%, as a buffer.
- ***Break up long-term goals into short-term ones.*** Instead of waiting for large blocks of time, use short amounts of time to start a project or keep it moving.
- ***Visualize achieving your goal.*** By mentally rehearsing a task, you will be able to do it more smoothly.
- ***Keep track of the tasks you put off.*** Analyze the reasons you procrastinate. If the task is difficult or unpleasant, look for ways to make it easier or more fun. For example, if you find the readings for one of your classes particularly difficult, choose an especially nice setting for your reading, and then reward yourself each time you complete a section or chapter.
- ***Consider doing your least favorite tasks first.*** Once you have the most unpleasant ones out of the way, you can work on the tasks you enjoy more.
- ***Consolidate tasks when possible.*** For example, try walking to the store so that you run your errands and exercise in the same block of time.
- ***Identify quick transitional tasks.*** Keep a list of 5- to 10-minute tasks you can do while waiting or between other tasks, such as watering your plants, doing the dishes, or checking a homework assignment.
- ***Delegate responsibility.*** Asking for help when you have too much to do is no cop-out; it's good time management. Just don't delegate the jobs you know you should do yourself.
- ***Say no when necessary.*** If the demands made on you don't seem reasonable, say no—tactfully, but without guilt or apology.
- ***Give yourself a break.*** Allow time for play—free, unstructured time when you can ignore the clock. Don't consider this a waste of time. Play renews you and enables you to work more efficiently.

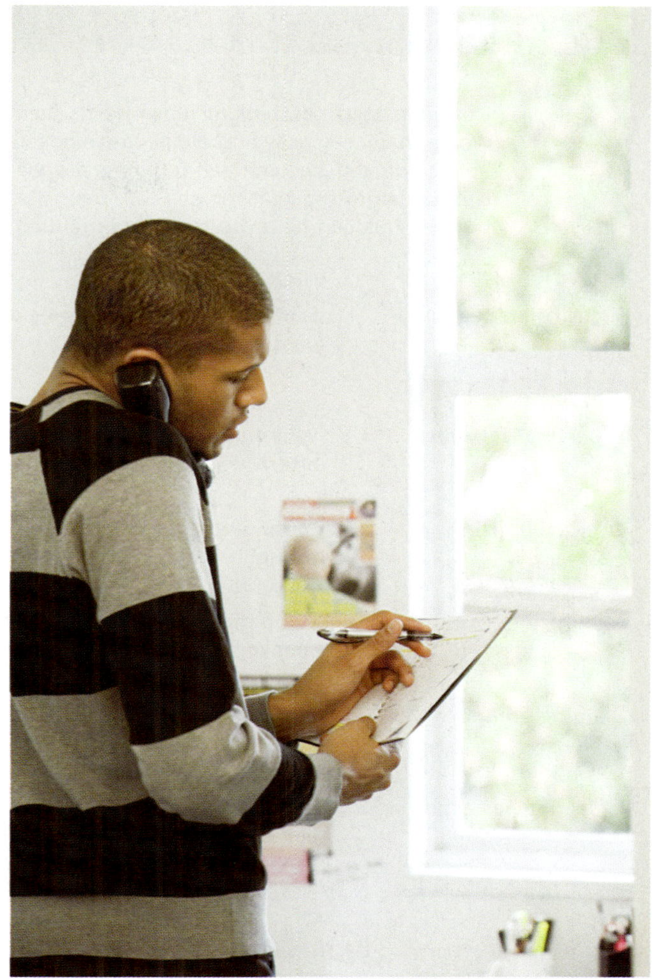
Time-management skills, including careful scheduling with a datebook or computer, can help people cope with busy days.

- ***Avoid your personal "time sinks."*** You can probably identify your own time sinks—activities like watching television, surfing the Internet, or talking on the phone that consistently use up more time than you anticipate and put you behind schedule. Some days, it may be best to avoid problematic activities altogether; for example, if you have a big paper due, don't sit down for a 5-minute TV break if it is likely to turn into a 2-hour break. Try a 5-minute walk if you need to clear your head.
- ***Stop thinking or talking about what you're going to do, and just do it!*** Sometimes the best solution for procrastination is to stop waiting for the right moment and just get started. You will probably find that things are not as bad as you feared, and your momentum will keep you going.

TAKE CHARGE

Realistic Self-Talk

Do your patterns of thinking make events seem worse than they truly are? Do negative beliefs about yourself become self-fulfilling prophecies? Substituting realistic self-talk for negative self-talk can help you build and maintain self-esteem and cope better with the challenges in your life. Here are some examples of common types of distorted, negative self-talk, along with suggestions for more accurate and rational responses.

COGNITIVE DISTORTION	NEGATIVE SELF-TALK	REALISTIC SELF-TALK
Focusing on negatives	School is so discouraging—nothing but one hassle after another.	School is pretty challenging and has its difficulties, but there certainly are rewards. It's really a mixture of good and bad.
Expecting the worst	Why would my boss want to meet with me this afternoon if not to fire me?	I wonder why my boss wants to meet with me? I guess I'll just have to wait and see.
Overgeneralizing	[*After getting a poor grade on a paper*] Just as I thought—I'm incompetent at everything.	I'll start working on the next paper earlier. That way, if I run into problems I'll have time to talk to the TA.
Minimizing	I won the speech contest, but none of the other speakers was very good. I wouldn't have done as well against stiffer competition.	It may not have been the best speech I'll ever give, but it was good enough to win the contest.
Blaming others	I wouldn't have eaten so much last night if my friends hadn't insisted on going to that restaurant.	I overdid it last night. Next time I'll make different choices.
Expecting perfection	I should have scored 100% on this test. I can't believe I missed that one problem through a careless mistake.	Too bad I missed one problem through carelessness, but overall I did very well on this test. Next time I'll be more careful.

SOURCE: Based on W. Schafer. 1999. *Stress Management for Wellness,* 4th ed. Copyright © 2000 Wadsworth, a part of Cengage Learning, Inc. Reproduced by permission. www.cengage.com/permissions.

For more help with time management, complete Activity 10 in the Behavior Change Workbook.

Cognitive Techniques

Certain thought patterns and ways of thinking, including ideas, beliefs, and perceptions, can contribute to stress and have a negative impact on health. But other habits of mind, if practiced with patience and consistency, can help break unhealthy thought patterns. Below are some suggestions for changing destructive thinking:

- Monitor your self-talk and try to minimize hostile, critical, suspicious, and self-deprecating thoughts (see the box "Realistic Self-Talk").
- Modify your expectations. They often restrict experience and lead to disappointment. Try to accept life as it comes.
- Live in the present. Clear your mind of old debris and fears so you can enjoy life as it is now.
- Go with the flow. Accept what you can't change, forgive others for their faults, and be flexible.

Cultivating your sense of humor is another key cognitive stress-management technique. Even a fleeting smile produces changes in your autonomic nervous system that can lift your spirits. Hearty laughter triggers the release of endorphins, and after a good laugh, your muscles go slack and your pulse and blood pressure dip below normal; you are relaxed.

Relaxation Techniques

The **relaxation response** is a physiological state characterized by a feeling of warmth and quiet mental alertness. This state is the opposite of the fight-or-flight response. When you induce the relaxation response by using a relaxation technique, your heart rate, breathing, and metabolism slow down. Blood pressure and oxygen consumption decrease. At the same time, blood flow to the brain and skin increases, and brain waves shift from an alert beta rhythm to a relaxed alpha rhythm.

The techniques described in this section are among the most popular techniques and the easiest to learn; also, see

Solving Problems

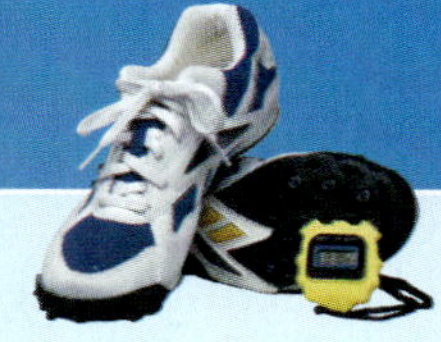

PERSONAL CHALLENGE

Got a problem that's stressing you out? Solve it! Problem solving is a skill—one that requires practice and patience, but one that can pay off in a more balanced, less stressful life. Think of a problem that's bugging you right now, and take the following steps to solve it:

1. Define the problem in a sentence or two. Write it down.
2. List the problem's cause. There may be more than one.
3. List some potential solutions. Don't stop with one or the most obvious one. Write down several options.
4. For each solution, list the potential positive and negative consequences. Be thorough.
5. Choose the solution you think will work best, or will have the fewest negative consequences.
6. List the steps you'll need to take to carry out your solution.
7. Get started with the list of steps you just made. Don't delay unless you have to.
8. As you work on solving the problem, pause occasionally and reevaluate. Revise your approach, if necessary.

If you can't seem to solve a problem on your own, get help. Talk to someone who knows you well, or get help from a counselor, and work through these steps again. Any problem can be solved, but some may just be too big to handle on your own.

the box "Relaxing Through Meditation." All these techniques take practice, so it may be several weeks before the benefits become noticeable in everyday life.

Progressive Relaxation In this simple relaxation technique, you tense and then relax the muscles of the body one group at a time. Also known as deep muscle relaxation, this technique addresses the muscle tension that occurs when the body is experiencing stress. Consciously relaxing tensed muscles sends a message to other body systems to reduce the stress response.

To practice progressive relaxation, begin by inhaling as you contract your right fist. Then exhale as you release your fist. Repeat. Contract and relax your right bicep. Repeat. Do the same using your left arm. Then, working from forehead to feet, contract and relax other muscles. Repeat each contraction at least once, inhaling as you tense and exhaling as you relax. To speed up the process, tense and relax more muscles at one time—for example, both arms simultaneously. With practice, you'll be able to relax quickly just by clenching and releasing only your fists.

Visualization Also known as imagery, visualization is so effective in enhancing sports performance that it has become part of the curriculum at training camps for U.S. Olympic athletes. This same technique can be used to induce relaxation, to help change habits, and to improve performance on an exam, on stage, or on a playing field.

To practice visualization, imagine yourself floating on a cloud, sitting on a mountaintop, or lying in a meadow. Try to identify all the perceptible qualities of the environment—sight, sound, temperature, smell, and so on. Your body will respond as if your imagery were real.

An alternative is to close your eyes and imagine a deep purple light filling your body. Then change the color to a soothing gold. As the color lightens, so should your distress. Imagery can also enhance performance: Visualize yourself succeeding at a task that worries you.

Deep Breathing Your breathing pattern is closely tied to your stress level. Deep, slow breathing is associated with relaxation. Rapid, shallow, often irregular breathing occurs during the stress response. With practice, you can learn to slow and quiet your breathing pattern, thereby

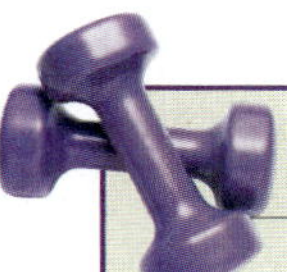

Fitness Tip

Activities like yoga and tai chi are well known for their relaxing, meditative aspects. But they're great workouts, too. If you're looking for a way to improve your flexibility and muscle tone while exercising in a quiet, pressure-free environment, check out a local yoga or tai chi class. Be sure the class is led by a qualified professional.

KEY TERM

relaxation response A physiological state characterized by a feeling of warmth and quiet mental alertness.

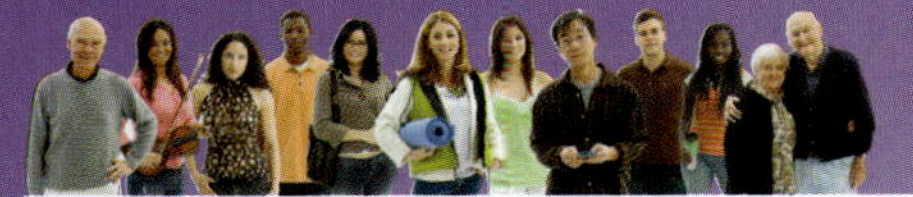

Relaxing Through Meditation

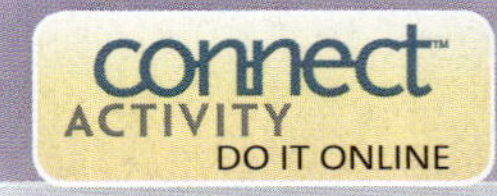

DIMENSIONS OF DIVERSITY

Techniques for managing stress by inducing the relaxation response have been developed in many cultures over the centuries. One such technique is yoga, described in Chapter 5. Another technique that has become popular in the United States is meditation.

At its most basic level, meditation, or self-reflective thought, involves quieting or emptying the mind to achieve deep relaxation. Some practitioners of meditation view it on a deeper level as a means of focusing concentration, increasing self-awareness, and bringing enlightenment to their lives. Meditation has been integrated into the practices of several religions—Buddhism, Hinduism, Confucianism, Taoism—but it is not a religion itself, nor does its practice require any special knowledge, belief, or background.

There are many styles of meditation, based on different ways of quieting the mind. Here is a simple, practical technique for eliciting the relaxation response using one style:

1. Pick a word, a phrase, or an object to focus on. You can choose a word or phrase that has a deep meaning for you, but any word or phrase will work. Some meditators prefer to focus on their breathing.
2. Sit comfortably in a quiet place. Close your eyes if you're not focusing on an object.
3. Relax your muscles.
4. Breathe slowly and naturally. If you're using a focus word or phrase, silently repeat it each time you exhale. If you're using an object, focus on it as you breathe.
5. Keep your attitude passive. Disregard thoughts that drift in.
6. Continue for 10–20 minutes once or twice a day.
7. After you've finished, sit quietly for a few minutes with your eyes closed, then open. Then stand up.

Allow relaxation to occur at its own pace; don't force it. Don't be surprised if you can't tune your mind out for more than a few seconds at a time. It's nothing to get angry about. The more you ignore the intrusions, the easier it will become. If you want to time your session, peek at a watch or clock occasionally, but don't set a jarring alarm.

Although you'll feel refreshed even after the first session, it may take a month or more to get noticeable results. Be patient. Eventually, the relaxation response becomes so natural that it occurs spontaneously or on demand when you sit quietly for a few moments.

also quieting your mind and relaxing your body. Try one of the breathing techniques described in the box "Breathing for Relaxation" for on-the-spot tension relief, as well as for long-term stress reduction.

Listening to Music Music can relax us. It influences pulse, blood pressure, and the electrical activity of muscles. Listening to soothing, lyrical music can lessen depression, anxiety, and stress levels. To experience the stress-management benefits of music, set aside a period of at least 15 minutes to listen quietly. Choose music you enjoy and selections that make you feel relaxed.

Other Stress-Management Techniques

Techniques such as biofeedback, hypnosis and self-hypnosis, and massage require a partner or professional training or assistance. As with the relaxation techniques presented, all take practice, and it may be several weeks before the benefits are noticeable.

Biofeedback helps people reduce their response to stress by enabling them to become more aware of their level of physiological arousal. In biofeedback, some measure of stress—perspiration, heart rate, skin temperature, or muscle tension—is electronically monitored, and feedback is given using sound (a tone or music), light, or a meter or dial. With practice, people begin to exercise conscious control over their physiological stress responses. The point of biofeedback training is to develop the ability to transfer the skill to daily life without the use of electronic equipment.

GETTING HELP

You can use the principles of behavioral self-management described in Chapter 1 to create a stress-management program tailored specifically to your needs. The starting point of a successful program is to listen to your body. When you learn to recognize the stress response and the emotions and thoughts that accompany it, you'll be in a position to begin handling stress. Labs 10.1 and 10.2 can guide you in identifying and finding ways to cope with stress-inducing situations.

If you feel you need guidance beyond the information in this text, excellent self-help guides can be found in bookstores or the library; helpful Web sites are listed in For Further Exploration at the end of the chapter. Some people also find it helpful to express their feelings in a journal. Grappling with a painful experience in this way provides an emotional release and can help you develop more constructive ways of dealing with similar situations in the future.

Peer Counseling and Support Groups

If you still feel overwhelmed despite efforts to manage your stress, you may want to seek outside help. Peer counseling, often available through the student health

Breathing for Relaxation

IN FOCUS

Controlled breathing can do more than just help you relax. It can also help control pain, anxiety, and other conditions that lead to or are related to stress. There are many methods of controlled breathing. Two of the most popular are belly breathing and tension-release breathing.

Belly Breathing

1. Lie on your back and relax.
2. Place one hand on your chest and the other on your abdomen. Your hands will help you gauge your breathing.
3. Take in a slow, deep breath through your nose and into your belly. Your abdomen should rise significantly (check with your hand); your chest should rise only slightly. Focus on filling your abdomen with air.
4. Exhale through your mouth, gently pushing out the air from your abdomen.

Tension-Release Breathing

1. Lie down or sit in a chair and get comfortable.
2. Take a slow, deep breath into your abdomen. Inhale through your nose. Try to visualize the air moving to every part of your body. As you breathe in, say to yourself, "Breathe in relaxation."
3. Exhale through your mouth. Visualize tension leaving your body. Say to yourself, "Breathe out tension."

These techniques have many variations. For example, sit in a chair and raise your arms, shoulders, and chin as you inhale; lower them as you exhale. Or slowly count to 4 as you inhale, then again as you exhale.

Many yoga experts suggest breathing rhythmically, in time with your own heartbeat. Relax and listen closely for the sensation of your heart beating, or monitor your pulse while you breathe. As you inhale, count to 4 or 8 in time with your heartbeat, then repeat the count as you exhale. Breathing in time with soothing music can work well, too.

Experts suggest inhaling through the nose and exhaling through the mouth. Breathe slowly, deeply, and gently. To focus on breathing gently, imagine a candle burning a few inches in front of you. Try to exhale softly enough to make the candle's flame flicker, not hard enough to blow it out.

Practice is important, too. Perform your chosen breathing exercise two or more times daily, for 5–10 minutes per session.

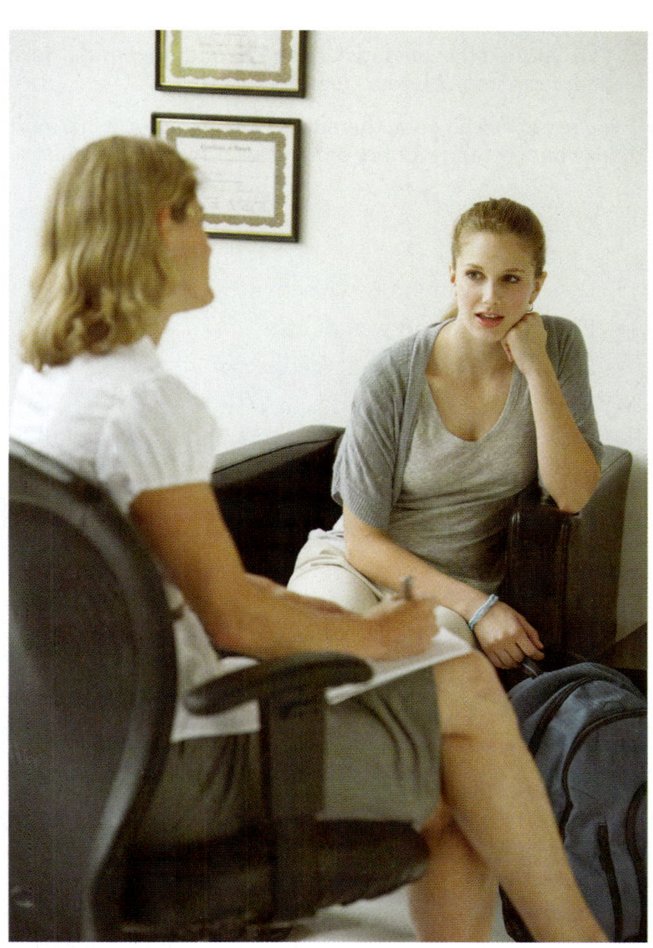

Many people seek help from professional therapists when dealing with stress-related problems.

center or counseling center, is usually staffed by volunteer students with special training that emphasizes maintaining confidentiality. Peer counselors can steer those seeking help to appropriate campus and community resources or just offer sympathetic listening.

Support groups are typically organized around a particular issue or problem: All group members might be entering a new school, reentering school after an interruption, struggling with single parenting, experiencing eating disorders, or coping with particular kinds of trauma. Simply voicing concerns that others share can relieve stress.

Professional Help

Psychotherapy, especially a short-term course of sessions, can also be tremendously helpful in dealing with stress-related problems. Not all therapists are right for all people, so it's a good idea to shop around for a compatible psychotherapist with reasonable fees. (See the box "Choosing and Evaluating Mental Health Professionals.")

Is It Stress or Something More Serious?

Most of us have periods of feeling down when we become pessimistic, anxious, less energetic, and less able to enjoy life. Such feelings and thoughts can be normal responses to the ordinary challenges of life. Symptoms that may indicate a more serious problem include the following:

- Depression, anxiety, or other emotional problems begin to interfere seriously with school or work performance or in getting along with others.

CRITICAL CONSUMER

Choosing and Evaluating Mental Health Professionals

College students are usually in a good position to find convenient, affordable mental health care. Larger schools typically have health services that employ psychiatrists and psychologists as well as counseling centers staffed by professionals and peer counselors. Resources in the community may include a school of medicine, a hospital, and a variety of professionals who work independently. It's a good idea to get recommendations from physicians, friends who have been in therapy, or community agencies, rather than to pick a counselor or therapist at random.

Financial considerations are also important. Find out the cost of different services and what your health insurance will cover. If you're not adequately covered by a health plan, don't let that stop you from getting help; investigate low-cost alternatives on campus and in your community. The cost of treatment is linked to how many therapy sessions will be needed, which in turn depends on the type of therapy and the nature of the problem. Psychological therapies focusing on specific problems may require eight or ten sessions at weekly intervals. Therapies aiming for psychological awareness and personality change can last months or years.

Deciding whether a therapist is right for you requires meeting the therapist in person. Before or during your first meeting, find out about the therapist's background and training:

- Does she or he have a degree from an appropriate professional school and a state license to practice?
- Has she or he had experience treating people with problems similar to yours?
- How much will therapy cost?

You have a right to know the answers to these questions and should not hesitate to ask them. After your initial meeting, evaluate your impressions:

- Does the therapist seem like a warm, intelligent person who would be able to help you and is interested in doing so?
- Are you comfortable with the personality, values, and beliefs of the therapist?
- Is the therapist willing to talk about the techniques he or she will use? Do these techniques make sense to you?

If you answer yes to these questions, this therapist may be satisfactory for you. If you feel uncomfortable—and if you are not in need of emergency care—it's worthwhile to set up one-time consultations with one or two others before you make up your mind. Take the time to find someone who feels right for you.

Later in your treatment, evaluate your progress:

- Are you being helped by the treatment?
- If you are displeased, is it because you aren't making progress or because therapy is raising difficult, painful issues you don't want to deal with?
- Can you express dissatisfaction to your therapist? Such feedback can improve your treatment.

If you're convinced your therapy isn't working or is harmful, thank your therapist for her or his efforts and find another.

- Suicide is attempted or is seriously considered.
- Symptoms such as hallucinations, delusions, incoherent speech, or loss of memory occur.
- Alcohol or drugs are used to the extent that they impair normal functioning, finding or taking drugs occupies much of the week, or reducing the dosage leads to psychological or physical withdrawal symptoms.

Depression is of particular concern because severe depression is linked to suicide, one of the leading causes of death among college students. In some cases, depression, like severe stress, is a clear-cut reaction to a specific event, such as losing a loved one or failing in school or work. In other cases, no trigger event is obvious. Symptoms of depression include the following:

- Negative self-concept
- Pervasive feelings of sadness and hopelessness
- Loss of pleasure in usual activities
- Poor appetite and weight loss
- Insomnia or disturbed sleep
- Restlessness or fatigue
- Thoughts of worthlessness and guilt
- Trouble concentrating or making decisions
- Thoughts of death or suicide

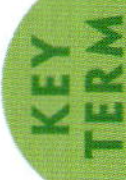

depression A mood disorder characterized by loss of interest, sadness, hopelessness, loss of appetite, disturbed sleep, and other physical symptoms.

Not all of these symptoms are present in everyone who is depressed, but most experience a loss of interest or pleasure in their usual activities. Warning signs of suicide include expressing the wish to be dead, revealing contemplated suicide methods, increasing social withdrawal and isolation, and exhibiting a sudden, inexplicable lightening of mood (which can indicate the person has finally decided to commit suicide).

If you are severely depressed or know someone who is, expert help from a mental health professional is essential. Most communities and many colleges have hotlines and/or health services and counseling centers that can provide help. The National Suicide Prevention Lifeline can be reached at 1-800-273-TALK. Treatments for depression and many other psychological disorders are highly effective.

Ask yourself

QUESTIONS FOR CRITICAL THINKING AND REFLECTION

What percentage of your daily stress is time related? How effective are your time-management skills? Identify one thing you can start doing right now to manage your time better, and describe how you can apply it to one aspect of your daily routine.

TIPS FOR TODAY AND THE FUTURE

For the stress you can't avoid, develop a range of stress-management techniques and strategies.

RIGHT NOW YOU CAN

- Practice deep breathing for 5–10 minutes.
- Visualize a relaxing, peaceful place and imagine yourself experiencing it as vividly as possible. Stay there as long as you can.
- Do some stretching exercises.
- Get out your datebook and schedule what you'll be doing the rest of today and tomorrow. Pencil in a short walk and a conversation with a friend.

IN THE FUTURE YOU CAN

- Take a class or workshop, such as one in assertiveness training or time management, that can help you overcome a source of stress.
- Find a way to build relaxing time into every day. Just 15 minutes of meditation, stretching, or deep breathing can induce the relaxation response.

SUMMARY

- Stress is the collective physiological and emotional response to any stressor. Physiological responses to stressors are the same for everyone.
- The autonomic nervous system and the endocrine system are responsible for the body's physical response to stressors. The sympathetic nervous system mobilizes the body and activates key hormones of the endocrine system, causing the fight-or-flight reaction. The parasympathetic system returns the body to homeostasis.
- Behavioral responses to stress are controlled by the somatic nervous system and fall under a person's conscious control.
- The general adaptation syndrome model and research in psychoneuroimmunology contribute to our understanding of the links between stress and disease. People who have many stressors in their lives or who handle stress poorly are at risk for cardiovascular disease, impairment of the immune system, and many other problems.
- Potential sources of stress include major life changes, daily hassles, college- and job-related stressors, and interpersonal and social stressors.
- Positive ways of managing stress include regular exercise, good nutrition, support from other people, clear communication, spiritual wellness, effective time management, cognitive techniques, and relaxation techniques.
- If a personal program for stress management doesn't work, peer counseling, support groups, and psychotherapy are available.

FOR FURTHER EXPLORATION

BOOKS

Greenberg, J. 2010. *Comprehensive Stress Management,* 12th ed. New York: McGraw-Hill. *Provides a clear explanation of the physical, psychological, sociological, and spiritual aspects of stress and offers numerous stress-management techniques.*

Kabat-Zinn, J. 2006. *Coming to Our Senses: Healing Ourselves and the World Through Mindfulness.* New York: Hyperion. *Explores the connections among mindfulness, health, and physical and spiritual well-being.*

Pennebaker, J. W. 2004. *Writing to Heal: A Guided Journal for Recovering from Trauma and Emotional Upheaval.* Oakland, Calif.: New Harbinger Press. *Provides information about using journaling to cope with stress.*

Seaward, B. L. 2009. *Managing Stress: Principles and Strategies for Health and Well-Being,* 6th ed. Boston: Jones and Bartlett. *A comprehensive textbook for college students.*

ORGANIZATIONS AND WEB SITES

American Headache Society. Provides information for consumers and clinicians about different types of headaches, their causes, and their treatment.
http://www.americanheadachesociety.org/

The American Institute of Stress. A resource of in-depth information on stress, its causes, and its treatments.
http://www.stress.org

American Psychiatric Association: Healthy Minds, Healthy Lives. Provides information on mental wellness especially for college students.
http://www.healthyminds.org

American Psychological Association. Provides information on stress management and psychological disorders.
http://www.apa.org
http://apa.org/helpcenter

Association for Applied Psychophysiology and Biofeedback. Provides information about biofeedback and referrals to certified biofeedback practitioners.
http://www.aapb.org

Benson-Henry Institute for Mind Body Medicine. Provides information about stress-management and relaxation techniques.
http://www.massgeneral.org/bhi

National Institute of Mental Health (NIMH). Publishes informative brochures about stress and stress management as well as other aspects of mental health.
http://www.nimh.nih.gov

National Sleep Foundation. Provides information about sleep and how to overcome sleep problems such as insomnia, apnea, and jet lag.
http://www.sleepfoundation.org

COMMON QUESTIONS ANSWERED

Q Are there any relaxation techniques I can use in response to an immediate stressor?

A Yes. Try the deep breathing techniques described in the chapter, and try some of the following to see which work best for you:

- Do a full-body stretch while standing or sitting. Stretch your arms out to the sides and then reach them as far as possible over your head. Rotate your body from the waist. Bend over as far as is comfortable for you.
- Do a partial session of progressive muscle relaxation. Tense and then relax some of the muscles in your body. Focus on the muscles that are stiff or tense. Shake out your arms and legs.
- Take a short, brisk walk (3–5 minutes). Breathe deeply.
- Engage in realistic self-talk about the stressor. Mentally rehearse dealing successfully with the stressor. As an alternative, focus your mind on some other activity.
- Briefly reflect on something personally meaningful. In one study of college students, researchers found that self-reflection on important personal values prior to a stressful task reduces the hormonal response to the stressor.

Q Can stress cause headaches?

A Stress is one possible cause of the most common type of headache, the tension headache. About 90% of headaches are tension headaches, characterized by a dull, steady pain, usually on both sides of the head. It may feel as though a band of pressure is tightening around the head, and the pain may extend to the neck and shoulders. Acute tension headaches may last from hours to days, while chronic tension headaches may occur almost every day for months or even years. Stress, poor posture, and immobility are leading causes of tension headaches. There is no cure, but the pain can be relieved with over-the-counter painkillers; many people also try such therapies as massage, relaxation, hot or cold showers, and rest. Stress is also one possible trigger of migraine headaches, which are typically characterized by throbbing pain (often on one side of the head), heightened sensitivity to light and noise, visual disturbances such as flashing lights, nausea, and fatigue.

If your headaches are frequent, keep a journal with details about the events surrounding each one. Are your tension headaches associated with late nights, academic deadlines, or long periods spent sitting at a computer? Are migraines associated with certain foods, stress, fatigue, specific sounds or odors, or (in women) menstruation? If you can identify the stressors or other factors that are consistently associated with your headaches, you can begin to gain more control over the situation. If you suffer persistent tension or migraine headaches, consult your physician.

For more Common Questions Answered about stress, visit the Online Learning Center at www.mhhe.com/fahey.

SELECTED BIBLIOGRAPHY

American College Health Association. 2010. *American College Health Association–National College Health Assessment II Reference Group Executive Summary Spring 2010.* Linthicum, Md.: American College Health Association.

American Psychological Association. 2010. *How Does Stress Affect Us?* (http://www.apa.org/helpcenter/stress-effects.aspx; retrieved March 20, 2011).

American Psychological Association. 2010. *Learning to Deal with Stress* (http://www.apa.org/helpcenter/stress-learning.aspx; retrieved March 20, 2011).

American Psychological Association. 2010. *Mind/Body Health: Stress* (http://www.apa.org/helpcenter/stress.aspx; retrieved March 20, 2011).

American Psychological Association. 2010. *Stress in America 2010.* Washington, D.C.: American Psychological Association.

Caldwell, K., et al. 2010. Developing mindfulness in college students through movement-based courses: Effects on self-regulatory self-efficacy, mood, stress, and sleep quality. *Journal of American College Health* 58(5): 433–442.

Centers for Disease Control and Prevention. 2010. *Coping with a Disaster or Traumatic Event: Information for Individuals and Families* (http://emergency.cdc.gov/mentalhealth/general.asp; retrieved March 20, 2011).

Cohen, S., W. J. Doyle, and A. Baum. 2006. Socioeconomic status is associated with stress hormones. *Psychosomatic Medicine* 68(3): 414–420.

Freedman, N. 2010. Treatment of obstructive sleep apnea syndrome. *Clinics in Chest Medicine* 31(2): 187–201.

Hefner, J., and D. Eisenberg. 2009. Social support and mental health among college students. *American Journal of Orthopsychiatry* 79(4): 491–499.

Hook, J. N., et al. 2010. Empirically supported religious and spiritual therapies. *Journal of Clinical Psychology* 66(1): 46–72.

Institute of Medicine Committee on Sleep Medicine and Research. 2006. *Sleep Disorders and Sleep Deprivation: An Unmet Public Health Problem*, ed. H. R. Colton and B. M. Altevogt. Washington, D.C.: National Academies Press.

Mayo Foundation for Medical Education and Research. 2008. *Stress: Win Control over the Stress in Your Life* (http://www.mayoclinic.com/health/stress/SR00001; retrieved March 20, 2011).

National Sleep Foundation. 2011. *2011 Sleep in America Poll.* Washington, D.C.: National Sleep Foundation.

Nordboe, D. J., et al. 2007. Immediate behavioral health response to the Virginia Tech shootings. *Disaster Medicine and Public Health Preparedness* 1(Suppl. 1.): S31–S32.

Roddenberry, A., and K. Renk. 2010. Locus of control and self-efficacy: Potential mediators of stress, illness, and utilization of health services in college students. *Child Psychiatry and Human Development* 41(4): 353–370.

Telles, S., et al. 2009. Effect of a yoga practice session and a yoga theory session on state anxiety. *Perceptual and Motor Skills* 109(3): 924–930.

The New York Times. 2010 Update. *Times Topics: School Shootings* (http://topics.nytimes.com/top/reference/timestopics/subjects/s/school_shootings/index.html; retrieved March 20, 2011).

Torpy, J. M. 2008. Chronic stress and the heart. *Journal of the American Medical Association* 298(14): 1722.

U.S. Department of Health and Human Services, National Institutes of Health. 2009. *Stress* (http://www.nlm.nih.gov/medlineplus/stress.html; retrieved March 20, 2011).

Name ______________________ Section ______________ Date ______________

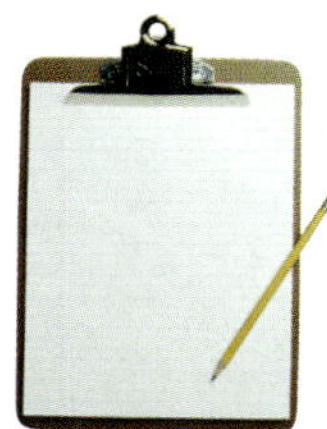

LAB 10.1 Identifying Your Stress Level and Key Stressors

How Stressed Are You?

To help determine how much stress you experience on a daily basis, answer the following questions.

How many of the symptoms of excess stress in the list below do you experience frequently? ______________

Symptoms of Excess Stress

Physical Symptoms	*Emotional Symptoms*	*Behavioral Symptoms*
Dry mouth	Anxiety	Crying
Excessive perspiration	Depression	Disrupted eating habits
Frequent illnesses	Edginess	Disrupted sleeping habits
Gastrointestinal problems	Fatigue	Harsh treatment of others
Grinding of teeth	Hypervigilance	Increased use of tobacco, alcohol, or other drugs
Headaches	Impulsiveness	Problems communicating
High blood pressure	Inability to concentrate	Sexual problems
Pounding heart	Irritability	Social isolation
Stiff neck or aching lower back	Trouble remembering things	

Yes	No	
_____	_____	1. Are you easily startled or irritated?
_____	_____	2. Are you increasingly forgetful?
_____	_____	3. Do you have trouble falling or staying asleep?
_____	_____	4. Do you continually worry about events in your future?
_____	_____	5. Do you feel as if you are constantly under pressure to produce?
_____	_____	6. Do you frequently use tobacco, alcohol, or other drugs to help you relax?
_____	_____	7. Do you often feel as if you have less energy than you need to finish the day?
_____	_____	8. Do you have recurrent stomachaches or headaches?
_____	_____	9. Is it difficult for you to find satisfaction in simple life pleasures?
_____	_____	10. Are you often disappointed in yourself and others?
_____	_____	11. Are you overly concerned with being liked or accepted by others?
_____	_____	12. Have you lost interest in intimacy or sex?
_____	_____	13. Are you concerned that you do not have enough money?

Experiencing some stress-related symptoms or answering yes to a few questions is normal. However, if you experience a large number of stress symptoms or you answered yes to a majority of the questions, you may be experiencing a high level of stress. Take time out to develop effective stress-management techniques. Many coping strategies that can aid you in dealing with college stressors are described in this chapter. Additionally, your school's counseling center can provide valuable support.

LABORATORY ACTIVITIES

Weekly Stress Log

Now that you are familiar with the signals of stress, complete the weekly stress log to map patterns in your stress levels and identify sources of stress. Enter a score for each hour of each day according to the ratings listed below.

	A.M.							P.M.												
	6	7	8	9	10	11	12	1	2	3	4	5	6	7	8	9	10	11	12	*Average*
Monday																				
Tuesday																				
Wednesday																				
Thursday																				
Friday																				
Saturday																				
Sunday																				
Average																				

Ratings: 1 = No anxiety; general feeling of well-being
2 = Mild anxiety; no interference with activity
3 = Moderate anxiety; specific signal(s) of stress present
4 = High anxiety; interference with activity
5 = Very high anxiety and panic reactions; general inability to engage in activity

To identify daily or weekly patterns in your stress level, average your stress rating for each hour and each day. For example, if your scores for 6:00 A.M. are 3, 3, 4, 3, and 4, with blanks for Saturday and Sunday, your 6:00 A.M. rating would be 17 ÷ 5, or 3.4 (moderate to high anxiety). Then calculate an average weekly stress score by averaging your daily average stress scores. Your weekly average will give you a sense of your overall level of stress.

Using Your Results

How did you score? How high are your daily and weekly stress scores?

Are you satisfied with your stress rating? If not, set a specific goal:

What should you do next? Enter the results of this lab in the Preprogram Assessment column in Appendix C. If you've set a goal for improvement, begin by using your log to look for patterns and significant time periods in order to identify key stressors in your life. Below, list any stressors that caused you a significant amount of discomfort this week; these can be people, places, events, or recurring thoughts or worries. For each, enter one strategy that would help you deal more successfully with the stressor. Examples of strategies might include practicing an oral presentation in front of a friend or engaging in positive self-talk.

Next, begin to put your strategies into action. In addition, complete Lab 10.2 to help you incorporate lifestyle stress-management techniques into your daily routine.

Name ______________________ Section ______________ Date ______________

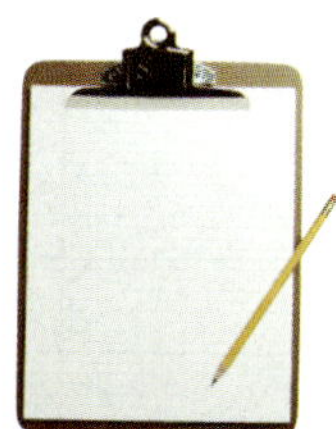

LAB 10.2 Stress-Management Techniques

Part I Lifestyle Stress Management

For each of the areas listed in the table below, describe your current lifestyle as it relates to stress management. For example, do you have enough social support? How are your exercise and nutrition habits? Is time management a problem for you? For each area, list two ways that you could change your current habits to help you manage your stress. Sample strategies might include calling a friend before a challenging class, taking a short walk before lunch, and buying and using a datebook to track your time.

	Current lifestyle	Lifestyle change #1	Lifestyle change #2
Social support system			
Exercise habits			
Nutrition habits			
Time-management techniques			
Self-talk patterns			
Sleep habits			

LABORATORY ACTIVITIES

Part II Relaxation Techniques

Choose two relaxation techniques described in this chapter (progressive relaxation, visualization, deep breathing, meditation, listening to music). If a recording is available for progressive relaxation or visualization, these techniques can be performed by your entire class as a group.

List the techniques you tried.

1. ______________________________

2. ______________________________

How did you feel before you tried these techniques?

____

____

____

What did you think or how did you feel during each of the techniques you tried?

1. ______________________________

____

____

2. ______________________________

____

____

How did you feel after you tried these techniques?

____

____

____

Name ______________________ Section ______________ Date ____________

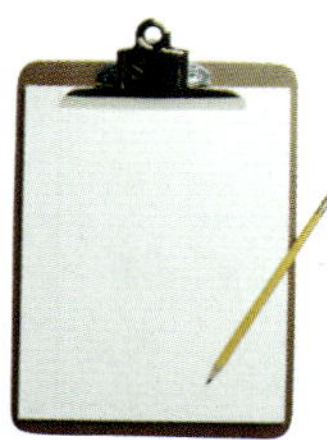

LAB 10.3 Developing Spiritual Wellness

To develop spiritual wellness, it is important to take time out to think about what gives meaning and purpose to your life and what actions you can take to support the spiritual dimension of your life.

Look Inward

This week, spend some quiet time alone with your thoughts and feelings. Slow the pace of your day, remove your watch, turn your phone off, and focus on your immediate experience. Try one of the following activities or develop another that is meaningful to you and that contributes to your sense of spiritual well-being.

- ***Spend time in nature.*** Experience continuity with the natural world by spending solitary time in a natural setting. Watch the sky (day or night), a sunrise, or a sunset; listen to waves on a shore or wind in the trees; feel the breeze on your face or raindrops on your skin; smell the grass, brush, trees, or flowers. Open all your senses to the beauty of nature.
- ***Experience art, architecture, or music.*** Spend time with a work of art or architecture or a piece of music. Choose one that will awaken your senses, engage your emotions, and challenge your understanding. Take a break and then repeat the experience to see how your responses change the second time.
- ***Express your creativity.*** Set aside time for a favorite activity, one that allows you to express your creative side. Sing, draw, paint, play a musical instrument, sculpt, build, dance, cook, garden—choose an activity in which you will be so engaged that you will lose track of time. Strive for feelings of joy and exhilaration.
- ***Engage in a personal spiritual practice.*** Pray, meditate, do yoga, chant. Choose a spiritual practice that is familiar to you or try one that is new. Tune out the outside world and turn your attention inward, focusing on the experience.

In the space below, describe the personal spiritual activity you tried and how it made you feel—both during the activity and after.

LABORATORY ACTIVITIES

Reach Out

Spiritual wellness can be a bond among people and can promote values such as altruism, forgiveness, and compassion. Try one of the following spiritual activities that involve reaching out to others.

- ***Share writings that inspire you.*** Find two writings that inspire, guide, and comfort you—passages from sacred works, poems, quotations from literature, songs. Share them with someone else by reading them aloud and explaining what they mean to you.
- ***Practice kindness.*** Spend a day practicing small acts of personal kindness for people you know as well as for strangers. Compliment a friend, send a card, let someone go ahead of you in line, pick up litter, do someone else's chores, help someone with packages, say please and thank you, smile.
- ***Perform community service.*** Foster a sense of community by becoming a volunteer. Find a local nonprofit group and offer your time and talent. Mentor a youth, work at a food bank, support a literacy project, help build low-cost housing, visit seniors in a nursing home. You can also work on national or international issues by writing letters to your elected representatives and other officials.

In the space below, describe the spiritual activity you performed and how it made you feel—during the activity and after. Include details about the writings you chose or the acts of kindness or community service you performed.

Keep a Journal

One strategy for continuing on the path toward spiritual wellness is to keep a journal. Use a journal to record your thoughts, feelings, and experiences; to jot down quotes that engage you; to sketch pictures and write poetry about what is meaningful to you. Begin your spiritual journal today.

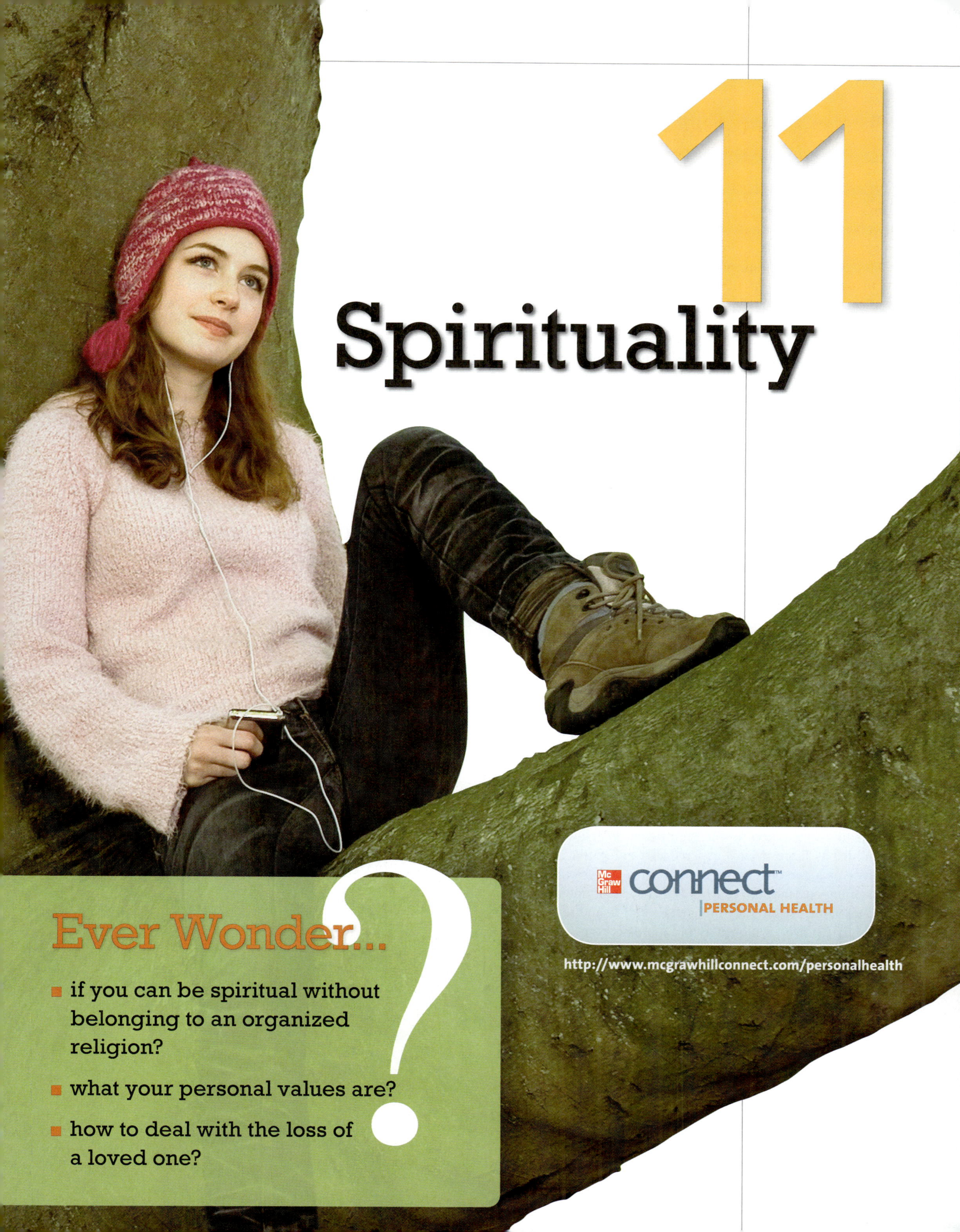

11 Spirituality

Ever Wonder...

- if you can be spiritual without belonging to an organized religion?
- what your personal values are?
- how to deal with the loss of a loved one?

Someone once said that the longest journey is the journey inward. The spiritual journey is deeply personal and individual. It may begin as a yearning for connection with what is universal and timeless or a belief in a power in the universe that is greater than oneself. It often involves a search for meaning and purpose or a desire for a more intense participation in life. Many people now believe that spiritual health enhances their psychological and physical well-being, and they pursue spiritual wellness as one of the important dimensions of total wellness.

It seems that all people in all times have experienced spiritual aspirations. Worldwide, there are more than 20 major religions and thousands of other forms of spiritual expression. In the spirit of modern genetics, some scientists have been searching for a biological basis for human spirituality—a gene or genes that would account for our spiritual experiences and yearnings—and one researcher, Dean Hamer of the National Cancer Institute, believes he has found such a gene.[1] No matter what the role of biology, however, spiritual experience and expression are clearly the product of complex interactions between individuals and their cultures.

Your spiritual health affects your **capacity for love, compassion, forgiveness, and fulfillment.** *It can be an antidote to stress, cynicism, fear, self-absorption, and pessimism.*

What Is Spirituality?

Because spirituality may involve different paths for different people, it has been defined in many ways. In health promotion literature, **spirituality** is commonly defined as a person's connection to self, significant others, and the community at large. Many experts also agree that spirituality involves a personal belief system or value system that gives meaning and purpose to life.[2] For some individuals this personal value system may include a belief in and reverence for a higher power, which may be expressed through an organized religion. For example, according to recent surveys, more than 8 in 10 Americans identify with a religion and believe in God or a universal spirit or higher power.[3] For others the spiritual dimension is nonreligious and centers on a personal value system that may be reflected in activities such as volunteer work. In either case, spirituality provides a feeling of participation in something greater than oneself and a sense of unity with nature and the universe.

SPIRITUALITY IN EVERYDAY LIFE

All of us have questions about our existence: Am I connected to something, or am I alone, isolated, and cut off? Is my life guided by my values, or am I drifting without a moral compass? What gives my life meaning? Searching for answers to these questions is part of life's spiritual journey.

Connection to Self and Others Being connected to yourself involves knowing who you are, developing self-awareness, and building self-esteem. Growth in these areas is an incremental process in which you develop a reservoir of inner strengths through such practices as becoming more compassionate or learning to be a better listener.

spirituality The experience of connection to self, others, and the community at large, providing a sense of purpose and meaning.

Spirituality also includes being responsible for yourself and taking charge of your life. Your spiritual health affects your capacity for love, compassion, joy, forgiveness, altruism, and fulfillment. It can be an antidote to stress, cynicism, anger, fear, anxiety, self-absorption, and pessimism.

Connection with significant others through positive relationships is also essential to spiritual health and growth.

Participating in activities that reinforce feelings of connectedness with others is a way of enhancing spirituality in everyday life.

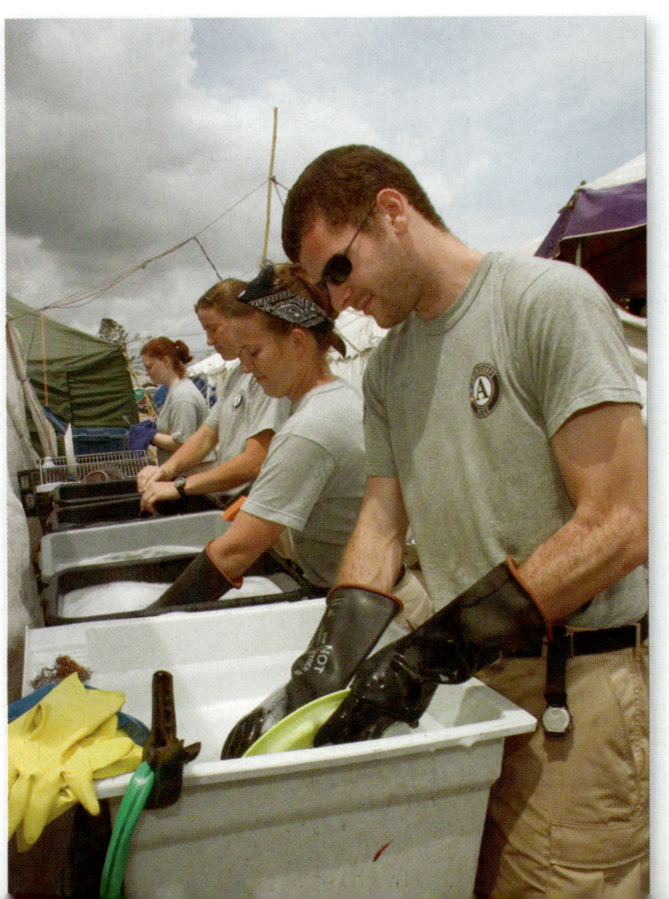

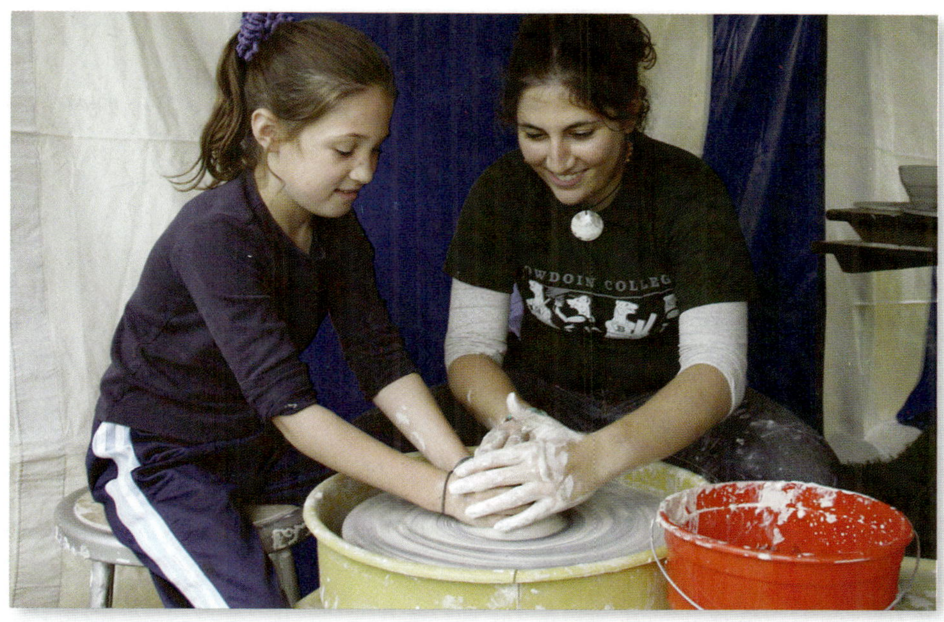

■ Engagement in meaningful activities—such as sharing one's expertise and passion with a younger person—is a major source of happiness and satisfaction for most people.

Healthy relationships involve a balance between closeness and separateness and are characterized by mutual support, respect, good communication, and caring actions. Having strong personal relationships improves health and self-esteem and gives greater meaning to life.[4,5]

Connection with the community includes enjoying constructive relationships at school, in the workplace, or in the neighborhood. Several studies have demonstrated links between social connectedness and positive outcomes for individual health and well-being.[5–7] Evidence shows that social participation and engagement are related to the maintenance of cognitive function in older adulthood and to lowered mortality rates. In general, the size of a person's social network and his or her sense of connectedness are inversely related to risk-related behaviors such as alcohol and tobacco consumption, physical inactivity, and behaviors leading to obesity.[5,6,8]

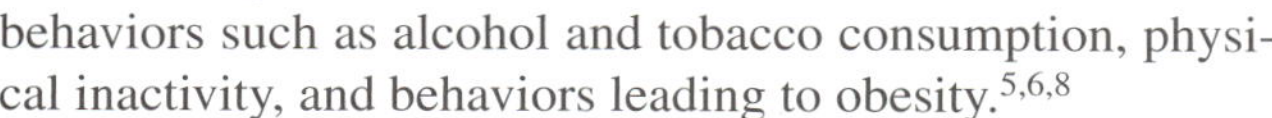

A Personal Value System Another aspect of spirituality involves developing a personal **value system**, a set of guidelines for how you want to live your life. *Values*, the criteria for judging what is good and bad, underlie moral principles and behavior. Your value system shapes who you are as a person, how you make decisions, and what goals you set for yourself. When you develop a way of life that makes sense and enables you to navigate the world effectively, the many choices you face each day become much less complex and easier to handle. Your value system becomes your map, providing a structure for decision making that allows flexibility and the possibility of change.

value system Set of criteria for judging what is good and bad that underlies moral decisions and behavior.

Meaning and Purpose in Life Why am I here? This question has been asked by people all over the world, in all eras, and at all stages of life. For young people, the answer may involve developing relationships and connections. For adults, the answer may be caring for others. For older adults, it may be working for a healthier planet. Positive psychology contributes the idea that meaning in life comes from using one's personal strengths to serve some larger end.

HAPPINESS AND LIFE SATISFACTION

The study of happiness is part of the positive psychology movement, with its focus on what makes life worth living. Surveys indicate that happiness is typical rather than unusual—9 out of 10 Americans report being very happy or pretty happy.[9] According to one poll, wealth, education, IQ, and youth have little impact on happiness; instead, the top source of happiness is connections with family and friends (Figure 11.1).[10] Other sources of happiness include contributing to the lives of others, having a sense of control over one's life, and having a religious or spiritual life.

In their research, positive psychologists have found that happiness involves three components: positive emotion and pleasure (savoring sensory experiences); engagement (depth of involvement with family, work, romance, and hobbies); and meaning (using personal strengths to serve some larger end).[8] The happiest people are those who orient their lives toward all three, but the latter two—engagement and meaning—are much more important in giving people satisfaction and happiness.

Happiness research has found that people can increase their level of happiness by practicing certain "happiness exercises":[11]

- *Three Good Things in Life.* Write down three things that went well each day and their causes every night for a week.
- *Using Signature Strengths in a New Way.* Using the classification of character strengths and virtues, take inventory of your character strengths and identify your top five strengths, your "signature strengths." Use one of these top strengths in a new and different way every day for a week.

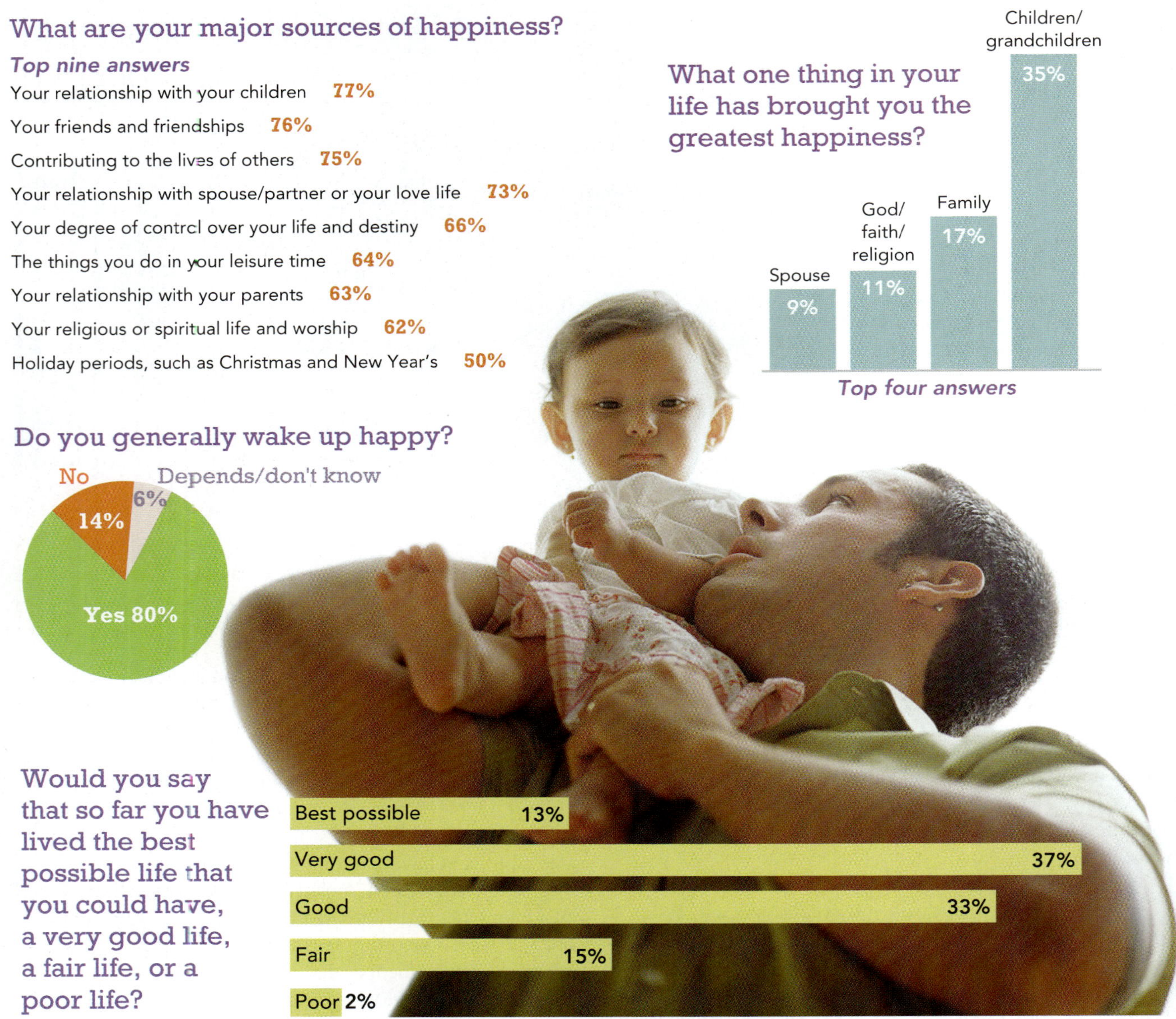

figure 11.1 **Sources of happiness and other happiness facts reported by Americans.**
Source: Adapted from "The New Science of Happiness," by C. Wallis, January 17, 2005, Time.

- *Gratitude Visit.* Write a letter of gratitude and then deliver it in person to someone who has been especially kind to you but whom you have never thanked properly.

Research found that two of these exercises—Three Good Things and Using Signature Strengths in a New Way—increased happiness and decreased depressive symptoms for 6 months. The Gratitude Visit caused large positive changes for 1 month.

Related research has identified other ways to increase happiness and life satisfaction, including performing acts of kindness, savoring life's joys, and learning to forgive (see the box "Steps to a More Satisfying Life"). Positive psychologists say that happiness exercises give meaning to life by helping people feel more connected to others. Almost everyone feels happier when they are with other people, even those who think they want to be alone.

The down side is that people may have a happiness "set point," determined largely by genetics. That is, no matter what happens in life, people may have a tendency to return to their norm. The notion that people can increase their happiness reinforces Western cultural biases about how individual initiative and a positive attitude can solve complex problems.[7] In addition, because happiness research focuses

Challenges & Choices

Steps to a More Satisfying Life

Want to be happier? Here are some practical suggestions, based on research findings by psychologist Sonia Lyubomirsky and other positive psychologists:

1. *Count your blessings.* Keep a gratitude journal in which you write down three to five things for which you are grateful once a week.
2. *Practice acts of kindness.* Being kind to others has many positive effects, including a greater sense of connection with the people around you.
3. *Savor life's joys.* Pay attention to moments of pleasure and wonder; keep a store of such memories so that you can call on them in less happy times.
4. *Thank a mentor.* Express your appreciation to those who have been kind to you.
5. *Learn to forgive.* Write a letter of forgiveness to anyone who has hurt or wronged you. Letting go of anger and resentment allows you to move on.
6. *Invest time and energy in friends and family.* Strong personal relationships are the biggest factor in life satisfaction.
7. *Take care of your body.* Practicing good self-care—getting enough sleep, exercising, smiling and laughing—makes your daily life more satisfying.
8. *Develop strategies for coping with stress and hardship.* For some people, religious faith offers help. For others, secular beliefs—even "this too shall pass"—serve as coping tools.

Sources: "Positive Psychology Progress: Validation of Interventions," by M. Seligman, T. Steen, N. Park, and C. Peterson, 2005, American Psychologist,*60(5), pp. 410–421; "The New Science of Happiness," by C. Wallis, January 17, 2005,* Time.

on internal processes, little or no attention is paid to the very real sources of unhappiness in people's lives that are connected to their social and economic circumstances.

Health Benefits of Spirituality

According to a *Newsweek* poll, 73 percent of Americans believe that prayer holds the power to heal,[12] and according to a 2004 study, one-third of Americans use prayer, in addition to conventional medical treatments, for health concerns.[13]

The connection between spirituality and health is gaining serious attention from the medical and scientific communities.[14,15] Hundreds of studies have been conducted on spirituality and health, and more than half the nation's medical schools now offer courses on spirituality and medicine, whereas only three did 20 years ago. The National Institutes of Health have spent millions of dollars on "mind-body" medicine.[16] The pursuit is not without its skeptics, however, and the connection between spirituality and health remains an area of controversy and debate.

PHYSICAL BENEFITS

Can prayer cure cancer or slow its progression? Can it lower blood pressure? Does spirituality speed healing after accidents or help people recover from surgery? Do religious people live longer?

There are no definitive answers to these questions, but a majority of 350 studies of physical health and 850 studies of mental health suggest a direct relationship between religious involvement and spirituality, on the one hand, and better health outcomes, on the other.[17] Research has found that religious involvement and spirituality are associated with lower blood pressure, decreased risk of substance abuse, less cardiovascular disease, less depression, less anxiety, enhanced immune function, and longer life.[18] Meditation and prayer in combination with traditional medical treatments are reported to relieve medical problems such as chronic pain, depression, anxiety, insomnia, and premenstrual syndrome.[19] There are enough positive results to spur further inquiry.

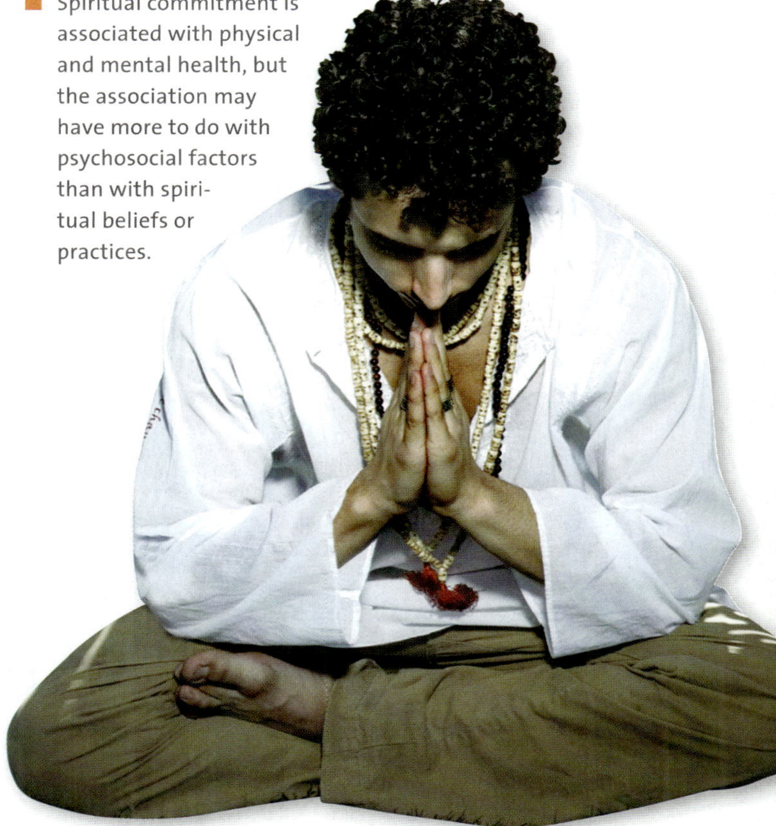

Spiritual commitment is associated with physical and mental health, but the association may have more to do with psychosocial factors than with spiritual beliefs or practices.

One of the most consistent research findings is that spiritually connected persons stay healthier and live longer than those who are not connected.[18,20] One study found that people who attend church regularly live an average of seven years longer than their non-churchgoing counterparts.[21] An important reason for this outcome is that people who are religious or spiritually connected generally have healthier lifestyles. They smoke less, drink less alcohol, have better diets, exercise more, and are more likely to wear seat belts and to avoid drugs and unsafe sex. However, these factors don't seem to account for all of the health-related benefits of religious and spiritual commitment. Studies find that the positive differences in death rates persist even after controlling for factors such as age, health, habits, demographics, and other health-related variables.[18]

Another explanation for better health among people who are spiritually involved is that they react more effectively to health crises. People who are religious or spiritual seem to be more willing than those who are not spiritually connected to alter their health habits, to be proactive in seeking medical treatment, and to accept the support of others. People who have strong ties to a religious group or another community segment may receive help and encouragement from that community in times of crisis.[22] Friends may transport them to the doctor and to church, shop for them, prepare meals, arrange child care, and encourage them to get appropriate medical treatment.

MENTAL BENEFITS

People who are spiritually involved tend to enjoy better mental health as well as physical health. One reason may be that religious people tend to be more forgiving, and recent research has linked forgiveness with lower blood pressure, less back pain, and overall better personal health.[23]

In addition, spiritual practices such as meditation, prayer, and worship seem to promote positive emotions such as hope, love, contentment, and forgiveness, which can result in lower levels of anxiety. This in turn may help to minimize the stress response, which suppresses immune functioning.[24–26] Many people may even turn to religion in times of stress.[27] Studies have also shown that prayer and certain relaxation techniques, such as meditation, yoga, and hypnotherapy, reduce the secretion of stress hormones and their harmful side effects.

Depression may also be mediated by spiritual involvement. Some studies indicate that people who are religiously involved suffer less depression and recover faster when they are depressed.[28,29] Religious people are also less likely to consider suicide.[12]

Studies have shown that spiritual connectedness appears to be associated with high levels of *health-related quality of life*, the physical, psychological, social, and spiritual aspects of a person's daily experience. Spiritual connectedness is especially important when a person is coping with serious health issues such as cancer, HIV infection, heart disease, limb amputation, or spinal cord injury.[18] This positive relationship persists even as physical health declines with serious illness.[30]

A DIFFERENT VIEW

Although the majority of studies indicate that spiritual connectedness has health benefits, many studies have found no relationship between health and spirituality. Some researchers have even suggested that spirituality can have negative outcomes for physical and mental health. For example, several studies indicate that when people experience a spiritual conflict in association with a health crisis, there is a

One of the most consistent research findings is that **spiritually connected persons stay healthier and live longer** *than those who are not connected.*

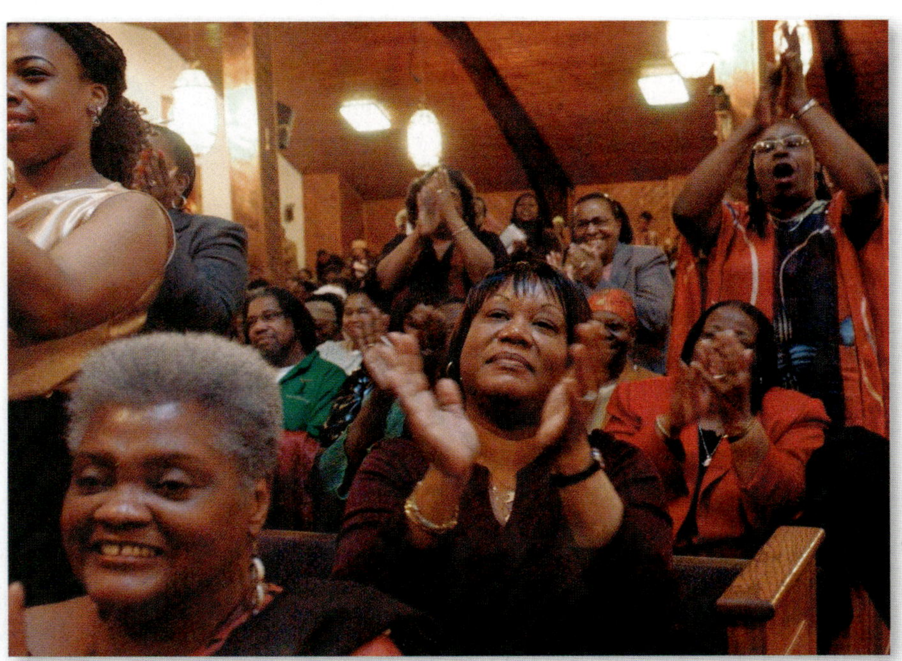

People who have strong ties to a religious or community group are more likely to have a network of people who can support and help them in time of need.

Who's at Risk?

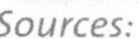

Spirituality and Health

Do people with spiritual or religious beliefs and practices have better health outcomes than people without such beliefs and practices? Many research studies have been conducted to investigate various aspects of this question, with contradictory and inconsistent results. The findings of a few of them are described here:

- A combination of frequent religious attendance, prayer, Bible study, and strong beliefs predicted a faster recovery from depression.[a]
- HIV-positive patients who underwent spiritual transformation (the development of spirituality or an increase in the level of spirituality) had a higher survival rate than those who did not undergo spiritual transformation.[b]
- Attendance and public participation in religion did not affect hypertension rates among adults; however, prayer was associated with an increased likelihood of hypertension, and forgiveness was associated with a lower risk of hypertension.[c]
- Cardiac patients who received intercessory prayer (prayer by strangers) fared no better than patients who did not receive such prayer.[d]
- Religious struggles and negative religious coping (for example, "questioning God's love") were correlated with higher risk of death in hospitalized older adults.[e]
- Among older adults (66–95 years old), men received more mental health benefits from religion than did women, and women with high, moderate, and low levels of organizational involvement in religion received similar levels of benefits regardless of their level of involvement.[f]
- Neither self-reported spirituality, frequency of church attendance, nor frequency of prayer was associated with recovery from heart attack.[g]
- An increase in religiosity/spirituality after a diagnosis of HIV infection was correlated with slower disease progression after 4 years.[h]

Sources:

[a] *"Religion and Remission of Depression in Medical Inpatients with Heart Failure/Pulmonary Disease," by H.G. Koenig, 2007,* Journal of Nervous and Mental Disease, 195, *pp. 389–395.*

[b] *"Spiritual Transformation, Psychological Well-Being, Health, and Survival in People With HIV," by G. Ironson and H. Kremer, 2009,* International Journal of Psychiatry in Medicine, 39*(3), pp. 263–281.*

[c] *"An Examination of the Relationship Between Multiple Dimensions of Religiosity, Blood Pressure and Hypertension," by A.C. Buck et al. 2008,* Social Science and Medicine, 68*(2), pp. 314–422.*

[d] *"Music, Imagery, Touch, and Prayer as Adjuncts to Interventional Cardiac Care," by M.W. Krucoff et al., 2005,* Lancet, 366, *pp. 211–217.*

[e] *"Religious Struggles as a Predictor of Mortality Among Medically Ill Elderly Patients," by K.I. Pargament et al., 2001,* Archives of Internal Medicine, 161, *pp. 1881–1885.*

[f] *"Religion and Mental Health Among Older Adults: Do the Effects of Religious Involvement Vary by Gender?" by M.J. McFarland, 2009,* Journal of Gerontology: Social Sciences, *10, p. 1093.*

[g] *"Spirituality, Religion, and Clinical Outcomes in Patients Recovering From an Acute Myocardial Infarction," by J.A. Blumenthal et al., 2007,* Psychosomatic Medicine, 69, *pp. 501–508.*

[h] *"An Increase in Religiousness/Spirituality Occurs After HIV Diagnosis and Predicts Slower Disease Progression Over 4 Years in People With HIV," by G. Ironson, R. Stuetzie, and M.A. Fletcher, 2006,* Journal of General Internal Medicine, 21, *pp. S62–S68.*

negative impact on their health status.[18,31–34] And one study concluded that people who knew they were receiving intercessory prayer (prayer by strangers) may have experienced increased anxiety and more complications than those who were unsure they were being prayed for.[35] It seems that the connection between spirituality and health can have both positive and negative implications and needs more study (see the box "Spirituality and Health").

Enhancing Your Spirituality: Looking Inward

How do you build a spiritual life? Greater connectedness and meaning can be found through a variety of practices, especially if they are done on a regular basis.

MEDITATION

Human beings are engaged in a constant inner monologue, reviewing the past, commenting on the present, and speculating about the future. This inner chatter can keep us from being fully present in our lives. **Meditation** is a way to slow your racing thoughts and quiet your mind by focusing on a word, an object (such as a candle flame), or a process (such as breathing). With practice, meditation can help you become calmer as you go about your daily routines. There are many ways to meditate, but all involve introspection and attention to your inner life.

meditation Technique for quieting the mind by focusing on a word, an object (such as a candle flame), or a process (such as breathing).

If you are interested in trying meditation as a way to build a spiritual life, follow the guidelines in the box

Challenges & Choices

Learning to Meditate

Meditation is an ancient technique with modern adaptations. Various forms of meditation have been developed, but their common goals are to calm the mind, raise awareness, and increase attention to what is happening in the present moment. Here are some guidelines for a type of meditation in which you focus on your breathing:

- Sit in a comfortable place—on a pillow on the floor or in a chair, for example—in a quiet room where you won't be disturbed. Close your eyes.
- Breathe deeply. Feel the breath as it enters your nostrils and fills your chest and abdomen; then release it.
- Focus your attention on your breathing and awareness of the moment. Try to be silent and still.
- Remain passive and relaxed as your thoughts come and go, noticing them without judging them. At first, your mind will fill with memories, worries, and random thoughts. Let go of the thoughts and feelings and return to the awareness of breath. Eventually, you will be able to concentrate for longer periods of time, and these periods of concentration may be accompanied by feelings of great tranquility.

Meditate for brief periods of time each day. Start out with 5 minutes and gradually build up to 15 minutes or more. Make a commitment to continue meditating for 3 months; you will not experience any changes or benefits unless you practice. Experiment until you find a place, time, and approach that work for you. If you would like more information about techniques, contact a meditation center, consult a teacher or book, search online, talk with more experienced meditators, or listen to a tape.

"Learning to Meditate." Although meditation may not appeal to everyone, the practice can offer many benefits. It is widely used in stress management and stress reduction programs. Proponents claim that meditation provides deep relaxation, promotes health, increases creativity and intelligence, and brings inner happiness and fulfillment.

Mindfulness is both a form of meditation and the practice of living fully in the moment. By learning to be conscious of your thoughts as they pass by—observing them, not judging them—you develop your ability to control and stop habitual, impulsive, or undesirable reactions. You become more capable of responding in a "thoughtful" and "mindful" way rather than becoming overwhelmed with negative emotions or self-criticism.[36] As you learn to focus on the present moment, you can be more in touch with your life as it is happening.

■ Meditation is a calming and centering spiritual practice.

When people learn to live fully in the moment, they sometimes experience a phenomenon known as **flow**, a feeling of being completely absorbed in an activity and a moment. In this state, people forget themselves, lose track of time, and feel as if they have become one with what they are doing. Writers describe times when words seem to come through them; athletes refer to being "in the zone." Flow has been described as one of the most enjoyable and valuable experiences a person can have.[37] When you learn to be mindful and live in the moment, you are more likely to experience flow in your daily activities.

mindfulness Awareness and acceptance of living fully in the moment.

flow Pleasurable experience of complete absorption and engagement in an activity.

Mindfulness is celebrated by the noted Vietnamese monk Thich Nhat Hanh in these words:

> Our true home is in the present moment.
> To live in the present moment is a miracle.
> The miracle is not to walk on water.
> The miracle is to walk on the green Earth in the present moment,
> To appreciate the peace and beauty that are available now.[38]

JOURNALING

Another approach to building a spiritual life is *journaling*. As you record your feelings, thoughts, breakthroughs, and desires in a private journal, you will begin to understand yourself more clearly.

Psychologist James Pennebaker has found that writing about emotional upheavals can improve physical and mental health. He suggests writing about any of the following:

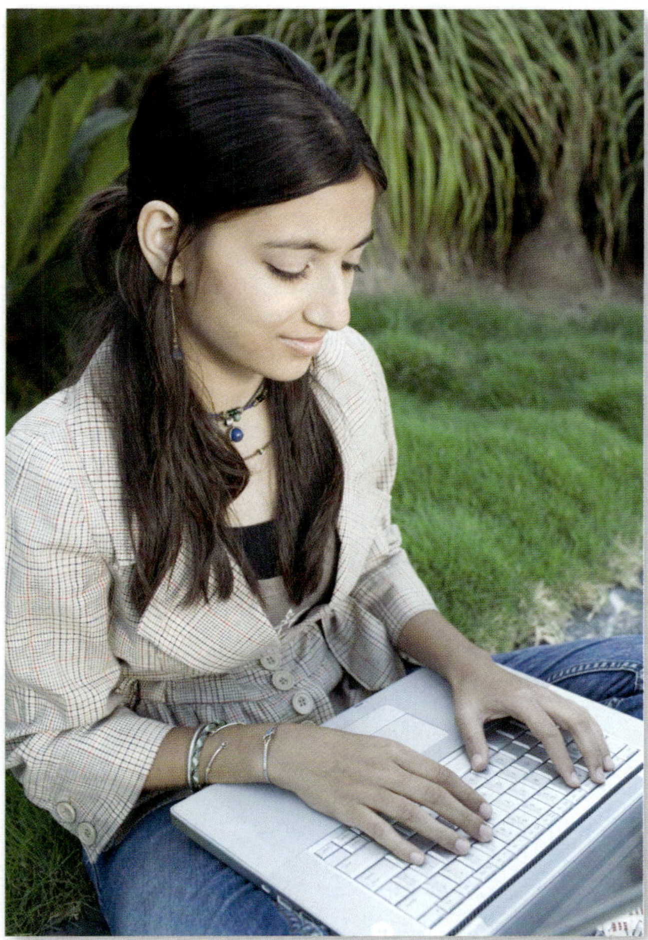

Journaling offers a way to explore your feeelings, deepen your self-understanding, and discover what is important to you.

- Something that you are thinking or worrying about too much.
- Something that you are dreaming about.
- Something that you feel is affecting your life in an unhealthy way.
- Something that you have been avoiding for days, weeks, or years.[39]

The more honest you are, the better. Don't censor yourself as you write; just let your thoughts flow. Try to move beyond the superficial telling to asking yourself, Why am I feeling this way?

Journaling is an effective way to learn about who you are and where you have been. Listening to your inner dialogue may offer you a sense of peace and a positive outlook on your experiences. In some cases, journaling can be painful, stirring up emotions that may be difficult to handle on your own. If you find yourself feeling overwhelmed, consider contacting a professional for counseling.[40]

RETREAT

A *retreat* is a period of seclusion, solitude, or group withdrawal for prayer, meditation, or study. Retreats are intended to reenergize your life and restore your zest for living. A spiritual retreat might offer a balance of activities that encourage growth, foster learning, and restore energy, so that when you return to your normal surroundings, you may live life to the fullest in a purposeful way.

Many kinds of facilities offer retreats, workshops, and programs for spiritual growth, but you can use your home for a retreat as well. Set aside a weekend and plan to give up all social events, phone calls, errands, television, newspapers, Internet, and all nonessential housework. Then prepare for exploration. You might meditate, journal, draw, write poetry, take walks to enjoy the beauty of nature, listen to music, read—whatever you want to do that you find deepening and centering. At their best, retreats stimulate the mind, enhance self-awareness, and refresh the spirit. They provide food for the body, mind, and spirit.

THE ARTS

Scholar Joseph Campbell once asserted, "The goal of life is rapture. Art is the way we experience it. Art is the transforming experience." Experiencing the arts—whether sculpture, painting, music, poetry, literature, theater, storytelling, dance, or some other form—is another way to build a spiritual life. Experiencing great art can inspire you, through felt experience, to think about the purpose of life and the nature of reality.[41] By engaging your heart, mind, and spirit, art can give you fresh insights, challenge preconceptions, and trigger inner growth.

When you enjoy and appreciate the arts, you embrace diverse cultures past and present and frequently discover in them the universal themes of human existence—love, loss, birth, death, isolation, community, continuity, change. When you express yourself creatively, you may be able to experience a spiritual connection between your inner core and the natural world beyond yourself. Both experiences—art appreciation and artistic expression—can be transforming. If the visual or performing arts are not part of your life right now, try to schedule time to visit a museum or attend a concert. Make notes or sketches in a journal reflecting on your experiences. Doing so may stimulate new spiritual connections in your life.

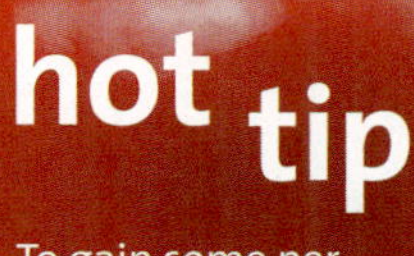

hot tip

To gain some perspective on values and meaning in life, go to YouTube and watch Randy Pausch's inspiring "Last Lecture," delivered after the popular professor had been given a prognosis of 3–6 months left to live.

LIVING YOUR VALUES

Building a spiritual life also means bringing your deepest beliefs and intentions into the world—that is, living your values. A 2010 report conducted by the Pew Research Center found that students of the Millennial generation (ages 18–29) have values similar to those of older generations. Although Millennials set themselves apart by their racial diversity, immersion in technology, and love of self-expression and social media, like older generations, they rate being a good parent as one of the most important things in life (see Figure 11.2).[42] And although this generation has grown up in an age where almost anyone can become a YouTube star, gain a large following writing a blog, or exchange tweets with minor celebrities, 86 percent say that becoming famous is not important to them.[42]

Can you articulate what is most important to you in life? Are you living and acting in accordance with it? (See the box "Understanding Your Personal Values.") Try writing a "purpose statement" that will remind you of who you truly are and why you believe you are here on earth. Then ask yourself, Do I stay "on purpose" in my daily interactions and activities? Commit your purpose statement to memory, and read or recite it daily. It may be "to live and learn" or "to know my higher being and teach and express love."

Adopting a new habit, such as putting your best intentions into practice, takes time and work. Experts say that you have to continue to take action for 60 to 90 days to make a behavior change stick. As Aristotle

What is important in life?
Having a successful career is important 47%
Being a good parent is one of the most important things in life 52%
Having a successful marriage is very important 52%
Helping others in need is very important 60%
Becoming famous is not important 86%

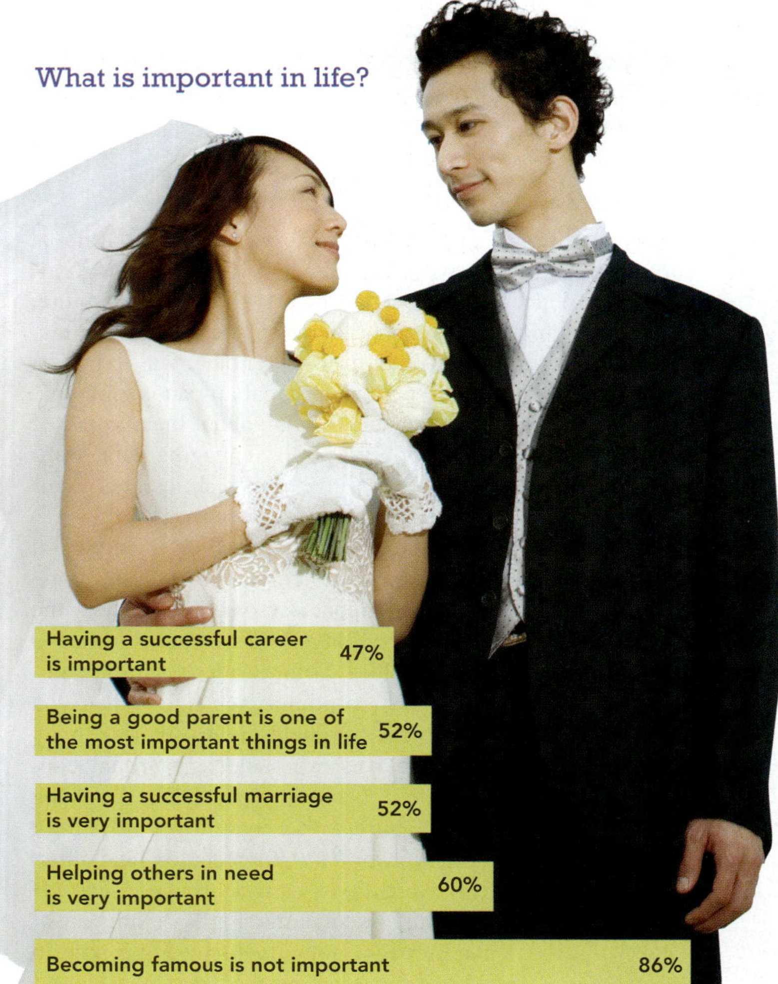

figure **11.2** **The Millennial generation and their values.**
Source: "Millennials: A Portrait of Generation Next." *Pew Research Center, accessed February 24, 2010, from http://pewsocialtrends.org/assets/pdf/millennials-confident-connected-open-to-change.pdf.*

Challenges & Choices

Understanding Your Personal Values

Many people are unaware of their core values and the guiding principles by which they live their lives. We seldom think through our values until we are faced with a difficult choice, and even then we may make a choice without being aware of our values. For inspiration we can look to people who stood up for their values despite enormous pressure to conform and foreseeable negative consequences. A prime example is Rosa Parks, who sparked the civil rights movement when she refused to sit in the back of the bus.

How would you articulate your own core values? Consider the following list of major life values and check off the ones that are important to you:

- ☐ achievement
- ☐ autonomy
- ☐ compassion
- ☐ connectedness
- ☐ creativity
- ☐ education
- ☐ family
- ☐ financial well-being
- ☐ freedom
- ☐ health
- ☐ home
- ☐ honesty
- ☐ integrity
- ☐ learning
- ☐ love
- ☐ personal growth
- ☐ prestige
- ☐ relationships
- ☐ service
- ☐ social justice
- ☐ spirituality
- ☐ status

Which of these (or others) are most important and meaningful to you? Write your top three here:

____

____

____

What guiding principles can you derive from them? How can you embody them in your life?

understood almost 2,500 years ago, "We are what we repeatedly do. Excellence is not an act, then, but a habit."

Enhancing Your Spirituality: Looking Outward

Many believe that people can develop their spirituality by participating in their communities in a positive way. Unpaid work directly promotes community well-being through the services provided, whether that means caring for an elderly relative or working on a community project. It also has indirect benefits by building the social networks that contribute to optimal well-being.

SERVICE LEARNING

One way that people can connect classroom activities to community service and community building is through **service learning**. The purpose of integrating community service with academic study is to enrich learning, teach civic responsibility, and strengthen communities. Students are encouraged to take a positive role in their community, such as by tutoring, caring for the environment, or conducting oral histories with senior citizens. All of these activities are meant to teach people how to extend themselves beyond their enclosed world, taking a risk to get involved in the lives of others. In this way they learn about caring and taking care of—two particularly important concepts for personal growth.

service learning Form of education that combines academic study with community service.

VOLUNTEERING

Volunteering is another way to be connected with other people. Volunteers may experience a "helper's high," similar to a "runner's high."[43] Research shows that people who give time, money, and support to others are likely to be more satisfied with their lives and less depressed.[44]

Not all kinds of volunteering have the same effect, however. One-on-one contact and direct involvement significantly influence the effect of volunteering on the volunteer. Working closely with strangers appears to increase the potential health benefits of the experience. Liking the volunteer work, performing it consistently, and having unselfish motives further increase the feelings of helper's high and the health benefits associated with it.[45,46] Simply donating money or doing volunteer work in isolation does not seem to have the same positive effect.

Just as the high of helping may create enjoyable immediate benefits, the calm of helping may result in significant long-term health benefits. For example, volunteering may reduce the negative health effects of living with high levels of stress for long periods of time. Those who have experienced a helper's high have noted specific improvements in their physical well-being. These improvements included a reduction in arthritis pain, lupus symptoms, asthma attacks, migraine headaches, colds, and episodes of the flu. Volunteering may even result in longer life for the volunteer.[47,48]

SOCIAL ACTIVISM AND THE GLOBAL COMMUNITY

Some people connect with their communities—local, national, and global—through social activism. A social cause, such as overcoming poverty or fighting illiteracy, can unite people from diverse backgrounds for a common good. Many people find it meaningful to participate in global citizenship by joining organizations such as those described in the box "Global Activism."

If you are interested in social activism, look for ways to participate through your school, your religious community, or groups you locate on the Internet. When you volunteer for such an organization, you commit yourself to building a foundation for a better world, making a contribution through service to others, and creating opportunities for mutual understanding.

How is spirituality related to community involvement? Some claim that when we attend to our inner life, we nurture our compassionate responses to human need and develop a passion for social justice. Others believe that contributing to community welfare and striving for justice are the ways to a rich inner life.

Some people turn away from social activism because they think it's "just politics." We hear news stories that use

Volunteers benefit others and themselves when they serve their communities. President Obama has emphasized the importance of volunteering by participating in several community service projects since his inauguration, and his administration has created a Web site, www.serve.gov, to put people in touch with volunteer opportunities in their communities.

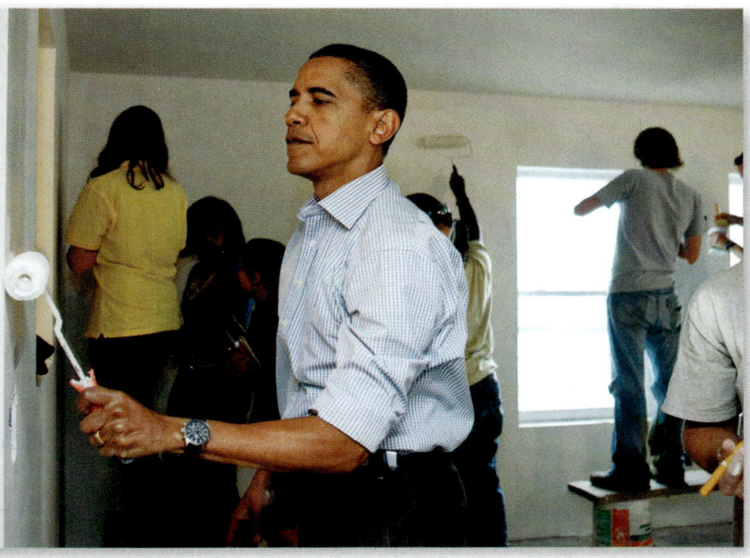

Highlight on Health

Global Activism

Many organizations help individuals put their values into practice in the world. Here are a few:

- The Peace Corps was inspired by President John F. Kennedy's call to college students to give two years of their lives to help people in developing nations. Today, it is still sending people to developing nations like Ecuador, Ghana, and Ukraine with the goal of promoting world peace and friendship. Its volunteers do everything from helping teachers develop their teaching methodologies, to raising awareness about health issues like HIV/AIDS, to teaching environmental conservation strategies, to teaching computer skills.
- Habitat for Humanity is widely known for its work providing housing for needy people in the United States, but it also works on its goal of eliminating poverty and homelessness on a global level. So far, the organization has built more than 350,000 houses in more than 90 countries.
- Greenpeace focuses on the most crucial worldwide threats to the planet's biodiversity and environment. Greenpeace has been campaigning against environmental degradation since 1971, bearing witness in a nonviolent manner.
- The Earth Charter Initiative is an international organization dedicated to building a sustainable world based on respect for nature, universal human rights, economic justice, and peace. A basic premise of the Earth Charter is that these attributes must be cultivated at the local community level before they can emerge at the national and global levels.

catchphrases associating traditional values with the religious right and social justice with the liberal left. Any action can be cloaked in the guise of religiosity, and distinguishing politics with a religious flavor from the practice of authentic spiritual values can be difficult. The former is designed to manipulate people's feelings for political gain; the latter has no hidden agenda or ulterior motive.

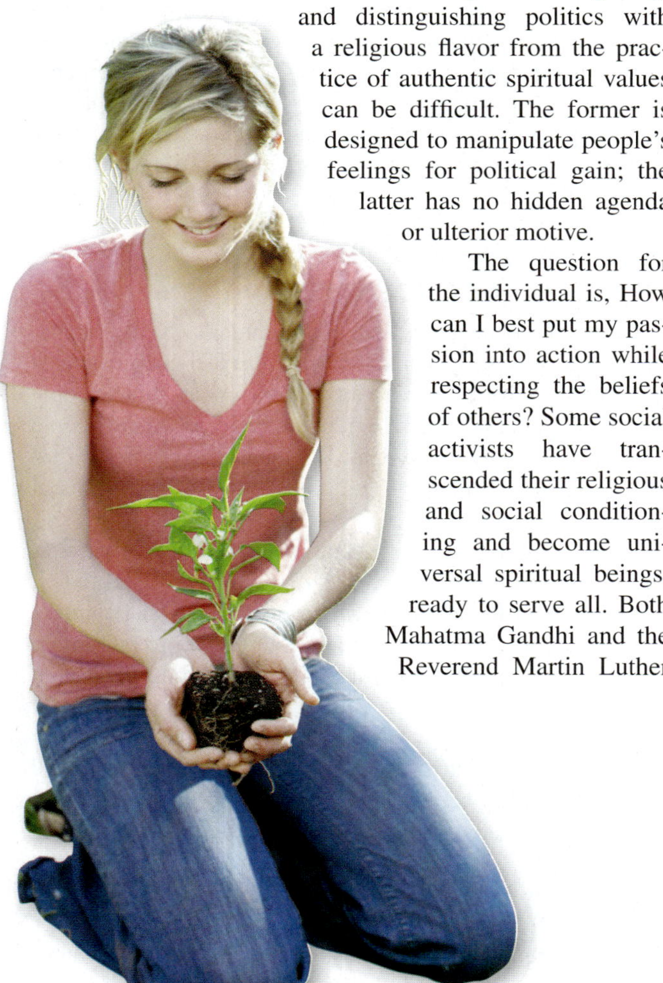

The question for the individual is, How can I best put my passion into action while respecting the beliefs of others? Some social activists have transcended their religious and social conditioning and become universal spiritual beings, ready to serve all. Both Mahatma Gandhi and the Reverend Martin Luther King, Jr., developed an integrated worldview and worked to create global community.

NATURE AND THE ENVIRONMENT

The impulse that propels people to the mountains or seashore for their holidays is the same impulse that drives pilgrims to sites of religious importance—the need to reconnect with the natural world. Many cultures in history, including many Native American cultures, did and do have a strong spiritual connection to nature or "Mother Earth." These cultures promote reverence for the universe, which results in a strong spiritual connection to nature.

Some people combine ecological, ethical, and spiritual interests and beliefs into what has been called *eco-spirituality*. They may participate in retreats or periods of reflection to deepen their connections to the earth. They may advocate respect for the sacredness of creation and the concept of tending (caring for, nurturing, and participating in nature). Daily activities that incorporate environmental values might include recycling, composting, and walking or riding a bike instead of driving. As with volunteerism and social activism, when you are environmentally active, the benefits flow back to you, sustaining your spirituality and adding meaning to life.

Death and Dying

Death and dying have great spiritual significance for people of all cultures. In one study, 89 percent of Americans described a "good death" as one that included making peace with God.[49] Many also included prayer and discussing the meaning of death in their description of a good death.

When someone you love dies, the experience is extremely personal, yet it is one that you also share with others. Life and death are part of the cycle of existence and the natural order of things. Many report that because of their personal faith, they do not fear death, since they know that their lives have had meaning within the context of a larger plan.

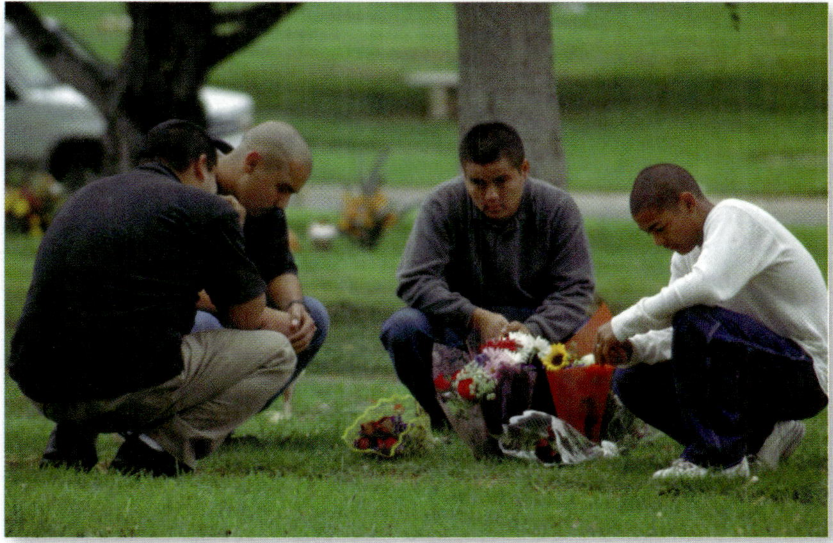

Spiritual beliefs and rituals can help people deal with grief and pain when a loved one dies.

STAGES OF DYING AND DEATH

In 1969 Elisabeth Kübler-Ross published *On Death and Dying*, one of the first books to propose a set of stages that people go through when they believe they are in the process of dying.[50] The five stages are (1) denial and isolation, (2) anger, (3) bargaining, (4) depression, and (5) acceptance. Over time, further study has shown that these stages are not linear—individuals may experience them in a different order or may return to stages they have already gone through—nor are they necessarily universal—individuals may not experience some stages at all.

Many believe that life is full of transitions, with death being the last. A shared sense of mortality can be the basis for feeling connected with other human beings. Recently, health care professionals have begun to describe ways to *live* with an illness rather than simply looking at the diagnosis as the point at which one begins to prepare for death. As medical care has improved, many individuals diagnosed with cancer or HIV infection have recovered or lived with the disease for many years. The critical thing to remember is that one need not go on a "death watch" after a diagnosis; usually, there is time to repair relationships, to build memories, and to review one's life. The dying person may find comfort and strength in talking through the process with family and friends or with a spiritual advisor.

Research has found that terminally ill persons derive strength and hope from spiritual and religious beliefs. In fact, terminally ill adults report significantly greater religious involvement and depth of spiritual perspective than do healthy adults. Studies suggest that, unrelated to belief in an afterlife, religiously involved people at the end of life are more accepting of death than those who are less religiously involved. In addition, religious involvement and spirituality are associated with less death anxiety.[18]

HEALTHY GRIEVING

Grief is a natural reaction to loss. Besides the loss of loved ones to death, we grieve many kinds of losses throughout our lives: divorce, relocation, traumatic experiences, loss of health and mobility, and even expected life transitions such as having the last child leave home. Grief is often expressed by feelings of sadness, loneliness, anger, and guilt. These feelings are part of the process of healing, since we do not begin to feel better until we have acknowledged and felt sorrow over our loss.

Physical symptoms of grief may include crying and sighing, aches and pains, sleep disturbances, headaches, lethargy, reduced appetite, and stomach upset. The intense emotions you feel at the time of a loss can have a negative impact on immune system functioning, reducing your ability to fight off illness. Studies have shown that surviving spouses may have increased risk for heart disease, cancer, depression, alcoholism, and suicide.[51,52] Ten to 15 percent of bereaved people struggle for several years or longer with grief reactions that interfere with their ability to function.[53] Everyone has higher risk for disease after the loss of a loved one, but those who are more resilient may cope with the loss better. Resilient people seem to be more likely to find comfort in talking and thinking about the deceased and are flexible enough to either suppress or express emotions about a death.[53]

Bereavement after the loss of a loved one typically involves four phases:

- *Numbness and shock*. This phase occurs immediately after the loss and lasts for a brief period. The numbness protects you from acute pain.
- *Separation*. As the shock wears off, you start to feel the pain of loss, and you experience acute yearning and longing to be reunited with your loved one.
- *Disorganization*. You are preoccupied and distracted; you have trouble concentrating and thinking clearly. You may feel lethargic and indifferent. This phase can last much longer than you anticipate.
- *Reorganization*. You begin to adjust to the loss. Your life will never be the same without your loved one, but your feelings have less intensity and you can reinvest in life.

If you experience the death of a loved one, it is important to take care of yourself while you are grieving. There

Public Health in Action: End-of-Life Decision Making

Many physicians believe it is important to discuss end-of-life decisions with their patients—to talk about whether a patient wants anything and everything done to prolong life or whether, in certain circumstances, the patient would prefer comfort over invasive treatments. Research has found that when physicians have end-of-life discussions with their patients, the quality of care increases while costs decrease. Overall, it appears that palliative or hospice care leads to more comfortable deaths, while aggressive care does not necessarily prolong life. There will always be isolated "miracle" situations where life is prolonged due to an aggressive intervention, but overall the data indicate that the quality of life and life itself are not prolonged through extreme measures.

However, like any health care service or treatment, having an end-of-life discussion with a physician costs money. In 2003, Congress passed a law that covered these discussions for terminally ill people with Medicare, the national insurance plan for people 65 and older. This meant that terminally ill patients would not have to pay out of pocket to have end-of-life discussions with their doctors and that doctors would be fairly compensated for their time spent on these discussions, thus increasing the likelihood that these conversations would occur.

In 2009, a congressional committee in the House of Representatives proposed that as part of health care reform Medicare's coverage of end-of-life discussions be expanded to include such discussions for older people who were not terminally ill. Every five years, Medicare would pay for a doctor to discuss with the patient issues like setting up a living will, designating a health care proxy, or obtaining hospice care. The goal of the legislation, as with the 2003 bill, was to improve the quality of life for older Americans and decrease rapidly rising health care costs. However, some opponents of the bill termed these optional conversations "death panels" that would force people to die early and against their will. Because of this widespread misunderstanding, the proposal was ultimately stripped from the final House bill.

Even though coverage for end-of-life discussions has not yet been expanded to senior citizens who are not terminally ill, those who have been diagnosed with a terminal illness can still have their end-of-life conversations with their doctors covered by Medicare. And under a 1991 act passed during George H.W. Bush's Administration, hospitals are required to ask all adult patients whether they have an advanced directive and to inform them of their right to refuse treatment.

Although discussions about end-of-life care are never easy, having them improves the quality of life for a patient and provides peace of mind for the patient's family. When not being mislabeled as "death panels," government advocacy and support for end-of-life advance decision making appears to make good sense.

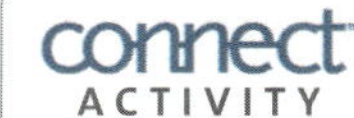

Sources: "Oh, Those Death Panels," by A. Sullivan, 2009, Time, *accessed February 24, 2010, from www.time.com; "Health Care Costs in the Last Week of Life: Associations with End-of-Life Conversations," by B. Zhang et al., 2009,* Archives of Internal Medicine 169(5), *pp. 480–488.*

is no right or wrong way to grieve and no specific timetable. Friends who suggest that it's time to move on need to understand that you are on your own journey and cannot be rushed. You need to give yourself permission to feel the loss and take time to heal. Some people seem to cope better if they talk about the death rather than internalizing their feelings. During the grieving process it is vital that you eat a balanced diet, exercise regularly, drink plenty of fluids, and get enough rest. Keeping a journal and talking about the person who has died can also be part of the healing process. Finally, you should not hesitate to ask friends for support, since having a nurturing social network is particularly helpful in coping with loss.

If intense grief persists for more than a year, or if you find yourself losing or gaining weight or not sleeping, consult a health professional to get a treatment referral. Treatment options might include support groups, family therapy, individual counseling, or a psychiatric evaluation.

RITUALS AROUND DEATH

Beliefs about death and rituals for marking the loss of loved ones vary across cultures. In some cultures, mourners have wakes and parties that last for days; in others, they sing and play music; in still others, they cover mirrors so they cannot see what they look like during times of grief.

Many rituals that surround death and dying are actually for the living, to help people cope with the loss of a loved one. Rituals help mourners move through the emotional work of grieving. When a person has been important to us, we never forget that person or lose the relationship. Instead, we find ways of "emotionally relocating" the deceased person in our lives, keeping our bonds with them while moving on. Cultural rituals can facilitate this process.

END-OF-LIFE DECISIONS

Many people dread a situation in which they or those they trust will have no say in decisions about their end-of-life treatment[50] (see the box "End-of-Life Decision Making"). To avoid this situation, they can make known their preferences through the use of formal legal documents that grant a **durable power of attorney for health care (DPOAHC)**

durable power of attorney for health care (DPOAHC) Formal legal power to make health care decisions for someone who is no longer able to do so for himself or herself.

Consumer Clipboard

How to Create an Advanced Directive

No matter how healthy you feel, it is wise to create an official document that outlines your wishes in the case that you are unable to make medical decisions for yourself—an advanced directive. Even if you have no current health problems, a sudden injury (e.g., from a motor vehicle accident) could leave you unable to communicate your wishes with regard to your medical treatment.

The main types of advanced directives are a living will and a durable power of attorney for health care, though they are sometimes referred to by different names in various states. It's a smart idea to have both. These need not be complicated documents, and you do not need a lawyer to have them created, though you should check your state's laws and guidelines before creating one. There are software packages you can buy to create these documents, but your state should have forms that you can download and fill out yourself.

Living Will

- This document outlines the kind of care you do or do not want to receive in the event you are unable to voice your preferences yourself.
- It does not allow someone else to make decisions for you.
- A living will is only for health care. It is not the same thing as a conventional will.
- When writing a living will, consider the kinds of treatments that are commonly administered to very ill patients and in what circumstances you do or do not wish to receive them. For example, if you fall into a permanent coma, do you want to continue to be kept alive with a feeding tube?
- Some treatments to consider: life-prolonging medical care (dialysis, blood transfusions, medical tests, use of a respirator, CPR), food and water (and whether you want these continued if you are in a vegetative state), and palliative care.

Durable Power of Attorney for Health Care

- This document designates someone to be your health care proxy. This person will be able to make medical decisions for you in the event you are unable to make them yourself.
- You can give the person as much or as little decision-making power as you would like.
- In general, your health care proxy will be able to take the following actions unless you specifically prohibit them: allow or refuse treatment, hire or fire medical personnel, access your medical records, choose medical personnel and facilities, and visit you.
- You should discuss with your health care proxy your treatment wishes (see suggested topics in the "End-of-Life Decisions" section).

After you create your advanced directive, have the document notarized and distribute copies to your doctor and family members.

Sources: Adapted from "The Living Will and Power of Attorney for Health Care: An Overview," by Shae Irving, Nolo Press, retrieved March 3, 2010, from www.nolo.com/legal-encyclopedia/article-29595.html; "End-of-Life Decisions: Advance Directives," National Hospice and Palliative Care Organization, retrieved March 3, 2010, from www.caringinfo.org/UserFiles/File/PDFs/AdvanceDirectives/ENGLISH_Advance_Dir.pdf.

to someone they trust or through a **living will**, in which they outline what types of medical treatment they do or don't want to receive (see the box "How to Create an Advanced Directive"). These directives may cover any issue the patient considers important.

living will
Formal legal document that outlines the medical treatment a person does or doesn't want to receive when he or she is no longer able to make such decisions.

hospice
Program that provides care for the terminally ill and their loved ones.

A common concern is whether life-sustaining treatment should be withdrawn when there is no hope of recovery. These decisions should be made in supportive consultation with family members, close friends, a spiritual advisor, and health care professionals. Such decisions must take into account the patient's values, the most common ones being family and interpersonal relationships, spiritual beliefs or religion, and independence.[54]

When terminally ill patients do decide to have treatment withdrawn, they often turn to **hospice**. Hospice is not a place but a concept of care. The goal is to improve the quality of life in a patient's last days by providing *palliative care*—pain management, comfort, and attention to the person's physical, spiritual, emotional, and social needs. Hospice programs also provide support for family members, including help with caring for their loved one.

Beyond medical decisions, there are also practical concerns to take care of at the end of life. Organ donation is one consideration, especially since there are more people who need organ donations than there are organ donors. Over 100 people die every week in the United States from the lack of available organs for transplant.[55] Organ donors need not be in perfect health at the time of death, and all costs associated with organ donation are paid by the recipient, not the donor. Anyone over the age of 18 can become an organ donor by indicating so on his or her driver's license, but this decision should also be discussed with family members as they may be asked to sign a consent form before the donation can be carried out. People also need to let their loved ones know whether they want to be buried or cremated, what kind of funeral or memorial service they prefer, and who will administer their financial and legal affairs.

There are also profound emotional issues to work through, including the grief of both the dying person and the loved ones who will be left behind.

LIFE AFTER DEATH

Belief in an afterlife is a tenet of most faith traditions. Although some investigators say no proof of life after death exists, other researchers argue that there is empirical evidence from individuals who have been resuscitated following a near-death experience.[56,57] It would be comforting to know that there is some afterlife and that we will be reunited with our loved ones in another state of existence. However, such comforts cannot be provided by science; they remain in the realm of faith and belief.

You Make the Call

Do You Have the Right to Choose?

Ethical questions about the right to die have become more prominent since the 1975 case of Karen Ann Quinlan. She was brought to the hospital in a coma and subsequently declared to be in a persistent vegetative state. After many years of court battles, her parents were finally granted their request to have her life support discontinued. Since then, similar cases have been fought in the public spotlight, including the case of Terri Schiavo, who was taken off life support in 2005 after 2 years in a persistent vegetative state.

It is now generally acknowledged that patients have the right to refuse life-sustaining treatment, and all states authorize written advance directives by means of which individuals can state their wishes. More controversial than withdrawing treatment is the practice of actively hastening a person's death, referred to as *active euthanasia* or *physician-assisted suicide*. In this case, a physician helps a terminally ill patient administer a lethal dose of drugs to himself or herself.

Oregon is currently the only state that permits physician-assisted suicide. The Oregon Death with Dignity Act requires that a patient be terminally ill with less than 6 months to live, be judged mentally competent by two physicians, and make two oral requests and one written request at least 2 weeks apart. Since its passage, more than 200 people have taken advantage of the provisions of the bill. The legality of the act was upheld by the U.S. Supreme Court in 2006.

Proponents of physician-assisted suicide, sometimes referred to as the right to die, believe that individuals have the right to choose how they will die, just as they have the right to choose how they will live. The rights of patients to refuse life support and to sign do-not-resuscitate orders are currently protected, and they are not so different from the right to actively choose how and when to die, according to this view.

Opponents of the right to die argue that human life is unconditionally valuable and that allowing physician-assisted suicide opens the door to abuse. They believe that if more attention were paid to palliative care at the end of life, people would not need to request physician-assisted suicide.

Do terminally ill people have the right to end their lives on their own terms, or is assisted suicide a violation of our cultural values? You make the call.

PROS

- Although life should be protected, people should be allowed to die with dignity when they are terminally ill or in unbearable pain. It is the humane thing to do.
- Loss of autonomy and control are among the most feared aspects of dying. Allowing people the right to die lets them maintain their sense of personal identity until the end of their lives.
- Medical and financial resources are used, keeping people alive who are ready to die. These resources could be freed up for other uses if terminally ill patients were allowed to choose to die.

CONS

- Life is unconditionally valuable, and commitment to life is a value of virtually all societies. Physician-assisted suicide undermines this value, legitimizes suicide, and gives "permission" to more people to commit suicide.
- The vow to "do no harm" is part of the physician's oath. Any compromise in this commitment would undermine the public's faith in the medical profession.
- The practice opens the door to abuse. Some people may feel pressured to end their lives to relieve financial or emotional strains on their families, and in some cases, family members may apply such pressure.
- If attention is paid to pain management and palliative care, people can live out their days and die a natural death. Pain should be managed and depression treated so that people don't feel the need to end their lives.

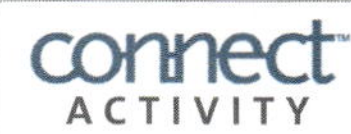

IN REVIEW

How is spirituality defined?
Spirituality is often defined as a person's connection to self, others, and the community at large. It usually involves a personal belief system or a value system that gives meaning and purpose to life. It provides a feeling of participation in something greater than oneself and a sense of unity with nature and the universe.

How does a person build a spiritual life?
Anyone can develop a regular spiritual practice. Examples include meditation, mindfulness, journaling, retreat, experiencing the arts, and developing a daily routine that embodies one's values. Some people develop their spirituality through community involvement, such as volunteering or social activism, and others find their spiritual connection in nature.

What health benefits are associated with spirituality?
Spiritually connected people tend to enjoy better mental and physical health than those who do not describe themselves as spiritually connected, although the reasons for these differences are a matter of debate. Spiritual connectedness appears to be related to higher levels of health-related quality of life—the physical, psychological, social, and spiritual aspects of a person's daily experiences.

What kinds of experiences are associated with death and dying?
Death is a natural part of the cycle of existence, but most people experience anxiety when facing the prospect of their own death or the death of a loved one. People with spiritual beliefs tend to derive strength and hope from their beliefs and may be more accepting of death. Hospice care can make the end of life a more comfortable and peaceful experience.

Web Resources

A Campaign for Forgiveness Research: This organization is dedicated to promoting forgiveness around the world as a way of improving the human condition. The site features myths and truths about forgiveness and offers ways to make forgiveness a part of your life.
www.forgiving.org

American Meditation Institute for Yoga Science and Philosophy: As an introduction, this Web site describes a systematic procedure for meditation. For those interested in learning meditation, the organization advocates finding a qualified teacher for personal instruction.
www.americanmeditation.org

Hospice Foundation of America: Focusing on hospice as a concept of care, this site describes the growth of the hospice movement and explains its goals. Hospice is presented as a unique source of comfort for patients and families facing death.
www.hospicefoundation.org

Organ Donation: This official U.S. government Web site for organ donation and transplantation describes the myths and facts associated with organ donation. It features a donor card that you can sign and carry.
www.organdonor.gov

12 Environmental Issues

Ever Wonder...
about the environmental cost of a fast-food burger?
what the effects of climate change will be?
what you should do with your old computer when you get a new one?
Mc Graw Hill
connect
PERSONAL HEALTH
http://www.mcgrawhillconnect.com/personalhealth

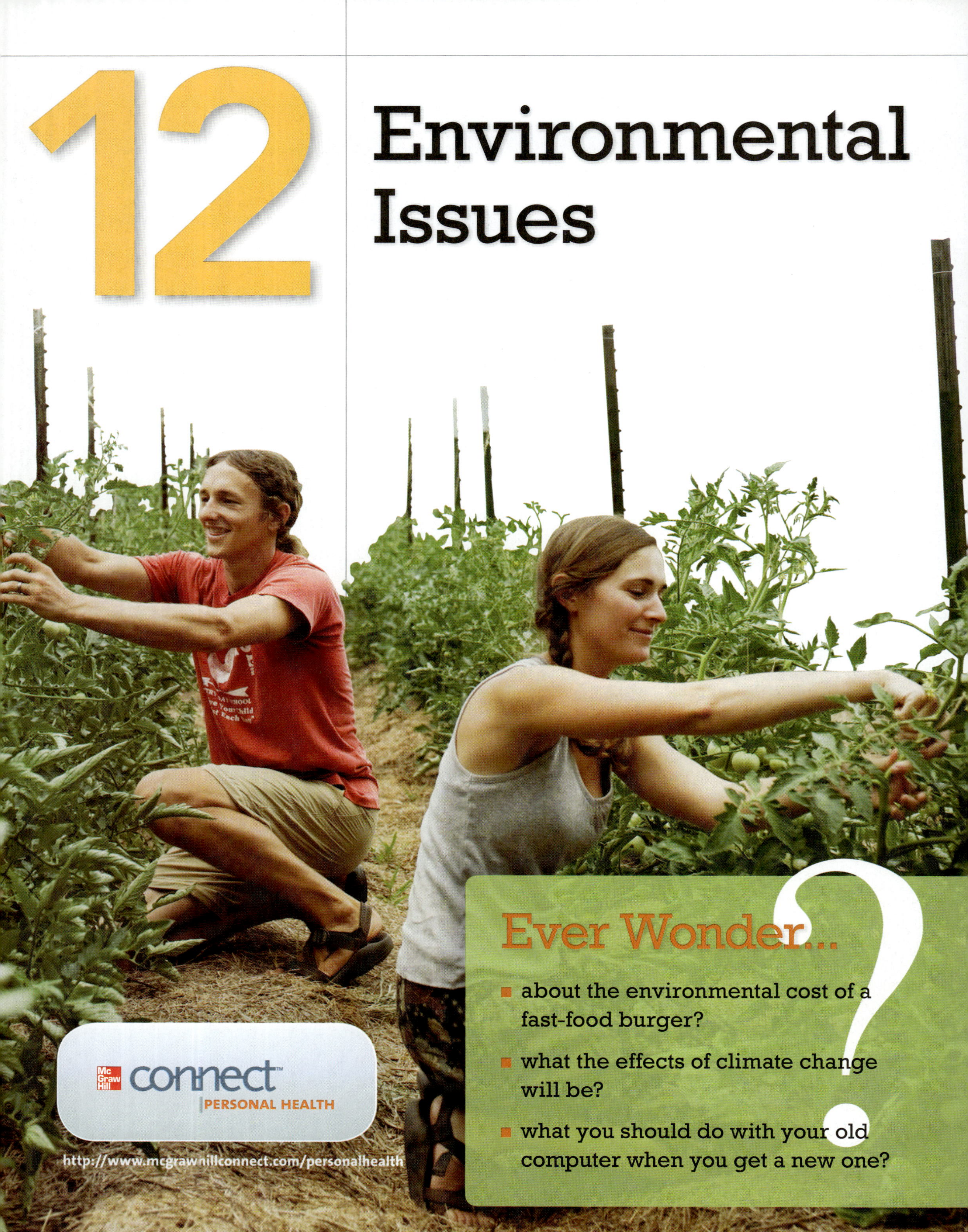

When we look at environmental health issues, we become aware that our lives are part of the intricate web of living organisms and nonliving natural resources that make Earth a single, vital ecosystem. Only recently have people come to realize that the planet's resources are not infinite. We have also realized that many human activities have damaged the integrity of our ecosystem and threatened our own health. The possible enormity of this damage leaves many of us overwhelmed.

There are actions that can be taken, however, if individuals and societies recognize that resources are limited and if they take responsibility for protecting and preserving these resources. For example, colleges and universities are "going green," and students are becoming proactive in driving their schools to adopt environment-friendly policies and programs.

The field of **environmental health** has traditionally been concerned with infectious diseases associated with contaminated water, food, waste, and other pollutants. Recently, the field has expanded to encompass pollutants that result from human and industrial activities and that cause chronic diseases and global environmental damage. Major issues today include climate change, the depletion of resources, especially energy resources, and world overpopulation—the issue that underlies and amplifies all our environmental concerns (see the box "Global Climate Change and Health").

Water and Water Quality

Scientists estimate that only about 14 one-thousandths (0.014 percent) of the earth's water is readily available for human use.[1] Usable water supplies are further diminished by human activities that destroy or pollute natural ecological systems.

WATER SUPPLIES AND SHORTAGES

The earth's supply of water is continuously collected, purified, and distributed in a natural process called the *water cycle*. The water we use has two sources: surface water and groundwater. *Surface water* is precipitation that is stored in lakes, reservoirs, and wetlands (swamps, marshes, bogs) on the surface of the earth. It is renewed fairly rapidly in areas where precipitation occurs 12 to 20 days a year.

Groundwater is precipitation that sinks into the ground. This water is stored in giant underground reservoirs called *aquifers* and slowly moves to areas where it is discharged, such as a stream, a river, a lake, or an ocean, as part of the water cycle. Groundwater makes up 95 percent of the world's supply of freshwater.[2] In North America, about half of the drinking water comes from groundwater supplies.

environmental health The area of health concerns that focuses on the interactions of humans with all aspects of their environment.

Withdrawal rates of surface water are projected to double in the next 20 years and exceed reliable sources in a growing number of areas. In the United States and Canada, water supplies are abundant, but much of our water is contaminated by industrial and agricultural wastes or is in the wrong place at the wrong time.[1,2] Conflicts between regions and states over water supplies have existed throughout U.S. history and are likely to intensify in the future, especially as people migrate and industries relocate to the West and Southwest.[3] The United States Geological Survey projects that 36 states will face water shortages by 2013 due to droughts, rising

Conflicts *between regions and states over water supplies have existed throughout U.S. history and are likely to* **intensify in the future.**

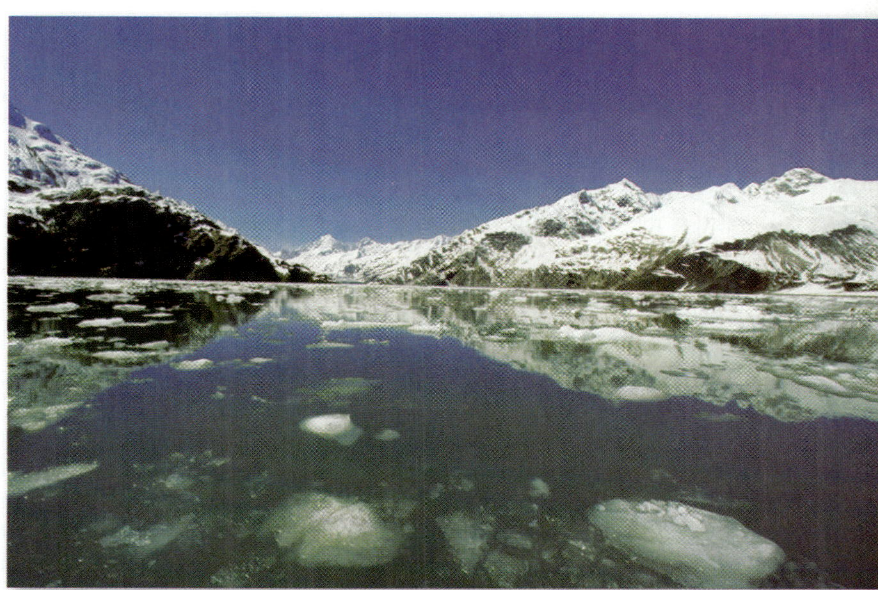

Melting ice and shrinking glaciers are just some of the signs of global warming and climate change.

Who's at Risk? Global Climate Change and Health

- Scientists project that global temperatures could rise by 1.0–4.5° F by 2050 and by 2.2–10.0° F by the close of the 21st century. This rise in temperatures would significantly increase heat-related deaths. Older adults, obese individuals, and children are at highest risk for heat-related deaths.
- As a result of global warming, pollen blooms will occur 10 days earlier in 2017 than they did in 2007 and be more severe. Tropical diseases like West Nile virus, malaria, yellow fever, and dengue fever may become more prevalent and expand to new areas in the United States.
- The Environmental Protection Agency projects that seawater in the United States will rise by 39 inches by the end of the 21st century. The rise in seawater would place 22,000 square miles of the United States under water. The most vulnerable areas are southern Florida, the Chesapeake Bay region, New Orleans, and San Francisco.
- One-sixth of the world's population does not have access to safe water. Half of the world's population suffers from a waterborne disease at any given moment. Problems with safe water are especially prevalent in developing nations.
- According to the United Nations Environment Programme, a 10 percent thinning of the ozone layer of the atmosphere would cause an additional 300,000 cases of non-melanoma skin cancer worldwide, 4,500 cases of malignant melanoma, and 1.5 million cases of cataracts each year.
- Analysts project that global carrying capacity—the number of people the earth can support at subsistence level—is 50 billion people. However, cultural carrying capacity—the number of people the earth can support at an optimum standard of living—is about 9 billion people. World population is expected to hit this number by about 2050. Because there are not enough energy resources to meet the optimal standard of living needs for everyone, we can expect to see continuing conflict over world resources, especially between developed and developing nations.

Sources: Climate Change 2007: The Physical Science Basis, *Intergovernmental Panel on Climate Change, 2007, Geneva, Switzerland; "Global Warming: Early Signs," Intergovernmental Panel on Climate Change, 1999, retrieved June 18, 2008, from www.climatehotmap.org; "Get Out Your Handkerchief," by S. Begley, June 4, 2007,* Newsweek, *p. 62; "Future Sea Level Changes," U.S. Environmental Protection Agency, retrieved June 18, 2008, from www.epa.gov/climatechange/science/futureslc.html.*

earth surface temperatures, urban sprawl, and wasteful use of water.

Individuals can play an important role in water conservation. Most of our "drinking water" in the United States is used for toilet flushing, bathing, cooking, lawn watering, clothes and dish washing, and cleaning. For tips on reducing your personal use of water, see the box "You Can Help Conserve Water."

Water resource experts say the main cause of water waste is the artificially low cost of water. Government subsidies to agriculture and industry have led to limited financial incentives to invest in water-saving technologies. Many water utility companies charge residences a flat fee for water usage rather than a fee based on how much water is used, and thus residences that use a lot of water pay the same amount as those who use less. Water resource experts, however, predict that local governments will need to make unpopular decisions to significantly raise water prices or to adopt systems that charge consumers according to the amount of water they use. Such a system is in place in Brazil, where residents use pay-as-you-go cards that are loaded with water credits. A resident enters a card code into a water manager device that then gives a specific amount of water. This system has resulted in significant reductions in water use.

water pollution Any chemical, biological, or physical change in water quality that has a harmful impact on living organisms or makes water unsuitable for desired use.

WATER POLLUTION

Water pollution refers to any chemical, biological, or physical change in water quality that has a harmful impact on living organisms or makes water unsuitable for desired use.[4] The U.S. Environmental Protection Agency (EPA) claims that all but a few of the surface-water reservoirs in the United States are contaminated by discharge pollutants at specific locations through sewers, pipes, or ditches. Sources for these pollutants include factories, sewage treatment plants that remove some but not all pollutants, active and abandoned mines, oil spills, and agricultural feedlots. Runoff from large land areas such as croplands, golf courses, lawns, and parking lots also pollutes surface water.[1]

Cleaning up pollutants that reach aquifers lying deep in the ground is very difficult. The main sources of groundwater contamination are storage lagoons, septic tanks, landfills, hazardous waste dumps, and underground storage tanks filled with gasoline, oil, solvents, and hazardous waste. Such tanks can corrode and leak after 25 to 40 years. Groundwater is also contaminated when individuals dump or spill oil, gasoline, paint thinners, or other organic solvents onto the ground.[1,2]

Challenges & Choices

You Can Help Conserve Water

Americans use about 100 gallons of water per person a day for domestic purposes. This rate is three times the per capita average for the world as a whole. Here are some tips to help you conserve water:

Bathroom About 65 percent of residential water is used in the bathroom. The toilet accounts for 40 percent of all water used in the home.

- Install a low-flow toilet, which saves about 30 gallons of water per day.
- Install water-saving showerheads and flow restrictors on all faucets. If you can fill a 1-gallon bucket in 15 seconds, you need a more efficient fixture.
- Turn off sink faucets when brushing your teeth, shaving, or washing. An open faucet sends about 7 gallons of water down the drain every minute.
- Repair leaks promptly. A faucet that leaks one drop a second can waste 200 gallons of water in a month. You can test for toilet leaks by adding a few drops of food coloring to the water in the toilet tank. If you have a leak, some color will show up in the toilet bowl within minutes.
- Take shorter showers. Cutting your shower time by 1 minute saves about 500 gallons of water a year.

Laundry About 15 percent of residential water is used in the laundry room.

- When buying a new washing machine, purchase a front-loading machine that fills at different levels for loads of different sizes.
- Wash your clothes only when you have a full load. If you must wash small loads, select the lowest possible water-level setting.
- Buy appliances with an "Energy Star" label. An Energy Star washing machine can save up to 7,000 gallons of water a year.

Kitchen About 10 percent of residential water is used for drinking and cooking.

- Run your dishwasher only when you have a full load. Use the short cycle and let your dishes air-dry.
- If you wash your dishes by hand, do not let the water run continuously.
- Start a compost pile instead of using a garbage disposal. Garbage disposals and water softener systems use large amounts of water.

Outdoors About 10 percent of residential water is used outdoors. This percentage is as much as 65 percent in desert climates.

- Water your lawn and plants early in the morning and in the evening, minimizing loss of water through evaporation in the midday heat.
- Install drip irrigation systems for gardens and flower beds.
- Xeriscape—landscape with native plants, which adapt to local annual precipitation.
- Wash your car using a bucket for soapy water; use the hose only for rinsing. If you use a commercial car wash, choose one that recycles water.

Sources: One Makes the Difference, *by J.B. Hill, 2002, New York: HarperCollins;* Living in the Environment, *by G.T. Miller, 2002, Belmont, CA: Wadsworth/ Thomson Learning;* Water on Tap: A Consumer's Guide to the Nation's Drinking Water, *U.S. Environmental Protection Agency, Washington, DC: Office of Water, 1997.*

SAFE DRINKING WATER

In the United States, the Safe Drinking Water Act of 1974 established many health standards for drinking water. About 8 percent of people in the United States, primarily farmers and rural residents, rely on their own private drinking water supplies. Owners of private wells are not required to comply with EPA health standards, but people using private water supplies must take special precautions to ensure water safety.[1]

About 1 in 15 households in the United States uses bottled water as the main source of drinking water.[2] Bottled water is just as vulnerable to contamination as tap water, however. If you use bottled water, look for the trademark International Bottled Water Association for assurance of contaminant-free water.[2]

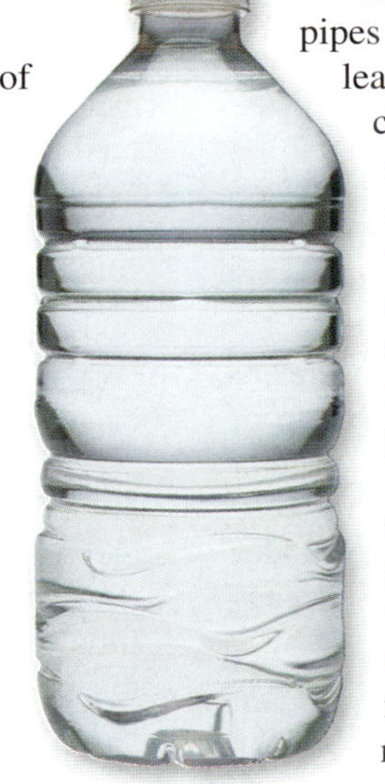

In some older homes, contamination from lead water pipes or lead solder on pipes is a concern. Exposure to lead can cause serious health problems, especially in children. To minimize lead exposure, let the water run for a minute or so after turning on the tap; this can flush away lead that may have leached into the water.[2] Cold water is less likely to contain lead that has been leached from supply pipes, so use only cold water for cooking and preparing infant formula. Both lead water pipes and lead solder on pipes have been banned in the United States.

Ensuring a sustainable water supply for ourselves and future generations will require several strategies. Consumers and businesses need to use water-saving technologies; farmers and the agriculture industry need to develop ways to irrigate crops more efficiently; and government and policy makers must manage water basins and groundwater fairly

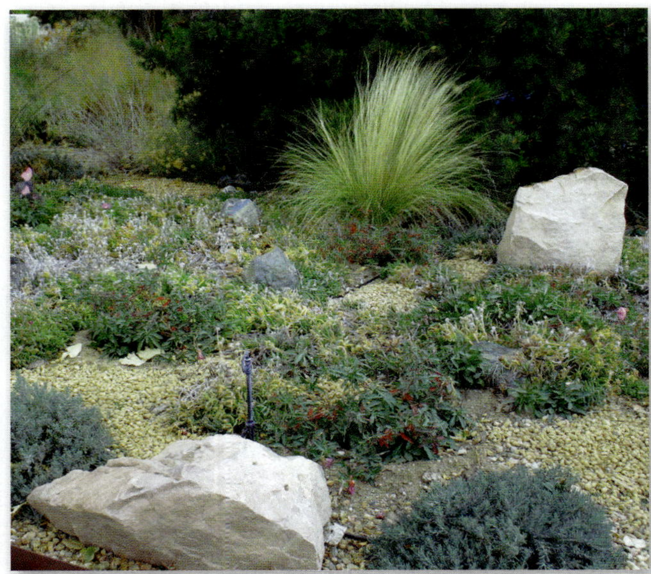

Xeriscaping saves water by using native plants, avoiding supplemental irrigation, and preventing the loss of water to evaporation and run-off—without sacrificing the aesthetic appeal of a beautiful garden.

and effectively. Such strategies are likely to be controversial and difficult to implement, but failure to address our water-related problems will lead to economic and health problems, increased environmental degradation, and loss of biodiversity.

Air and Air Quality

Like water, air is an essential resource that many of us take for granted until it becomes polluted and hazardous to our health. According to the EPA, one in three Americans live in an area where the air is unhealthy to breathe at least part of the year.

EARTH'S ATMOSPHERE

The atmosphere is the whole mass of air surrounding the earth. The innermost layer of atmosphere is called the *troposphere*, or lower atmosphere. This layer contains about 80 percent of the earth's air and extends 11 miles above sea level at the equator and about 5 miles above the poles. The second layer is the *stratosphere*, or upper atmosphere. It extends from 11 to 30 miles above Earth's surface.

The presence of certain gases in the lower atmosphere helps regulate the earth's temperature by trapping heat from the sun and preventing it from radiating back into space, a process called the **greenhouse effect**. Without the greenhouse effect, the surface of the earth would be much colder and less hospitable to life.[6,7] The two most important **greenhouse gases** are carbon dioxide and water vapor.

An important component of the upper atmosphere is **ozone**, an odorless, colorless gas composed of three atoms of oxygen. Ozone forms naturally in the upper atmosphere and provides a protective layer that shields us from the sun's harmful ultraviolet (UV) radiation waves. This shield prevents about 95 percent of the sun's UV rays from reaching the earth's surface.[1] Although it is protective in the upper atmosphere, ozone in the lower atmosphere is hazardous to health; ground-level ozone is discussed in the next section.

AIR POLLUTION

Air pollution is the presence of one or more chemicals in the atmosphere of sufficient quality and in sufficient quantity to cause harm to life.[1] A few hundred years ago, most air pollution occurred as a result of natural events, such as dust storms and sandstorms, forest fires, and volcanic eruptions. These natural pollutants still exist today, but since the Industrial Revolution in the 18th century, human activities have become the primary source of air pollutants.

The EPA designates the six air pollutants of greatest concern as "criteria pollutants"; they are carbon monoxide, sulfur dioxide, nitrogen dioxide, suspended particulate matter, ground-level ozone, and metal and metal compounds. All of these pollutants cause respiratory problems; some of them also cause cancer, heart disease, and birth defects.[1,8]

The EPA uses a measure of air pollution called the **Air Quality Index (AQI)** to provide the public with a daily report on air conditions and any associated health warnings. The AQI measures five individual pollutants in local communities on a scale of 0 to 500 and provides an overall air quality value and recommendations for outdoor activity levels. The higher the number, the less healthy the air. For example, at 30, air quality is considered good; at 100 or higher, air is considered unhealthy for sensitive groups, such as people with asthma; at 200, air is considered very unhealthy; and at 300 or higher, it is considered hazardous. (Levels above 300 almost never occur in U.S. communities.)

The EPA provides charts for four pollutants: ozone, particle pollution, carbon monoxide, and sulfur dioxide. (Levels of nitrogen dioxide are usually so low that they pose little direct threat to health, so a chart is not provided for this pollutant.) The AQI chart for carbon monoxide is shown in Figure 12.1. Levels of health concern are associated with

greenhouse effect
Warming of the earth's surface by heat trapped by gases in the lower atmosphere.

greenhouse gases
Gases that help trap heat in the lower atmosphere and radiate it back to the earth; they include carbon dioxide, water vapor, and others.

ozone
Odorless, colorless gas composed of three atoms of oxygen; in the upper atmosphere, ozone forms a protective shield blocking UV radiation from the sun; at ground level, ozone is a dangerous pollutant.

air pollution
Presence of one or more chemicals in the atmosphere of sufficient quality and in sufficient quantity to cause harm to life.

Air Quality Index (AQI)
Measure of air pollution issued daily by the EPA.

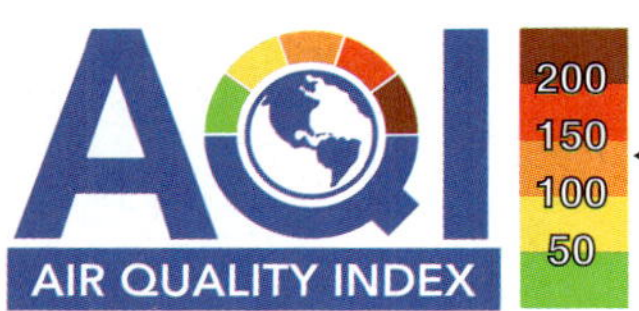

Pollutant: Particles

Today's Forecast: 130

Quality: Unhealthy for Sensitive Groups

People with heart or lung disease, older adults, and children are at risk.

(a)

Air Quality Index (AQI): Carbon Monoxide (CO)

Index Values	Levels of Health Concern	Cautionary Statements
0 - 50	Good	None
51 - 100*	Moderate	None
101 - 150	Unhealthy for Sensitive Groups	People with heart disease, such as angina, should reduce heavy exertion and avoid sources of CO, such as heavy traffic.
151 - 200	Unhealthy	People with heart disease, such as angina, should reduce moderate exertion and avoid sources of CO, such as heavy traffic.
201 - 300	Very Unhealthy	People with heart disease, such as angina, should reduce exertion and avoid sources of CO, such as heavy traffic.
301 - 500	Hazardous	People with heart disease, such as angina, should reduce exertion and avoid sources of CO, such as heavy traffic. Everyone else should reduce heavy exertion.

*An AQI of 100 for carbon monoxide corresponds to a CO level of 9 parts per million (averaged over 8 hours)

(b)

figure **12.1** **The EPA's Air Quality Index. (a) A sample AQI report in a newspaper. (b) An AQI chart for carbon monoxide.**

Source: Air Quality Index: A Guide to Air Quality and Your Health, *U.S. EPA, 2004, www.epa.gov.*

different colors so that the public can quickly understand air quality warnings.[1] The AQI is available in newspapers, on television broadcasts, and on state or local pollution agency Web sites. The EPA also provides maps on its Web site that track and forecast ozone levels in cities and regions.

Ozone Ground-level ozone is a hazard. Ozone is a highly reactive gas that is poisonous to most living organisms. It causes respiratory irritation, aggravates respiratory and heart disease, and damages the lungs. Physical activity or outdoor work requiring exertion and deep breathing results in deeper penetration of ozone into the lungs. For unknown reasons, about one in three people has an unusual susceptibility to ozone. Also at greater risk are active children with respiratory disorders (such as asthma), adults with respiratory diseases (such as emphysema), and older adults (because respiratory function declines with age).[1,9] In response to findings from an EPA panel of independent science advisers, the agency decided in 2010 to lower the acceptable level of ground-level ozone to better protect public health and welfare.

Particulate Matter Another hazardous component of air pollution is **particulate matter**, particles or droplets of dust, soot, oil, metals, or other compounds suspended in the air. The measurement unit for these particles is the micron (a human hair is about 70 microns in diameter), and the smaller the particle, the more likely it is to cause health damage. Scientists believe that small particles that remain in the lungs for a long time irritate and damage alveoli, the tiny air sacs in the lungs.[1] Ultrafine particles may also trigger an immune system response that alters blood chemistry and blood pressure, contributing to heart disease and lung disease.[8] You can check levels of ozone and particulate matter for your city at www.airnow.gov.

particulate matter Particles or droplets of dust, soot, oil, metals, or other compounds suspended in the air.

smog Mixture of pollutants in the lower atmosphere that makes the air hazy.

industrial smog Type of air pollution that forms mostly in cold weather and is caused primarily by burning large amounts of coal and oil.

Smog One of the primary sources of outdoor air pollutants is **smog**, a mixture of pollutants in the lower atmosphere that makes the air hazy. There are two types of smog: industrial smog and photochemical smog. **Industrial smog** is caused primarily by the burning of large amounts of coal and oil for heating, manufacturing, and the production of electrical power.[10] This type of smog occurs mostly in cold weather and produces a low-lying layer of pollution close to the earth's surface. Industrial smog is no longer a major problem in most developed countries. Coal and heavy oil are burned only in large furnaces or boiler systems that maintain strict pollution control, and waste gases are removed via tall smokestacks that transfer

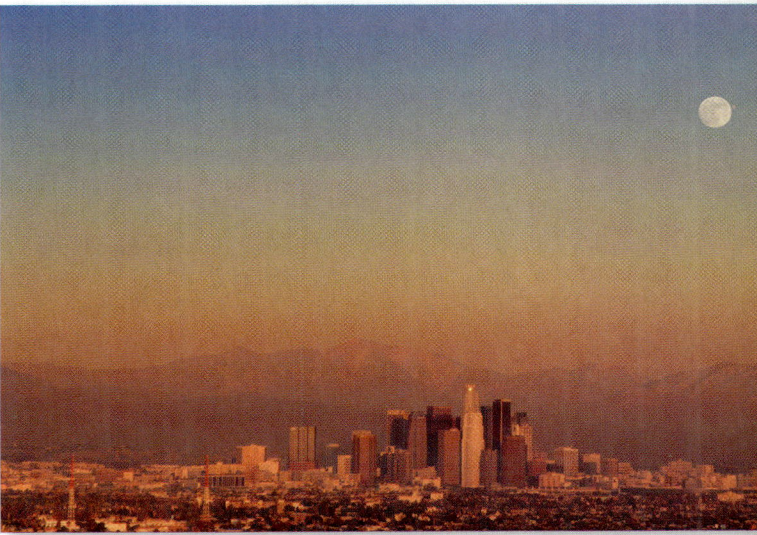

Photochemical smog and poor air quality plague Los Angeles not only because of motor vehicle exhaust but also because of the city's climate, shifting wind and weather conditions, and topographical features.

pollutants to downwind areas. This type of smog is still very much a problem in developing countries, however.

Photochemical smog is the type of smog that sits as a thick haze over many cities in the summer. It forms when pollutants from motor vehicle exhaust, industry, and other sources combine in the presence of sunlight and heat, producing large amounts of ozone and more than 100 other chemicals. All modern cities have photochemical smog, but it is much more prevalent in sunny, warm, dry climates with high population density and high use of **fossil fuels** (oil, coal, and natural gas) in transportation and industry.

photochemical smog
Type of air pollution that forms when pollutants from motor vehicle exhaust, industry, and other sources combine in the presence of sunlight and heat, producing ozone and more than 100 other chemicals.

fossil fuels
Oil, coal, and natural gas—fuels that were produced over the course of millions of years by the pressure and heat of the earth acting on the buried remains of plants and animals containing carbon; they are typically extracted from the earth by drilling.

temperature inversion
Weather condition in which a warm layer of air moves in over a cooler layer, trapping pollutants in the air near the earth's surface.

acid deposition
Depositing of acidic pollutants from the atmosphere on the earth's surface, in either dry or wet form.

Photochemical smog problems can be amplified by a temperature inversion.[1] Under normal conditions, the air at the earth's surface is heated by the sun and rises to mix with cool air above it. Surface air is replaced by cooler air that in turn is heated and rises, creating a natural circulation process. In a **temperature inversion**, a warm layer of air moves in over a cooler layer, trapping it so that the air cannot circulate. Pollutants at ground level can build up to dangerous levels if the inversion lasts more than a few days. Very large cities with mountains on three sides and the ocean on the other side, extensive automobile use, and a sunny climate with light winds have ideal conditions for temperature inversions and smog.

The Clean Air Act of 1990 required the EPA to set national emission standards for more than 100 different air pollutants. These standards have led to continued improvements in air quality by encouraging use of public transportation, non-gas-burning automobiles, the use of scrubbers to clean polluted air from smokestacks, reduced use of fossil fuels, and increased use of renewable energy.[1]

In addition, the 2002 Clear Skies Initiative amendment to the 1990 Clean Air Act set mandatory caps that substantially reduce emissions of sulfur dioxide, nitrogen oxide, and mercury from coal-fired electric power generation.[5] Individuals can also take steps to improve outdoor air quality (see the box "You Can Help Improve Outdoor Air Quality").

Acid Deposition and Precipitation Another major source of outdoor air pollutants is **acid deposition**, which occurs when acidic pollutants drop out of the atmosphere onto the earth's surface. The two major pollutants involved in

Challenges & Choices

You Can Help Improve Outdoor Air Quality

Small changes in individual behaviors and lifestyles can add up to big changes in greenhouse gas emissions.

- Walk, bike, skate, carpool, or use public transportation instead of driving your car. Each gallon of gas used by a car contributes about 20 pounds of carbon dioxide to the atmosphere. If all Americans between the ages of 10 and 74 replaced 30 minutes of driving with walking or biking, they would cut carbon dioxide emissions by 64 million tons a year.
- Get regular tune-ups for your car. A well-running car produces about 475 fewer pounds of carbon dioxide than a poorly tuned car.
- Check your tires to make sure they are inflated to the right pressure. When tires are properly inflated, your car uses less gas.
- Make sure your car's air conditioner isn't leaking chemicals, and limit your use of it to only the hottest days.
- If you are buying a car, consider an electric or a hybrid car that does not rely heavily on gasoline. If you don't get a hybrid, look for a car that gets good gas mileage.
- Turn down your home heating thermostat by at least 1 degree. You can cut energy consumption by as much as 10 percent for each degree.
- Buy the most energy-efficient homes, lights, and appliances available. Use compact fluorescent bulbs in lamps. Lighting accounts for about 20 percent of the total electricity used in the United States; refrigerators consume about 7 percent of total electricity.
- Turn down the thermostat on your water heater to between 110° and 120° F. Insulate hot water pipes. Hot water heaters consume about 20 percent of all energy used in a home.
- Keep houseplants to help clean the air in your home, and plant shade trees outside.

Sources: Living in the Environment, *by G.T. Miller, 2002, Belmont, CA: Wadsworth/Thomson Learning; Clear Skies Initiative, U.S. EPA, www.epa.gov; "Driving Up the Cost of Clean Air," by D.C. Holzman, 2005,* Health Perspectives, 113 *(4), pp. A246–A249.*

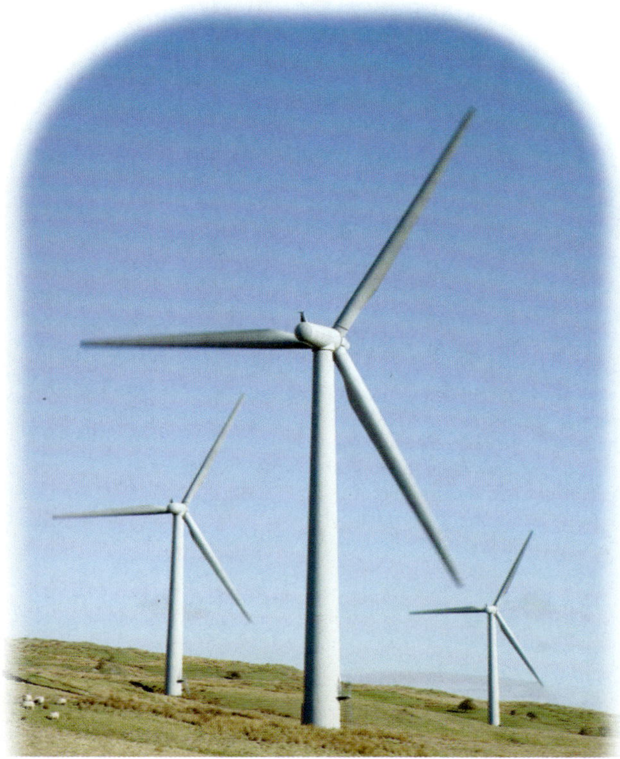

The primary contributors to acid deposition are sulfur dioxide from coal-burning power plants and carbon dioxide from motor vehicle emissions. Clean-energy sources like windmill farms do not release harmful chemicals into the air.

acid deposition are sulfur dioxide from coal-burning power plants and nitrogen dioxide from motor vehicle emissions.

Acid deposition can be dry or wet. Dry deposition occurs when acidic gases and particulate matter are blown by winds onto buildings, homes, cars, and trees or washed from surface areas by rainstorms. Dry deposition causes damage to stone, metal, and paint and necessitates repair to public monuments and buildings totaling millions of dollars every year. Dry deposition accounts for nearly half of the acid deposition falling from the atmosphere.[10]

Wet deposition, or **acid precipitation**, occurs when acidic pollutants mix with moisture in the atmosphere and fall to earth as acid rain, snow, sleet, hail, or fog. This type of acid deposition has devastated lakes, streams, and forests in certain parts of the world, killing trees, fish, and aquatic wildlife. The pollutants in acid precipitation also cause respiratory problems in vulnerable individuals.

The degree of environmental damage from acid deposition depends on the ability of the soil to neutralize acid. Where soils are alkaline, such as in parts of the U.S. Midwest, there is less damage. Where soils are neutral or acidic, as in the northwestern United States, northeastern North America, and many parts of Canada and Europe, damage is extensive.

Although prevention strategies offer the most promise, they are politically difficult to implement since the people and ecosystems affected are often distant from the actual source of acid deposition. Wind, hydropower, and natural gas are cleaner energy sources than coal, and environmentalists argue they would be more politically popular choices if the hidden environmental and health costs of coal's contribution to acid deposition and precipitation were widely recognized.

THINNING OF THE OZONE LAYER OF THE ATMOSPHERE

Every spring and early summer, a massive "hole" appears in the ozone layer of the atmosphere over Antarctica. This thinning of the ozone layer is caused by **chlorofluorocarbons (CFCs)**, chemicals used as coolants in refrigeration and air-conditioning units, as propellants in aerosol sprays, as solvents in cleaning products, and as foaming agents in some rigid foam products.[11] When these chemicals are released or leak into the air, they slowly rise into the upper atmosphere, where chlorine atoms destroy ozone.

Without the protection of the ozone layer, humans are at risk for more severe sunburns, more skin cancers, more cataracts (clouding of the lens in the eye, causing blindness), and suppression of the immune system, which increases the risk for infectious diseases.[1,11]

International agreements under the 1989 Montreal Protocol and subsequent treaties called for the reduction and eventual elimination of CFC production by 2000. This protocol is currently supported by 160 nations. However, because it takes CFCs 11 to 20 years to reach the upper atmosphere, it will be at least 50 years before the ozone layer begins to recover.[1] In the meantime, the hole continues to grow. During certain times of the year, it extends into populated areas of South America and Australia, and people living there are advised to stay indoors during critical periods and wear sunscreen and hats when they go outdoors.

acid precipitation Mixing of acidic pollutants in the atmosphere with moisture and their precipitation in the form of rain, snow, sleet, hail, or fog.

chlorofluorocarbons (CFCs) Chemicals used as coolants, propellants, solvents, and foaming agents that destroy ozone in the upper atmosphere.

global warming Gradual rise in the average temperature of the earth's surface, caused by an increase in greenhouse gases in the lower atmosphere.

GLOBAL WARMING AND CLIMATE CHANGE

For the past few hundred years, human activities have increased the amount of greenhouse gases in the lower atmosphere. These activities—burning fossil fuels, burning forests, cultivating cropland, raising cattle and other livestock on a mass basis, producing fertilizers, creating landfills—have significantly increased levels of carbon dioxide, methane, nitrous oxide, ozone, and other greenhouse gases. The intensification of the greenhouse effect has led to **global warming**, a gradual rise in the average temperature of the earth's surface (Figure 12.2).

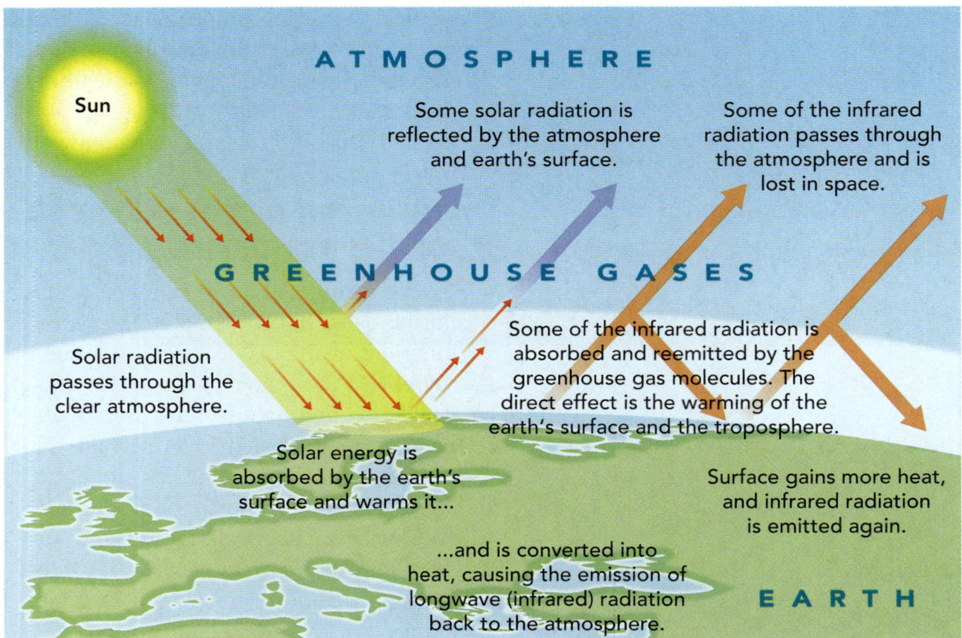

figure 12.2 **The greenhouse effect.** About two-thirds of the sun's radiation is absorbed by the earth and then reflected back into the atmosphere. Greenhouse gases—water vapor, carbon dioxide, ozone, methane, nitrous oxide, and others—trap infrared radiation from the earth, warming the atmosphere. Human activities are causing greenhouse gas levels in the atmosphere to increase, which in turn increases the temperature of the earth.

Source: Reprinted with permission from Information on Climate Change, *United Nations Environment Programme (UNEP).*

According to the National Academy of Sciences, the surface temperature of the earth has risen 1.1–1.3° F in the past century, but research suggests that most global warming has taken place in the past 50 years. Signs of global warming include melting of the ice caps and of glaciers, northward migration of some warm-climate fish, the bleaching of coral found in tropical areas, and the rise of sea levels by 4 to 8 inches over the past century.[1,11–14]

A 2007 report by the Intergovernmental Panel on Climate Change (IPCC), a network composed of more than 2,500 climate experts from more than 130 countries, concluded that it is very likely that the earth's surface temperature will rise in the range of 3.6° F to 8.1° F between 2005 and 2100. The most likely increase is about 5.4° F unless significant cuts are made in greenhouse gas emissions. An increase of less than this amount is likely only if greenhouse gas emissions decrease from 59 to 85 percent by 2050. The IPCC further concluded that a 3.6° F increase is likely inevitable but manageable. A temperature increase of 5.4° F would be catastrophic.

Some analysts and public policy makers believe global warming is a naturally occurring event and is not primarily due to human activities. They also argue that potential consequences are remote, worst-case scenarios that lead to unnecessary worries and measures. These analysts do not believe we will experience significant global warming in this century.

Predicted Effects of Climate Change Agriculture, water resources, forests, wildlife, and coastal areas are all vulnerable to the effects of global warming and climate change. Melting glaciers and polar ice sheets may cause sea levels to rise by 39 inches by the end of the 21st century. Seawater would encroach on Wall Street in New York City and many of the major airports and interstates in Louisiana, Florida, North Carolina, Texas, and New Jersey.

Without the protection of the ozone layer, humans are at risk for **more severe sunburns, more skin cancers, more cataracts, and suppression of the immune system.**

As climate changes, storms are expected to become more frequent and intense; some areas are likely to receive more rain while others become drier. These changes will affect the kinds of food that can be grown and shift the

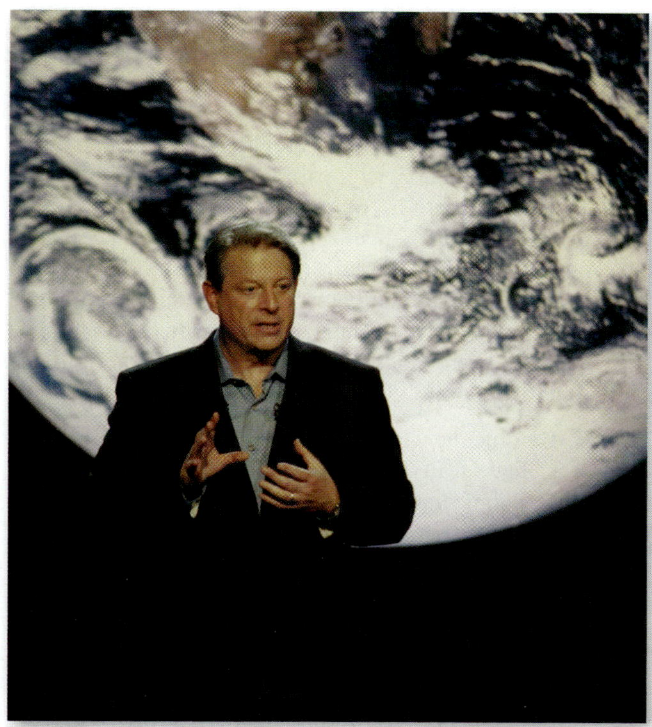

Al Gore spoke out for the environment in his 2006 documentary film about global warming, *An Inconvenient Truth*. The former vice president won the 2007 Nobel Peace Prize for his role in increasing public awareness about climate change.

nature of agriculture throughout the world. Crop damage may increase because agricultural pests and diseases flourish in warmer weather.[1,15–17]

Climate change is likely to have many adverse impacts on health, with significant loss of life. More frequent and severe heat waves would cause more heat-related deaths and illnesses. Heat causes more deaths in the United States than hurricanes, lightning, tornadoes, and floods combined. Mosquito-borne illnesses would increase, especially in the southern parts of the United States. Air quality would decline, because pollution is worse in warmer weather. Older adults and people with cardiovascular and respiratory disorders would be particularly vulnerable to adverse health effects of global warming.[17]

What Can Be Done? To address global climate change, 38 nations signed the Kyoto Protocol, a United Nations–sponsored international agreement, in 1997. The protocol called for nations to cut their emissions of greenhouse gases, particularly carbon dioxide, by about 5.2 percent below 1990 levels by 2012. This market-based treaty allows for *cap-and-trade* systems, in which countries and private companies trade and sell their greenhouse gas emission allowances to other countries and businesses. It also encourages private companies to develop new technologies that reduce greenhouse gas emissions.

Although the United States was the greatest producer of greenhouse gases at the time, it chose not to sign the Kyoto agreement, citing insufficient evidence of global warming and potential strain on the economy, including job losses. Instead, the United States introduced a voluntary emission reduction plan across all sectors of the economy.

The 2009 Copenhagen Accord at the United Nations Climate Change Conference endorsed the continuation of the Kyoto Protocol. The conference did not produce an official, legally binding agreement but did produce a nonbinding pledge to keep global warming below 3.6° F. The pledge will require industrialized nations like the United States to reduce greenhouse emissions by 25 to 40 percent below 1990 levels by 2020. China and India pose the greatest threat to any progress made by the Copenhagen Accord. China has surpassed the United States in greenhouse gas emissions and will almost double its emissions by 2020. India is projected to have about the same emissions as the United Sates by 2050. However, China and India collectively pledged to reduce their emissions by only 4 percent. This means the greenhouse gas emissions of China and India by 2020 would more than overshadow the proposed cuts pledged by other signatories of the Copenhagen Accord. Developed nations such as the United States are not likely to sign on to legally binding greenhouse gas reduction agreements until cuts are also legally binding for China, India, and other developing nations. (For more discussion of this issue, see "You Make the Call" at the end of this chapter.)

Substantial reduction in carbon dioxide emissions will require massive changes in industrial processes, transportation, energy sources, and personal lifestyles.[3] Cost estimates to meet standards run into the billions of dollars, to be shouldered not just by businesses but also by consumers through higher car prices, higher gas prices, and costlier car maintenance to meet federal emission controls.

Institutions, communities, and individuals can take steps to prevent climate change. Some have already begun the work of greenhouse gas reduction. The presidents of many of the leading higher education institutions in the United States met in 2007 to pledge their schools to the "green college campus" movement. By reducing the "carbon footprint" of their campuses and promoting energy conservation, colleges and universities can have a significant impact on climate change. According to the EPA, schools that use more energy-efficient equipment, lighting, and mechanical systems in residences, classrooms, offices, and laboratories can reduce their carbon footprint as well as lower their operating costs.

The next generation of campus buildings, including sports stadiums, will most likely be built with reusable materials, be designed to conserve water, and be powered by alternative energy. More important, the next generation of students will understand the significance of climate change and be ready to take the green movement with them when they leave campus. You can assess how environmentally friendly your lifestyle is with this chapter's Personal Health Portfolio.

INDOOR AIR POLLUTION

Levels of air pollution indoors can be higher and more hazardous than levels of air pollution outside. On average, Americans spend between 80 and 90 percent of their time indoors.[18] Spending extensive time indoors magnifies health risks from indoor air pollutants, possibly to 50 times the health risks experienced outdoors. Eleven of the most common air pollutants are usually two to five times higher inside the home than outside.[1] The EPA estimates that exposure to indoor air pollutants causes 6,000 cases of cancer every year in the United States.[18]

Pollutants inside the home include allergens, such as dust mites and animal dander; mold and mildew; and chemicals, usually as fumes or vapors. You can reduce many of the biological pollutants (allergens, mold, bacteria) by keeping the house clean, keeping pets clean, washing bedding weekly, and maintaining the relative humidity between 30 and 50 percent. Removing shoes when entering the house can also keep residues from pesticides and lead from collecting on carpets. According to the EPA, the most dangerous indoor air pollutants are environmental tobacco smoke, formaldehyde, radon, carbon monoxide, mold, and polybrominated diphenyl ethers.[18,19]

Formaldehyde Formaldehyde is a colorless gas that is commonly used in the construction of household materials, such as those used in furniture, drapes, and fiberboard. Vapors can seep out of these materials into the home. Daily exposures to this irritating gas can cause chronic breathing problems, dizziness, skin rash, headaches, sore throat, sinus infections, and eye irritation.[20] The EPA estimates that 1 in every 5,000 people who lives in a mobile or other manufactured home for 10 or more years will develop cancer from formaldehyde exposure.

Radon Colorless, odorless, and tasteless, **radon** is a radioactive gas that occurs naturally in some soils, rocks, and building materials. It can seep into homes through dirt floors and cracks in foundations. When it becomes attached to dust particles, radon can be inhaled. It has been definitively linked to lung cancer but not other respiratory diseases, such as asthma.[1] Your chances of getting lung cancer from radon exposure depend on the level of radon in your home, the amount of time you spend in your home, and whether you are a smoker or an ex-smoker. Smokers and ex-smokers already have lung tissue damage that makes them more susceptible to radon-related lung cancer.[1] If you are interested in finding a qualified radon professional to test levels in your home, contact your state radon office or the National Environmental Health Association.

radon Radioactive gas that occurs naturally in some soils, rocks, and building materials and is hazardous to human health.

solid waste Any unwanted or discarded material that is not a liquid or gas; garbage.

Carbon Monoxide Carbon monoxide is produced by the incomplete burning of fuels containing carbon. This gas impairs the transport of oxygen in the blood. Symptoms of carbon monoxide poisoning include mental confusion, irregular heartbeat, dizziness, blurred vision, mild nausea, and headache. Severe poisoning can cause seizures, coma, and death. Fetuses and very young children are especially vulnerable to the toxic effects of carbon monoxide.

High concentrations of carbon monoxide indoors are very dangerous. Gas stoves, space heaters, furnaces, fireplaces, wood-burning stoves, and cigarette smoke are common sources. If you or family members experience symptoms of carbon monoxide poisoning, turn off combustion appliances and leave the contaminated area immediately. If the symptoms are serious, go to a hospital emergency center.[21]

Mold Basements with relative humidity above 60 percent often have walls and floors blackened by mold colonies. Some people have an allergic reaction to airborne mold spores; symptoms include coughing, sneezing, wheezing, eye irritation, and headaches. Mold can also bother people without allergies; mold spores inflame lung tissues and produce chemicals called mycotoxins that are hazardous when inhaled. If you regularly sneeze, cough, or have trouble breathing when you are in certain parts of your home, mold may be the problem. You may need to consult an expert to identify and remove sources of mold.[19]

Polybrominated Diphenyl Ethers (PBDEs) PBDEs are flame retardant chemicals used in plastic and foam products, such as furniture cushions and carpet pads; hard casings for televisions, telephones, computers, and other electronic equipment; and insulation for cables and wires.[20] PBDEs seep or leach out of these products and enter the environment, showing up in house dust, soil, and plants and animals. They have been found in human breast milk, tissue, and blood.

The major health concern is that PBDEs can accumulate in human tissue and may cause chromosome abnormalities. Children who spend a lot of time at floor level are at greater risk for exposure by ingestion and inhalation.[22] PBDEs are under study by government-sponsored scientific endeavors, and some manufacturers of computers and office equipment have voluntarily stopped using them in their products.

Waste Management

Waste products are a natural outcome of the process of living on earth, but humans tend to generate large quantities of waste that must be managed in safe and satisfactory ways. Industrial processes and a "throwaway" attitude among consumers both contribute to the problem of excessive waste in our society.

SOLID WASTE

Solid waste is any unwanted or discarded material that is not a liquid or gas. The United States generates nearly 12 billion tons of solid waste each year. Ninety-nine percent of this waste is produced by mining, oil and natural gas production, agriculture, and industrial activities. The remaining

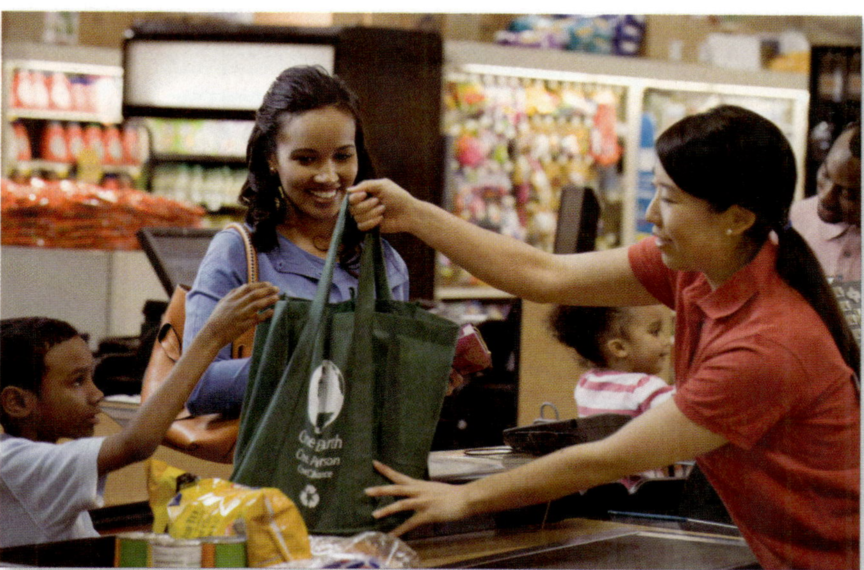

Both paper and plastic take energy to produce and burden landfills when discarded. The best choice for shopping is a reusable cloth bag.

1 percent is municipal solid waste, commonly called garbage and refuse, from businesses and homes.

The United States leads the world in garbage production, generating about 1,600 pounds per person per year. Canada ranks third.[1,23] The main components of garbage are paper products (including packaging and junk mail), yard waste, plastics, metals, glass, and wood. Food waste is not a major contributor to garbage because most is processed in garbage disposals and directed into sewage systems. *E-waste* (discarded computers, printers, TVs, and other electronic products) is the fastest-growing solid waste disposal problem (see the box "The Global Problem of E-Waste").

sanitary landfills Carefully selected sites where waste is buried, sometimes in plastic-lined containers or pits; they are designed to prevent leaching into water supplies and soil for at least 10 to 40 years.

hazardous waste Any discarded solid or liquid material that contains a toxic, carcinogenic, or mutagenic compound at levels that exceed EPA safety standards; catches fire easily; is reactive or unstable enough to explode or release toxic fumes; or corrodes metal containers.

Methods of managing solid waste have traditionally included burning, burying, and shipping wastes to other states or countries. Most of these methods were problematic and are now subject to numerous regulations. The principal method of dealing with solid waste today is burying it in sanitary landfills; this method is used to dispose of 54 percent of municipal solid waste in the United States and 80 percent in Canada.[1] **Sanitary landfills** are carefully selected sites where waste is buried, sometimes in plastic-lined containers or pits; they are designed to prevent leaching into water supplies and soil for at least 10 to 40 years.

A second method of dealing with solid waste is burning it in large city incinerators. Temperatures inside these incinerators exceed 1800° F, which prevents air pollution. In some cases, energy generated by the burning of refuse is sold as electricity to offset the cost of the incinerators, a waste management technique called waste-to-energy recovery.[1]

HAZARDOUS WASTE

Hazardous waste is any discarded solid or liquid material that meets one or more of four criteria: (1) the material contains a toxic, carcinogenic, or mutagenic compound at levels that exceed EPA safety standards (for example, solvents, pesticides); (2) it catches fire easily (for example, gasoline, oil-based paints); (3) it is reactive or unstable enough to explode or release toxic fumes (for example, chlorine, chlorine bleach); or (4) it corrodes metal containers (for example, drain cleaners, industrial cleaners).[1]

The top five chemical compounds of concern are arsenic, lead, mercury, vinyl chloride, and polychlorinated biphenyls, or PCBs (used to insulate electrical transformers). Nearly 75 percent of the world's hazardous waste is generated by the United States.[1]

Direct exposure to hazardous waste poses health hazards, whether it is touched, inhaled, or ingested. Safe handling measures have significantly reduced direct exposure to hazardous waste, but indirect exposure occurs when wastes leak from sanitary landfills and contaminate water supplies. Such leaks are suspected of causing cancer, respiratory

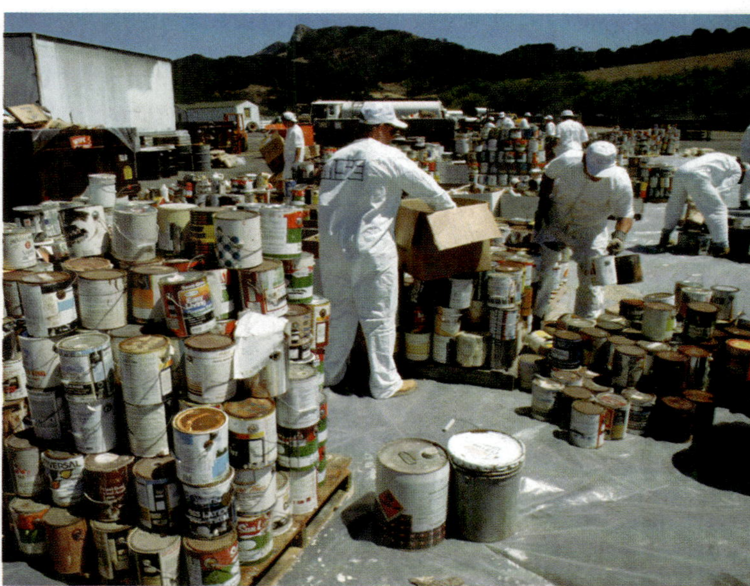

There is no good way to dispose of some hazardous materials. Experts recommend buying fewer products containing toxic contaminants.

Highlight on Health

The Global Problem of E-Waste

Americans purchase about 50 percent of the world's electronic devices—laptops, monitors, printers, cell phones, and so on—but recycle only 10 to 15 percent of them. While not classified as hazardous waste, e-waste can contain toxic elements like lead, mercury, and cadmium, and it is thus important that people dispose of it properly. Many of the components of electronic products are valuable resources that can be recycled and reused. For example, the various metals used in cell phones can be reused in the electronics and automotive industries. Rechargeable cell phone batteries can also be recycled into new batteries.

California is currently the only state that has passed laws requiring manufacturers to bear the cost of collecting, transporting, and recycling electronic devices, and many other states have taken action to facilitate e-waste recycling. You can find out whether your state has an electronic recycling program by visiting www.eiatrack.org. Independent of state laws, some electronics manufacturers and retailers, including Apple and Costco, provide drop-off locations for their products or accept discarded items via mail. Visit www.mygreenelectronics.com for more information on specific manufacturers and programs.

A major problem associated with e-waste is the actual recycling process. In the past, many developed countries sent their hazardous waste to less developed countries for disposal. This practice was banned in 1989 by the Basel Convention (an international environmental agreement) out of concern that less developed countries were not properly equipped to dispose of the waste and were suffering ecological damage as a result. The United States is one of three countries (along with Haiti and Afghanistan) that signed the agreement but did not ratify it. The United States currently sends most of its e-waste to Afghanistan and Haiti for disposal and recycling. It should be noted that much e-waste is classified as solid waste rather than hazardous waste.

The Basel Action Network (BAN) is a non-profit organization named for the Basel Convention and formed to confront the global "toxic trade" in e-waste and other pollutants from rich to poor countries. This organization has launched a certification program for responsible recyclers of e-waste called e-Stewards. Certified e-Steward recyclers use responsible means of disposal and recycling—they do not ship e-waste to poor communities, use prison labor, or dispose of e-waste in landfills or incinerators. Some major corporations, including Samsung and Bank of America, have signed up with the program, pledging to use only e-Steward recyclers for their e-waste. You can find your closest e-Steward-certified recycler at http://e-stewards.org. If your cell phone, computer, or camera is still in good working order, donating it to charity is another option. Visit www.recyclingforcharities.com for more information.

Sources: Living in the Environment, *by G. T. Miller and S. E. Spoolman, 2008, Belmont, CA: Pearson; "Where to Recycle Electronics, Free,"* Consumer Reports, *2009,* Consumer Reports, *June, p. 11; "Do the Right Thing: Use Only E-Stewards," Basel Action Network, retrieved June 2, 2010, from www.ban.org.*

diseases, neurological damage, developmental deficits, and other health problems in people in neighboring communities.

Today, federal laws drastically restrict the storage of hazardous waste in sanitary landfills.[23] Much of it is stored in ponds, pits, buildings, and specialized hazardous landfills or disposed of by injection into deep underground wells.

Household Hazardous Waste Hazardous waste is also generated in the home. It is estimated that the average home accumulates about 100 pounds of household hazardous waste (HHW) annually.[23] This waste includes batteries, paints, cleaners, oils, and pesticides, often stored in closets, basements, and garages. These products pose serious health threats.

> **medical waste** Any solid or liquid waste generated in the medical diagnosis, treatment, or immunization of human beings or animals.

Disposal of HHW is also a problem. Hazardous waste should not be poured down the drain, onto the ground, or into storm drains, nor should it be disposed of in the trash. Many communities have special collection days or permanent collection facilities for such waste. The best strategy is to limit your purchase of these items.

Emergent Contaminants A growing concern today is *emergent contaminants*, products that are showing up in local rivers and other water sources. They include pharmaceuticals, cosmetics, antibacterial soap, shampoo, shaving lotion, skin cream, dishwashing liquids, plastic, flame retardants, and many other chemical compounds. It is not clear whether these contaminants have health effects. Alone, they occur in minute quantities—you would have to drink 17,000 gallons of contaminated water to ingest the equivalent of one 200-mg ibuprofen tablet—but collectively they can form a "cocktail" of chemicals. Some experts believe these compounds can disrupt the endocrine system and play havoc with hormones, including estrogen, androgen, and thyroid hormones.

Medical Waste The EPA has specific regulations pertaining to **medical waste**, any solid or liquid waste that is generated in the medical diagnosis, treatment, or immunization of human beings or animals. It includes used needles and syringes, used culture dishes and other glassware, discarded surgical gloves, blood and blood products, tissue samples, and any materials contaminated by contact with such products. Medical waste disposal is strictly regulated by the states to prevent the spread of bloodborne pathogens and infectious disease. Public exposure to medical waste is very rare due to these regulations.

Radiation and Radioactive Waste Low-level radiation is used in medical and dental procedures, such as chest X-rays, dental X-rays, nuclear medicine diagnosis, and radiation therapy. Although these uses have contributed to improvements in health in some areas, exposure to X-rays should be limited. Recently, concern has grown about other sources of low-level radiation, such as televisions, computer monitors, microwave ovens, and cell phones. These devices do emit low levels of radiation, but research has so far been inconclusive on their health effects, if any.[1]

Today, the United States has the **highest recycling rate of any industrialized country.**

Disposal of radioactive waste is problematic. Waste with low levels of radioactivity, such as radioactive isotopes used in medicine, is often disposed of in landfills and near-surface burials, an approach that may lead to contamination of groundwater. High-level radioactive waste, generated by the production of nuclear weapons and the operation of nuclear power plants, is dangerous for tens of thousands of years; developing deposit sites that can offer this kind of protection is a challenge that has to be faced by the United States and other world powers.

APPROACHES TO WASTE MANAGEMENT: RECYCLING AND MORE

Most citizens do not want landfills, incinerators, and hazardous waste repositories located in their communities. This understandable "not in my backyard" attitude frustrates waste management operators and government officials. Many citizens argue that the real problem is not where to dispose of waste but how to stop producing so much of it.[1]

Some studies have found that factories, landfills, and hazardous and solid waste dumps are disproportionately located in low-income communities and those populated by Blacks, Latinos, Asians, and Native Americans. Living near a hazardous waste dump increases risk for respiratory disorders and cancer. The environmental justice movement advocates protection from environmental hazards regardless of race, gender, age, national origin, income, or social class and seeks to prevent environmental discrimination in these communities.

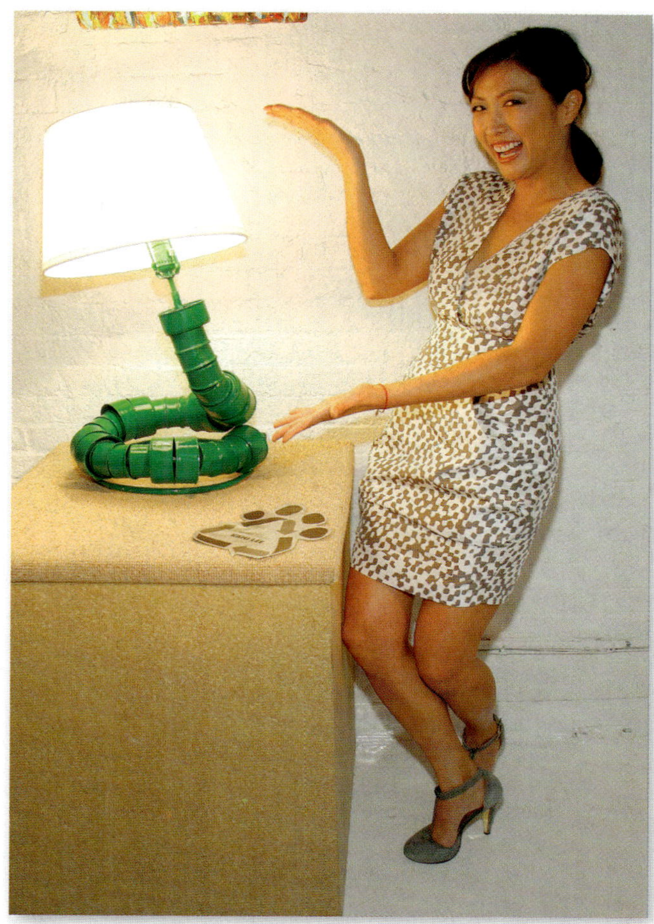

As part of Earth Day 2010 activities in New York City, the RePURRposed Art Gallery displayed art made from recycled cat food cans. Recycling one 3 oz can saves enough energy to power a 60-watt lightbulb for two hours.

Many communities have established recycling programs to help address the problem of excessive waste. **Recycling** is a circle, or loop, program in which materials that would otherwise be discarded are collected, sorted, cleaned, and processed into raw materials to make new products. Today, the United States has the highest recycling rate of any industrialized country. Americans recycle 28 percent of their waste.[1]

recycling Circle, or loop, program in which materials that would otherwise be discarded are collected, sorted, cleaned, and processed into raw materials to make new products.

Many communities provide curbside pickup of paper, glass, metals, and certain types of plastics (see Figure 12.3). Many states have deposit/refund programs to encourage recycling of beverage containers made of glass or aluminum. Communities with these laws report that 90 percent of glass and can beverage containers are returned.[24]

Besides recycling household items, individuals can take many other actions to help control and prevent waste. These include buying recyclable, reusable, or compostable

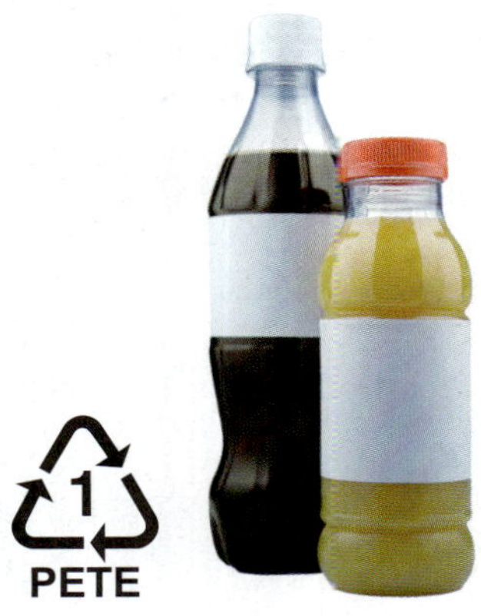

Recyclable, without lids.

Includes most soft drink and juice bottles. Do not reuse since bottles can accumulate bacteria.

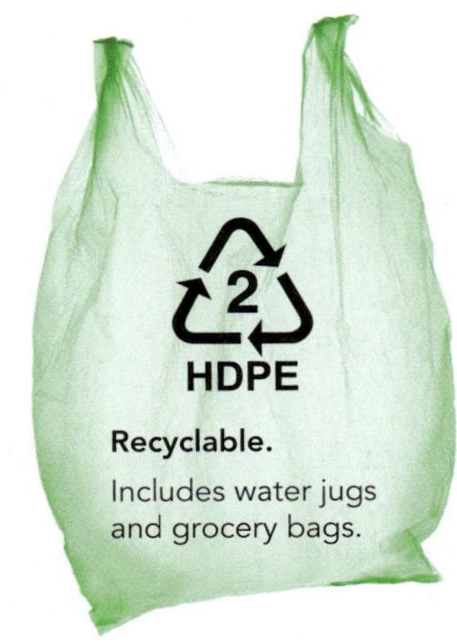

Recyclable.

Includes water jugs and grocery bags.

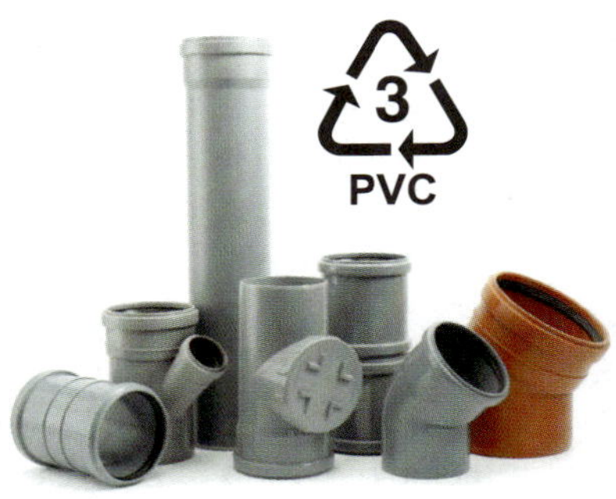

Recyclable.

Includes PVC pipes.

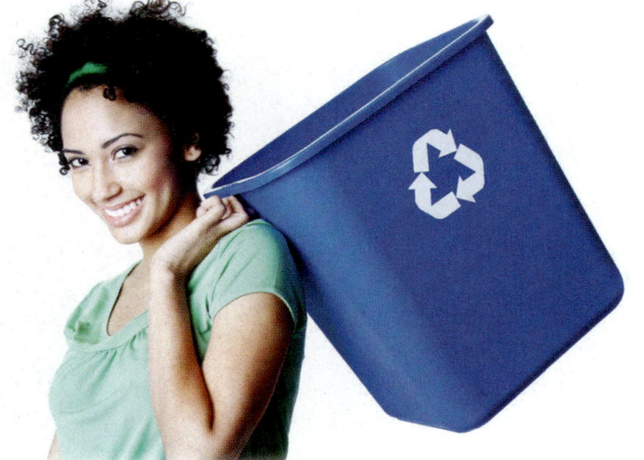

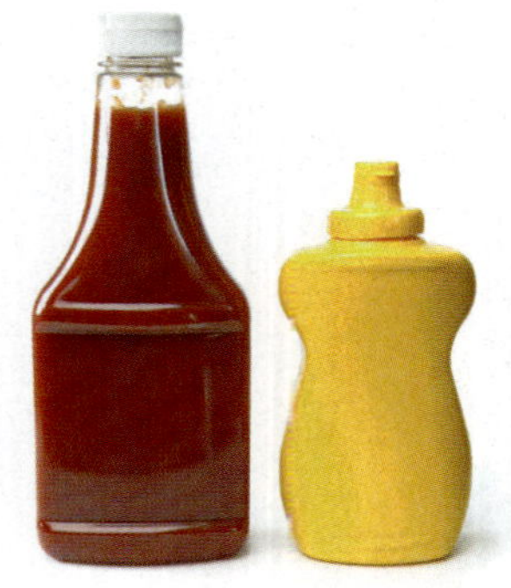

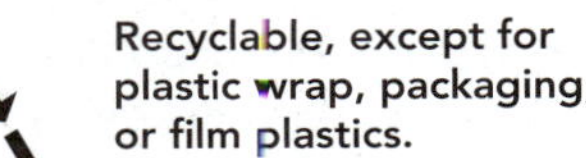

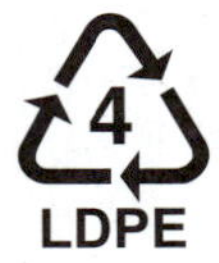

Recyclable, except for plastic wrap, packaging, or film plastics.

Includes squeezable containers like ketchup or mustard bottles.

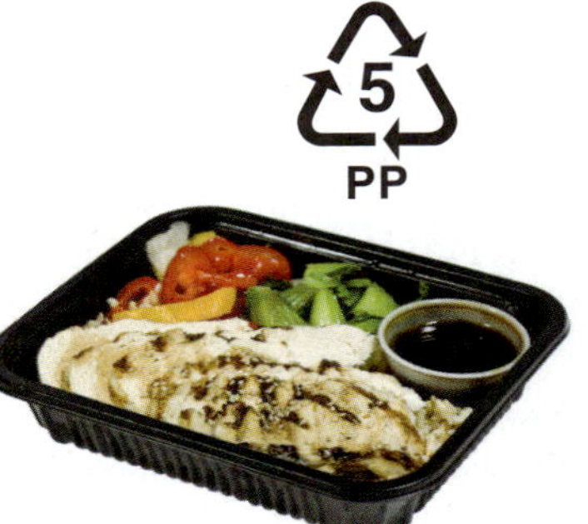

Recyclable.

Includes microwaveable meals.

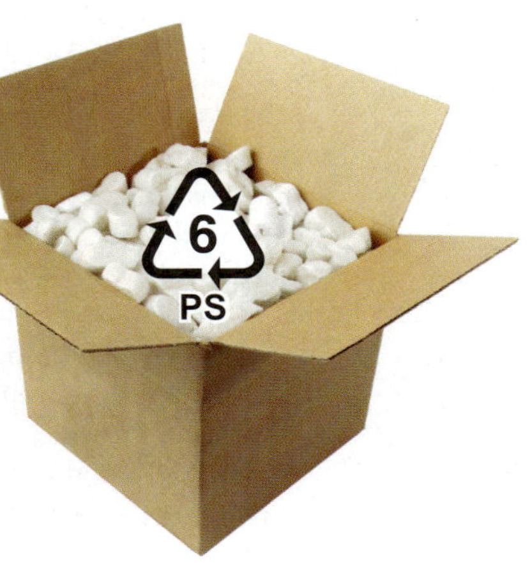

Generally not recyclable.

Includes items made of Styrofoam, such as egg cartons, packing peanuts, and Styrofoam cups. When possible, choose items made of paper instead. Some shipping stores may accept packing peanuts for reuse.

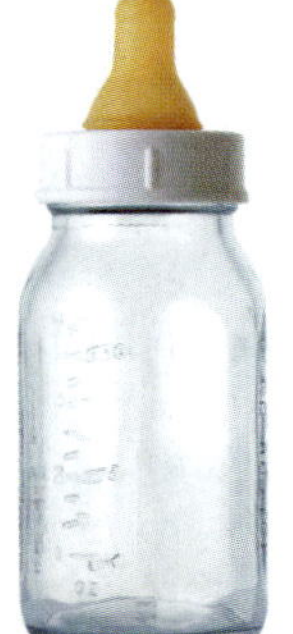

7
OTHER

Difficult to recycle.

Includes shatterproof bottles like baby bottles and reusable water bottles. Some include Bisphenol A, which has been approved by the FDA, but which has also been linked to health issues in lab animals.

figure **12.3** **What plastic can and can't be recycled.** The number inside a triangle that you see on the bottom of beverage and food containers indicates what type of plastic the product is made of—not all of which are recyclable. Community and campus recycling programs can vary in the types of materials accepted and in whether they accept materials with no numbers at all, so check with your own local recycling program to see what is and isn't accepted.

Source: Adapted from "Plastic Rap," by C. Weber, August 2008, The Gazette.

products; composting yard trimmings; using rechargeable batteries; using reusable cloth bags for grocery shopping; reducing use of paper towels and other paper products; buying products with as little Styrofoam, cardboard, or paper packaging as possible; and stopping junk mail by contacting the Direct Marketing Association (www.thedma.org).

hot tip

Buy furniture and other wood products that have a certification label from the Forest Stewardship Council, which means the wood has come from a well-managed forest.

Ecosystems and Biodiversity

An **ecosystem** is an interconnected community of organisms living together in a physical environment as a balanced, mutually supportive system. A frog pond in a meadow is an ecosystem; so is our planet. **Biodiversity**, or biological diversity, is the variety of different animal and plant species on earth, numbering in the millions, and the genetic variation in their gene pools—the material used in the process of evolution when changing environmental conditions require that species adapt or die out.[3]

An ecologically and biologically diverse planet offers innumerable benefits to humans. Twenty-five percent of medicines used in North America are derived from natural substances contained in plants and animals.[25] Choices in food, fuel, and lumber are enhanced by the variety of life-forms on the planet. Wild areas provide abundant opportunities for recreation, retreat, and refreshment. Most important, natural ecosystems promote the health of the planet, playing a role in climate maintenance, water cycling, soil production, waste disposal, and pest control.

Unfortunately, human activities have significantly disrupted these ecosystems and caused a decline in biodiversity. Nearly 50 percent of the earth's land surface has been disturbed or degraded by human activities.[1] Forests, grasslands, and wetlands have been converted for urban expansion and agricultural, industrial, and recreational use. Every year, hundreds of plant and animal species become extinct, and thousands more are at risk of extinction. The processes involved in this pattern of disruption include deforestation, desertification, and loss of freshwater resources.

ecosystem Interconnected community of organisms living together in a physical environment as a balanced, mutually supportive system.

biodiversity Variety of different animal and plant species on earth and the genetic variation in their gene pools.

deforestation Removal of trees from a forested area without adequate replanting.

DEFORESTATION

Deforestation is the removal of trees from a forested area without adequate replanting. When trees are cut down faster than they are replaced, forests become a non-renewable resource. In the past 8,000 years, human activity has reduced the world's forests by about 46 percent, mostly in the past 3 decades.[1]

In North America, the size and health of forests have been slightly improved since 1920 by reforestation. Some ecologists believe, however, that replacing *old-growth forests* (those that have flourished for several hundred years without interference from human activities or natural disasters) with *second-growth forests* (those that have been replanted following human activities or natural disasters) causes an overall reduction in biodiversity. Others claim that national parks and forests, tree farms, and lumber companies' reforestation programs are sufficient to preserve forest biodiversity. Year-round recreational use of national forests, including use of snowmobiles and all-terrain vehicles, hiking, mountain biking, cross-country skiing, camping, swimming, and hunting, also threatens the natural habitats of animals and plants. Heavy use of national forests results in noise, litter, pollution, and vandalism.[1]

Wetlands are biologically diverse habitats that are also sensitive to climate change and pollutants. The oil spill that occurred in April 2010 off the coast of Louisiana seriously damaged the wetlands on the coast, which are home to nesting birds, spawning fish, and endangered sea turtles, among many other species of plants and animals.

In tropical areas of the world—in Africa, Asia, and Central and South America—deforestation has resulted in significant declines in tropical forests. About 90 percent of forest loss is occurring in tropical forests. Although tropical forests make up only 6 percent of the world's land, they are home to between 50 and 90 percent of all terrestrial species. At present deforestation rates, 50 percent of tropical species could be extinct by 2042.[1,3,25] Such an extinction could carry a heavy price, because tropical plants play an important role in removing some of the excess carbon dioxide that human activity puts into the atmosphere.

DESERTIFICATION

Another process of environmental degradation is **desertification**, the conversion of once fruitful land into infertile wasteland, or desert. A desert is a terrestrial region in which evaporation exceeds precipitation and the average annual precipitation is less than 10 inches.[26] Every day, on average, 40 square miles of land are turned into desert by droughts in combination with human activities, such as livestock grazing, poor irrigation techniques, and overplanting of crops.[1] Unlike natural deserts, human-created deserts are associated with worldwide famines. Some scientists believe that global warming contributes to desertification, because climate change produces droughts in areas that once had adequate rainfall.[1]

desertification Conversion of once-fruitful land into desert.

LOSS OF FRESHWATER RESOURCES

Many rivers in North America are threatened by industrial, agricultural, and city wastes as well as disruption of water flow by dams, channelization, and diversion of water for agricultural irrigation. The National Wild and Scenic Rivers Act (NWSRA) of 1968 protects rivers with outstanding scenic, recreational, geological, wildlife, historical, or cultural values from development, but only 0.2 percent of the 3.5 million miles of waterways in the United States are protected by the NWSRA. Environmentalists have lobbied Congress to increase designated waterway lengths to 2 percent, a proposal opposed by many developers and some local communities.[1,27]

Lakes are threatened by acid precipitation and pollution, which kill plant and animal life. Sewage and agricultural runoff also pollute lakes and deplete oxygen in the water. Some lakes shrank or dried up when humans withdrew more water from them than could be replaced by rainfall. Another threat is the intentional or unintentional introduction of nonnative species of fish and other organisms into lakes, which disrupts the balance of the ecosystem and usually results in the extinction of native species.

Wetlands are vulnerable as well. Swamps, marshes, and bogs are vital ecological resources for wildlife and the environment. They provide breeding areas and habitats for wildlife, store enormous amounts of water, keep the water table high during droughts, and help prevent flooding.[27] Despite their vital ecological roles, wetlands are often viewed as wasteland and considered fair game for draining, building, and agriculture. They are also vulnerable to industrial and agricultural runoff and human sewage, all of which destroy animal and plant life. The U.S. Fish and Wildlife Service estimates that more than 50 percent of wetlands in the United States have been destroyed in the past two centuries.[1]

PROTECTING ECOSYSTEMS

Stringent federal and state protection of animal and plant habitats in forests, deserts, and wetlands is a component of sustainable land management programs. The United States has several laws in place protecting endangered species, and many species are protected by international agreements. Genetically improved trees and tree farms can be part of a successful forest management program. Business and industry can help preserve forests by recycling paper, using fiber that does not come from trees to make paper, and using wood efficiently.

Individuals can help preserve forests by reusing and recycling paper products, refusing to buy products or materials made from endangered or threatened species, purchasing wood products with the Good Wood Seal, and stopping junk mail. Individuals can also let their elected representatives know that they are in favor of environmental protections, and they can support groups taking action to preserve natural habitats.[28]

Energy Resources

Although the United States contains 4.5 percent of the world's population, it uses 24 percent of the world's commercial energy. Energy use per person in North America is nearly 50 percent

Public Health in Action

Reducing Automobile Emissions

About 70 percent of oil consumption is used for transportation and more than 65 percent of transportation oil is used in personal vehicles. The Corporate Average Fuel Economy (CAFE) is federal regulations intended to improve the average fuel economy of new cars and light trucks (which include sports utility vehicles and vans). The United States and Canada currently have the weakest CAFE standards among developed nations—27.5 miles per gallon (mpg) for cars and 20.7 mpg for light trucks.

In 2010, the National Highway Traffic Safety Administration (NHTSA) and the EPA released new regulations that will increase CAFE standards to 35.5 mpg by 2016. The heighted fuel standards will save an estimated 8.1 billion barrels of oil over the lifetime of model year 2012–2016 vehicles. While consumers will see an increase in the price of vehicles conforming to these standards, it will be more than offset by fuel savings over the life of the vehicle.

Ironically, government subsidies, including tax breaks for oil companies and car manufacturers, have played a pivotal role in the slow movement toward higher CAFE standards. These subsidies, in turn, have kept gas prices in the United States lower than those in most other developed nations and have served as a disincentive for consumers to move toward more fuel-efficient cars.

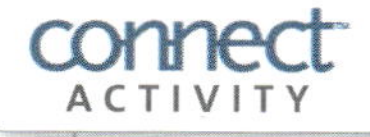

The hidden costs, however, have been increased illness and deaths from air and water pollution, loss of biodiversity from acid precipitation, and potential catastrophic impacts associated with global warming. The dependency of the United States on foreign oil also weakens national energy security since much of the imported oil comes from regions with unstable or unfriendly political regimes.

The removal of government subsidies that soften the price of gas for consumers and the implementation of tax rebates for fuel-efficient cars could play major roles in the movement toward less dependence on oil. California is already moving in this direction. It has introduced a fee-rate program that places a higher tax on fuel-inefficient cars. The revenue from the tax will be used to provide rebates for fuel-efficient vehicles. If the present fleet of cars, trucks, and SUVs were replaced with plug-in hybrids, oil consumption would be reduced by 70 to 90 percent by 2030 and carbon dioxide emissions would be reduced by 27 percent. While such a drastic move is unlikely, the increase in CAFE standards will reduce emissions from vehicles by 21 percent by 2030. We are also likely to see more regulation at the federal and state levels in the coming years that will reduce emissions even further.

Sources: "Emissions Limits, Greater Fuel Efficiency for Cars, Light Trucks Made Official," by J. Eilperin, April 2, 2010. The Washington Times; *"NHTSA and EPA Establish New National Program to Improve Fuel Economy and Reduce Greenhouse Gas Emissions for Passenger Cars and Light Trucks," National Highway Traffic Safety Administration, retrieved May 31, 2010, from www.nhtsa.gov/staticfiles/rulemaking/pdf/cafe/CAFE-GHG_Fact_Sheet.pdf;* Living in the Environment, *by G. T. Miller and S. E. Spoolman, 2009, Belmont, CA: Brooks/Cole.*

Pesticides used in the Midwest to raise beef have washed into the Mississippi River, creating **a large, oxygen-depleted "dead zone" where bottom-dwelling water life cannot survive.**

higher than in Germany, France, Japan, or the United Kingdom and 100 times higher than in India or China. Nonrenewable energy resources provide 91 percent of the commercial energy used in the United States, 84 percent from fossil fuels and 7 percent from nuclear power.[1] Dependence on oil, coal, and natural gas is the primary cause of air pollution, water pollution, and global warming.[25]

The United States has only 2 percent of world oil reserves and thus is heavily dependent on foreign oil to meet its energy needs.[29] Environmentalists believe the solution lies not in the relentless pursuit of fossil fuels but in energy conservation (see the box "Reducing Automobile Emissions"). They argue that our efforts should focus on reducing the ecological effects of current energy practices, diminishing energy waste, and shifting toward renewable, nonpolluting energy sources such as water, wind, geothermal, and solar power.[1] When we conserve energy, they point out, we lower the demand on commercial energy sources, which in turn reduces the emission of air pollutants and greenhouse gases (see the box "Eating Green").

World Population Growth

Overpopulation increases the severity of every environmental problem on our planet. The world's population grew

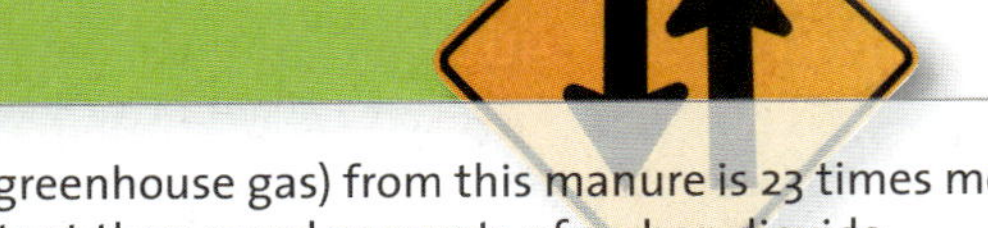

Challenges & Choices

Eating Green

The United Nations Food and Agriculture Organization reports that the meat sector of agriculture is responsible for 18 percent of the world's greenhouse gas emissions. The production of large amounts of red meat also takes a significant toll on the environment by requiring large amounts of land, the diversion of huge quantities of water for irrigation, and the use of toxic chemicals as pesticides and fertilizers. Much of the land in the Midwest is now used to grow grain for animal feed to meet Americans' demand for beef. Here are some of the costs:

- It takes 1,600 calories from oil, gas, and other fossil fuels to produce 100 calories worth of grain-fed beef. In comparison, it takes only 500 calories of fossil fuels to produce 100 calories worth of chicken.
- 14 trillion gallons of irrigation water are used each year to produce feed for livestock.
- A large feedlot of 50,000 cattle produces as much manure as a city of several million people. Methane (a greenhouse gas) from this manure is 23 times more potent than equal amounts of carbon dioxide.
- Pesticides used in the Midwest to raise beef have washed into the Mississippi River, creating a large, oxygen-depleted "dead zone" where bottom-dwelling water life cannot survive.

In contrast, greater reliance on a plant-based diet—a "green" diet—can help preserve the integrity of the environment:

- It takes only 50 calories from fossil fuels to produce 100 calories worth of plant foods.
- A low-meat diet uses 41 percent less energy and generates 37 percent fewer greenhouse gas emissions than a high-meat diet.
- If the typical American switched to an all-plant diet, the estimated reduction in carbon dioxide emitted each year would be 430 million tons, or 6 percent of the nation's greenhouse gas emissions.

Source: "Eating Green," by J. Jacobson, September 2007, Nutrition Action Newsletter, *pp. 3–7.*

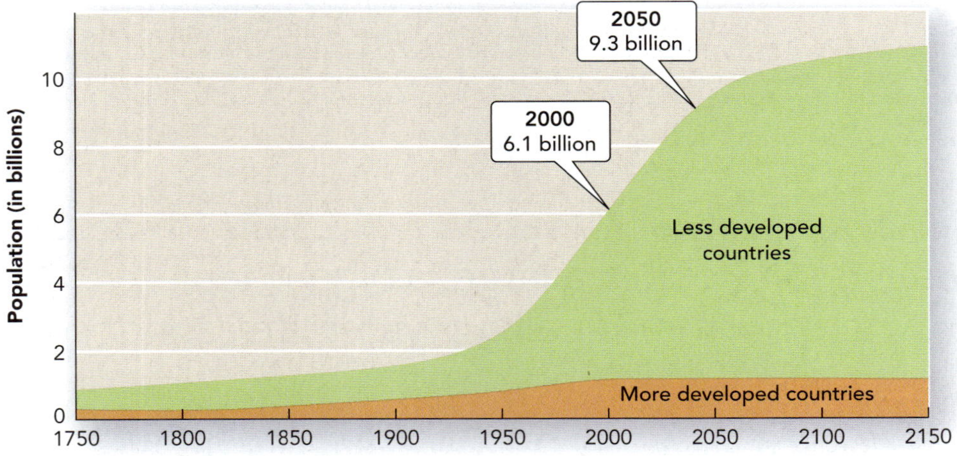

figure **12.4** **World population growth, 1750–2150.**

Sources: World Population Prospects: The 2004 Revision, *United Nations Population Division, 2005, New York: United Nations;* Human Population: Fundamentals of Growth, *Population Reference Bureau, www.prb.org/;* Historical Estimates of World Population, *U.S. Census Bureau, 2005, www.census.gov.*

slowly until about 1750, when living conditions began to improve as a result of the Industrial Revolution. Since then, it has grown exponentially (Figure 12.4). World population reached 1 billion in about 1800, 1.6 billion in 1900, 2 billion in 1930, and 3 billion in 1960. A billion people were added between 1960 and 1975 and another billion between 1975 and 1987.[30] By the year 2000, world population stood at 6.1 billion, and by 2010, it had reached 6.8 billion. The United Nations predicts that world population will reach 9.3 billion by 2050 and stabilize at about 10 billion in 2200.[31] Much of the population growth will take place in the less developed countries of Africa, Asia, and Latin America.

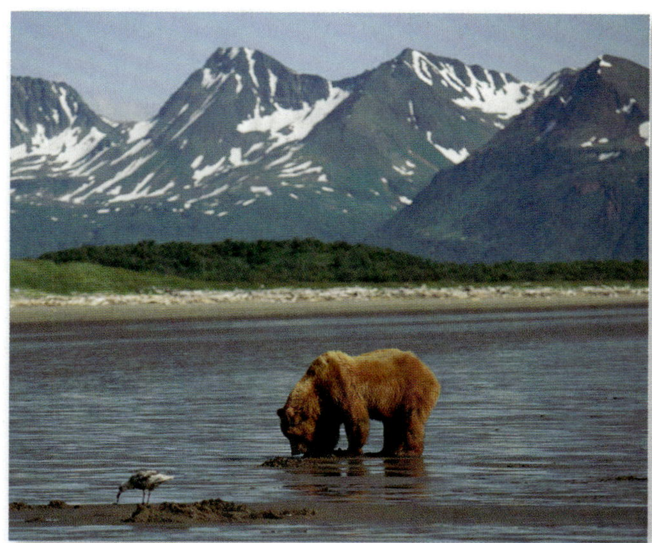

People are becoming more aware that the planet is a single, intricate, and sometimes fragile ecosystem that includes plants, animals, water, air, and all the interdependent patterns of life on earth.

HOW MANY PEOPLE CAN THE PLANET SUPPORT?

The projected growth in the world's population has raised a vital question: How many people can the planet support? The answer depends on whether we are talking about the number of people the earth can support at subsistence levels—referred to as *global carrying capacity*—or the number the earth can support at an optimum standard of living—referred to as *cultural carrying capacity*. Subsistence living includes enough food, water, land, and energy to survive. An optimum standard of living includes the luxuries that are part of life in the developed world, such as plentiful food, indoor plumbing, cars, and air conditioning.

As noted earlier, analysts estimate that the global carrying capacity of the earth is 50 billion people,[32] but the cultural carrying capacity is much less. If luxuries are minimized, the cultural carrying capacity could be well above the population of 9 billion projected for 2050. If luxuries are maximized, it is probably lower than the current population of 6.8 billion. In other words, there are probably not enough resources, especially energy resources, to extend an optimum standard of living to everyone alive on the planet right now.

These global inequities may only be magnified in the future, with the world's 200-some nations coexisting in a finite global environment with very different standards of living. Currently, at least 2 billion people in the world are poorer than the 34 million people living below the official poverty line in the United States. This discrepancy increases by a million people every year.[1]

APPROACHES TO POPULATION CONTROL

If standards of living are to be improved for all the people on the planet, population growth has to be slowed. Approaches to population control include extending **family planning** resources, which help people make informed decisions about the number and spacing of their children, to women and couples around the world; empowering women and increasing their access to educational and employment opportunities; reducing poverty and infant mortality and improving access to health care, all of which encourage parents to have fewer, healthier children; and offering incentives (such as salary bonuses, free education) and disincentives (such as higher taxes) to promote smaller families.

family planning Informed decisions that individuals and couples make about the number and spacing of their children; most family planning programs provide information on birth control, birth spacing, breastfeeding, and prenatal care.

Family planning programs alone could have a significant effect if implemented in developing countries, according to the United Nations. The success of family planning programs in developing nations has been mixed, however. Minimal success has been attained in some very populous countries, including many countries in Africa and Latin America, primarily for cultural and religious reasons.[1]

A SUSTAINABLE PLANET

A resource management tool called the *ecological footprint* can be used to compare human consumption of natural resources with the planet's ecological capacity to regenerate used resources. In other words, it provides a comparison of a lifestyle and pattern of consumption with the earth's ability to provide for this pattern. Ecological footprints can reveal how sustainable a particular lifestyle is and can point out inequities of resource use and consumption.

Currently the ecological footprint of the United States is the largest in the world. Americans consume more resources, generate more pollution, and discard more waste than any other people on the globe. If China and India were to catch up to the United States in ecological footprint, a second planet Earth would be needed to meet world resource requirements.

Even though environmental health involves human activities all over the globe, each of us can take actions today to reduce the size of the American ecological footprint (see the box "What College Students Can Do"). The Earth Day organization (www.earthday.net/footprint2/flash.html) provides an ecological footprint quiz that estimates how much productive land and water you need to support what you use and what you discard. This quiz will enable you to compare your personal ecological footprint to the footprints of other people and what is available on planet Earth. You can use this information to shift your personal lifestyle toward a more sustainable and earth-friendly one.

Consumer Clipboard

What College Students Can Do

College students can do their part for planetary health by living an environmentally conscious lifestyle. Here are a few examples:

- Recycle or donate computers, cell phones, CDs, iPods, MP3 players, and other electronic equipment to help solve the electronic waste problem.
- Use fewer personal care items (cosmetics, toothpaste, deodorant) that spill down the drain. Cosmetics that contain fewer solvents are less harmful to the environment. To find out more about the ingredients in cosmetics that you use, visit the Campaign for Safe Cosmetics (www.safecosmetics.org).
- Plug your electronic devices into a power strip and turn off the power strip when not in use. Turned-off electronic devices still use energy, called phantom electricity. Phantom electricity is responsible for more than 75 million tons of carbon dioxide emissions each year in the United States.
- Buy an energy-efficient car or truck. One gallon of gas produces 20 pounds of carbon dioxide. The American Council for an Energy-Efficient Economy's *Green Book* will help you evaluate the carbon dioxide impact of your current vehicle or a vehicle you are planning to buy.
- Paper or plastic? Plastic bag production produces less water pollution, air pollution, and solid waste than does that of paper bags, but plastic bags take more than 1,000 years to degrade. Paper is biodegradable and is a renewable resource, but paper bags take more energy to produce than plastic bags. Your best choice is reusable cloth bags for grocery shopping.
- Buy more of your food from local markets. A typical meat travels about 22,000 miles to reach the U.S dinner plate. A California lettuce travels 2,973 miles to reach New York City, and a Hawaiian pineapple travels 3,943 miles to reach the Midwest. The energy resources used for food transportation and the pollution generated contribute to many of our environmental problems. Many college campuses are now placing a priority on locally grown food. Learn more at www.localharvest.org and www.foodroutes.org.
- Know your labels. Earth Friendly and ECO-SAFE labels are unregulated and do not guarantee a product is environmentally safe. The government does regulate label use of organic food, recycled products, and Energy Star appliances. Green Seal, Eco Logo, Greenguard, and Forest Stewardship are independent groups that certify environmentally friendly products.

Sources: Global Warming Survival Handbook, *by D.E. Rothschild, 2007, United Kingdom: Live Earth;* Wake Up and Smell the Planet, *edited by B. Davis, 2007, Seattle: Skipstone.*

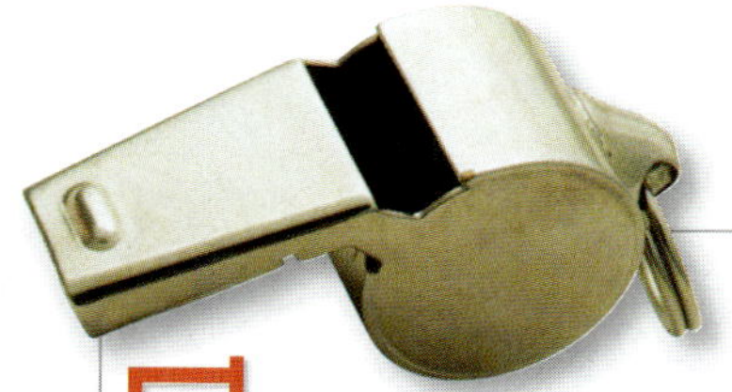

You Make the Call

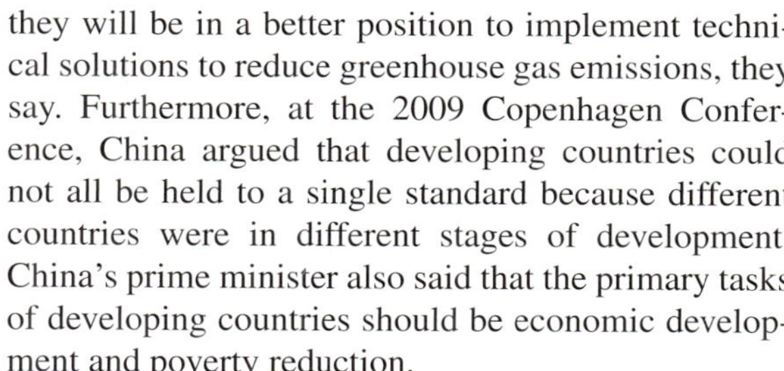

Should Developing Nations Share an Equal Burden With Developed Nations in Reducing Greenhouse Gas Emissions?

A global effort is under way to curb greenhouse gas emissions, but there is a debate over whether all countries should share the burden equally. While industrialized nations like the United States have generated the most emissions in the past, developing nations like China and India will be major contributors in the future.

People who want developing nations to drastically cut their emissions along with industrialized nations argue that developing nations have the most to lose from the negative effects of global warming and therefore should participate along with developed countries in reversing this trend. Developing countries have fewer resources to defend themselves against rising sea levels, increased intensity of storms, and other effects of climate change. Proponents also argue that developing nations will have greater long-term success if they do not become dependent on fossil fuels and instead begin using sustainable energy sources early in their development. Secretary of State Hillary Clinton told the prime minster of India in 2009 that "climate change would not be solved even if developed countries stopped emitting greenhouse gas emissions today, unless action is taken across the world." She pointed out that although India has one of the lowest per capita greenhouse-gas emissions rates currently, developing countries will contribute over 80 percent of the growth in future emissions. China's emissions have doubled since 2003, and it is now the world's largest emitter of greenhouse gases.

Those who think developing nations should not have to make the same emissions reductions as industrialized nations argue that industrialized nations have caused the majority of global warming and therefore have more of a responsibility to reverse it. Developing nations say they do not have as much money as developed nations to fight global warming and that spending a large amount of money in this area would hinder their economic growth. Once their economies have grown, they will be in a better position to implement technical solutions to reduce greenhouse gas emissions, they say. Furthermore, at the 2009 Copenhagen Conference, China argued that developing countries could not all be held to a single standard because different countries were in different stages of development. China's prime minister also said that the primary tasks of developing countries should be economic development and poverty reduction.

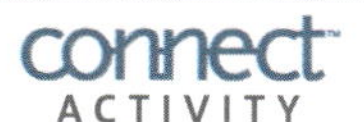

Differences in opinion on this issue contributed to the failure of the Copenhagen Conference to produce a legally binding treaty. Industrialized nations were unwilling to ratify an agreement unless developing nations set more stringent greenhouse gas emission reduction goals. Developing nations resisted the proposed cuts, citing a need to protect economic growth. The issue of whether developing countries should have to reduce emissions as much as developed countries will continue to be debated during future international climate change talks. What do you think?

PROS

- Developing nations will be responsible for more than 80 percent of the growth in future greenhouse gas emissions. China, a developing country, has doubled its greenhouse gas emissions since 2003 and is now the world's largest emitter of greenhouse gases.
- Developing nations will be the least able to protect themselves from the ill effects of climate change and thus have the most to gain from curbing global warming.
- Developing countries will be better able to sustain their economic growth if their economies are not dependent on fossil fuels.

CONS

- Industrialized nations, particularly the United States, have emitted and continue to emit far more greenhouse gases than do developing nations.
- Rich nations have the wealth to finance emissions-reducing technology both for themselves and for developing nations.
- Per capita greenhouse gas emissions in developing countries are still relatively low; thus, it is unfair to ask developing nations to reduce emission levels at the same rates as developed nations.

Sources. "*Clinton Accepts Blame for 'Global Warming' Role, Ponders Link Between Climate Change and Family Planning,*" *by P. Goodenough, 2009, www.cbsnews.com;* "*China Plays Key Role Making Copenhagen Talks Successful,*" *by Y. Zhixiao, 2009,* Xinhua News Agency, *retrieved May 31, 2010, from http://news.xinhuanet.com/english/2009-12/25/content_12704224.htm.*

IN REVIEW

What is environmental health?

Traditionally, environmental health focused on the conditions that contributed to infectious diseases, such as contaminated food and water, insects and rodents, and the disposal of waste. Today the field encompasses a broad range of issues, from global climate change to overpopulation. The key principle underlying environmental health is that we inhabit a small planet with infinite interconnections and finite resources.

What are the key issues in environmental health today?

Key issues include water quality and quantity; air pollution, global warming, and climate change; management of waste, including hazardous and radioactive waste; loss of biodiversity and ecosystems; depletion of energy resources; and world overpopulation.

What can people do to make a difference?

There are innumerable small and large steps individuals can take every day to make a difference in the environment, from recycling to conserving energy to reducing their ecological footprint. Information is widely available on how individuals can move toward a more sustainable and earth-friendly lifestyle.

Web Resources

CDC National Center for Environmental Health: This Web site provides information on environmental topics such as the elimination of chemical weapons, earthquakes, lead poisoning, and cancer clusters. The organization offers fact sheets, brochures, and other publications.
www.cdc.gov/nceh

Natural Resources Defense Council: This Web site features weekly Web picks and a current legislative watch. Its Guide to Green Living includes ideas for green gifts, how to live green, and buying energy-efficient appliances.
www.nrdc.org

U.S. Environmental Protection Agency: The EPA site offers news and information on topics such as acid rain, environmental laws, hazardous waste, oil spills, ozone, radon, and wetlands. Click on "where you live," enter your zip code, and find out environmental information about your community.
www.epa.gov

U.S. Geological Survey: Focusing on the study of our landscape, natural resources, and natural hazards, USGS provides information on a variety of science topics, including climate, oceans and coastline, water resources, and plants and animals.
www.usgs.gov

World Watch Institute: This independent research organization focuses on critical global issues, looking for practical solutions. It offers a wide range of publications and online features on such topics as global security, population, and climate change.
www.worldwatch.org

World Wildlife Fund: This organization is dedicated to protecting endangered wildlife and preserving wild places. Its Global 200 is a scientific ranking of critical terrestrial, freshwater, and marine habitats that must be protected to preserve the "web of life."
www.wwfus.org

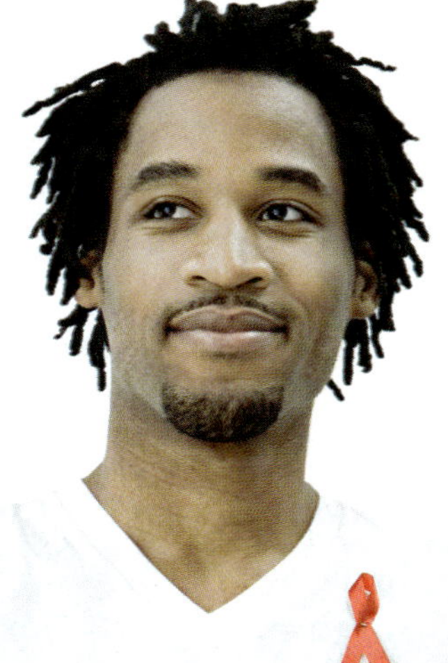

13 Infectious Diseases

COMING UP IN THIS CHAPTER

Discover the major types of organisms that cause infections and how your body protects you from disease › Learn about common infections—how they are transmitted and their symptoms and treatments › Understand common sexually transmitted infections › Take steps to prevent infections and limit the impact they have on you

Wellness Connections

How do infectious diseases relate to your overall wellness? If you're a young adult, they are probably one of the most obvious causes of temporary illness and discomfort in your life. Physical wellness is diminished in the short term by even minor infections, such as head colds. However, good physical wellness and intellectually sound health choices can help protect you from infections. Are you using your critical thinking skills to try to avoid and to safely treat infectious diseases? Do you wash your hands regularly? Are your immunizations up-to-date?

Emotional, social, and spiritual wellness, especially as they affect your stress levels, can make you less susceptible to infections, or more. Along with intellectual wellness, these wellness dimensions also influence the decisions you make about sexual behavior, which in turn affect your risk for contracting a sexually transmitted infection. How are your communication and relationship skills? If you're sexually active, do you always practice safer sex?

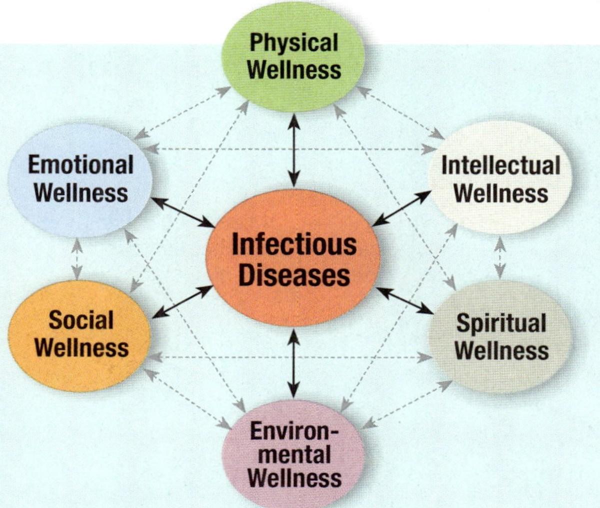

Your environment also plays an important role in your risk for infection. Water and food can spread infectious diseases, as can insects and rodents. You can help by promoting environmental wellness and by preparing for emergencies, such as natural disasters that cause a breakdown of the public health measures that protect us from many infections that plagued past generations.

Infectious diseases were the leading cause of death in the United States before 1900, and they remain a leading killer worldwide. Although U.S. death rates have dropped dramatically, infectious diseases are still a major cause of illness and lost work and school time. This chapter provides an introduction to infectious diseases, including those that are sexually transmitted. You'll learn how to recognize and treat common diseases—and most importantly, how to prevent them.

Infection and Immunity

An **infectious disease** is one that can be passed among people. Common infections include colds, flu, bronchitis, mononucleosis, and the many sexually transmissible infections. Some infections are easy to catch and relatively mild; others are much more serious—but often more difficult to catch.

infectious disease A disease that is transmissible from person to person through direct or indirect means; infection refers to invasion and multiplication of an organism; symptomatic disease follows if the body cannot quickly eliminate the pathogen.

pathogen A specific causative agent of infectious disease; examples include virus, bacteria, protozoa, and fungi.

Pathogens

What causes infectious diseases?

Infections are caused by **pathogens,** disease-causing agents that can be passed among people. Pathogens fall into a number of categories (Figure 13-1). Most pathogens are tiny, including the viruses and bacteria that cause many familiar

Pathogen	Effects	Diseases
Viruses Tiny microbes consisting of one or more molecules of DNA or RNA surrounded by a protein coat	Viruses can enter and take over body cells, using them to rapidly produce more copies of the virus while at the same time damaging or destroying the cells.	Common cold, influenza, mononucleosis, hepatitis, cold sores, genital herpes, HIV/AIDS, genital warts, measles, mumps, rabies, polio
Bacteria Single-celled organisms that may be in the shape of rods, balls, or spirals	Bacteria may secrete toxins or enzymes that destroy cells or interfere with cell functioning.	Lyme disease, pneumonia, peptic ulcers, tuberculosis, boils, toxic shock syndrome, strep throat, meningitis, gonorrhea
Fungi A primitive form of plant that may be single- or multi-celled	Fungi may release enzymes that destroy cells.	Yeast infections, thrush, athlete's foot, jock itch, certain types of pneumonia and meningitis
Protozoa Microscopic single-celled animals that can live independently of a host	In the human body, protozoa may release toxins and enzymes that destroy cells or interfere with their functioning.	Malaria, giardia, toxoplasmosis, African sleeping sickness
Prions Specific types of abnormal proteins	Prions accumulate in the central nervous system and cause degenerative diseases.	Bovine spongiform encephalopathy ("mad cow disease"), Creutzfeldt-Jakob disease
Helminths Parasitic worms that live in or on a host	Worms compete with body cells for nutrients and can block blood and lymph vessels or the digestive tract.	Tapeworm infection, pinworm infection, hookworm infection, swimmer's itch
Ectoparasites Complex organisms that may live in or on a host's skin	Infestations may cause local irritation; in some cases, ectoparasites also transmit other types of pathogens.	Lice, scabies, ticks, fleas

Figure 13-1 Pathogens, effects, and associated diseases

infections; these are often referred to as microbes or microorganisms. However, infections can also be caused by larger organisms, including lice and parasitic worms, although these infections may also be referred to as infestations.

It's important to note that many microbes live in a healthy human body and are needed to keep the body functioning normally. For example, your intestines contain types of bacteria that help digest food, destroy disease-causing microbes, and provide needed vitamins. However, even these helpful organisms can cause illness if their numbers become unbalanced or if they gain entry into a part of the body that is normally microbe-free. For example, healthy people usually carry *Staphylococcus aureus* bacteria on their skin and in their nasal passages without suffering any illness. But *S. aureus* can cause a number of different diseases if it enters the body through a cut or sore. Similarly, antibiotics can kill friendly bacteria in the mouth, which allows fungi to grow out of control and cause a disease known as thrush.

In some cases, it's important to distinguish between *infection,* meaning a disease-causing organism invades your body and starts to multiply, and *disease,* meaning you're experiencing obvious signs and symptoms. In some cases, you can have an infection—and be capable of transmitting the responsible pathogen to someone else—without ever experiencing symptoms. Your body may also be able to destroy an infectious agent before it ever causes symptoms, meaning you had an infection but not a disease. An infectious disease with symptoms occurs when your body's defenses cannot quickly and completely fight off an invading pathogen.

Q Why are some infections more serious than others?

Many factors determine the severity of an infectious disease. Pathogens vary in their *virulence*—their innate ability to cause intense or severe symptoms. The viruses responsible for colds typically cause only mild, temporary infections affecting the upper respiratory system; the viruses that cause AIDS and smallpox, on the other hand, usually cause severe symptoms. Pathogens can also infect different parts of the body; for example, a bacterial infection confined to a small area of skin is likely to be less severe than an infection by the same bacteria if it gains access to the bloodstream and therefore the entire body. The amount of the pathogen you are initially exposed to can also have an impact—it's easier for your body to destroy a smaller number of pathogens.

And of course, your health status is also important. Just because a pathogen is present doesn't mean you'll become ill. Think about the times you've been around someone who was sick but you didn't become ill yourself. Many pathogenic organisms are present on and in your body at all times, but if the agent isn't too virulent, and if your own resistance is strong, then you won't become ill. A strong immune system can fight off more infectious agents than a weak one. Some groups of people are at more risk for serious effects from infections, including infants, older adults, and pregnant women; infections that pose little risk to a healthy adult may be dangerous to people in these groups.

Mind Stretcher
Critical Thinking Exercise

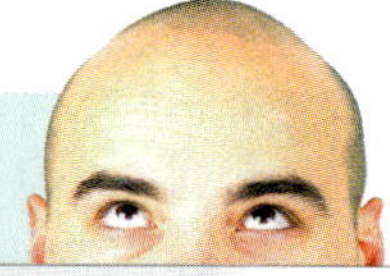

Does the government have the right to quarantine people who have a particularly virulent infectious disease? Which do you think should take precedence: concerns about public safety or the rights of individuals? Are there characteristics of an illness, such as the mode of transmission or the severity of the effects, that should be taken into consideration in making this decision? Under what circumstances, if any, do you feel it is appropriate to quarantine an infectious person?

The Cycle of Infection

Q How do you actually catch an infectious disease?

In order for an infectious disease to occur, a pathogen must gain entry into a host's body and start to replicate and cause symptoms. The transmission of an infection requires (1) a source of pathogens, (2) a susceptible host, and (3) a mode of transmission. Whether a person gets a disease depends on the relationship among these three factors.

MYTH or FACT
You should avoid cat litter boxes if you are pregnant.
WATCH ONLINE

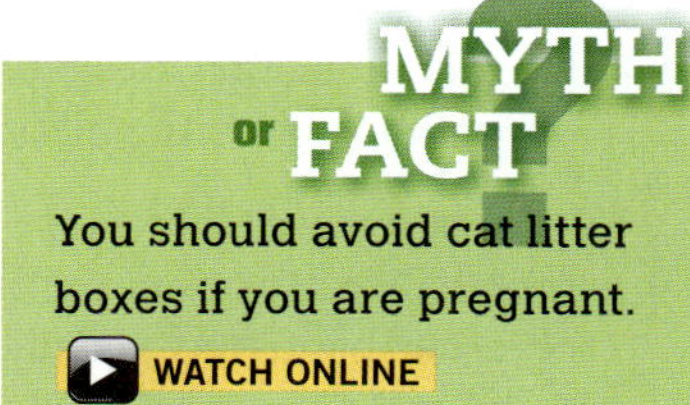

- **Source of pathogens:** Infectious agents can come from another person, an animal, water, or even soil. The environment that supports a pathogen's survival and growth is called its *reservoir,* and reservoirs often contain a large community of the pathogen. For many common infectious diseases, the reservoirs are the bodies of people who are already infected. Many disease-causing organisms can survive only a short time once they leave their usual reservoir or host.
- **Susceptible host:** People are more susceptible to infection if their immune system is weak or one of their natural physical defenses is compromised—such as by a cut in the skin. For example, very young children, older adults, and people with underlying health problems are all more susceptible to infections. Factors such as stress, smoking, use of antibiotics or other drugs, and vaccination history all affect a person's risk of infection.

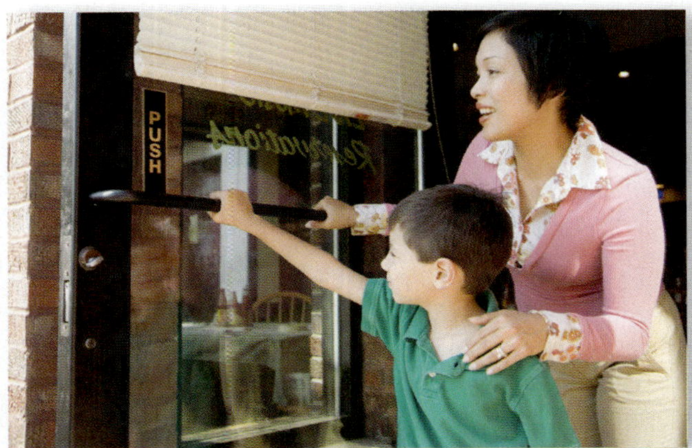

Many viruses and bacteria can be easily transmitted through direct and indirect contact. You can pick up pathogens by shaking hands or by touching shared surfaces such as doorknobs and keyboards.

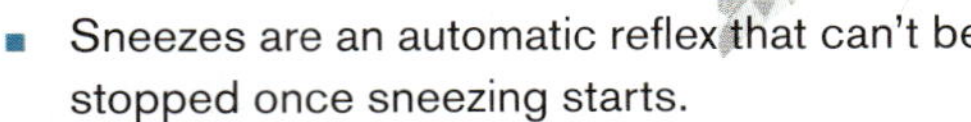

Fast Facts

Achoo!

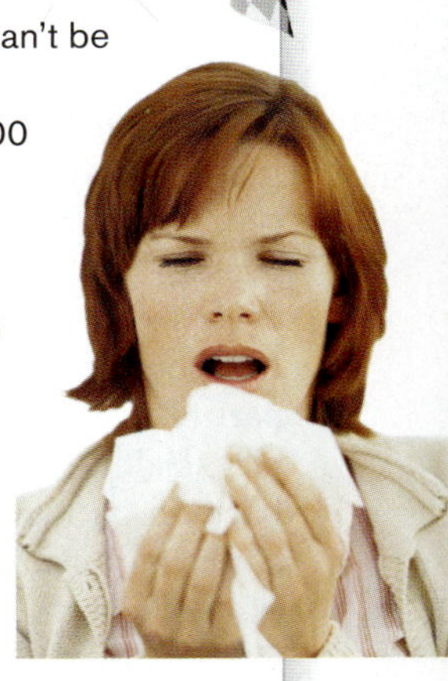

- Sneezes are an automatic reflex that can't be stopped once sneezing starts.
- Sneezes can travel at speeds up to 100 miles per hour, and the wet spray can radiate as far as five feet.
- People don't sneeze when they're asleep because the nerves involved in the reflex are also resting.
- Up to 35% of all people sneeze when exposed to sudden bright light.
- Some people sneeze when plucking their eyebrows because the nerve endings in the face are irritated and then fire an impulse that reaches the nasal nerve.

Source: Library of Congress (2010). Does your heart stop when you sneeze? *Everyday Mysteries* (http://www.loc.gov/rr/scitech/mysteries/sneeze.html).

- **Mode of transmission:** Understanding how pathogens are transmitted can help you identify ways to break the cycle. To cause an infection, a pathogen must exit its reservoir and then reach and enter a new host. There are different modes of transmission: direct and indirect contact, inhalation, and contact with a disease *vector* such as a mosquito or tick. Different pathogens have different typical modes of transmission. People can transfer pathogens from their hands, mouth, or genitals by coming into direct contact with another person—through touching, kissing, or sexual activity. Sexually transmitted infections such as chlamydia, gonorrhea, and herpes are usually transmitted through direct contact. Injection drug use can also directly transmit a pathogen into the bloodstream of a new host.

The viruses that cause the common cold may be transmitted directly or indirectly. If a person with a cold sneezes onto her hand and her phone, a potential new host could pick up the virus from shaking her hand or borrowing her phone—and then touching his own eyes or nose and transferring the virus.[1]

The flu virus is most often transmitted through inhalation: A person sneezes or coughs, and the virus is sprayed into the air in tiny droplets, which other people can breath in. These droplets can also land on surfaces in the environment. Although some pathogens die quickly after leaving their hosts, cold and flu viruses are viable after many hours on surfaces such as desks and doorknobs.[2] Indirect contact can also occur when a person ingests contaminated water or food.

Finally, some pathogens are transmitted through insect or animal vectors. Malaria is an example of a vector-borne disease. A mosquito picks up the protozoa by biting an infected person and then can pass the protozoa on to the next person it bites. Lyme disease is another example of an infection transmitted through an insect vector. The Lyme disease bacterium normally lives in mice and other small animals, but it is transferred to humans through the bite of a tick.

How do the pathogens enter the new host? Typically, they enter through any of the body's natural openings (mouth, nose, genitals, and so on), as well as through cuts and scrapes on the surface of the skin.

The Body's Defenses

Q | Do I start out with any resistance to disease?

Each of us is born with a specific capacity to resist certain diseases, but there is little consistency from one person to the next. This is why some people seem to never get colds, some people who have inhaled tuberculosis bacteria never get the disease, and some people do not become sick in the midst of an epidemic. Scientists are still trying to determine the exact causes for differences in disease resistance. Some of it seems to be present from birth, yet it remains to be determined how much of our resistance is inherited and how much is determined by factors such as age, illness, and nutritional status.

We all have built-in defenses against infectious diseases. Physical barriers are the first line of protection. Your skin is your body's largest organ, and most pathogens cannot get through your skin unless it is damaged in some way. Thus, you are more likely to get an infection if your skin has been scraped, cut, or burned, or if passage

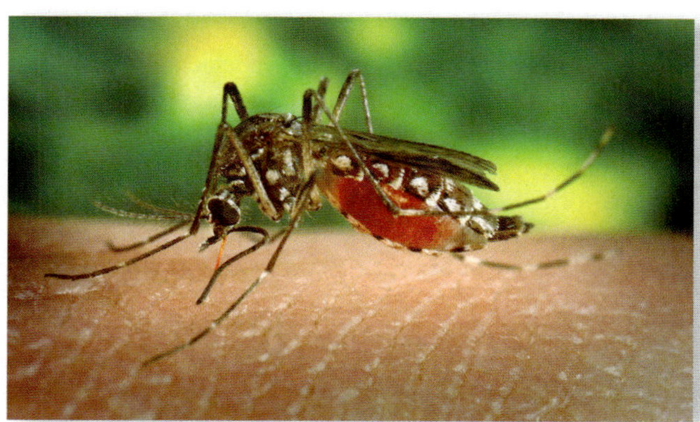

Your skin provides an effective physical barrier, but pathogens can be transmitted through cuts, scrapes, and burns, and via injection drug use or the bites of certain animal or insect vectors. Female mosquitoes can penetrate the skin and potentially transmit infections such as malaria and West Nile virus.

through the skin is aided by something like an injection or a bite from a mosquito.

Many of the openings in the human body—mouth, nostrils, eyelids, lungs, and genitals—are lined with mucous membranes. Although these linings seem delicate, they provide significant protection by secreting mucus that traps pathogens. The hairs in your nose and ears also trap many pathogens. Any foreign substances that enter the lungs may be expelled through the cough reflex or by the actions of hairlike cilia in your lungs that help push particles up and out.

Just as damage to the skin increases your risk of infection, so does damage to these other physical barriers. One reason that smoking increases your risk of infection is that it destroys the cilia in the lungs. If you have a sexually transmitted infection that causes sores or blisters, you are more likely to contract another infection. For example, having genital warts or herpes infection increases your risk for contracting HIV infection.[3]

Your body also has chemical barriers to pathogens. Your digestive tract contains acids, proteins, enzymes, and friendly bacteria that can all discourage the entry and spread of pathogens. Substances in tears can dissolve the outer coating of certain bacteria. Vaginal secretions normally produce a slightly acidic environment, which encourages the growth of some microbes and discourages the growth of others.

You can help out your body's physical defenses through actions such as washing your hands and limiting contact with objects and surfaces used by a person who is ill.

The Immune System

Q | How do I develop my immunity?

Your immunity can come from several sources. Your **immune system** comes into play if a pathogen gets through the physical and chemical barriers. Your immune system is a complex network of specialized organs, tissues, and cells that defends the body from disease-causing microbes and helps repair damaged tissue. A complete description of the immune system and the immune response is beyond the scope of this text, but here are a few key concepts to keep in mind:

immune system A complex network of organs, tissues, and cells that produce the immune response and defend the body from disease-causing agents.

antigen Protein molecules on the surface of infectious agents that the immune system recognizes as foreign, triggering the immune response.

antibody Molecule produced by the immune system that binds to a specific antigen, marking it for destruction.

- Immune cells constantly circulate through your body, ready to recognize foreign substances and take action. All cells carry protein markers on their surface; protein markers on pathogens, known as **antigens,** are recognized as being foreign and trigger the immune response.
- Some cells of the immune system respond to the damage and toxins a pathogen produces. They move to the site of the infection, "eat" the invading microbes, and destroy infected body cells. Pain and swelling at the site of an infection are often the result of the body's battle to keep the infection from spreading.
- If an infection persists or spreads, other cells of the immune system produce large numbers of **antibodies.** These specialized proteins bind to the pathogen's specific antigen and help mark it for destruction.
- The fever (elevated body temperature) that often accompanies an infection can help speed up parts of the immune response. It may also make the host a less hospitable environment for the pathogen. Fevers of 100°F or less are usually not harmful and don't need to be treated.
- For certain pathogens, once you've been exposed, the body produces specialized "memory" cells. These cells are able to recognize the antigen associated with the pathogen and respond quickly if you ever become infected with the same microbe again. In this way, you can essentially become immune to the pathogen—if you are infected, your body will quickly kill the pathogens and no disease will develop.

In addition to the natural immunity that develops after an infection, you can also acquire immunity without actually experiencing the infection. This occurs following a vaccination (see p. 372) or through direct injection of antibodies. Babies can also temporarily acquire immunity from their mothers through breast-feeding, because breast milk contains protective maternal antibodies.[4]

Q | What causes swollen lymph glands?

Swollen lymph glands, also called lymph nodes, usually indicate an active immune response to an infection.

lymphatic system Network of vessels and organs that returns fluid to the circulatory system; produces, activates, and transports infection-fighting cells and plays a role in disposing of foreign material and cellular debris.

vaccine A preparation of weakened or killed microorganisms or inactivated toxins that is administered to stimulate immunity; it elicits an immune response that offers long-lasting protection against that particular antigen.

acute infection An infection that develops rapidly and lasts for a short period; characterized by incubation, prodrome (beginning of symptoms), illness, and convalescence and recovery.

chronic infection A prolonged infection that continues beyond the time when the immune system would usually clear the infection from the body.

latent infection An infection that lies dormant in the body for a period of time but may recur under certain circumstances.

Your lymph glands are part of the **lymphatic system,** a collection of vessels and organs that carry out several different functions in the body. Lymph vessels pick up fluid lost from capillaries and return it to the circulatory system. The lymph vessels are similar to blood vessels, but to move fluid, they rely on compression from muscle contractions rather than the pumping action of the heart.

The lymphatic system also plays a key role in the defense against invading pathogens. The spleen, thymus, and bone marrow help produce and activate infection-fighting cells. Lymph vessels transport fluid containing foreign material and cellular debris to lymph nodes for disposal. The lymph nodes are located at intervals throughout the body; they contain many immune cells, which during an infection ingest and destroy invading pathogens.

The lymph nodes that most often become swollen are those in your neck, armpits, and groin. The location of a swollen gland can provide clues to the source or location of an infection. The swelling usually subsides within a few days, but it can take up to several weeks after an infection has cleared for lymph nodes to return to normal size.

The Role of Immunizations

Q | Do vaccines weaken my immune system?

No. **Vaccines** strengthen your immune system by preparing your body to fight infection. They create immunity against infections you haven't had. Vaccines are made from killed, weakened, or incomplete pathogens. They work by exposing the body to foreign antigens from the microbe, which the immune system responds to by producing antibodies. Vaccines do not cause the infectious disease, but they do prime your body to respond to the pathogen if you are ever infected. A vaccine may also include an inactive version of a bacterial toxin so that the body can develop a defense against it.

No vaccine is completely effective, and some people have a stronger immune response to a vaccine than others. The effects of some vaccines fade so that regular booster shots are needed to maintain immunity. Figure 13-2 shows the immunizations recommended for U.S. adults; for additional information and the recommendations for children, visit the "Vaccines and Immunizations" page of the Centers for Disease Control (http://www.cdc.gov/vaccines).

Stages and Patterns of Infectious Diseases

Q | Can all infections be cured?

No. There are different kinds of infections, and the ones most likely to resolve on their own or be cured quickly with treatment are **acute infections,** which are characterized by a short duration and a fairly typical series of stages (Figure 13-3):

- *Incubation:* Time between infection with the pathogen and the first appearance of symptoms. The immune system is able to stop some infections during this stage and clear the pathogen from the body, meaning no disease develops.
- *Prodrome:* Initial appearance of general signs and symptoms of illness. An individual might begin to feel unwell.
- *Illness:* Signs and symptoms of the specific infection develop and become more severe.
- *Convalescence:* Acute symptoms of the infection subside. The time required for recovery depends on the severity of the infection and the underlying health of the individual.

These stages occur for many infectious diseases, including the common cold. However, infections can follow other patterns. In a **chronic infection,** the illness persists or recurs over a long period. Hepatitis can become a chronic liver infection, slowly causing cirrhosis or liver cancer. Up to 10,000 Americans die from chronic hepatitis each year.[5] HIV infection can be a chronic progressive disease, meaning the infection persists and often worsens over time, with more and more of the virus produced in the body.

In a **latent infection,** the pathogen lies dormant in the body but retains the ability to replicate. Illness can recur if immunity weakens due to aging, poor health habits, hormonal imbalance, or another infection. Chicken pox is an example of a latent infection: People can harbor the virus throughout their life without experiencing symptoms. But at some later point, if immunity weakens, they can develop shingles, a painful infection of the nerves.

DOLLAR STRETCHER
Financial Wellness Tip

Wash your hands often and thoroughly to prevent illnesses that can be costly in terms of both time and money. You don't need fancy soaps or chemicals; plain old soap and water is just as effective. If you use liquid soap, get a refillable dispenser that squirts out just enough soap for a single use.

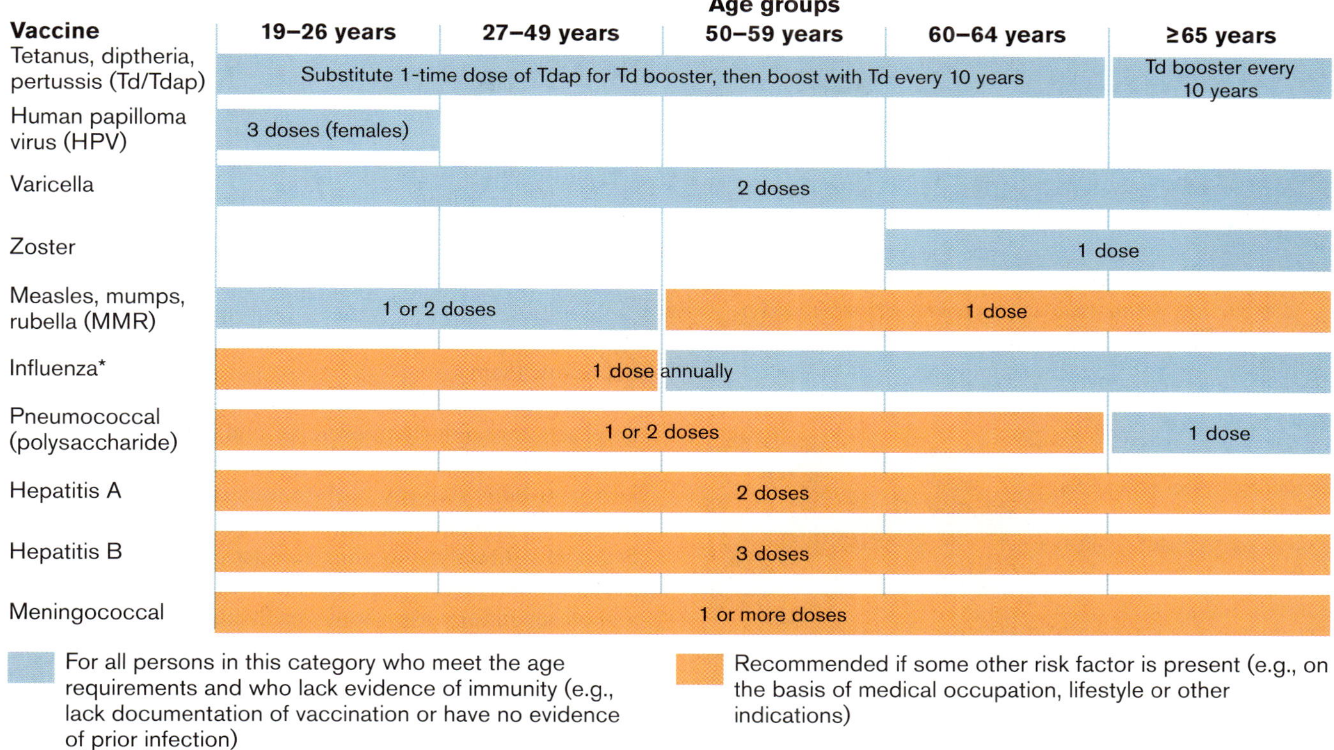

** In 2010, the CDC recommended that all persons 6 months and older receive the seasonal influenza vaccine for the 2010–2011 season.*

Figure 13-2 **Recommended immunizations for adults.** For more information and additional recommendations, visit http://www.cdc.gov/vaccines.

Sources: Centers for Disease Control and Prevention. (2010). Recommended adult immunization schedule—United States, 2010. *Morbidity and Mortality Weekly Report, 59*(1), 1–4. Centers for Disease Control and Prevention. (2010). Prevention and control of influenza with vaccines. *Morbidity and Mortality Weekly Report, 59,* 1–62.

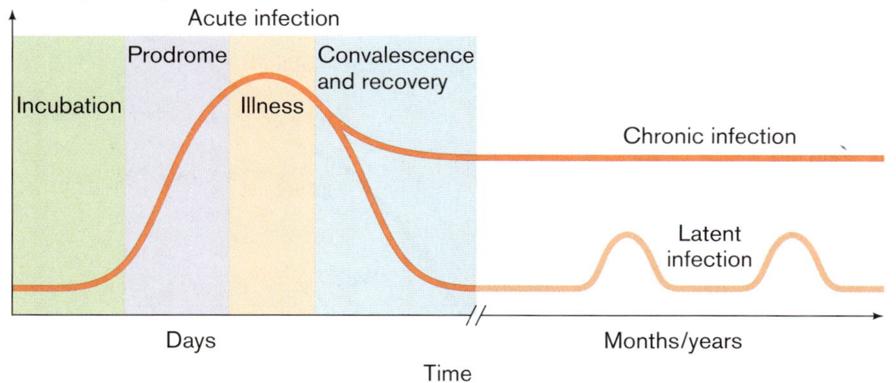

Figure 13-3 **Stages and patterns of infections.** Acute infections follow a typical four-stage pattern and usually resolve in days or weeks. Chronic infections persist over a longer period, whereas latent infections can recur if an individual's immunity weakens.

Prevention and Treatment of Infectious Diseases

Q | How can I keep from getting sick?

Your two best strategies for preventing infectious diseases are to keep pathogens out of your body and to maintain a strong immune system.

What can you do to avoid infectious agents? Your best defense is hand washing—do it often and do it thoroughly (Figure 13-4). If soap and water aren't available, use an alcohol-based hand sanitizer. Many common infectious diseases are transmitted through touch: An infected person transfers microbes directly (handshake) or indirectly (doorknob) to your hands. When you touch your eyes, nose, or mouth, the pathogen gains access to your body. Studies

When to wash

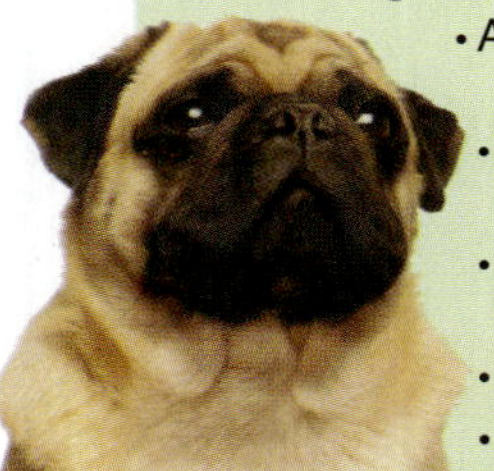

- Before and after preparing food
- Before and after eating food
- After using the toilet
- After changing diapers or cleaning up a child who has used the toilet
- Before and after tending to someone who is sick
- After blowing your nose, coughing, or sneezing
- After handling an animal or animal waste
- After handling garbage
- Before and after treating a cut or wound

How to wash

- Wet your hands with clean running water and apply soap
- Use warm water if it is available
- Rub hands together to make a lather and scrub all surfaces
- Continue rubbing hands for 20 seconds; if you need a timer, hum the "Happy Birthday" song from beginning to end twice
- Rinse hands well under running water
- Dry your hands using a paper towel or air dryer; if possible, use your paper towel to turn off the faucet

When using hand sanitizer

- If soap and water are not available, use alcohol-based gel (at least 60% alcohol) to clean hands
- Apply product to the palm of one hand, using the amount of product indicated on the label
- Rub hands together
- Rub the product over all surfaces of hands and fingers until hands are dry

Figure 13-4 Hand washing guidelines. When and how to wash your hands may seem simple and obvious—but the majority of people do not follow the recommendations. Consistently and thoroughly washing your hands is one of the best ways to help reduce your risk of many common infectious diseases.

Source: Centers for Disease Control and Prevention. (2010). *Clean hands save lives* (http://www.cdc.gov/cleanhands).

have linked good hand hygiene with reduced rates of upper respiratory and gastrointestinal illnesses.[6] However, most college students do not follow recommendations for hand washing.[7] Remember to wash your hands often—it works!

For infections like influenza that are transmitted through airborne droplets, your best strategy is to avoid people who are sneezing and coughing or stand at least three feet away—six or more feet is even better. If you're the one who is sick and sneezing or coughing, you can help stop the spread of infections by keeping your germs to yourself:

- Cover your mouth and nose with a tissue when you cough or sneeze.
- Throw out your used tissue.
- If you don't have a tissue, cough or sneeze into your upper sleeve or elbow, not your hands.
- Wash your hands often; if soap and water are not available, use an alcohol-based hand rub.

These strategies may sound obvious, but many people do not follow them.

To help keep your immune system strong, practice good self-care. Eat right, exercise, and get plenty of sleep.[8] Avoid behaviors like smoking and excessive drinking that hurt your body's ability to fight infection. Never inject illicit drugs; contaminated injection equipment can transmit pathogens directly into your bloodstream. If you plan to get a tattoo or piercing, go to a facility that is clean and has a good reputation; ask about sterilization practices and be sure to follow the instructions you're given on caring for your skin.

Also pay special attention to emotional wellness: High levels of stress and poor mental health are associated with higher rates of infectious diseases (Figure 13-5).[9] On the flip side, many of the strategies to reduce stress also help boost the immune system. For example, a study that looked at stress levels, humor, and immune function found that laughing at a humorous video reduced stress and improved the activity of immune cells.[10] Your emotional wellness can have a powerful effect on how well your body responds to infec-

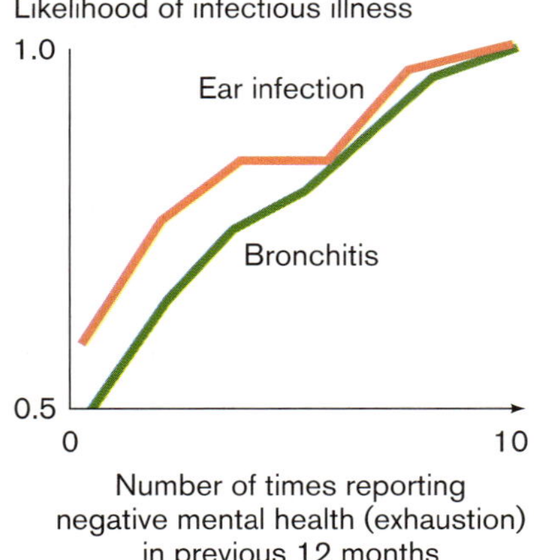

Figure 13-5 Mental health and risk of infectious disease in college students. Students who reported negative mental health—feelings of depression, anxiety, exhaustion, or hopelessness—also experienced higher rates of infectious disease.

Source: Adams, T. B., Wharton, C. M., Quilter, L., & Hirsch, T. (2008). The association between mental health and acute infectious illness among a national sample of 18- to 24-year-old college students. *Journal of American College Health, 56*(6), 657–663.

Research Brief

Hand Hygiene and Illness Rates in College Students

Most people, college students included, do not follow the recommendations for hand washing: They don't wash at all the recommended times or for the recommended duration. But does it really make a difference? Researchers recently studied students in four college residence halls, comparing a study group and a control group. For the study group, alcohol-gel hand-sanitizer dispensers were installed in every room, bathroom, and dining hall. The groups were followed for eight weeks and compared in terms of hand-hygiene behavior, symptom and illness rates, and absenteeism from class.

What did the researchers find? The study group showed improvements over the control group in all areas.

- Improved hand-hygiene practices: both hand washing frequency and the use of hand sanitizers were significantly higher in the study group; the increase in hand washing was thought to be due to increased awareness of the importance of hand hygiene.
- Reduced symptoms of upper respiratory illness: for example, students in the study group were 15% less likely to experience sore throat and stuffy nose and 30% less likely to develop cough or fever.
- Reduced rates of illness: the study group showed a 20% improvement in illness rate.
- Fewer missed school/work days: the study group missed 40% fewer days than the control group.

This study clearly showed the power of just a little more attention to hand hygiene. If you'd like to be sick less often and miss fewer days of school and work due to upper respiratory illness, wash your hands!

Source: White, C., Kolble, R., Carlson, R., et al. (2003). The effect of hand hygiene on illness rates among students in university residence halls. *American Journal of Infection Control, 31*(6), 364–370.

tion. See the box "Keeping Yourself Well" for a summary of actions you can take to help support your immune system.

Q | I'm confused about antibiotics—when do they really work?

Antibiotics are powerful medications that have saved many lives. At the same time, they are often misused, which can also lead to problems. Antibiotics primarily fight bacterial infections, although they may also be prescribed for certain conditions caused by fungi and parasites. They act by killing bacteria or preventing them from reproducing. They don't work against any infections caused by viruses, including colds, flu, and most sore throats and coughs. Sometimes a person with a viral infection will develop a secondary bacterial infection as a complication; antibiotics may be prescribed to destroy the bacteria, but they won't treat the initial viral infection.

Most bacteria die when exposed to antibiotics, but some develop resistance to the drug's effects. If these resistant bacteria spread, they are more difficult to treat. Every time you take antibiotics, you increase the chances that some bacteria in your body will develop resistance.[11] So, it's important to take antibiotics no more often than necessary. In addition, when antibiotics are prescribed for an infection, you should take them for the recommended duration—not just until your symptoms disappear. Stopping treatment too soon can allow an infection to return and also contributes to the development of resistance.

antibiotic A compound that is used to treat bacterial infections by killing the bacteria or inhibiting its growth.

Although beneficial, antibiotics also have side effects, including upset stomach, diarrhea, and, in women, vaginal yeast infections. Some antibiotics can also impair the functioning of the liver or kidneys.

DOLLAR STRETCHER
Financial Wellness Tip

Treat minor infections at home—you don't need to pay for a doctor visit or antibiotics, which don't treat viral infections like colds and flu. For upper respiratory infections, rest and drink plenty of warm liquids. If symptoms are bothersome, try inexpensive, generic medications.

Q | How are infections treated?

Treatment depends on the type of pathogen, the severity of the infection, and the person's underlying health status. Many minor infections don't need to be treated—your immune system can successfully eliminate the pathogen. If symptoms are uncomfortable during the acute phase the illness, over-the-counter medications are available to relieve nasal congestion, body aches, and other minor symptoms. If your symptoms are

Wellness Strategies

Keeping Yourself Well

- Get regular, moderate exercise.
- Eat a healthy diet.
- Get plenty of sleep.
- Control stress.
- Don't smoke, avoid secondhand smoke, and consume alcohol moderately, if at all.
- Wash your hands frequently and thoroughly.
- Don't rub your eyes, touch your nose, or eat with your fingers without washing your hands first.
- Avoid people with obvious signs of illness.
- Clean shared environmental surfaces (desks, phones, doorknobs), especially if you live or work with someone who is ill.
- Handle and prepare foods safely.
- Avoid disease carriers like mosquitoes, ticks, and rodents. To protect yourself from insect bites, wear long pants and long-sleeved shirts when you hike or work outdoors; you can also apply an insect repellent (for more information, visit http://www.nlm.nih.gov/medlineplus/insectbitesandstings.html).
- Abstain from sex or consistently practice safer sex.
- Don't inject drugs.
- Keep immunizations up to date.
- Stock an emergency kit to use in case of a breakdown in public health services, such as after a natural disaster (for advice about kits, visit http://www.ready.gov).

unusually severe or your illness persists, check with your health care provider.

Antimicrobial drugs exist for several categories of pathogens. For bacterial infections, antibiotics may be prescribed (see above). Specific antiviral drugs are available for few infections, including herpes, hepatitis, influenza, and HIV. Similarly, there are drugs that specifically target fungal and protozoal infections.

Infectious Diseases on Campus

For college students, even minor infectious diseases can impact academic performance. Students should also be alert to signs and symptoms that may indicate more serious conditions.

Colds and Influenza

Q How do you tell if you have a cold or the flu?

Colds and **influenza** ("the flu") are both caused by viruses and have some of the same symptoms, but there are differences (Table 13-1). Influenza is the more serious disease, although colds are more common and probably responsible for more lost days at school and on the job than any other infectious disease. For all the misery a cold can cause, in the vast majority of cases it will resolve without treatment—and nothing you do will shorten its duration.

There are hundreds of viruses that can cause the common cold. They are thought to be transmitted primarily by indirect contact—you touch a contaminated surface or object and then rub your eyes. Cold viruses can enter the body through the mucous membrane of the eyes. It takes about 48 hours from the time of exposure for symptoms to appear, and colds generally last two to seven days. Weather doesn't affect your risk for a cold, although being forced indoors into more crowded conditions increases your chance for exposure. Cold viruses pass easily from person to person. Colds are more frequent in children, becoming fewer with age. Complications are fairly unusual but are more likely among older adults.

influenza A highly infectious respiratory disease caused by an influenza virus; the "flu."

Influenza viruses are more likely to be transmitted through respiratory droplets that infected people release when they cough, sneeze, or talk. People with influenza can probably pass the virus to others up to about six feet away. They are contagious and able to infect others beginning about a day before symptoms develop and up to five to seven days after becoming ill.[12] Symptoms of influenza usually come on suddenly and typically include fever, body aches, and severe fatigue. The flu typically lasts longer than a cold. It also carries a greater risk of serious complications, including pneumonia, bronchitis, and sinus and ear infections. Older adults, pregnant women, young children, and people with chronic medical conditions are more likely to have serious problems. Thousands of Americans die from influenza and its complications every year.

Q Why is there a new flu vaccine every year?

Most cases of the flu are caused by influenza A and influenza B viruses. Influenza A viruses are further divided into subtypes based

TABLE 13-1 IS IT A COLD OR THE FLU?

SYMPTOM	COLD	FLU
FEVER	Rare	Usual; high (100°–102°F or higher); lasts 3–4 days
HEADACHE	Rare	Common
GENERAL ACHES, PAINS	Slight	Usual, often severe
FATIGUE, WEAKNESS	Sometimes	Usual; can last up to 2–3 weeks
EXHAUSTION	Never	Usual; typically at the beginning of the illness
STUFFY NOSE	Common	Sometimes
SNEEZING	Usual	Sometimes
SORE THROAT	Common	Sometimes
CHEST DISCOMFORT, COUGH	Mild to moderate	Common; can be severe
COMPLICATIONS	Sinus congestion, middle-ear infection, worsening of asthma symptoms	Bronchitis, pneumonia; worsening of chronic conditions; can be life-threatening

Source: National Institute of Allergy and Infectious Diseases. (2008). *Is it a cold or the flu?* (http://www.niaid.nih.gov/topics/Flu/understandingFlu/Pages/publications.aspx).

on proteins on their surface (H and N); recall the H1N1 virus that caused a flu *pandemic* (worldwide outbreak of disease) in 2009–2010. Influenza viruses continually change over time—sometimes slightly, sometimes significantly—and when they do, the immune system no longer recognizes the new version of the virus. Any immunity to other strains you had from past infections or vaccinations no longer protects you. So, the flu vaccine is reformulated every year to target the strains most likely to be circulating.

Infectious Mononucleosis

Q Does mono only come from kissing?

Epstein-Barr virus (EBV), a member of the **herpes** family of viruses, is the pathogen that causes infectious mononucleosis, or "mono." It is transmitted via saliva, which is how it got nicknamed the "kissing disease." Although it can be transmitted through kissing, any activity that brings someone in contact with the saliva of an infected person can transfer the virus—for example, sharing a drinking glass. The primary symptoms are fever, sore throat, swollen glands, and fatigue; some people also develop a swollen spleen. Serious complications are rare, but the fatigue associated with the infection can sometimes last for several months. People who develop an enlarged spleen will be advised to avoid certain physical activities as well as contact sports to reduce the risk of rupturing the spleen.

By age 40, it's estimated that 95 percent of American adults have been infected with EBV.[13] Not everyone develops symptoms, but EBV is a latent infection, so the virus remains dormant in the body (see p. 372). The infection can reactivate, but it usually causes no symptoms even though it can be passed on to someone else. Because the virus can be carried in the saliva of otherwise healthy people, transmission is nearly impossible to prevent.

herpes A family of viruses that includes those responsible for chicken pox, cold sores, mononucleosis, and genital herpes; herpes viruses have the ability to establish lifelong latent infections.

meningitis Inflammation of the meninges, the membranes that surround the brain and the spinal cord.

Meningitis

Q Which is the infection that causes stiff neck?

You are probably thinking of **meningitis,** which is inflammation of the membranes that surround the brain and spinal

Wellness Strategies

Starve a Fever, Feed a Cold?

Although popularized by Mark Twain, this old adage—and its exact opposite—dates back to the 1500s. Today's medical experts will tell you that neither of these is prudent advice, but it is hard for many to turn away from medical myths. Your body always needs energy, regardless of the type of infection, so make sure to eat to satisfy your appetite. Even though the common cold has no cure, there are treatments that can make the suffering more tolerable. Many of these strategies are also good for home treatment of influenza.

- Drink plenty of liquids: Water, juice, clear broth, or warm lemon water with honey help loosen congestion and prevent dehydration. Avoid alcohol.
- Rest: Colds can tire you out, but influenza is especially associated with severe fatigue and body aches.
- Try a saltwater gargle: Dissolve 1/2 teaspoon salt in 8 ounces of warm water and gargle to temporarily relieve a sore or scratchy throat.
- Try saline nasal spray: Over-the-counter saline nasal sprays can combat stuffiness and congestion. Avoid or limit use of nasal decongestant sprays, which can lead to a worsening of symptoms when the medication is discontinued.
- Use over-the-counter cold medicines cautiously: Decongestants may relieve some of your symptoms but will not shorten the length of your cold; some also have side effects including drowsiness and upset stomach. Choose single-ingredient products, and don't exceed the recommended dosages. Antihistamines may provide some relief from cold symptoms, but they are more appropriate for treating allergies.
- Use pain relievers cautiously: Aspirin, acetaminophen, or ibuprofen can all reduce a fever and bring some relief from the aches and pains, but they won't make your symptoms go away any faster. Aspirin and ibuprofen can cause stomach irritation, and if taken for a long period or in higher-than-recommended doses, acetaminophen can be toxic to your liver. Talk to your doctor before giving acetaminophen to children, and don't give aspirin to children or teens because of the risk of Reye's syndrome, a rare but potentially fatal disease.
- Limit or avoid over-the-counter cough medicines: Don't take a cough suppressant if you have a productive cough. Soothing your throat with warm liquids and throat lozenges and humidifying the air in your residence can be more effective than any drugs. (The Food and Drug Administration recommends that nonprescription cough medicines *not* be given to children under age 2.)

And remember, antibiotics are not effective at treating viral infections like colds and the flu.

cord. Symptoms in adults typically include high fever, severe headache, stiff neck, and sensitivity to bright light. The most common cause is a viral infection, and viral meningitis usually resolves on its own after about 7–10 days. However, bacterial meningitis, which has the same symptoms, is a much more severe infection that can lead to disability or even death. Anyone experiencing meningitis symptoms needs to see a physician immediately (Table 13-2); if treated early with antibiotics, bacterial meningitis can be cured.

Bacterial Skin Infections

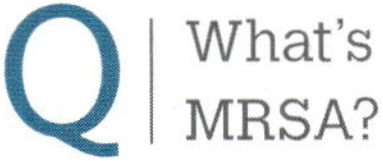

The acronym MRSA stands for methicillin-resistant *Staphylococcus aureus*. It's a type of staph bacteria that is resistant to many antibiotics and therefore difficult to treat. MRSA used to be a common cause of hospital-acquired pneumonia and bloodstream infections, but it is now also a major cause of skin infections outside medical settings. Risk factors for the spread of MRSA include close skin-to-skin contact, skin cuts or abrasions, crowded living conditions, and contaminated items and surfaces. Places where these risk factors are common include athletic facilities, dormitories, military barracks, and daycare centers. See the box "Avoiding Infections from the Gym" for more information.

Skin infections usually start out as red, swollen, painful lumps; they may initially look like pimples, boils, or insect bites. If the infection spreads, you may also become generally ill with fever, swollen glands, and so on. If you experience these symptoms, you should contact your health care provider for a diagnosis and appropriate treatment; MRSA skin infections require professional treatment. Skin infections can also be caused by other pathogens, including *Streptococcus* bacteria. Athlete's foot, herpes, and impetigo are all examples of other common skin infections.

TABLE 13-2 COMMON INFECTIONS: SYMPTOMS AND TREATMENTS

ILLNESS (PATHOGEN)	SYMPTOMS	HOME TREATMENT	WHEN TO SEEK MEDICAL CARE
COMMON COLD (over 200 different viruses)	Runny nose, nasal congestion, mild cough, sore throat, low-grade fever, sneezing	Usually resolves on its own; fluids, rest, and over-the-counter medications to treat symptoms; avoid alcohol and tobacco	Worsening symptoms after third day, difficulty breathing, stiff neck
INFLUENZA (influenza A or B virus)	Sudden-onset fever, extreme fatigue, headache, body aches, cough	Usually resolves on its own; same home treatment as for colds; prescription antivirals available	Difficulty breathing, severe headache or stiff neck, confusion, fever lasting more than 3 days; new, localized pain in ear, chest, sinuses; people at high risk for complications should contact a health care provider if they develop flu symptoms
BRONCHITIS (different viruses or bacteria)	Cough that may start out dry and later produce mucus; sore throat, fever	Usually resolves on its own; same home treatment as for colds	Shortness of breath, high fever, shaking chills (signs of pneumonia); wheezing and cough that last more than 2 weeks; people at high risk for complications should check with a health care provider
MONONUCLEOSIS (Epstein-Barr virus)	High fever, swollen glands, severe sore throat, fatigue; nausea, vomiting, and loss of appetite can occur	Usually resolves on its own; rest, fluids; avoid contact sports until symptoms resolve due to risk of spleen rupture	Fever lasting more than 3 days; symptoms lasting longer than 7–10 days; severe abdominal pain (possibly indicating ruptured spleen)
MENINGITIS (several different viruses or bacteria)	High fever, stiff and painful neck, headache; vomiting, sleepiness, confusion, seizures	Requires medical evaluation; if determined to be a viral infection, home treatment to relieve symptoms is appropriate	Immediately; bacterial meningitis requires treatment with antibiotics to avoid serious or deadly complications
STREP THROAT (*Streptococcus* bacteria)	Sudden-onset sore throat and fever; swollen glands; red and white pus on tonsils; absence of cold symptoms	A visit to health care provider is appropriate; saltwater gargles, throat lozenges, over-the-counter medications to treat symptoms	Strep throat is treated with antibiotics to reduce duration of symptoms and risk of complications
BACTERIAL SKIN INFECTION (*Staphylococcus aureus* or *Streptococcus*)	Skin sore or rash; red, swollen, warm, and painful areas of skin; if infection spreads, general symptoms of fever, chills, swollen glands	A visit to health care provider is appropriate; warm compresses; keep infected area clean and dry; topical antibiotics if advised by health care provider	Bacterial skin infections are usually treated with antibiotics; stay alert for worsening symptoms or infection on the face
URINARY TRACT INFECTIONS (different bacteria)	Cloudy, bloody, or strong-smelling urine; frequent urination; pain or burning with urination; low fever; pain in lower abdomen	Requires medical evaluation; drink plenty of water; in women, drinking cranberry juice has been shown to help prevent but not treat urinary tract infections	Bacterial urinary tract infections are usually treated with antibiotics; stay alert for worsening symptoms, which may indicate the infection has spread to the kidneys

Wellness Strategies

Avoiding Infections from the Gym

Skin infections in athletes are very common and can also affect recreational athletes and anyone who works out at a gym. Here are some steps you can take to reduce your risk:

- Ask your gym or exercise facility about its cleaning procedures—what is cleaned and how often? Does it provide cleansers and wipes for people to use?
- If facility exercise mats aren't cleaned between each class, bring your own exercise mat, and clean your mat after each workout.
- Use clothing or a towel to act as a barrier between exercise equipment and your bare skin; if you use a towel, wash it after each workout.
- If you have any skin abrasions or cuts, cover them with a sterile bandage.
- Wash your hands before and after working out; hand hygiene is important in all settings.
- Shower after a workout. Wash all parts of your body, including your feet. Athletes in sports with high rates of skin infection should wash with antibacterial cleanser.
- Dry your feet, armpits, and groin area thoroughly after using a locker room or public shower. Consider wearing shower shoes in shared showering facilities—but don't skip washing your feet.
- Change all your clothes (including socks and underwear) after a workout and shower. Keep your dirty and clean clothes in separate gym bags.
- Don't borrow or share water bottles, towels, razors, bar soap, deodorant, or other personal hygiene items.
- If you notice any symptoms, see a doctor, follow the recommended treatment, and don't go back to the gym until the doctor says your infection is no longer contagious.

Sources: Zinder, S. M., Basler, R. S. W., Foley, J., Scarlata, C., & Vasily, D. B. (2010). National Athletic Trainers' Association position statement: Skin diseases. *Journal of Athletic Training, 45*(4), 411–428. American Academy of Family Physicians. (2009). *Tinea infections: Athlete's foot, jock itch, and ringworm* (http://familydoctor.org/online/famdocen/home/common/infections/common/fungal/316.html).

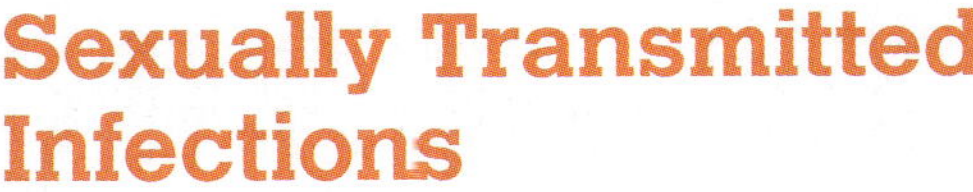

Sexually Transmitted Infections

Sexually transmitted infections (STIs) are among the most common types of infections in the United States, with an estimated 19 million new cases each year (Table 13-3). About half of all new infections occur among people ages 15–24. STIs are primarily spread through person-to-person sexual contact—vaginal, oral, or anal sex—although some can also be transmitted in other ways. Some STIs can be easily treated and cured, but others are chronic, incurable, and even life threatening. All STIs are preventable.

Q | Do women get more STIs than men?

Yes, women are more likely to have STIs and more likely to experience serious complications from them. Transmission of many STIs, including genital herpes and HIV, is more likely to occur from an infected male to his female partner than from an infected female to her male partner. Approximately one in five women between 14 and 49 has genital herpes infection compared with one in nine men in the same age group.[14] Young women are also more likely than older women to contract STIs and to experience serious effects; the cervix of young women is covered with cells that are especially susceptible to STIs.

sexually transmitted infection (STI) An infection that is primarily spread through person-to-person sexual contact.

Most STIs affect both men and women, but in many cases, they cause more severe problems in women, including infertility. Having an STI during pregnancy can cause early labor, infection of the uterus, and in some cases dangerous infections in the baby.

Q | Do STIs show up immediately?

Not necessarily. Many sexually transmitted infections are asymptomatic, meaning people are unaware they are infected and can pass the infection on to others. Some STIs have very minor symptoms that can be overlooked or mistaken for other conditions. It's important to realize that anyone who is sexually active can have an STI—even if they've never had any signs or symptoms of disease. It doesn't matter who you are, it's what you do that counts.

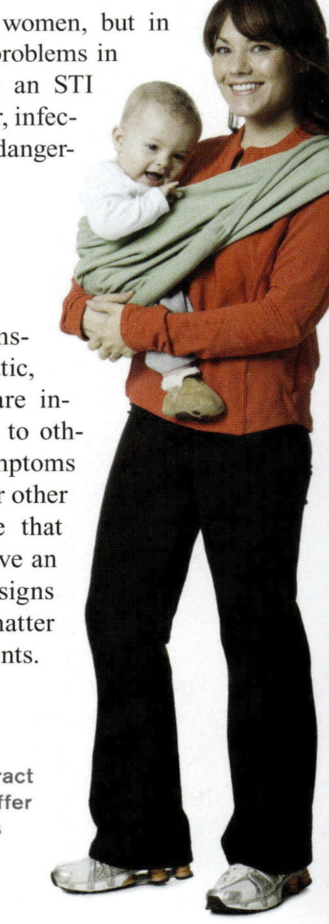

Women are more likely than men to contract sexually transmitted infections and to suffer serious complications from them. Infants can also be at risk for contracting infections from their mothers during pregnancy, childbirth, and breast-feeding.

TABLE 13-3 **STIs IN THE UNITED STATES: A SNAPSHOT**

	ESTIMATED ANNUAL INCIDENCE	ESTIMATED PREVALENCE*	OUTLOOK IF DIAGNOSED
TRICHOMONIASIS	7.4 million	n/a	Curable with antibiotics
HPV INFECTION	6.2 million	20 million	Vaccine-preventable; incurable but often resolves on its own; can cause cancer
CHLAMYDIA	2.8 million	1.9 million	Curable with antibiotics
GENITAL HERPES	1.6 million	45 million	Chronic and incurable; treatments can reduce symptoms and outbreaks
GONORRHEA	700,000	n/a	Curable with antibiotics
SYPHILIS	60,000	n/a	Curable with antibiotics
HIV INFECTION	56,000	1.1 million	Chronic and potentially fatal; treatable but incurable
HEPATITIS B	43,000	1.25 million	Vaccine-preventable; incurable but often resolves on its own; can cause fatal liver disease

*Because viral STIs can be persistent and incurable, the number of currently infected people capable of transmitting the infection (prevalence) greatly exceeds the annual number of new cases (incidence).

Sources: Centers for Disease Control and Prevention. (2010). Fact sheet: HIV in the United States (http://www.cdc.gov/hiv/resources/factsheets/us.htm). Centers for Disease Control and Prevention. (2010). HCV FAQs for health professionals (http://www.cdc.gov/hepatitis/HCV/HCVfaq.htm). Weinstock, H., Berman, S., & Cates, W. (2004). Sexually transmitted diseases among American youth: Incidence and prevalence estimates, 2000. *Perspectives on Sexual and Reproductive Health, 36*(1), 6–10. Additional data from the Kaiser Family Foundation and the Guttmacher Institute.

Trichomoniasis

Q | What's the most common sexually transmitted infection?

In terms of new cases each year, **trichomoniasis,** or "trich," is the most common. The protozoa *Trichomonas vaginalis* causes vaginal infections in women and infections of the urethra (urine canal) in men. Most infected women have symptoms such as vaginal discharge and painful urination, but most infected men do not have symptoms. Trichomoniasis is diagnosed with lab tests and treated with prescription medication. If a woman develops trichomoniasis, she and her partner both need to be treated because it's likely he is infected even if he has no symptoms. Treatment should be completed before resuming sexual activity. Trichomoniasis has two serious complications if untreated: It significantly increases the risk of HIV transmission, and, in pregnant women, it can lead to premature labor and delivery.

Chlamydia

Q | How often should I get checked for chlamydia?

Annual screening for **chlamydia** is recommended for sexually active women 25 years of age and younger, as well as older women with risk factors (many sex partners or a new sex partner). Testing is also recommended for pregnant women.

Chlamydia is caused by *Chlamydia trachomatis,* a bacterium that can be transmitted during vaginal, oral, or anal sex or from an infected mother to her baby during childbirth. About 70 percent of those who are infected have no symptoms, but among those who do, abnormal discharge from the vagina or penis and pain while urinating are most common.

Untreated, chlamydia can cause serious infections of the fallopian tubes in women and the urethra and epididymis (curved tube on the back of the testicle) in men. People infected through oral sex may have symptoms in the throat.

Chlamydia can be treated with antibiotics, but reinfection is possible—and even likely, if a woman's partner isn't also treated. In women, untreated chlamydia is a leading cause of serious and permanent damage to the reproductive organs, which can lead to infertility. Infected infants may develop pneumonia and eye infections that can potentially cause blindness.

Gonorrhea

Q | Can a person really get gonorrhea from oral sex?

Yes, unprotected oral sex can transmit the infection, although it's not as common as infection of the reproductive

trichomoniasis Sexually transmitted infection caused by the protozoa *Trichomonas vaginalis.*

chlamydia Sexually transmitted infection caused by the bacterium *Chlamydia trachomatis.*

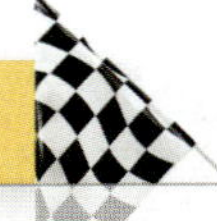

Fast Facts

No, Not Really: Top STI Myths

Myth: If someone has an STI, you can tell because you can see the signs.

Fact: Many STIs have no signs or symptoms; someone without any symptoms can have an STI and transmit it to a partner.

Myth: Only people who have a lot of sex partners get STIs.

Fact: Anyone who has sexual contact of any kind can contract an STI.

Myth: You can't get an STI from oral sex.

Fact: The pathogens that cause STIs can enter the body through tiny cuts or tears in the mouth or in some cases through skin-to-skin contact with an infected area or sore.

Myth: Once you've had a particular STI, you can't get it again.

Fact: You do not become immune to STIs such as chlamydia and gonorrhea, so you can contract them multiple times. Infections such as herpes and HIV are chronic and incurable.

Myth: You can't get an STI if you're on the pill.

Fact: Birth control pills do not protect against STIs.

Myth: Douching helps prevent STIs.

Fact: Douching increases the risk for several STIs as well as pelvic inflammatory disease. Douching alters the balance of organisms that live in the vagina in harmful ways and can also force pathogens to go from the vagina higher up into the reproductive system.

or urinary tract. Among young women, as many as 10–25 percent of infections may be in the throat.[15] **Gonorrhea** is a bacterial infection caused by *Neisseria gonorrhoeae.* It is spread through contact with the penis, vagina, mouth, or anus; it can also be spread from mother to baby during delivery. Most women have no symptoms, and those who do may have nonspecific symptoms that are mistaken for a bladder or vaginal infection. Men can also be asymptomatic, although sometimes discharge and painful urination occur.

As with chlamydia, untreated gonorrhea can damage a woman's reproductive organs and cause infertility and chronic pelvic pain. In men, an untreated infection can damage the epididymis and also potentially lead to infertility—although this is less likely than in women. If transmitted to an infant during childbirth, the bacteria can cause dangerous infections of the blood, joints, and eyes.

gonorrhea Sexually transmitted infection caused by the bacterium *Neisseria gonorrhoeae.*

Gonorrhea can be treated with antibiotics, but many strains of the bacteria have developed resistance, which can make treatment more difficult. Although the infection can be cured with antibiotics, treatment does not reverse the damage, and re-infection is possible.

Pelvic Inflammatory Disease (PID)

Q | If I have chlamydia, does that mean I also have PID?

Not necessarily, but you are at risk. **Pelvic inflammatory disease (PID)** is infection and inflammation of the uterus, ovaries, fallopian tubes, and other reproductive organs in women. It is usually the result of untreated chlamydia or gonorrhea; douching and use of an intrauterine device (IUD) can also increase the risk of PID.[16]

In PID, bacteria move up from the vagina and infect other reproductive organs. The infection may have no initial symptoms, or there may be severe symptoms, including sudden onset of fever and pain. Signs can include vaginal discharge, painful urination or intercourse, pain in the lower abdomen, and irregular menstrual bleeding.

PID damages the reproductive organs, and the resulting scar tissue can cause chronic pelvic pain, tubal (ectopic) pregnancy, and infertility from blocked fallopian tubes. More than 1 million women are treated for PID each year, and many others have the condition but don't know it. Each year, an estimated 100,000 women become infertile and more than 150 women die from PID.[17] Infertility is more likely to occur if you have prolonged or repeated bouts of PID.

If you think you have pelvic inflammatory disease, see your physician immediately: Early treatment with antibiotics can limit the damage and long-term complications. As with other sexually transmitted diseases, a woman's sex partners also need to be treated.

Syphilis

Q | How many stages of syphilis are there?

There are four separate but sometimes overlapping stages to **syphilis.** The disease is caused by the bacterium *Treponema pallidum,* which can be transmitted through infected skin and mucous membranes in the genitals, lips, mouth, or anus. Syphilis can also be passed from a pregnant woman to her infant during pregnancy, causing a disease called congenital syphilis.

Primary syphilis is the first stage, characterized by the appearance of a painless sore, called a chancre, at the point of infection. The sore is full of bacteria that can be transmitted to others, but it may go unnoticed. A chancre usually disappears within about three to six weeks regardless of whether the infection is treated.

pelvic inflammatory disease (PID) Infection of the reproductive system in women, typically caused by untreated chlamydia or gonorrhea; can result in reproductive system damage and infertility.

syphilis A multistage sexually transmitted infection caused by the bacterium *Treponema pallidum.*

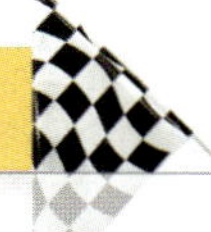
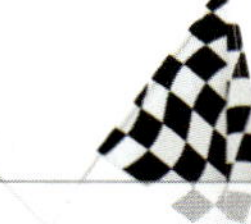

Fast Facts

Sex Is . . . ?

How do you define *sex*? Surveys of college students show changing perceptions over time.

Behavior	Percentage of university students who classified behavior as sex 1991	2007
Penile-vaginal intercourse	99.5%	97.5%
Penile-anal intercourse	81.0%	78.4%
Partner's oral contact with your genitals	40.2%	19.9%
Oral contact with partner's genitals	39.9%	18.7%

Does it matter? For prevention of infections, the important point to remember is that the pathogens that cause STIs don't care how you define *sex*. Any of the activities on this list can transmit microbes and cause disease.

Source: Hans, J. D., Gillen, M., & Akande, K. (2010). Sex redefined: The reclassification of oral-genital contact. *Perspectives on Sexual and Reproductive Health, 42*(2).

TABLE 13-4 PREVALENCE OF HERPES SIMPLEX VIRUS TYPE 2 AS MEASURED BY BLOOD TESTS*

	PREVALENCE (%)
TOTAL	16.2%
AGE GROUP (YEARS)	
14–19	1.4%
20–29	10.5%
30–39	19.6%
40–49	26.1%
REPORTED NUMBER OF LIFETIME SEX PARTNERS	
1	3.9%
2–4	14.0%
5–9	16.3%
≥10	26.7%

*Over 80% of those whose blood test was positive for HSV 2 had never received a diagnosis of genital herpes.

Source: Centers for Disease Control and Prevention. (2010). Seroprevalence of herpes simplex virus type 2 among persons aged 14–49 years—United States, 2005–2008. *Morbidity and Mortality Weekly Report, 59*(15), 456–459.

genital herpes A chronic or latent sexually transmitted infection caused by the herpes simplex virus (HSV) and characterized by genital sores.

Secondary syphilis develops two to ten weeks later. The most common symptom is a non-itchy skin rash, usually on the palms of the hands and soles of the feet. Other signs include swollen lymph glands, headache, fatigue, sore throat, and hair loss. Symptoms of secondary syphilis usually disappear with or without treatment, although they may recur.

Latent syphilis develops in people who haven't been treated. Symptoms of the disease disappear, but the bacteria remains in the body. Early in the latent stage a person can still infect others, but this risk fades over time.

A small percentage of people with latent syphilis go on to develop the fourth stage, *tertiary syphilis*. In this stage, the syphilis bacteria damages major organs and can cause mental illness, heart disease, blindness, and death.

During pregnancy, syphilis can cause miscarriage, premature birth, stillbirth, and infant death. Babies born with congenital syphilis may have birth defects, seizures, development delays, and other problems. Syphilis can be cured with antibiotics in all stages, but organ damage cannot be reversed. A fetus can be cured in the womb if the mother is treated early enough in the pregnancy.

Genital Herpes

Q | Does everyone have herpes?

No, not everyone. But the infection is very common, and the majority of infected people don't know their status (Table 13-4). **Genital herpes** can be caused by herpes simplex virus type 1 (HSV 1) or type 2 (HSV 2), but in most cases HSV 2 is responsible. HSV 1 more often infects the lips and mouth, causing cold sores, but it can cause genital herpes if transmitted through

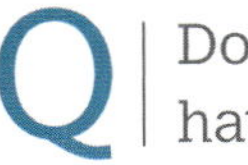

Latex condoms provide an essentially impermeable barrier to particles the size of STI pathogens and are highly effective in preventing STIs. Condoms cannot provide protection if sites of infection or potential exposure are not covered by condoms. Consistent and correct use of condoms can reduce but not eliminate the risk of STI transmission.

Living with . . .

Genital Herpes

Finding out you have genital herpes can be a shock—and you may feel angry and ashamed as well as worried about rejection. Remember that genital herpes is a very common infection and that although challenging, it can be successfully managed. In healthy adults, genital herpes usually doesn't cause any serious health problems. For most people, outbreaks become less frequent over time—perhaps four to five outbreaks during the first year after diagnosis and then fewer after that. Some helpful strategies for managing genital herpes include the following:

- Follow your physician's advice for managing the infection. Take all prescribed medications, even if the symptoms go away.
- Maintain a healthy lifestyle and manage stress to support your immune system and reduce outbreaks (see p. 374).
- Be aware of potential triggers for outbreaks, which can vary from person to person. For example, some people find outbreaks linked to certain other illnesses or to hormonal changes associated with the menstrual cycle.
- Avoid sexual activity when you feel an outbreak coming on or have symptoms. But remember, you can transmit the infection even if you have no symptoms.
- During an outbreak, keep the sores clean and dry; if you touch a sore, wash your hands thoroughly. Wear loose-fitting cotton underwear and don't wear pantyhose; heat and moisture can slow healing.
- Use latex condoms during sex. Used consistently and correctly, condoms are effective at significantly reducing the risk of spreading herpes; however, since they don't cover all potentially infectious areas, they do not completely eliminate risk.
- Tell your sexual partners so that they can be tested for herpes. Inform any new partners before you have sex.
- Find a counselor or a support group—in person or online.

human papillomavirus (HPV) infection A sexually transmitted viral infection that can cause genital warts and cellular changes that lead to cervical and other cancers; can be a chronic infection.

oral sex. HSV 2 can also infect the mouth. Overall, about 50–80 percent of American adults have oral herpes (primarily from HSV 1), and about 20 percent have genital herpes (primarily from HSV 2).

Most people contract genital herpes by having sex or close skin-to-skin contact with an infected person. The main symptom of herpes is sores at the site where the virus entered the body. The sores may start with a tingling feeling, erupt as red bumps, and then develop into small blisters or painful open sores. Some people also experience fever, headache, muscle aches, swollen glands, and other genital or urinary symptoms.

In most people, HSV is a latent infection; the virus remains in nerve cells for life and can become active and cause outbreaks several times a year. Recurrences often include visible sores and symptoms, but the virus can also be active without causing any signs. Although transmission of the virus is more likely when obvious sores are present, people with genital herpes can transmit the virus even if they have no symptoms and no idea they are infected.

There is no treatment or cure for genital herpes. There are antiviral drugs that help treat symptoms and prevent or reduce outbreaks. Using these drugs reduces but does not eliminate the chance of passing herpes to sexual partners. Because HSV can pass from mother to fetus and harm the baby, pregnant women who have herpes or whose sex partners have herpes should develop a plan with their physician to reduce the risk of the baby being infected. Having herpes also increases the likelihood of contracting HIV from an infected partner.

Genital Warts (HPV Infection)

Q | Do genital warts go away?

For many people, genital warts clear up over time. However, they can become a chronic infection or have other serious effects. Genital warts are caused by **human papillomavirus (HPV) infection.** However, many people have genital HPV infection without having genital warts. There are more than one hundred types of HPV, many of which are harmless. Of those that are sexually transmitted, some types cause genital warts and some can cause changes in cells that can lead to cancer of the cervix, vulva, vagina, penis, or anus. Genital warts can also cause problems during pregnancy; in rare cases, infants born to infected mothers can develop warts in their throats.

HPV infection is very common and easily transmitted through skin-to-skin contact. Close to 30 percent of young women acquire HPV from their first male sex partner, and that within three years of becoming sexually active, 50 percent of women have been infected.[18] Males are also infected at a high rate: In a two-year study of heterosexually active male university students, 62 percent of the study participants acquired new HPV infections.[19]

For many people, genital HPV infection has no symptoms. But even in these cases, complications can develop, and the virus can be transmitted to sexual partners. When warts do appear, they may be raise or flat, small or large;

they can appear anywhere on, in, or around the genitals. Women may unknowingly have warts on their cervix. Genital warts do not turn into cancer; the types of HPV that cause warts are different from those that cause cancer. However, an individual can be infected with both types.

There are treatments for visible genital warts, including creams, laser treatment, and freezing or burning; sometimes warts disappear without treatment. However, there is no treatment for the underlying viral infection. Because the virus remains in the body, warts can come back after treatment.

In about 90 percent of cases, the body's immune system clears HPV within two years of infection. But not all cases clear up, and because the infection can have no symptoms, it is difficult to determine who is and is not capable of transmitting it.

The primary complication of HPV infection is cervical cancer. The cellular changes associated with cervical cancer can be detected with regular Pap tests, which are recommended for all women starting within three years after they become sexually active.

Genital HPV infection is one of the two sexually transmitted viruses for which vaccines are available. There are two vaccines (Cervarix and Gardasil) that protect against the types of HPV that cause about 70 percent of cervical cancers. Gardasil also protects against the types of HPV that cause about 90 percent of cases of genital warts. The vaccines are recommended for all females when they are 11 or 12 as well as females between 13 and 26 who haven't already been fully vaccinated. Gardasil is also licensed for use in males ages 9 to 26 for the prevention of genital warts. The vaccines do not treat established HPV infections.

Along with the vaccine, consistent condom use can also protect against HPV infection.[20] However, condoms do not provide complete protection because not all skin surfaces that can carry the virus are covered by a condom. See the box "Preventing Sexually Transmitted Infections" for additional strategies.

Viral Hepatitis

Q | Are herpes and HIV the only incurable STIs?

No. Along with HPV infection, some forms of **viral hepatitis** can also develop into chronic, incurable infections. Hepatitis is inflammation of the liver, and the three most common causes are the following:

- *Hepatitis A virus (HAV),* which is usually transmitted through contaminated food and water. Hepatitis A usually resolves on its own, and a vaccine is available. There are about 25,000 U.S. cases per year.

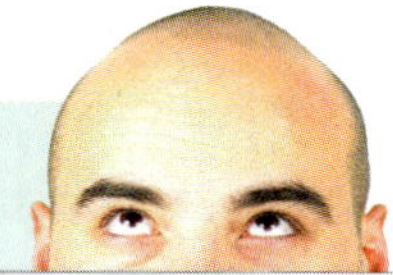

Mind Stretcher
Critical Thinking Exercise

Do you feel comfortable about having a frank discussion with a new partner about your sexual histories? Under what circumstances do you feel such a discussion would be appropriate or inappropriate? Develop several statements you could use to bring up the subject of STIs and safer sex with a potential sex partner.

- *Hepatitis B virus (HBV),* which is transmitted through semen, vaginal fluids, blood, and saliva. Hepatitis B is described in more detail below.
- *Hepatitis C virus (HCV),* which is primarily transmitted through blood. Most new U.S. infections occur through injection drug use. Hepatitis C leads to chronic infection in about 85 percent of those who are infected.

Hepatitis B is most commonly transmitted through sex with an infected partner, through contact with the blood of an infected person, or from a mother to infant during childbirth. Hepatitis is more easily transmitted than HIV and some other bloodborne infections, so there is some risk of infection from sharing razors or toothbrushes with an infected person. However, the virus isn't transmitted through shaking hands, coughing, or sharing utensils. There are about 43,000 new cases each year (see Table 13-3).

Symptoms of acute hepatitis B may include jaundice (yellowing of the skin and whites of the eyes), abdominal pain, nausea or vomiting, dark urine, and fatigue. The acute phase may last from several weeks to up to six months. There is no specific treatment for hepatitis B infection other than good self-care. In some people, the virus remains in the body after the acute stage of the infection, causing chronic disease. People with chronic hepatitis may exhibit no symptoms, but some develop serious and potentially fatal liver damage or liver cancer.

viral hepatitis Inflammation of the liver caused by infection with one of the hepatitis viruses; can become a chronic infection.

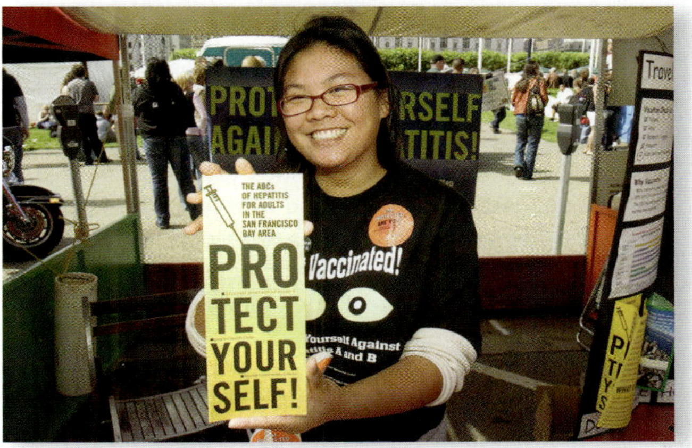

Wellness Strategies

Preventing Sexually Transmitted Infections

You can lower your risk of getting an STI with the following steps. The steps work best when used together. No single strategy can protect you from every single type of STI.

- **Don't have sex.** The surest way to keep from getting any STI is to practice abstinence. This means not having vaginal, oral, or anal sex. Keep in mind that some STIs, such as genital herpes, can be spread without having intercourse.
- **Be faithful.** Having a sexual relationship with one partner who has been tested for STIs and is not infected is another way to lower your risk of getting infected. Be faithful to each other. This means you only have sex with each other and no one else.
- **Limit your number of sex partners.** Choose partners who have also had few sex partners. The fewer partners you have, the less likely you are to encounter someone who is infected with an STI. Keep in mind, however, that even people with only one lifetime sexual partner can have an STI.
- **Use condoms correctly and every time you have sex.** Use condoms from the very start to the very end of each sex act and with every sex partner. A male latex condom offers the best protection. You can use a male polyurethane condom if you or your partner has a latex allergy. For vaginal sex, women should use a female condom if their partner won't wear a condom. For oral or anal sex, use a male latex condom. A dental dam might also offer some protection from some STIs.
- **Know that some methods of birth control—such as birth control pills, shots, implants, and diaphragms—will not protect you from STIs.** If you use one of these methods, be sure to also use a condom correctly *every time* you have sex.
- **Talk with your sex partners about STIs and using condoms before having sex.** It's up to you to set the ground rules and to make sure you are protected.
- **Don't assume you're at low risk for STIs if you're a woman who has sex only with women.** Some common STIs are spread easily by skin-to-skin contact. Also, most women who have sex with women have had sex with men, too.
- **Talk frankly with your doctor and each sex partner about any STIs you or your partner has or has had.** Talk about symptoms, such as sores or discharge. Try not to be embarrassed. Your doctor is there to help you with any and all health problems.
- **Have regular exams—get tested and insist your partners do, too.** Ask your doctor if you should be tested for STIs and how often you should be retested. Testing for many STIs is simple and often can be done during a checkup. The sooner an STI is found, the easier it is to treat.
- **Get vaccinated against HPV.** If you're age 26 or younger, ask if vaccination is appropriate for you.
- **Be alert for symptoms.** If you experience any genital or urinary symptoms, see your doctor. Don't have sex until you and your partners complete treatment.
- **Avoid using drugs or drinking too much alcohol.** These activities may lead to risky sexual behavior, such as not wearing a condom.

Source: National Women's Health Information Center. (2009). Overview. *Sexually Transmitted Infections* (http://www.womenshealth.gov/faq/sexually-transmitted-infections.cfm). Centers for Disease Control and Prevention. (2010). What patients should know when they are diagnosed with genital warts (http://www.cdc.gov/hpv/Signs-Symptoms.html).

There is a vaccine to prevent hepatitis B. It is routinely given to all infants and is also safe for children and adults.

HIV Infection and AIDS

In the United States, someone is infected with HIV every 10 minutes, and someone dies from HIV/AIDS every 45 minutes.[21] Worldwide, the statistics are even more dramatic, with 7,400 people infected every day, half of them under age 25.[22] Although medications developed to treat the infection have dramatically extended survival and greatly improved quality of life, HIV/AIDS remains an enormous global challenge.

HIV is not equally distributed across the population in the United States. Men have higher rates of HIV infection than women (Figure 13-6). Although African Americans make up about 13 percent of the U.S. population, they account for about half of all new HIV cases. However, it's important to remember that anyone can be infected with HIV. Recent surveys indicate that nearly 40 percent of young adults engage in high-risk HIV behavior.[23]

Q | Is there a difference between HIV and AIDS?

Yes. **Human immunodeficiency virus (HIV)** is the infectious agent that causes **acquired immune deficiency syndrome (AIDS).** HIV is a

human immunodeficiency virus (HIV) The virus that causes HIV infection and AIDS; infects and destroys cells of the immune system.

acquired immune deficiency syndrome (AIDS) A disease of the immune system characterized by a severe reduction in the number of CD4+ cells, leaving an individual susceptible to other infections and diseases; the final stage of HIV infection.

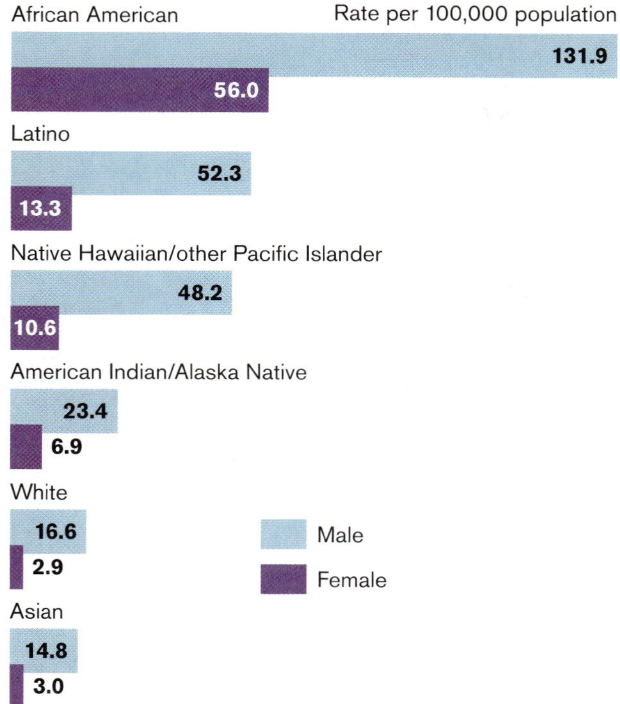

Figure 13-6 Estimated rates of diagnosis of HIV infection among U.S. adults and adolescents, by sex and race/ethnicity

Source: Centers for Disease Control and Prevention. (2010). Diagnoses of HIV infection and AIDS in the United States and dependent areas. *HIV Surveillance Report, 2008, 20* (http://www.cdc.gov/hiv/topics/surveillance/resources/reports).

pathogen, and AIDS is the late stage of HIV infection—a chronic infection that slowly destroys the body's immune system. People with HIV may look and feel healthy, experiencing no symptoms, for years after the initial infection. However, the virus is active in their body, infecting and destroying immune system cells as it reproduces. The specific type of blood cell that HIV destroys is called a CD4+ T cell, which is critical for the body to fight infection. Over time, HIV levels increase and CD4+ T cell levels decrease, leaving people less able to fight off other diseases and infections. Measurement of CD4+ T cell counts indicate the progress of the infection and aid in treatment decisions.

If damage to the immune system is severe, a person develops AIDS. This final stage of HIV infection is diagnosed when he or she develops an opportunistic infection—an infection a person without HIV infection would be unlikely to contract—or has a dangerously low number of CD4+ T cells. Prior to the development of treatments, people progressed from HIV infection to AIDS within a few years. With the new medications, people may live years or even decades with HIV infection without developing AIDS.

Q Where in the world is HIV/AIDS the biggest problem? 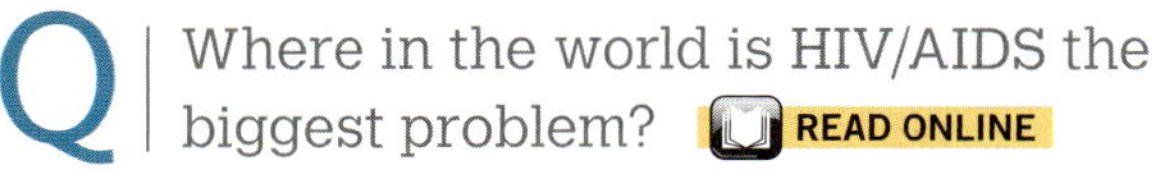

Q Do condoms really help prevent HIV infection?

TRANSMISSION AND SYMPTOMS. Yes. Use of condoms does not completely eliminate risk, but it greatly reduces the transmission of HIV.[24] Most problems with condom effectiveness relate to improper or inconsistent use. HIV is found in blood, semen, and vaginal secretions and can be transmitted by sharing of these body fluids. According to the Centers for Disease Control and Prevention, HIV is spread primarily in the following ways:[25]

- Not using a condom when having sex with a person who has HIV. All unprotected sex with someone who has HIV contains some risk. However, unprotected anal sex is riskier than unprotected vaginal sex. Unprotected oral sex can also be a risk for HIV transmission, but it is a much lower risk than anal or vaginal sex.
- Having multiple sex partners or the presence of other sexually transmitted infections (STIs) can increase the risk of infection during sex. As described earlier in the chapter, any breaks in the skin or mucous membranes can allow a virus to pass more easily into the body.
- Sharing needles, syringes, other equipment, or rinse water used to prepare illicit drugs for injection.
- Being born to an infected mother—HIV can be passed from mother to child during pregnancy, birth, and breast-feeding.

Among American adolescents and adults, the three most common modes of transmission are male-to-male sexual contact, heterosexual contact, and injection drug use (Figure 13-7). Less commonly, HIV may be transmitted

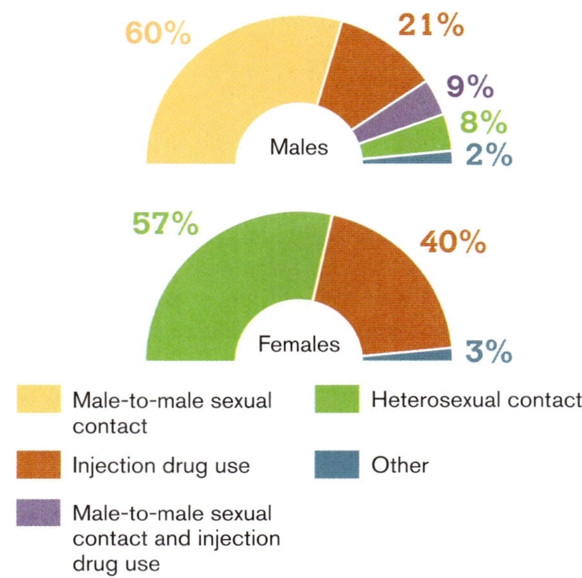

Figure 13-7 Transmission routes among U.S. adults and adolescents diagnosed with AIDS

Source: Centers for Disease Control and Prevention. (2010). Diagnoses of HIV infection and AIDS in the United States and dependent areas. *HIV Surveillance Report, 2008, 20* (http://www.cdc.gov/hiv/topics/surveillance/resources/reports).

Wellness Strategies

Using Condoms the Right Way for STI Prevention

Why Condoms Fail: The failure of condoms to protect against STI transmission usually results from inconsistent or incorrect use, rather than product failure.

- Inconsistent or nonuse can lead to STI acquisition because transmission can occur with a single sex act with an infected partner.
- Incorrect use diminishes the protective effect of condoms by leading to condom breakage, slippage, or leakage. Incorrect use more commonly entails a failure to use condoms *throughout* each entire sex act, from start (of sexual contact) to finish (after ejaculation).

How to Use a Condom Consistently and Correctly:

- Use a new condom for every act of vaginal, anal, and oral sex throughout the *entire* sex act (from start to finish).
- Before any genital contact, put the condom on the tip of the erect penis with the rolled side out.
- If the condom does not have a reservoir tip, pinch the tip enough to leave a half-inch space for semen to collect. Holding the tip, unroll the condom all the way to the base of the erect penis.
- After ejaculation and before the penis gets soft, grip the rim of the condom and carefully withdraw. Then gently pull the condom off the penis, making sure that semen doesn't spill out.
- Wrap the condom in a tissue and throw it in the trash where others won't handle it.
- If you feel the condom break at any point during sexual activity, stop immediately, withdraw, remove the broken condom, and put on a new condom.
- Ensure that adequate lubrication is used during vaginal and anal sex, which might require water-based lubricants. Oil-based lubricants (such as petroleum jelly, shortening, mineral oil, massage oils, body lotions, and cooking oil) should not be used because they can weaken latex, causing breakage.
- Do not use condoms lubricated with the spermicide nonoxynol-9; it can cause irritation and increase the risk of getting an STI from an infected partner.

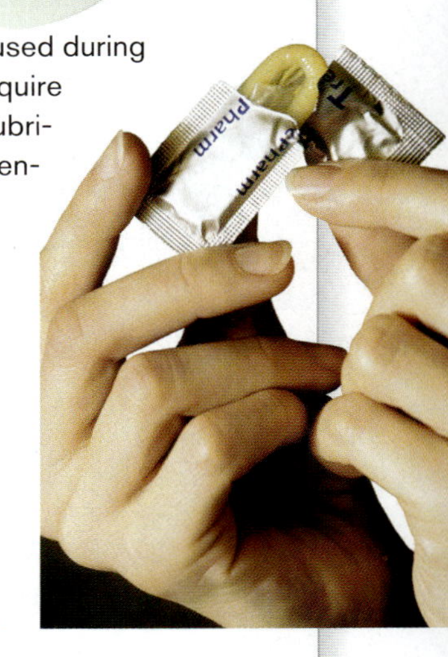

For more instructions on using condoms, as well as advice on talking to a partner about condoms and safer sex, visit the Web site for the American Social Health Association (http://www.ashastd.org/condom/condom_overview.cfm). For information on the use of condoms for pregnancy prevention—including combining condoms with other contraceptive methods and using over-the-counter emergency contraception in case of condom breakage—visit the Web sites for the American College of Obstetricians and Gynecologists' publications (http://www.acog.org/publications/patient-education) and Planned Parenthood (http://www.plannedparenthood.org).

Source: Centers for Disease Control and Prevention. (2010). *Male latex condoms and sexually transmitted diseases* (http://www.cdc.gov/condomeffectiveness/brief.html).

to health care workers through needle sticks. Before HIV blood tests, people could also be infected from a blood transfusion or organ transplant; however, the risk is now extremely small due to rigorous screening. HIV cannot survive outside the human body and is not transmitted through air, water, or insect bites; there are no documented cases of transmission through saliva, tears, sweat, or closed-mouth kissing.

To prevent the transmission of HIV infection, take steps to avoid or limit your risk behaviors. Refer to the box on p. 386 on preventing STIs for specific guidelines. Abstain from sex or practice safer sex consistently. Many people know what safer sex behaviors are but don't consistently practice them. Think about your own behavior, and if you act in risky ways, ask yourself why. In addition, if you inject drugs, get counseling and treatment; using clean needles and syringes reduces the risk of transmission, but it's much better to stop drug use and avoid all the associated risks. If you have a risky sexual encounter and believe you were exposed to HIV, see your health care provider immediately. In some cases, HIV medications can prevent infection if they are started shortly after exposure to the virus.

Q | Do any methods of birth control besides condoms help with STIs?

READ ONLINE

Q | What are symptoms of HIV and AIDS?

Most people infected with HIV are asymptomatic, although some develop nonspecific symptoms during the acute phase of the initial infection: fever, headache, fatigue, muscle aches, and enlarged lymph nodes. These symptoms typically resolve with no treatment and may be attributed to influenza or an-

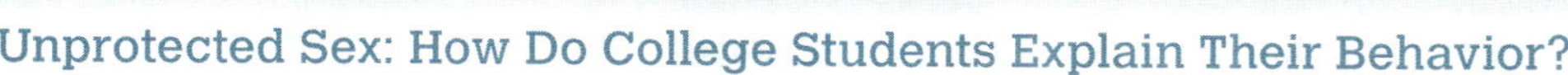

Research Brief

Unprotected Sex: How Do College Students Explain Their Behavior?

By the time young adults get to college, most have received vast amounts of information about the consequences of unprotected sex in terms of both pregnancy and STIs. Despite a lot of knowledge about the risks, many young adults still fail to consistently practice safer sex. How do they explain this inconsistency? In a recent study, researchers asked a group of young adults to keep diaries for several weeks to track their condom use and non-use during intercourse. Once the diaries were complete, the students were interviewed to explore their decision making.

Less than 25 percent of the students used condoms or oral contraceptives consistently. Most who did use condoms saw them as a means of preventing pregnancy rather than preventing disease. Their explanations for their risky behaviors fell into several categories:

- *Biased evaluation of risk:* Students equated the degree of closeness and intimacy they felt for their partner with reduced risk for STIs.
- *Biased evaluation of evidence:* Students believed that since their pattern of behavior (unsafe sex) had not in the past resulted in pregnancy or an STI, it must not be very risky.
- *Endorsement of poor alternatives:* Some students justified their choice to not use condoms with the use of an alternative prevention strategy—even though they recognized the alternative as a poor one (withdrawal, counting on luck).
- *False justifications:* Despite stating a strong desire to avoid STIs and pregnancy, students weighted short-term benefits of not using a condom as more important than the long-term negative consequences.
- *Dismissing or ignoring risk:* Some students felt invulnerable to the negative outcomes that other people might experience ("it won't happen to me"), and others felt that the negative outcomes could be easily solved (abortion, drug treatment).

Do any of these explanations or rationalizations sound familiar to you? What would you say to yourself or a peer to dispute these false beliefs? If you engage in unprotected sex, examine your own attitudes carefully. Challenge yourself—and others—to acknowledge the personal risks you face, and commit yourself to taking steps to reduce those risks.

Source: O'Sullivan, L. F., Udell, W., Montrose, V. A., Antoniello, P., & Hoffman, S. (2010). A cognitive analysis of college students' explanations for engaging in unprotected sexual intercourse. *Archives of Sexual Behavior,* 39, 1121–1131.

other minor illness. During this early acute phase, people are extremely infectious.

After the acute phase is over, any symptoms that occurred resolve. Although the virus remains in the body, replicating and destroying CD4+ T cells, infected people exhibit no symptoms and likely are completely unaware of the infection. However, they are capable of infecting others.

During the late stages of HIV infection, when the immune system has been severely weakened, people may experience a variety of symptoms. These include rapid weight loss, extreme fatigue, prolonged swelling of lymph nodes, sores in the mouth or genitals, and neurological disorders. The opportunistic infections that can occur in people with full-blown AIDS include pneumonia, cancer, liver disease, and many types of otherwise unusual viral, fungal, protozoan, and bacterial infections.

Q | Do you have to wait six months to find out if you have HIV?

TESTING AND TREATMENT. In most cases, no, although standard blood tests for HIV aren't accurate immediately following infection. These tests detect HIV antibodies, and it takes time for the immune system to produce enough antibodies to be detected by the test. In most cases, the body produces sufficient antibodies for detection within two to eight weeks following infection (the average is 25 days); 97 percent of infections can be detected within three months.[26] That means there is a small chance that it will take longer than three months—and in very rare cases up to six months—to get an accurate test result.

When you get a conventional test, it may take one or two weeks to get your results from the lab. However, some sites also offer rapid HIV testing, which provides results in twenty to thirty minutes. A positive HIV antibody test must be verified by a second test. More expensive tests that directly test for the presence of the virus in the body are available but are not typically used for screening purposes.

Current federal guidelines recommend HIV testing for every American ages 13 to 64 as part of routine medical care.[27] For anyone at high risk, yearly testing is recommended. Despite these guidelines, it's estimated that as many as one in five Americans with HIV are unaware of their status. If diagnosed early, an infected individual can get appropriate treatment and limit the spread of the virus to others. Routine testing is especially important for pregnant women. Babies born to untreated women with HIV infection have about a 25 percent chance of catching HIV; with treatment, the risk drops to about 2 percent.

Q | How long until someone with HIV dies?

With treatment, people can survive many years or even decades with HIV infection. The success of treatment depends on many factors, including an individual's underlying health status and how early in the course of infection treatment begins. Over thirty antiviral drugs are available to treat HIV infection. These medications do not cure the infection or eliminate the virus from the body, but they do suppress the virus, sometimes to undetectable levels. A person being treated for HIV must take antiviral drugs continuously; he or she can still transmit the virus, but the risk is much lower. The medications can have side effects, sometimes serious, and HIV can also become resistant to particular medications.

Researchers have worked for many years to design a vaccine, but HIV poses significant challenges. It directly attacks the immune system—the very cells that need to be activated by a vaccine. In addition, HIV frequently mutates to produce new strains. Although a vaccine remains elusive, there has been some success in developing microbicides that can be applied to the vagina prior to intercourse to help reduce the risk of transmission.[28] Microbicides may be particularly beneficial for women around the world who aren't able to negotiate mutual monogamy or condom use with their partners.

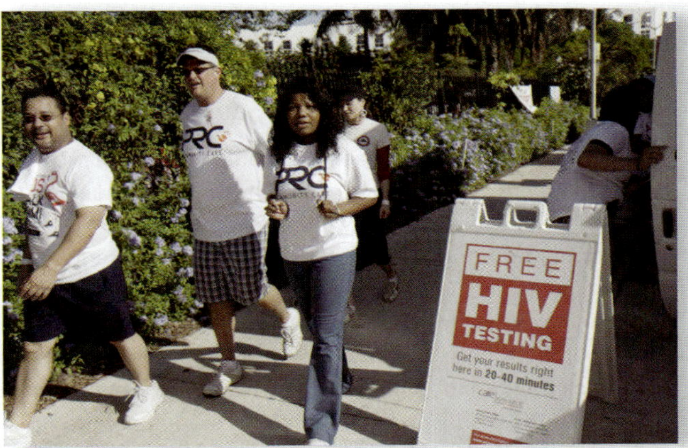

The CDC recommends HIV testing at least once for all Americans ages 13 to 64 as part of routine medical care. For anyone at high risk, annual testing is appropriate.

With no vaccine or cure on the horizon, it's important for everyone to take HIV prevention seriously.

Summary

Infectious agents are all around us and impossible to avoid. Fortunately, the body has many physical and chemical barriers to keep pathogens out and a complex immune system to tackle those microbes that do gain entry. Many infections are relatively mild and cause few problems in healthy individuals. For those that are more serious, many can be cured with medications and self-care. You can help limit the impact of infectious disease by engaging in wellness behaviors that support your immune system and by taking steps to avoid the transmission of pathogens. It's also important to keep your vaccinations up to date.

Although colds, influenza, and similar infections can be challenging to avoid, infections that are sexually transmitted have clear prevention strategies. Not having sex prevents all STIs, and if you are sexually active, you can greatly reduce your risk by using condoms and maintaining a mutually monogamous relationship with your partner. If diagnosed early, the bacterial STIs can be treated before any serious complications occur. The viral STIs are incurable, but there are vaccines for both HPV and hepatitis. HIV/AIDS is the most serious STI, and although treatments have improved, it remains an incurable and life-threatening infection.

More to Explore

American Social Health Association
http://www.ashastd.org

Centers for Disease Control and Prevention
http://www.cdc.gov

Joint United Nations Programme on HIV/AIDS
http://www.unaids.org

MedlinePlus: Infectious Diseases
http://www.nlm.nih.gov/medlineplus/infections.html

National Institute of Allergy and Infectious Diseases
http://www.niaid.nih.gov

LAB ACTIVITY 13-1 Infectious Disease Risk Checklist

SUBMIT ONLINE

NAME   DATE   SECTION

Equipment: None

Preparation: None

Instructions

Indicate whether each statement is true for you always, sometimes, or never; and fill in the additional information. Any statement for which you don't check "always" indicates an area where you could change your behavior to help reduce your risk for infectious diseases.

Avoiding Pathogens

Always	Sometimes	Never	
____	____	____	I frequently wash my hands with soap and water for at least 20 seconds.
____	____	____	I don't rub my eyes, touch my nose, or eat with my fingers without first washing my hands.
____	____	____	When soap and water aren't available, I use alcohol-based hand sanitizer.

If these statements aren't always true for you, describe your typical hand hygiene practices:

Always	Sometimes	Never	
____	____	____	I avoid close contact with people who have colds, flu, or other infectious diseases transmitted via touch or respiratory droplets.
____	____	____	I avoid disease carriers such as mosquitoes, ticks, and rodents. To avoid insect disease vectors, I use insect repellant and/or wear long sleeves and pants when necessary.
____	____	____	I never inject drugs (except if medically prescribed).
____	____	____	I follow food safety recommendations, including keeping foods at safe temperatures, not thawing foods on the counter, thoroughly cleaning all equipment, and using a food thermometer to check that foods are cooked to a safe temperature.
____	____	____	I have a kit prepared in case of emergencies that disrupt sanitation and other public health services.

Supporting Your Immune System

Always	Sometimes	Never	
____	____	____	I exercise regularly.
____	____	____	I eat a healthy diet.
____	____	____	I get plenty of sleep.
____	____	____	I manage my stress.
____	____	____	I don't smoke, and I avoid secondhand smoke.
____	____	____	I consume alcohol moderately, if at all.
____	____	____	My immunizations are up to date, including recommended booster shots.

LAB ACTIVITY 13-1

Check your immunization status against the recommendations in Figure 13-2 and note any vaccines recommended for you that you haven't had.

Assessing Your Risk for Sexually Transmitted Infections

Complete one of the following online assessments for STI risk. Then briefly comment on the experience.

The Body: http://www.thebody.com/surveys/sexsurvey.html

STD Wizard: http://www.stdwizard.org

Were you surprised by any of the questions or the results? Did you identify any risk areas that you had been unaware of?

Assessing Your Recent Experiences with Infectious Diseases

To help further identify infectious disease risks in your life, list and describe your three most recent infections. Note the symptoms and duration of your illness, and speculate on how you think you acquired the infection. For each, note one strategy you think might have reduced your risk for contracting the infection or lessened its effects on you.

Reflecting on Your Results

Are you doing all you can to prevent infectious diseases? Note at least three areas in which you could improve your behavior to reduce your risk. Then comment on what you think is holding you back. For example, if you know you should wash your hands more often, why don't you?

Planning Your Next Steps

Choose one behavior that you could change to help reduce your risk for infectious diseases, and develop at least three concrete strategies for making the change. For example, would putting hand washing reminders in your bathroom or hand sanitizer in your backpack help improve your hand hygiene?

APPENDIXES

NUTRITIONAL CONTENT OF COMMON FOODS

If you are developing a behavior change plan to improve your diet, or if you simply want to choose healthier foods, you may want to know more about the nutritional content of common food items. An appendix with this information is available on the *Fit and Well* Online Learning Center at **www.mhhe.com/fahey.**

You can track your daily food intake, calculate your nutrient intake from foods, and compare your intake with the U.S. Department of Agriculture's recommendations for your age, sex, height, and weight at the MyPlate Web site (**www.choosemyplate.gov**).

You can also look up the nutrient content of the foods you eat in the USDA Agricultural Research Service National Nutrient Database, which lists foods both by description and by nutrient content (**www.ars.usda.gov/Services/docs.htm?docid=17477**). For example, under "protein," you can find out how much protein there is in a chicken pot pie or what foods have the most protein per serving. Although cumbersome, the database is comprehensive.

Nutritional Content of Popular Items from Fast-Food Restaurants

Although most foods served at fast-food restaurants are high in calories, fat, saturated fat, cholesterol, sodium, and sugar, some items are healthier than others. If you eat at fast-food restaurants, knowing the nutritional content of various items can help you make better choices. Fast-food restaurants provide nutritional information both online and in print brochures available at most restaurant locations. To learn more about the items you order, visit the restaurants' Web sites:

Arby's:	**www.arbysrestaurant.com**
Burger King:	**http://www.bk.com/en/us/index.html**
Domino's Pizza:	**www.dominos.com**
Hardees:	**www.hardees.com**
KFC:	**www.kfc.com**
McDonald's:	**www.mcdonalds.com**
Papa John's Pizza:	**http://www.papajohns.com/index.html**
Pizza Hut:	**http://www.pizzahut.com**
Subway:	**http://www.subway.com/subwayroot/default.aspx**
Taco Bell:	**www.tacobell.com**
Wendy's:	**www.wendys.com**
White Castle:	**www.whitecastle.com**

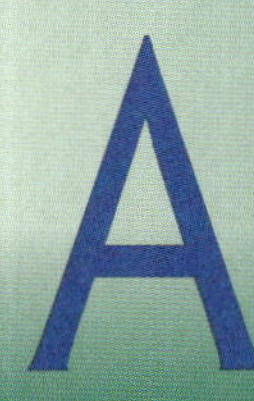

APPENDIX A

INJURY PREVENTION AND PERSONAL SAFETY

Unintentional injuries are the fifth leading cause of death among Americans overall and the leading killer of people under age 35. Injuries affect all segments of the population, but they are particularly common among minorities and people with low incomes, primarily due to social, environmental, and economic factors. The economic cost of injuries in the United States is high, with more than $650 billion spent each year for medical care and rehabilitation of injured people.

Injuries are generally classified into four categories, based on where they occur: motor vehicle injuries, home injuries, leisure injuries, and work injuries.

MOTOR VEHICLE INJURIES

According to the CDC, more than 36,000 Americans were killed and 2.3 million injured in motor vehicle crashes in 2009. Motor vehicle accidents are a leading cause of paralysis due to spinal injury and the leading cause of severe brain injury.

Factors in Motor Vehicle Injuries

Driving Habits Nearly 63% of motor vehicle injuries are caused by bad driving, especially speeding. As speed increases, momentum and force of impact increase and the time available for the driver to react decreases. Speed limits are posted to establish the safest ***maximum*** speed limit for a given area under ***ideal*** conditions. Aggressive driving—characterized by speeding, frequent and abrupt lane changes, tailgating, and passing on the shoulder—also increases the risk of crashes.

Distratcted driving contributes to 8000 crashes every day in the United States. Anything that distracts a driver—sleepiness, bad mood, children or pets in the car, use of a cell phone—can increase the risk of a crash. Sleepiness reduces reaction time, coordination, and speed of information processing and can be as dangerous as drug and alcohol use. Even mild sleep deprivation causes a deterioration in driving ability comparable to that caused by a 0.05% blood alcohol concentration.

Cell phone users respond to hazards about 20% slower than undistracted drivers and are about twice as likely to rear-end a braking car in front of them. According to 2011 statistics from the AAA Foundation for Traffic Safety, drivers who use cell phones are nearly four times as likely to be involved in a crash as drivers who don't. Hands-free devices do not help significantly; the mental distraction of talking is the factor in crashes rather than holding a phone. Newer research shows that text-messaging (texting) on a cell phone while driving is even more dangerous than talking. Several cities and states have outlawed the use of cell phones while driving; similar laws are being considered in many parts of the United States.

Safety Belts and Air Bags A person who doesn't wear a safety belt is twice as likely to be injured in a crash as a person who does wear one. Safety belts not only prevent occupants from being thrown from the car at the time of the crash but also provide protection from the "second collision," which occurs when the occupant of the car hits something inside the car, such as the steering column or windshield. The safety belt also spreads the stopping force of a collision over the body.

Since 1998, all new cars have been equipped with dual air bags—one for the driver and one for the front passenger seat. Air bags provide supplemental protection in a collision but are most useful in head-on collisions. (Many newer vehicles feature side air bags to offer protection in a side-impact crash.) They also deflate immediately after inflating and so do not provide protection in collisions involving multiple impacts. To ensure that air bags work as intended, follow these guidelines:

- Place infants in rear-facing infant seats in the back seat.
- Transport children age 12 and under in the back seat.
- Always use safety belts or appropriate safety seats.
- Keep at least 10 inches between the air bag cover and the breastbone of the driver or passenger.

If you cannot comply with these guidelines, you can apply to the National Highway Traffic Safety Administration for permission to install an on-off switch that temporarily disables the air bag.

Alcohol and Other Drugs Alcohol is involved in about 40% of all fatal crashes. Alcohol-impaired driving, defined by blood alcohol concentration (BAC), is illegal. The legal BAC limit is 0.08% in all states, but driving ability is impaired at much lower BACs. All psychoactive drugs have the potential to impair driving ability.

Preventing Motor Vehicle Injuries

About 75% of all motor vehicle collisions occur within 25 miles of home and at speeds lower than 40 mph. These crashes often occur because the driver believes safety measures are not necessary for short trips. Clearly, the statistics prove otherwise.

To prevent motor vehicle injuries:

- Obey the speed limit. If you have to speed to get to your destination on time, you're not allowing enough time.
- Always wear a safety belt and ask passengers to do the same. Strap infants and toddlers into government-approved

car seats in the back seat. Children who have outgrown child safety seats but who are still too small for adult safety belts alone (usually age 4–8) should be secured using booster seats. All children under 12 should ride in the back seat.
- Never drive under the influence of alcohol or other drugs or with a driver who is.
- Do not drive when you are sleepy or have been awake for 18 or more hours.
- Avoid using your cell phone while driving—your primary obligation is to pay attention to the road. If you do make calls, follow laws set by your city or state. Place calls when you are at a stop, and keep them short. Pull over if the conversation is stressful or emotional.
- Never text while driving.
- Keep your car in good working order. Regularly inspect tires, oil and fluid levels, windshield wipers, spare tire, and so on.
- Always allow enough following distance. Follow the "3-second rule": When the vehicle ahead passes a reference point, count out 3 seconds. If you pass the reference point before you finish counting, drop back and allow more following distance.
- Always increase following distance and slow down if weather or road conditions are poor.
- Choose major highways rather than rural roads. Highways are much safer because of better visibility, wider lanes, fewer surprises, and other factors.
- Always signal before turning or changing lanes.
- Stop completely at stop signs. Follow all traffic laws.
- Take special care at intersections. Always look left, right, and then left again. Make sure you have plenty of time to complete your maneuver in the intersection.
- Don't pass on two-lane roads unless you are in a designated passing area and have a clear view ahead.

Motorcycles and Scooters

About 1 out of every 10 traffic fatalities among people age 15–34 involves someone riding a motorcycle. Injuries from motorcycle collisions are generally more severe than those involving automobiles because motorcycles provide little, if any, protection. Scooter riders face additional challenges. Motorized scooters usually have a maximum speed of 30–35 mph and have less power for maneuverability.

To prevent motorcycle and scooter injuries:

- Make yourself easier to see by wearing light-colored clothing, driving with your headlights on, and correctly positioning yourself in traffic.
- Develop the necessary skills. Lack of skill, especially when evasive action is needed to avoid a collision, is a major factor in motorcycle and moped injuries. Skidding from improper braking is the most common cause of loss of control.
- Wear a close-fitting helmet, one marked with the symbol DOT (for Department of Transportation).
- Protect your eyes with goggles, a face shield, or a windshield.
- Drive defensively and never assume that other drivers see you.

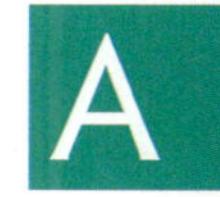

Pedestrians and Bicycles

Injuries to pedestrians and bicyclists are considered motor vehicle–related because they usually involve motor vehicles. About 1 in 8 motor vehicle deaths each year involves a pedestrian; more than 70,000 pedestrians are injured each year.

To prevent injuries when walking or jogging:

- Walk or jog in daylight.
- Make yourself easier to see by wearing light-colored, reflective clothing.
- Face traffic when walking or jogging along a roadway, and follow traffic laws.
- Avoid busy roads or roads with poor visibility.
- Cross only at marked crosswalks and intersections.
- Don't use headphones while walking or jogging.
- Don't hitchhike. Hitchhiking places you in a potentially dangerous situation.

Bicycle injuries result primarily from not knowing or understanding the rules of the road, failing to follow traffic laws, and not having sufficient skill or experience to handle traffic conditions. Bicycles are considered vehicles; bicycle riders must obey all traffic laws that apply to automobile drivers, including stopping at traffic lights and stop signs.

To prevent injuries when riding a bike:

- Wear safety equipment, including a helmet, eye protection, gloves, and proper footwear. Secure the bottom of your pant legs with clips and secure your shoelaces so they don't get tangled in the chain.
- Make yourself easier to see by wearing light-colored, reflective clothing. Equip your bike with reflectors and use lights, especially at night or when riding in wooded or other dark areas.
- Ride with the flow of traffic, not against it, and follow traffic laws. Use bike paths when they are available.
- Ride defensively; never assume that drivers can see you. Be especially careful when turning or crossing at corners and intersections. Watch for cars turning right.
- Stop at all traffic lights and stop signs. Know and use hand signals.
- Continue pedaling at all times when moving (don't coast) to help keep the bike stable and to maintain your balance.
- Properly maintain your bike.

Aggressive Driving

Aggressive driving, known as *road rage,* has increased more than 50% since 1990. Aggressive drivers increase the risk of crashes for themselves and others. They further increase the risk of injuries if they stop their vehicles and confront each other. Even if you are successful at controlling your own aggressive driving impulses, you may still encounter an aggressive driver.

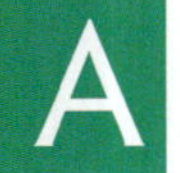

To avoid being the victim of an aggressive driver:

- Always keep distance between your car and others. If you are behind a very slow driver and can't pass, slow down to increase distance in case that driver does something unexpected. If you are being tailgated, do not increase your speed; instead, let the other driver pass you. If you are in the left lane when being tailgated, signal and pull over to let the other driver go by, even if you are traveling at the speed limit. When you are merging, make sure you have plenty of room. If you are cut off by a merging driver, slow down to make room.
- Be courteous, even if the other driver is not. Use your horn rarely, if ever. Avoid making gestures of irritation, even shaking your head. When parking, let the other driver have the space that both of you found.
- Refuse to join in a fight. Avoid eye contact with an angry driver. If someone makes a rude gesture, ignore it. If you think another car is following you and you have a cell phone, call the police. Otherwise, drive to a public place and honk your horn to get someone's attention.
- If you make a mistake while driving, apologize. Raise or wave your hand or touch or knock your head with the palm of your hand to indicate "What was I thinking?" You can also mouth the words "I'm sorry."

HOME INJURIES

Contrary to popular belief, home is one of the most dangerous places to be. The most common fatal home injuries are caused by falls, poisoning, fires, suffocation and choking, and incidents involving firearms.

Falls

About 90% of fatal falls involve people age 45 and older, but falls are a significant cause of unintentional death for people under age 25. Most deaths occurring from falls involve falling on stairs or steps or from one level to another. Falls also occur on the same level, from tripping, slipping, or stumbling. Alcohol is a contributing factor in many falls.

To prevent injuries from falls:

- Install handrails and nonslip surfaces in the shower and bathtub. Place skidproof backing on rugs and carpets.
- Keep floors, stairs, and outside areas clear of objects or conditions that could cause slipping or tripping, such as heavy wax coating, electrical cords, and toys.
- Put a light switch by the door of every room so no one has to walk across a room to turn on a light. Use night lights in bedrooms, halls, stairways, and bathrooms.
- Outside the house, clear dangerous surfaces created by ice, snow, fallen leaves, or rough ground.
- Install handrails on stairs. Keep stairs well lit and clear of objects.
- When climbing a ladder, use both hands. Never stand higher than the third step from the top. When using a stepladder, make sure the spreader brace is in the locked position. With straight ladders, set the base out 1 foot for every 4 feet of height. Don't stand on chairs to reach things.
- If there are small children in the home, place gates at the top and bottom of stairs. Never leave a baby unattended.

Poisoning

More than 2.4 million poisonings and over 30,000 poison-related deaths occur every year in the United States.

To prevent poisoning:

- Store all medicines out of the reach of children. Use medicines only as directed on the label or by a physician.
- Use cleaners, pesticides, and other dangerous substances only in areas with proper ventilation. Store them out of the reach of children.
- Never operate a vehicle in an enclosed space. Have your furnace inspected yearly. Use caution with any substance that produces potentially toxic fumes, such as kerosene. If appropriate, install carbon monoxide detectors.
- Keep poisonous plants out of the reach of children. These include azalea, oleander, rhododendron, wild mushrooms, daffodil and hyacinth bulbs, mistletoe berries, apple seeds, morning glory seeds, wisteria seeds, and the leaves and stems of potato, rhubarb, and tomato plants.

To be prepared in case of poisoning:

- Keep the number of the nearest Poison Control Center (or emergency room) in an accessible location. A call to the national poison control hotline (800-222-1222) will be routed to a local center.

Emergency first aid for poisonings:

1. Remove the poison from contact with eyes, skin, or mouth, or remove the victim from contact with poisonous fumes or gases.
2. Call the Poison Control Center immediately for instructions. Have the container with you.
3. Do not follow emergency instructions on labels. Some may be out-of-date and carry incorrect treatment information.
4. If you are instructed to go to an emergency room, take the poisonous substance or its container with you.

Guidelines for specific types of poisons:

- *Swallowed poisons.* Call the Poison Control Center or a physician for advice. Do not induce vomiting.
- *Poisons on the skin.* Remove any affected clothing. Flood affected parts of the skin with warm water, wash with soap and water, and rinse. Then call for advice.
- *Poisons in the eye.* For children, flood the eye with lukewarm water poured from a pitcher held 3–4 inches above the eye for 15 minutes; alternatively, irrigate the eye under a faucet. For adults, get in the shower and flood the eye with a gentle stream of lukewarm water for 15 minutes. Then call for advice.
- *Inhaled poisons.* Immediately carry or drag the person to fresh air and, if necessary, give rescue breaths (Figure A.1). If the victim is not breathing easily, call 9-1-1 for help. Ventilate the area. Then call the Poison Control Center for advice.

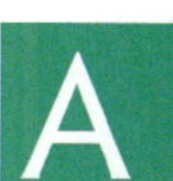

EMERGENCY CARE FOR CHOKING

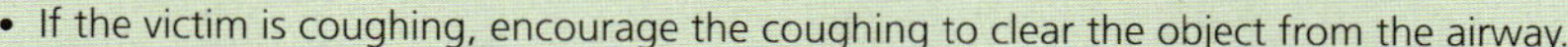

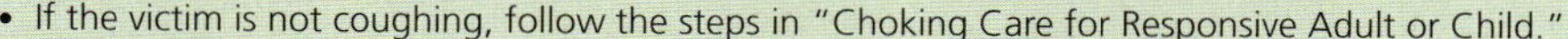

Choking Care for Responsive Adult or Child

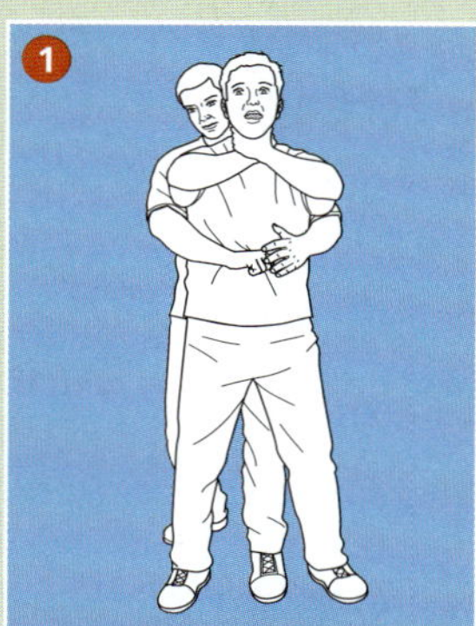

Stand behind an adult victim with one leg forward between the victim's legs. (With a child, kneel behind the victim.) Keep your head slightly to one side. Reach around the abdomen with both arms. Make a fist with one hand and place the thumb side of the fist against the abdomen just above the navel.

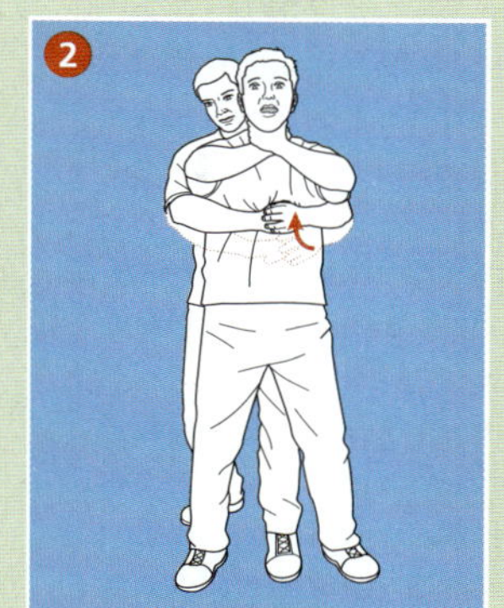

Grasp your fist with your other hand and thrust inward and upward into the victim's abdomen with quick jerks. Continue abdominal thrusts until the victim expels the object or becomes unresponsive. If the victim becomes unresponsive while you are administering abdominal thrusts, lower the victim to the floor onto his or her back, and follow the steps in "Choking Care for Unresponsive Adult or Child."

Choking Care for Unresponsive Adult or Child: CPR

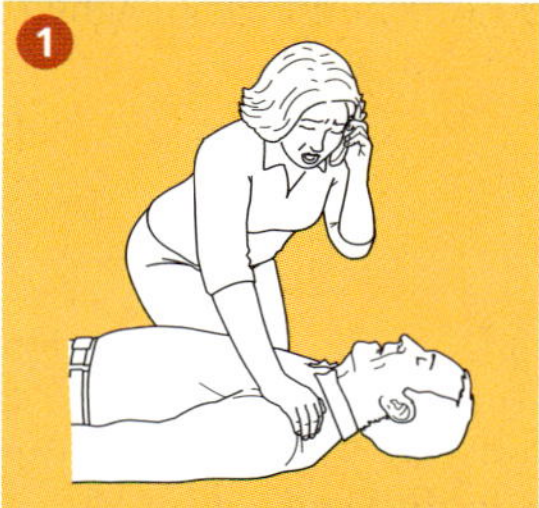

Call 911 and begin CPR.

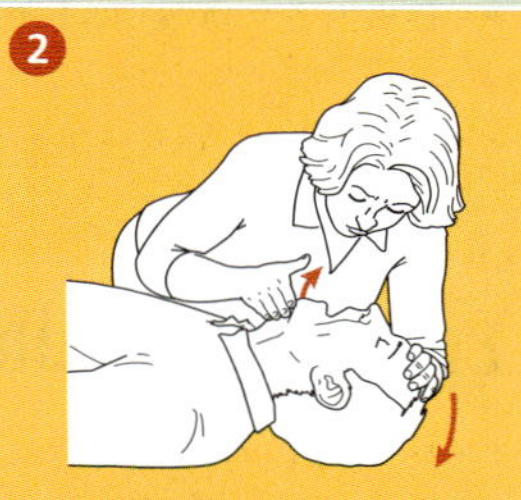

Open the airway to see if the victim is breathing. Use the "head tilt–chin lift" maneuver to open the airway: Push down on the forehead and lift the chin.

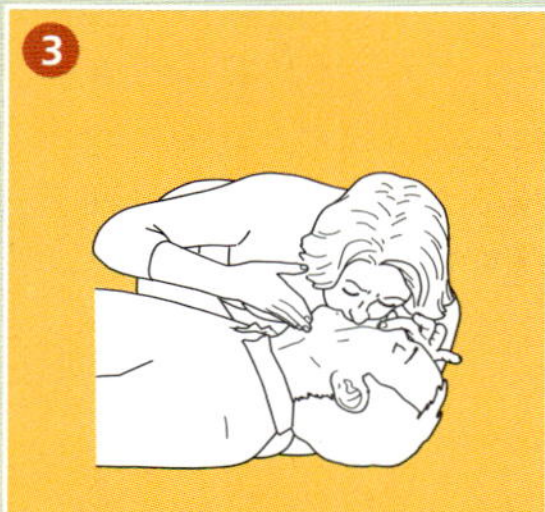

If the victim is not breathing, give two rescue breaths, each lasting 1 second. Pinch the victim's nose shut and blow a normal breath into the victim's mouth. If the first breath does not go in (the chest does not rise), reposition the head to open the airway and try again. Each time you give a rescue breath, look for an object in the victim's mouth and remove it if present.

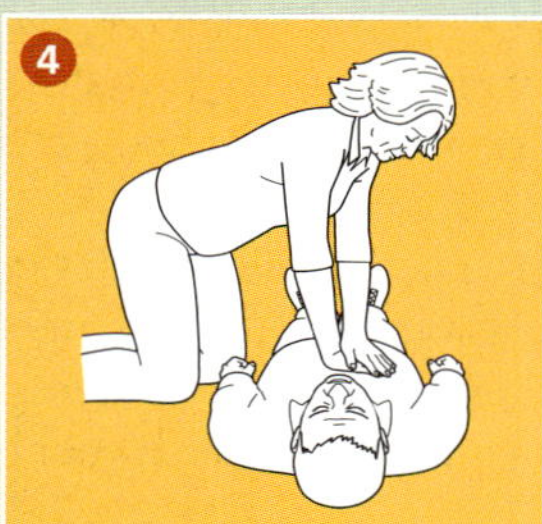

If the obstruction remains, begin chest compressions. Place the heel of one hand in the center of the chest between the nipples and the other hand on top of the first. Position your shoulders over your hands and lock your elbows. Give 30 chest compressions at a rate of 100 per minute. The chest should go down by 1 ½ to 2 inches. Then give two breaths, looking in the mouth for an expelled object. Continue chest compressions until help arrives. **Remember: Push hard and push fast at a rate of 100 compressions per minute.**

EMERGENCY CARE FOR CARDIAC ARREST

For cardiac arrest, the American Heart Association's revised (2005) Emergency Cardiac Care guidelines are as follows:

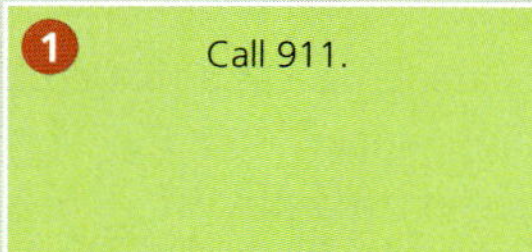

2 Start CPR (100 compressions per minute, stopping every 30 to 60 seconds to give two rescue breaths).

3 If an automated external defibrillator (AED) is available, or when one arrives, give one shock to restart the victim's heart.

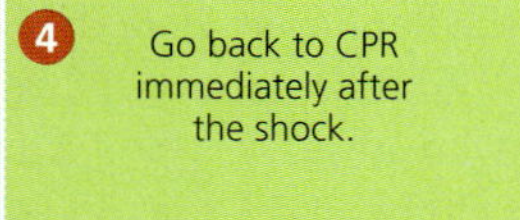

Hands-Only CPR

In 2008, the American Heart Association reported that hands-only (compression-only) CPR can be as effective as conventional CPR. There are only two steps:

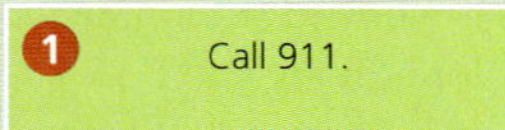

2 Push hard and fast in the center of the chest.

Don't wait for an emergency to learn how to use an AED or perform CPR.
To find a course in your area, contact the American Heart Association (800 242-8721) or the American Red Cross (202 303-4498).

FIGURE A. 1 Emergency care for choking and for cardiac arrest.

SOURCES: Adapted from American Heart Association. 2008. Hands-only (compression-only) cardiopulmonary resuscitation: A call to action for bystander response to adults who experience out-of-hospital sudden cardiac arrest. *Circulation* 117: 2162–2167; National Safety Council. 2007. *First Aid: Taking Action.* New York: McGraw-Hill; American Heart Association. 2005. Adult basic life support. *Circulation* 112: 19–34; New CPR guidelines: Simplicity to the rescue. 2006. *Harvard Health Letter,* March, Streamlined CPR guidelines a life-saving move. 2006. *Harvard Heart Letter,* February.

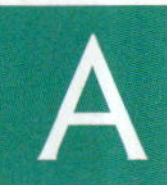

Fires

Each year, about 80% of fire deaths and 65% of fire injuries occur in the home. Careless smoking is the leading cause of home fire deaths. Cooking is the leading cause of home fire injuries.

To prevent fires:

- Dispose of all cigarettes in ashtrays. Never smoke in bed.
- Do not overload electrical outlets. Do not place extension cords under rugs or where people walk. Replace worn or frayed extension cords.
- Place a wire screen in front of fireplaces and woodstoves. Remove ashes carefully and store them in airtight metal containers, not paper bags.
- Properly maintain electrical appliances, kerosene heaters, and furnaces. Clean flues and chimneys annually.
- Keep portable heaters at least 3 feet away from curtains, bedding, towels, or anything that might catch fire. Never leave operating heaters unattended.

To be prepared for a fire:

- Plan at least two escape routes out of each room. Designate a location outside the home as a meeting place. Stage a home fire drill.
- Install a smoke detection device on every level of your home. Clean the detectors and test batteries once a month, and replace the batteries at least once a year.
- Keep a fire extinguisher in your home and know how to use it.

To prevent injuries from fire:

- Get out as quickly as possible and go to the designated meeting place. Don't stop for a keepsake or a pet. Never hide in a closet or under a bed. Once outside, count heads to see if everyone is out. If you think someone is still inside the burning building, tell the firefighters. Never go back inside a burning building.
- If you're trapped in a room, feel the door. If it is hot or if smoke is coming in through the cracks, don't open it; use the alternative escape route. If you can't get out of a room, go to the window and shout or wave for help.
- Avoid inhaling smoke. Smoke inhalation is the largest cause of death and injury in fires. To avoid inhaling smoke, crawl along the floor away from the heat and smoke. Cover your mouth and nose, ideally with a wet cloth, and take short, shallow breaths.
- If your clothes catch fire, don't run. Drop to the ground, cover your face, and roll back and forth to smother the flames. Remember: Stop-drop-roll.

Suffocation and Choking

Suffocation and choking account for about 5000 deaths annually in the United States. Children can suffocate if they put small items in their mouths, get tangled in their crib bedding, or get trapped in airtight appliances like old refrigerators. Keep small objects out of reach of children under age 3, and don't give them raw carrots, hot dogs, popcorn, peanuts, or hard candy. Examine toys carefully for small parts that could come loose; don't give plastic bags or balloons to small children.

Adults can also become choking victims, especially if they fail to chew food properly, eat hurriedly, or try to talk and eat at the same time. Many choking victims can be saved with abdominal thrusts, also called the Heimlich maneuver (see Figure A.1). Infants who are choking can be saved with blows to the upper back, followed by chest thrusts if necessary.

Incidents Involving Firearms

Firearms pose a significant threat of unintentional injury, especially to people between ages 5 and 29.

To prevent firearm injuries:

- Always treat a gun as though it were loaded, even if you know it isn't.
- Never point a gun—loaded or unloaded—at something you do not intend to shoot.
- Always unload a firearm before storing it. Store unloaded firearms under lock and key, away from ammunition.
- Inspect firearms carefully before handling them.
- If you own a gun, buy and use a gun lock designed specifically for that weapon.
- If you ever plan to handle a gun, take a firearms safety course first.

LEISURE INJURIES

Leisure injuries take place in public places but do not involve motor vehicles. Many injuries in this category involve such recreational activities as boating and swimming, playground activities, in-line skating, and sports.

Drowning and Boating Injuries

Although most drownings are reported in lakes, ponds, rivers, and oceans, more than half the drownings of young children take place in residential pools. Among adolescents and adults, alcohol plays a significant role in many boating injuries and drownings.

To prevent drowning and boating injuries:

- Develop adequate swimming skill and make sure children learn to swim.
- Make sure residential pools are fenced and that children are never allowed to swim without supervision.
- Don't swim alone or in unsupervised places.
- Use caution when swimming in unfamiliar surroundings or for an unusual length of time. To avoid being chilled, don't swim in water colder than 70°F.
- Don't swim or boat under the influence of alcohol or other drugs. Don't chew gum or eat while in the water.
- Check the depth of water before diving.
- When on a boat, use a life jacket (personal flotation device).

In-Line Skating and Scooter Injuries

Most in-line skating injuries occur because users are not familiar with the equipment and do not wear appropriate safety gear. Injuries to the wrist and head are the most common. To prevent injuries while skating, wear a helmet, elbow and knee pads, wrist guards, a long-sleeved shirt, and long pants.

Wearing a helmet and knee and elbow pads is also important for preventing scooter injuries. The rise in popularity of lightweight scooters has seen a corresponding increase in associated injuries. Scooters should not be viewed as toys, and young children should be closely supervised. Be sure that handlebars, steering column, and all nuts and bolts are securely fastened. Ride on smooth, paved surfaces away from motor vehicle traffic. Avoid streets and surfaces with water, sand, gravel, or dirt.

Sports Injuries

Since more people have begun exercising to improve their health, there has been an increase in sports-related injuries.

To prevent sports injuries:

- Develop the skills required for the activity. Recognize and guard against the hazards associated with it.
- Always warm up and cool down.
- Make sure facilities are safe.
- Follow the rules and practice good sportsmanship.
- Use proper safety equipment, including, where appropriate, helmets, eye protection, knee and elbow pads, and wrist guards. Wear correct footwear.
- When it is excessively hot and humid, avoid heat stress by following the guidelines given in Chapter 4.

WORK INJURIES

Many aspects of workplace safety are monitored by the Occupational Safety and Health Administration (OSHA), a federal agency. The highest rate of work-related injuries occurs among laborers, whose jobs usually involve extensive manual labor and lifting—two areas not addressed by OSHA safety standards. Back injuries are the most common work injury.

To protect your back when lifting:

- Don't try to lift beyond your strength. If you need it, get help.
- Get a firm footing, with your feet shoulder-width apart. Get a firm grip on the object.
- Keep your torso in a relatively upright position and crouch down, bending at the knees and hips. Avoid bending at the waist. To lift, stand up or push up with your leg muscles. Lift gradually, keeping your arms straight. Keep the object close to your body.
- Don't twist. If you have to turn with an object, change the position of your feet.
- Put the object down gently, reversing the rules for lifting.

Another type of work-related injury is damage to the musculoskeletal system from repeated strain on the hand, arm, wrist, or other part of the body. Such repetitive-strain injuries are proliferating due to increased use of computers. One type, carpal tunnel syndrome, is characterized by pain and swelling in the tendons of the wrists and sometimes numbness and weakness.

To prevent carpal tunnel syndrome:

- Maintain good posture at the computer. Use a chair that provides back support and place the feet flat on the floor or on a footrest.
- Position the screen at eye level and the keyboard so the hands and wrists are straight.
- Take breaks periodically to stretch and flex your wrists and hands to lessen the cumulative effects of stress.

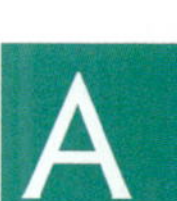

VIOLENCE AND INTENTIONAL INJURIES

According to the Federal Bureau of Investigation (FBI), nearly 1.3 million violent crimes occurred in the United States in 2009. Violence includes assault, sexual assault, homicide, domestic violence, suicide, and child abuse. Compared with rates of violence in other industrialized countries, U.S. rates are unusually high in two areas: homicide and firearm-related deaths.

Assault

Assault is the use of physical force to inflict injury or death on another person. Most assaults occur during arguments or in connection with another crime, such as robbery. Poverty, urban settings, and the use of alcohol and drugs are associated with higher rates of assault. The FBI estimates that about 807,000 aggravated assaults occurred in 2009, and 15,200 Americans were murdered that year. Homicide victims are most likely to be male, between ages 19 and 24, and members of minority groups. Most homicides are committed with a firearm; the murderer and the victim usually know each other.

To protect yourself at home:

- Secure your home with good lighting and effective locks, preferably deadbolts. Make sure that all doors and windows are securely locked.
- Get a dog, or post "Beware of Dog" signs.
- Don't hide keys in obvious places, and don't give anyone the chance to duplicate your keys.
- Install a peephole in your front door. Don't open your door to people you don't know.
- If you or a family member owns a weapon, store it securely. Store guns and ammunition separately.
- If you are a woman living alone, use your initials rather than your full name in the phone directory. Don't use a greeting on your answering machine that implies you live alone or are not home.
- Teach everyone in the household how to get emergency assistance.
- Know your neighbors. Work out a system for alerting each other in case of an emergency.
- Establish a neighborhood watch program.

To protect yourself on the street:

- Avoid walking alone, especially at night. Stay where people can see and hear you.

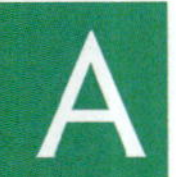

- Walk on the outside of the sidewalk, facing traffic. Walk purposefully. Act alert and confident. If possible, keep at least two arm lengths between yourself and a stranger.
- Know where you are going. Appearing to be lost increases your vulnerability.
- Carry valuables in a fanny pack, pants pocket, or shoulder bag strapped diagonally across the chest.
- Always have your keys ready as you approach your vehicle or home.
- Carry a whistle to blow if you are attacked or harassed. If you feel threatened, run and/or yell. Go into a store or knock on the door of a home. If someone grabs you, yell for help.

To protect yourself in your car:

- Keep your car in good working condition, carry emergency supplies, and keep the gas tank at least half full.
- When driving, keep doors locked and windows rolled up at least three-quarters of the way.
- Park your car in well-lighted areas or parking garages, preferably those with an attendant or a security guard.
- Lock your car when you leave it, and check the interior before opening the door when you return.
- Don't pick up strangers. Don't stop for vehicles in distress; drive on and call for help.
- Note the location of emergency call boxes along highways and in public facilities. Carry a cell phone.
- If your car breaks down, raise the hood and tie a white cloth to the antenna or door handle. Wait in the car with the doors locked and windows rolled up. If someone approaches to offer help, open a window only a crack and ask the person to call the police or a towing service.
- When you stop at a light or stop sign, leave enough room to maneuver if you need an escape route.
- If you are involved in a minor automobile crash and you think you have been bumped intentionally, don't leave your car. Motion to the other driver to follow you to the nearest police station.
- If confronted by a person with a weapon, give up your car.

To protect yourself on public transportation:

- While waiting, stand in a populated, well-lighted area.
- Make sure that the bus, subway, or train is bound for your destination before you board it. Sit near the driver or conductor in a single seat or an outside seat.
- If you flag down a taxi, make sure it's from a legitimate service. When you reach your destination, ask the driver to wait until you are safely inside the building.

To protect yourself on campus:

- Make sure that door and window locks are secure and that halls and stairwells have adequate lighting.
- Don't give dorm or residence keys to anybody.
- Don't leave your door unlocked or allow strangers into your room.
- Avoid solitary late-night trips to the library or laundry room. Take advantage of on-campus escort services.
- Don't exercise outside alone at night. Don't take shortcuts across campus that are unfamiliar or seem unsafe.
- If security guards patrol the campus, know the areas they cover and stay where they can see or hear you.

Sexual Assault—Rape and Date Rape

The use of force and coercion in sexual relationships is one of the most serious problems in human interactions. The most extreme manifestation of sexual coercion—forcing a person to submit to another's sexual desires—is rape. Taking advantage of circumstances that render a person incapable of giving consent (such as when drunk) is also considered sexual assault or rape. Coerced sexual activity in which the victim knows or is dating the rapist is often referred to as date rape.

An estimated 700,000 females are raped annually in the United States, and some males—perhaps 10,000 annually—are raped each year by other males. However, only a fraction of rapes are actually reported to authorities. For example, the FBI states that only 88,000 forcible rapes were reported to authorities in 2009. Rape victims suffer both physical and psychological injury. The psychological pain can be substantial and long-lasting.

To protect yourself against rape:

- Follow the guidelines listed earlier for protecting yourself against assault.
- Trust your gut feeling. If you feel you are in danger, don't hesitate to run and scream.
- Think out in advance what you would do if you were threatened with rape. However, no one knows what he or she will do when scared to death. Trust that you will make the best decision at the time—whether to scream, run, fight, or give in to avoid being injured or killed.

To protect yourself against date rape:

- Believe in your right to control what you do. Set limits and communicate them clearly, firmly, and early. Be assertive; men often interpret passivity as permission.
- If you are unsure of a new acquaintance, go on a group date or double date. If possible, provide your own transportation.
- Remember that some men think flirtatious behavior or sexy clothing indicates an interest in having sex.
- Remember that alcohol and drugs interfere with judgment, perception, and communication about sex. In a bar or at a party, don't leave your drink unattended, and don't accept opened beverages; watch your drinks being poured. At a party or club, check on friends and ask them to check on you.
- Use the statement that has proved most effective in stopping date rape: "This is rape and I'm calling the cops!"

If you are raped:

- Tell what happened to the first friendly person you meet.
- Call the police. Tell them you were raped and give your location.
- Try to remember everything you can about your attacker and write it down.
- Don't wash or douche before the medical exam. Don't change your clothes, but bring a new set with you if you can.
- Be aware that at the hospital you will have a complete exam. Show the physician any bruises or scratches.

- Tell the police exactly what happened. Be honest and stick to your story.
- If you do not want to report the rape to the police, see a physician as soon as possible. Be sure you are checked for pregnancy and STDs.
- Contact an organization with skilled counselors so you can talk about the experience. Look in the telephone directory under "Rape" or "Rape Crisis Center" for a hotline number.

Guidelines for men:

- Be aware of social pressure. It's OK not to score.
- Understand that "No" means "No." Stop making advances when your date says to stop. Remember that she has the right to refuse sex.
- Don't assume that flirtatious behavior or sexy clothing means a woman is interested in having sex, that previous permission for sex applies to the current situation, or that your date's relationships with other men constitute sexual permission for you.
- Remember that alcohol and drugs interfere with judgment, perception, and communication about sex.

Stalking and Cyberstalking

Stalking is characterized by harassing behaviors such as following or spying on a person and making verbal, written, or implied threats. It is estimated that 1 million U.S. women and 400,000 men are stalked each year; nearly 90% of stalkers are men. Cyberstalking, the use of electronic communications devices to stalk another person, is becoming more common. Cyberstalkers may send harassing or threatening e-mails or chat room messages to the victim, or they may encourage others to harass the victim by posting inflammatory messages and personal information on bulletin boards or chat rooms.

To protect yourself online:

- Never use your real name as an e-mail user name or chat room nickname. Select an age- and gender-neutral identity.
- Avoid filling out profiles for accounts related to e-mail use or chat room activities with information that could be used to identify you.
- Do not share personal information in public spaces anywhere online or give it to strangers.
- Learn how to filter unwanted e-mail messages.
- If you experience harassment online, do not respond to the harasser. Log off or surf elsewhere. Save all communications for evidence. If harassment continues, report it to the harasser's Internet service provider, your Internet service provider, and the local police.
- Don't agree to meet someone you've met online face-to-face unless you feel completely comfortable about it. Schedule a series of phone conversations first. Meet initially in a very public place and bring along a friend to increase your safety.

Coping After Terrorism, Mass Violence, or Natural Disasters

Certain areas of the United States are prone to natural disasters like Hurricane Irene, which wreaked havoc along the East Coast in 2011. Other natural disasters include tornadoes, floods, and earthquakes. Less frequent in the United States are episodes of mass violence or terrorist events such as those that occurred in Oklahoma in April 1995 and on September 11, 2001. When such events occur, some people suffer direct physical harm and/or the loss of relatives, friends, or possessions; many others experience emotional distress and are robbed of their sense of security.

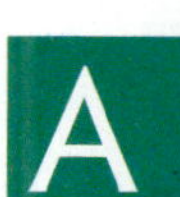

Each person reacts differently to traumatic disaster, and it is normal to experience a variety of responses. Reactions may include disbelief and shock, fear, anger and resentment, anxiety about the future, difficulty concentrating or making decisions, mood swings, irritability, sadness and depression, panic, guilt, apathy, feelings of isolation or powerlessness, and many of the behaviorial signs such as headaches or insomnia that are associated with excess stress (see Chapter 10). Reactions may occur immediately or may be delayed until weeks or months after the event.

Taking positive steps can help you cope with powerful emotions. Consider the following strategies:

- Share your experiences and emotions with friends and family members. Be a supportive listener. Reassure children and encourage them to talk about what they are feeling.
- Take care of your mind and body. Choose a healthy diet, exercise regularly, get plenty of sleep, and practice relaxation techniques. Don't turn to unhealthy coping techniques such as using alcohol or other drugs.
- Take a break from media reports and images, and try not to develop nightmare scenarios for possible future events.
- Reestablish your routines at home, school, and work.
- Find ways to help others. Donating money, blood, food, clothes, or time can ease difficult emotions and give you a greater sense of control.

Everyone copes with tragedy in a different way and recovers at a different pace. If you feel overwhelmed by your emotions, seek professional help. Additional information about coping with terrorism and violence is available from the Federal Emergency Management Agency (www.fema.gov), the U.S. Department of Justice (www. usdoj.gov), and the National Mental Health Association (www.nmha.org).

Emergency Preparedness

Most prevention and coping activities related to terrorism, mass violence, and natural disasters occur at the federal, state, and community levels. However, one step you can take is to put together an emergency plan and kit for your family or household that can serve for any type of emergency or disaster.

Emergency Supplies Your kit of emergency supplies should include everything you'll need to make it on your own for at least 3 days. You'll need nonperishable food, water, first-aid and sanitation supplies, a battery-powered radio, clothing, a flashlight, cash, keys, copies of important documents, and supplies for sleeping outdoors in any weather. Remember special-needs items for infants, seniors, and pets. Supplies for a basic emergency kit are listed in Figure A.2; add to your kit based on your family situation and the type of problems most likely to occur in your area.

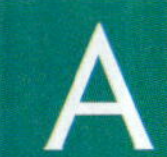

Basic emergency supplies

Map of the area for locating evacuation routes or shelters
Cash, coins, and credit cards
Copies of important documents stored in watertight container
Emergency contact list and phone numbers
Extra sets of house and car keys
Flashlights or lightsticks
Battery- or solar-powered radio
Battery-powered alarm clock
Extra batteries and bulbs
Cell phone or prepaid phone card
Signal flares
Fire extinguisher (small A-B-C type)
Whistle
Ladder
Tube tent and rope
Sleeping bags or warm blankets
Foam pads, pillows, baby bed
Complete change of warm clothing, footwear, outerware (jacket or coat, long pants, long-sleeved shirt, sturdy shoes, hat, gloves, raingear, extra socks and underwear, sunglasses)
Work gloves
Shutoff wrench for gas and water supplies
Shovel, hammer, pliers, screwdriver, and other tools
Compass
Matches in a waterproof container
Aluminum foil
Plastic storage containers, bucket
Duct tape, utility knife, and scissors
Paper, pens, pencils
Needles and thread

First aid kit

First aid manual
Thermometer
Scissors
Tweezers
Safety pins, safety razor blades
Needle
Latex or other sterile gloves
Sterile gauze pads
Cleansing agents (soap, isopropyl alcohol, antiseptic towelettes)
Sunscreen
Insect repellent
Antibiotic ointment
Burn ointment
Petroleum jelly or another lubricant
Sterile adhesive bandages, several sizes
Sterile rolled bandages and triangular bandages
Cotton balls
Eyewash solution
Chemical heat and cold packs
Aspirin or nonaspirin pain reliever
Anti-diarrhea medication
Laxative
Antacid
Activated charcoal (use if advised by Poison Control Center)
Potassium iodide (use following radiation exposure if advised by local health authorities)
Prescription medications and prescribed medical supplies
List of medications, dosages, and any allergies
Medicine dropper

Special needs items

Infant care needs (formula, bottles, diapers, powdered milk, diaper rash ointment)
Books or toys
Extra eyeglasses, contact lenses and supplies
Feminine hygiene supplies
Denture needs
Hearing aid or wheelchair batteries; other special equipment
Pet care supplies, including leash, pet carrier, copy of vaccination history, and tie-out stakes
Other (list)

Food and related supplies

Manual (nonelectric) can opener
Utility knife
Paper towels
Eating utensils: Mess kits, or paper cups and plates and utensils
Plastic garbage bags and resealing bags
Small cooking stove and cooking fuel (if food must be cooked)
Water purification tablets

Water: Three-day-supply, at least 1 gallon of water per person per day, stored in plastic containers:

Number of people: ______ x 1 gallon x 3 days = ______ total minimum gallons of water

Store additional water if you live in a hot climate or if your household includes infants, pregnant women, or people with special health needs. Don't forget to store water for pets. Containers can be sterilized by rinsing them with a diluted bleach solution (one part bleach to ten parts water). Replace your water supply every six months.

Food: At least a three-day supply of nonperishable foods—those requiring no refrigeration, preparation, or cooking and little or no water. Choose foods from the following list and add foods that members of your household will eat. Replace items in your food supply every six months.

Ready-to-eat canned meats, fruits, soups, and vegetables
Protein or fruit bars
Dry cereal or granola
Peanut butter
Sugar, salt, pepper
Dried fruit
Nuts
Crackers
Canned, powdered, or boxed juices
Nonperishable pasteurized milk or powered milk
Coffee, tea, sodas
High-energy foods
Comfort/stress foods
MREs (military rations)
Infant formula and baby foods
Pet foods

Sanitation

Plastic garbage bags (and ties)
Toilet paper
Moist towelettes or hand soap
Washcloth and towel
Personal hygiene items (toothbrush, shampoo, deodorant, comb, shaving cream, and so on)
Plastic bucket with tight lid
Household chlorine bleach, disinfectant
Powdered lime
Small shovel for digging latrine

For a clean air supply

Face masks or several layers of dense-weave cotton material (handkerchiefs, t-shirts, towels) that fit snugly over your nose and mouth.

Shelter-in-place supplies, to be used in an interior room to create a barrier between you and potentially contaminated air outside: Heavyweight plastic garbage bags or plastic sheeting; duct tape; scissors; and if possible, a portable air purifier with a HEPA filter.

Family emergency plan

Plan places where your family will meet; choose one location near your home and one outside your neighborhood.

Local ______________________ Outside neighborhood ______________________

Have one local and one out-of-state contact person for family members to call if separated during a disaster. (It may be easier to make long-distance calls than local calls.)

Local ______________________ Out-of state ______________________

FIGURE A.2 Sample emergency preparedness kit and plan.

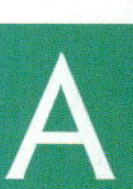

You may want to create several kinds of emergency kits. The primary one would contain supplies for home use. Put together a smaller, lightweight version that you can take with you if you are forced to evacuate your residence. Smaller kits for your car and your workplace are also recommended.

A Family or Household Plan You and your family or household members should have a plan about where to meet and how to communicate. Choose at least two potential meeting places—one in your neighborhood and one or more in other areas. Your community may also have set locations for community shelters. Where you go may depend on the circumstances of the emergency situation. Use your common sense, and listen to the radio or television for instructions from emergency officials about whether to evacuate or stay in place. In addition, know all the transportation options in the vicinity of your home, school, and workplace; roadways and public transit may be affected, so a sturdy pair of walking shoes is a good item to keep in your emergency kit.

Everyone in the family or household should also have the same emergency contact person to call, preferably someone who lives outside the immediate area and won't be affected by the same local disaster. Local phone service may be significantly disrupted, so long-distance calls may be more likely to go through. Everyone should carry the relevant phone numbers and addresses at all times.

It is also important to check into the emergency plans at any location where you or family members spend time, including schools and workplaces. For each location, know the safest place to be for different types of emergencies—for example, near load-bearing interior walls during an earthquake or in the basement during a tornado. Also know how to turn off water, gas, and electricity in case of damaged utility lines; keep the needed tools next to the shutoff valves.

Other steps you can take to help prepare for emergencies include taking a first-aid class and setting up an emergency response group in your neighborhood, residential building, or office. Talk with your neighbors: Who has specialized equipment (for example, a power generator) or expertise that might help in a crisis? Do older or disabled neighbors have someone to help them? More complete information about emergency preparedness is available from local government agencies and from the following:

American Academy of Pediatrics
(www.aap.org)

American Red Cross
(www.redcross.org)

Federal Emergency Management Agency
(www.fema.gov)

U.S. Department of Homeland Security
(www.ready.gov)

PROVIDING EMERGENCY CARE

You can improve someone else's chances of surviving if you are prepared to provide emergency help. A course in first aid offered by the American Red Cross and on many college campuses can teach you to respond appropriately when someone needs help. Emergency rescue techniques can save the lives of people who have stopped breathing, who are choking, or whose hearts have stopped beating. Pulmonary resuscitation (also known as rescue breathing, artificial respiration, or mouth-to-mouth resuscitation) is used when a person is not breathing (refer back to Figure A.1). Cardiopulmonary resuscitation (CPR) is used when a pulse can't be found. Training is required before a person can perform CPR. Significant changes were made to the guidelines for lay rescue CPR in 2005. Courses are offered by the American Red Cross and the American Heart Association.

When You Have to Provide Emergency Care Remain calm and act sensibly. The basic pattern for providing emergency care is *check-call-care*:

1. ***Check the situation.*** Make sure the scene is safe for both you and the injured person. Don't put yourself in danger; if you get hurt too, you will be of little help to the injured person.
2. ***Check the victim.*** Conduct a quick head-to-toe examination. Assess the victim's signs and symptoms, such as level of responsiveness, pulse, and breathing rate. Look for bleeding and any indications of broken bones or paralysis.
3. ***Call for help.*** Call 9-1-1 or a local emergency number. Identify yourself and give as much information as you can about the condition of the victim and what happened.
4. ***Care for the victim.*** If the situation requires immediate action (no pulse, shock, etc.), provide first aid if you are trained to do so (refer back to Figure A.1).

Selected Bibliography

Bren, L. 2005. Prevent your child from choking. *FDA Consumer,* September/ October.

Central Intelligence Agency. 2011. *The World Factbook.* Washington, D.C.: Central Intelligence Agency.

Federal Bureau of Investigation. 2009. *Hate Crime Statistics,* 2008. Washington, D.C.: U.S. Department of Justice.

Federal Bureau of Investigation. 2010. *Crime in the United States:* 2009. Washington, D.C.: U.S. Department of Justice.

Insurance Information Institute. 2007. *Road Rage* (http://www.iii.org/individuals/auto/lifesaving/roadrage; retrieved August 31, 2011).

Iudice, A., et al. 2005. Effects of prolonged wakefulness combined with alcohol and hands-free cell phone divided attention tasks on simulated driving. *Human Psychopharmacology* 20(2): 125–132.

National Center for Health Statistics. 2011. Deaths: Preliminary Data for 2009. *National Vital Statistics Reports* 59(4).

National Center for Health Statistics. 2011. *Health, United States,* 2010. Hyattsville, Md.: National Center for Health Statistics.

National Safety Council. 2011. *Injury Facts* 2011. Itasca, Ill.: National Safety Council.

U.S. Department of Homeland Security. 2005. *Ready America* (www.ready.gov; retrieved August 31, 2011).

B

APPENDIX B

EXERCISE GUIDELINES FOR PEOPLE WITH SPECIAL HEALTH CONCERNS

As explained in Chapters 2, 4, 6, 8, and 9, regular, appropriate exercise is safe and beneficial for many people with chronic conditions or other special health concerns. In fact, for many people with special health concerns, the risks associated with not exercising are far greater than those associated with a moderate program of regular exercise.

The fitness recommendations made throughout this book are intended for the general population and can serve as basic guidelines for any exercise program. If you have a chronic health condition, however, you may need to modify your exercise program to accommodate your situation. This appendix presents precautions and specialized recommendations for people with a variety of special health concerns.

These recommendations, however, are not intended to replace a physician's advice. If you have a special health concern, talk to your physician before starting any exercise program.

ARTHRITIS

- Begin an exercise program as early as possible in the course of the disease.
- Warm up thoroughly before each workout to loosen stiff muscles and lower the risk of injury.
- For cardiorespiratory endurance exercise, avoid high-impact activities that may damage arthritic joints. Consider swimming, water walking, or another type of exercise that can be done in a warm pool.
- Strength train the whole body. Pay special attention to muscles that support and protect affected joints. For example, build the quadriceps, hamstrings, and calf muscles to support and protect arthritic knees. Start with small amounts of weight and gradually increase the intensity of your workouts.
- Perform flexibility exercises daily to maintain joint mobility.

ASTHMA

- Exercise regularly. Acute attacks are more likely to occur if you exercise only occasionally.
- Carry medication during workouts and avoid exercising alone. Use your inhaler as recommended by your physician.
- Warm up and cool down slowly to reduce the risk of acute attacks.
- When starting an exercise program, choose self-paced endurance activities, especially those involving interval training (short bouts of exercise followed by a rest period). Gradually increase the intensity of your cardiorespiratory endurance workouts.
- Educate yourself about situations that can trigger an asthma attack and act accordingly when exercising. For example, cold, dry air can trigger or worsen an attack. Pollen, dust, and polluted air can also trigger an attack. To avoid attacks in dry air, drink water before, during, and after a workout to moisten your airways. In cold weather, cover your mouth with a mask or scarf to warm and humidify the air you breathe. Also, avoid outdoor activities during pollen season or when the air is polluted or dusty.

DIABETES

- Don't begin an exercise program unless your diabetes is under control and you have discussed exercise safety with your physician. Because people with diabetes have an increased risk for heart disease, an exercise stress test may be recommended.
- Don't exercise alone. Wear a bracelet that identifies you as someone with diabetes.
- If you take insulin or another medication, adjust the timing and amount of each dose as needed. Work with your physician and check your blood sugar level regularly so you can learn to balance your energy intake and output and your medication dosage.
- To prevent abnormally rapid absorption of injected insulin, inject it over a muscle that will not be exercised, and wait at least an hour before exercising.
- Check your blood sugar before, during, and after exercise. Adjust your diet and insulin dosage as needed. Keep high-carbohydrate foods on hand during a workout. Avoid exercise if your blood sugar level is above 250 mg/dl; if your blood sugar level is below 100 mg/dl, eat some carbohydrate-rich food before exercising.
- If you have poor circulation or numbness in your extremities, check your skin regularly for blisters and abrasions, especially on your feet. Avoid high-impact activities and wear comfortable shoes.
- For maximum benefit and minimum risk, choose moderate-intensity activities.

HEART DISEASE AND HYPERTENSION

- Check with your physician about exercise safety before increasing your activity level. Your doctor may recommend that you take an exercise stress test before starting your program.

- Exercise at moderate intensity rather than high intensity. Keep your heart rate below the level at which abnormalities appear on an exercise stress test.
- Warm up and cool down gradually. Every warm-up and cool-down session should last at least 10 minutes.
- Monitor your heart rate during exercise, and stop if you experience dizziness or chest pain.
- If your physician prescribes nitroglycerin, carry it with you during exercise. If you take a beta-blocker to manage hypertension, use RPE rather than heart rate to monitor your exercise intensity (beta-blockers reduce heart rate). Exercise at an RPE level of "fairly light" to "somewhat hard." Your breathing should be unlabored, and you should be able to talk during exercise.
- Don't hold your breath when exercising. Doing so can cause sudden, steep increases in blood pressure. Take special care during weight training and do not lift heavy loads. Exhale during the exertion phase of each lift.
- Increase exercise frequency, intensity, and time very gradually.

OBESITY

- For maximum benefit and minimum risk, begin by choosing low- to moderate-intensity activities. Increase intensity slowly as your fitness improves. Studies of overweight people show that exercising at moderate to high intensities causes more fat loss than training at low intensities.
- People who want to lose weight or maintain weight loss should exercise moderately for 60 minutes or more every day. To get the benefit of 60 minutes of exercise, you can exercise all at once or divide your total activity time into sessions of 10, 20, or 30 minutes.
- Choose non- or low-weight-bearing activities such as swimming, water exercises, cycling, or walking. Low-impact activities are less likely to cause joint problems or injuries.
- Stay alert for symptoms of heat-related problems during exercise (as described in Chapter 4). Obese people are vulnerable to heat intolerance.
- Ease into your exercise program and increase overload gradually. Increase time and frequency of exercise before increasing intensity.
- Include strength training in your fitness program to build or maintain muscle mass.
- Try to include as much lifestyle physical activity in your daily routine as possible.

OSTEOPOROSIS

- For cardiorespiratory endurance activities, exercise at the maximum intensity that causes no significant discomfort. If possible, choose low-impact, weight-bearing exercises to help safely maintain bone density. (See Chapter 4 for strategies for building and maintaining bone density.)
- To prevent fractures, avoid any activity or movement that stresses the back or carries a risk of falling.
- Include weight training in your exercise program to improve strength and balance and to reduce the risk of falls and fractures. Always use proper exercise technique and avoid lifting heavy loads.
- Include muscle-strengthening exercises 3 days per week.
- Include bone-strengthening exercises, such as jumping, at least 3 days per week.

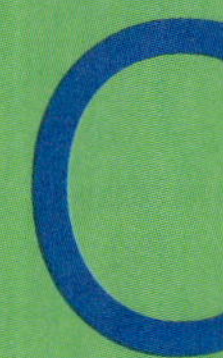

MONITORING YOUR PROGRESS

NAME ______________________ **SECTION** __________ **DATE** __________

As you completed the labs listed below, you entered the results in the Preprogram Assessment column of this appendix. Now that you have been involved in a fitness and wellness program for some time, do the labs again and enter your new results in the Postprogram Assessment column. You will probably notice improvement in several areas. Congratulations! If you are not satisfied with your progress thus far, refer to the tips for successful behavior change in Chapter 1 and throughout this book. Remember—fitness and wellness are forever. The time you invest now in developing a comprehensive, individualized program will pay off in a richer, more vital life in the years to come.

	Preprogram Assessment	**Postprogram Assessment**
LAB 2.3 Pedometer	Daily steps: _____	Daily steps: _____
LAB 3.1 Daily Diet		
Number of oz-eq	Grains: _____	Grains: _____
Number of cups	Vegetables: _____	Vegetables: _____
Number of cups	Fruits: _____	Fruits: _____
Number of cups	Milk: _____	Milk: _____
Number of oz-eq	Meat or beans: _____	Meat or beans: _____
Number of tsp	Oils: _____	Oils: _____
Number of g	Solid fats: _____	Solid fats: _____
Number of g or tsp	Added sugars: _____	Added sugars: _____
LAB 3.2 Dietary Analysis		
Percentage of calories	From protein: _____ %	From protein: _____ %
Percentage of calories	From fat: _____ %	From fat: _____ %
Percentage of calories	From saturated fat: _____ %	From saturated fat: _____ %
Percentage of calories	From carbohydrate: _____ %	From carbohydrate: _____ %
LAB 4.1 Cardiorespiratory Endurance		
1-mile walk test	$\dot{V}O_{2max}$: _______ Rating: _________	$\dot{V}O_{2max}$: _______ Rating: _________
3-minute step test	$\dot{V}O_{2max}$: _______ Rating: _________	$\dot{V}O_{2max}$: _______ Rating: _________
1.5-mile run-walk test	$\dot{V}O_{2max}$: _______ Rating: _________	$\dot{V}O_{2max}$: _______ Rating: _________
12-minute swim test	Rating: _____	Rating: _____

	Preprogram Assessment	Postprogram Assessment
LAB 5.1 Cardiovascular Health		
CVD risk assessment	Score: _____ Estimated risk: _____	Score: _____ Estimated risk: _____
Hostility assessment	Score: _____ Rating: _____	Score: _____ Rating: _____
LAB 6.1 Body Composition		
Body mass index	BMI: _____ kg/m2 Rating: _____	BMI: _____ kg/m2 Rating: _____
Skinfold measurements (or other methods for determining percent body fat)	Sum of 3 skinfolds: _____ mm % body fat: _____% Rating: _____	Sum of 3 skinfolds: _____ mm % body fat: _____% Rating: _____
Waist circumference	Circumf.: _____ Rating: _____	Circumf.: _____ Rating: _____
Waist-to-hip ratio	Ratio: _____ Rating: _____	Ratio: _____ Rating: _____
LAB 7.1 Daily Energy Needs	Daily energy needs: _____ cal/day	Daily energy needs: _____ cal/day
LAB 8.1 Muscular Strength		
Maximum bench press test	Weight: _____ lb Rating: _____	Weight: _____ lb Rating: _____
LAB 8.2 Muscular Endurance		
Curl-up test	Number: _____ Rating: _____	Number: _____ Rating: _____
Push-up test	Number: _____ Rating: _____	Number: _____ Rating: _____
Squat endurance test	Number: _____ Rating: _____	Number: _____ Rating: _____
LAB 9.1 Flexibility		
Sit-and-reach test	Score: _____ cm Rating: _____	Score: _____ cm Rating: _____
LAB 9.3 Low-Back Muscular Endurance		
Side bridge endurance test	Right: _____ sec. Rating: _____ Left: _____ sec. Rating: _____	Right: _____ sec. Rating: _____ Left: _____ sec. Rating: _____
Trunk flexors endurance test	Trunk flexors: _____ sec. Rating: _____	Trunk flexors: _____ sec. Rating: _____
Back extensors endurance test	Back extensors: _____ sec. Rating: _____	Back extensors: _____ sec. Rating: _____
LAB 10.1 Identifying Stressors	Average weekly stress score: _____	Average weekly stress score: _____

INDEX

Note: Page references in boldface type indicate pages with definitions.